Peripheral Lymphedema

Ningfei Liu
Editor

Peripheral Lymphedema

Pathophysiology, Modern Diagnosis and Management

Springer

Editor
Ningfei Liu
Department of Plastic and Reconstructive Surgery
Shanghai Ninth Peolple's Hospital
Shanghai Jiao Tong University
School of Medicine
Shanghai, China

ISBN 978-981-16-3483-3 ISBN 978-981-16-3484-0 (eBook)
https://doi.org/10.1007/978-981-16-3484-0

This Springer imprint is published by the registered company Springer Nature Singapore Pte Ltd.
The registered company address is: 152 Beach Road, #21-01/04 Gateway East, Singapore 189721, Singapore

Preface

This book, *Peripheral Lymphedema: Pathophysiology, Modern Diagnosis and Management*, was written during the global COVID-19 pandemic. It required the unrelenting efforts of all authors to finally complete this monograph on lymphedema. Thus, I would like to extend my heartfelt thanks to all the co-authors. Lymphedema cannot be controlled, and is unlike either a tumor, which grows fast and is life-threatening, or a virus infection, which spreads rapidly but can eventually be managed. Lymphedema is a chronic disease that affects patients throughout their lifetime and has severe complications in the late stage. It is currently an incurable disease that requires lifelong treatment and care. The authors of this book are all clinical lymphology professionals. They include internationally renowned experts who have been involved in the lymphology field for more than half a century as well as young clinicians who have made remarkable achievements in particular fields related to lymphedema treatments. The writing team has worked to provide readers with the latest research findings obtained in basic and clinical studies on clinical lymphology, with the aim of inspiring further research into the disease and exploration of new treatments. The book covers the following aspects: detailed anatomy of the lymphatic system, formation and transport of lymph, correlations between phenotype and genotype in primary lymphedema, pathophysiology of the lymphatic system during the onset and course of the disease, use of multimodal lymphatic imaging modalities in diagnosis of the disease and interpretation of their findings, lymphatic microsurgical treatments, and correct implementation of CDT treatments. In addition, many high-resolution color photographs and drawings are provided throughout the book to facilitate readers' clear understanding.

I would like to take the opportunity provided by the publication of this book to extend my gratitude to my family for their great and ongoing support and to my colleagues both at home and abroad for their valuable assistance.

Shanghai, China
October 17, 2020

Ningfei Liu

Contents

Part I

Overview of Lymphatic System

Physiology of Lymphatic System (Physiology of Capillary Filtrate Flow to Lymphatics)

1

Waldemar L. Olszewski

Abstract

The lymphatic system (LS) of human limbs (See Fig. 1.1).

Keywords

Lymph · Lymphatics · Lymphocytes · Lymphatic organs

1.1 The Lymphatic System in Connection with Tissue Fluid/Lymph Formation and Flow (Fig. 1.1) [1]

1.1.1 Structure and Function of the Lymphatic System Under Normal Conditions

The lymphatic system (LS) is composed of morphological and liquid compartments. It starts from the interstitial space and lymph vessel network to end up in the venous subclavian-jugular angle. The initial lymphatics are most dense in skin, gut, and lungs. These are the tissues with direct contact with the external environment. The initial lymphatics are present in all tissues and organs. Different organization of fluid drainage is found in the CNS (central nervous system). The other morphological component of LS is the resident and migrating lymphocyte pool contained in lymphatics, lymph nodes, spleen, bone marrow, and thymus. The liquid part of LS is the capillary filtrate/tissue fluid/lymph contained in the intercellular (interstitial, tissue) space and lymphatics [1] (Fig. 1.2).

The function of the lymphatic system is to maintain the proper chemical environment of cells and tissues, regulate the volume of water and stabilize the concentration of proteins at physiological concentration.

The "lymphatic space" consists of the intracellular and perivascular space, lymphatic vessels, recirculating immune cells, nutrients, and metabolic products of cells (Fig. 1.3). This space acts as a tank for excess tissue fluid in conditions of impaired lymphatic drainage or excessive capillary filtration (Starling's equation). The pliability of the lymphatic space is crucial in maintaining tissue homeostasis.

1.1.2 Important!

P_C—Increased blood capillary hydrostatic pressure will raise water movement to the interstitial space. However, obstruction of veins causing an increase in the venous capillary pressure will be immediately followed by arteriole contraction and decrease of venous capillary pressure, subsequently less filtration and lymph formation.

P_T—plasma concentration and oncotic pressure are stable and do not change unless in profound hypoproteinemia.

Q_P—plasma protein reflection coefficient depends on the degree of dilatation of endothelial junctions (pores or clefts) and thickness of the glycocalyx. It changes in inflammation of the tissue.

Π_C—capillary filtrate protein concentration is dependent upon the plasma filtration rate and expansion of the interstitial space. The more distensible is that space, as in the slow edema formation process, the longer remains the interstitial fluid protein concentration low. Water is rapidly diffusing into the interstitial space and diluting excess filtrated plasma protein. This is why even in long-lasting lymphedema we see LOW but NOT HIGH interstitial fluid/lymph protein concentration, unless there has been acute inflammation with high input of plasma proteins. The expansion of the interstitial space in human tissues is not included in Starling's equation.

Π_T—oncotic pressure depends on protein and protein-bound ions (Donnan formula) concentration and plays a basic role in the capillary filtration process in normal tissues but not so much in lymphedema where the distance between

W. L. Olszewski (✉)
Department of Vascular Surgery, Central Clinical Hospital, Ministry of Internal Affairs, Warsaw, Poland

N. Liu (ed.), *Peripheral Lymphedema*, https://doi.org/10.1007/978-981-16-3484-0_1

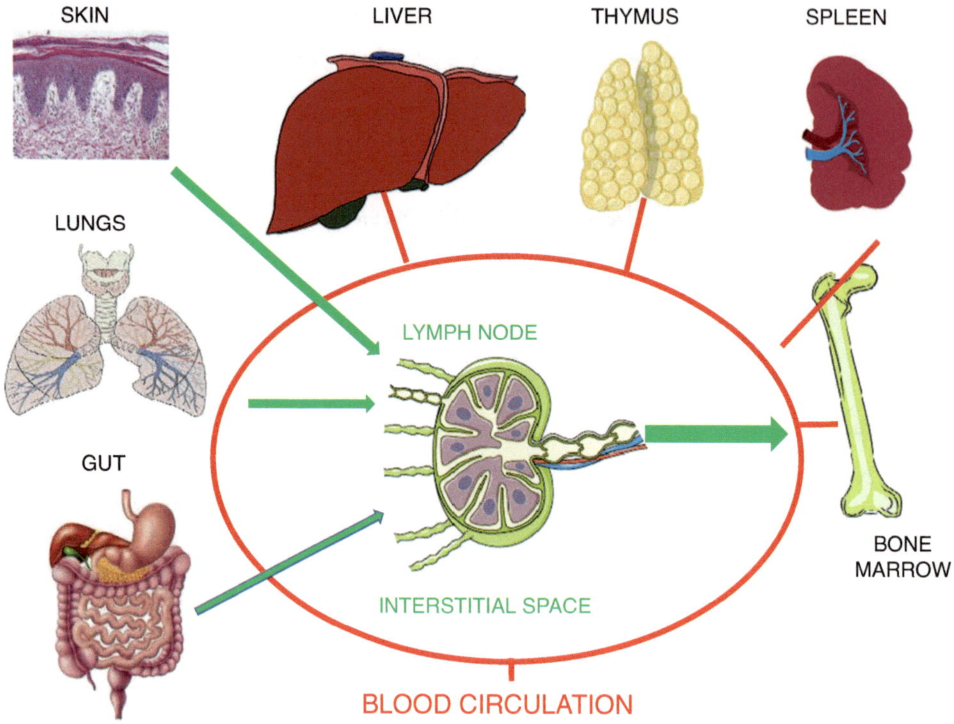

Fig. 1.1 The lymphatic system (LS) of human limbs consists of tissue fluid (TF) and lymph (L), interstitial space and lymph vessel network, lymphoid cells in organs as lymph nodes, spleen, bone marrow, thymus, gut, lungs, and liver, and freely migrating in fluids and tissues. Capillary filtrate becomes tissue fluid and flown to lymphatic is called lymph

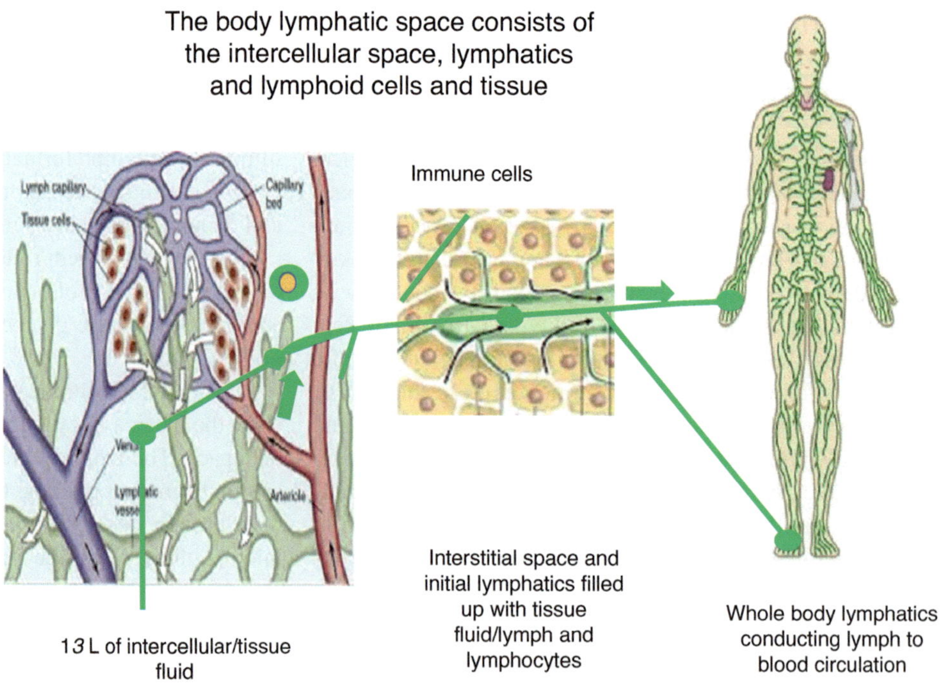

Fig. 1.2 Graphic representation of the events in the human lymphatic system. Follow the green line showing interstitial fluid and lymphocytes, initial and collecting lymphatics, and the whole body lymphatic network

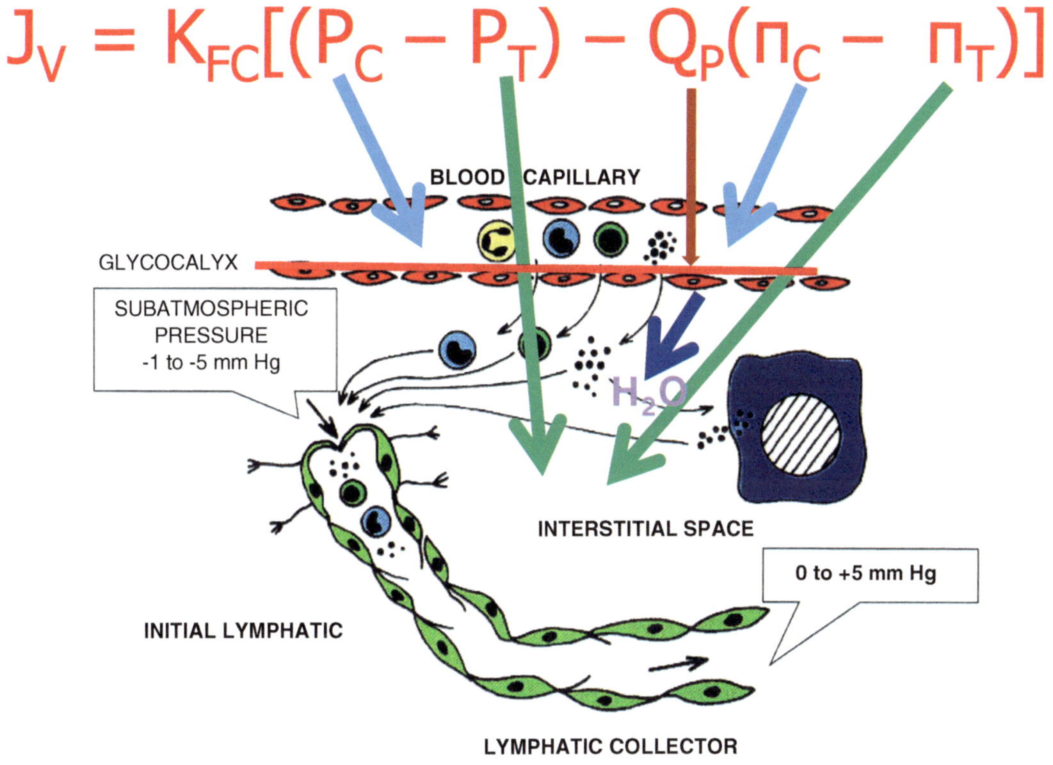

Fig. 1.3 The volume of plasma fluid filtered per unit time is described by the Starling equation for fluid filtration, where J_V is fluid volume, K is transcapillary permeability coefficient per surface unit, P is blood capillary (C), and tissue space (T) pressure, Q is protein reflection coefficient, Π is protein plasma (C) and tissue fluid (T) concentration. The leak passages are glycol-calyx-covered intercellular clefts, acting overall as a semi-permeable membrane. The hydrostatic pressure in the capillary blood vessels guides the fluid elements of blood through the vessel wall into the tissue space. At the same time, higher osmotic pressure in the vessel attracts water to the vessel lumen [2]

capillaries is increased, thus oncotic force becomes less effective.

The LS recognized the bacterial and viruses' antigens through PAMP (pathogen-associated molecular pattern). The cells with TLRs on their surface (dendritic cells, tissue macrophages, endothelial cells) are responsible for this (Fig. 1.4). After recognition of the bacterial antigens, they trigger a series of local anti-bacterial processes (production of cytokines, chemokines, and defensins) in the tissue.

The LS detects the tumor cells, carries them through the lymphatic vessels to lymph nodes, eliminates or promotes their proliferation (multiplication), generates tolerance to the tumor(?). It is still unknown whether LS responses to the necrotic cancer cells and the proteins they produce.

The LS removes own senescent and damaged cells from tissues and transports them to the lymph nodes. Does it preclude the expansion of autoimmune reaction? Are the specific cells derived from LNs involved in the healing and restoration of damaged tissue?

The LS vessels are the auto-reactive morphological fluid conductance structures (Fig. 1.5). They are independent under normal conditions from extrinsic forces as, e.g., heart, muscles, and respiration. The capillary filtrate/tissue fluid enters initial lymphatics when the hydrostatic pressure exceeds that of the intra-lymphatic lumen (Fig. 1.5a). In skin, contacting with the external environment, a dense network of lymphatics stands on alert (Fig. 1.5b). The collecting lymphatics have unidirectional valves and can contract actively (see dilated and contracted parts on Fig. 1.5c). In the lymph nodes, lymphatic sinuses comprise a large surface enabling slowing down lymph flow and filtering out cellular and soluble antigens (Fig. 1.5d).

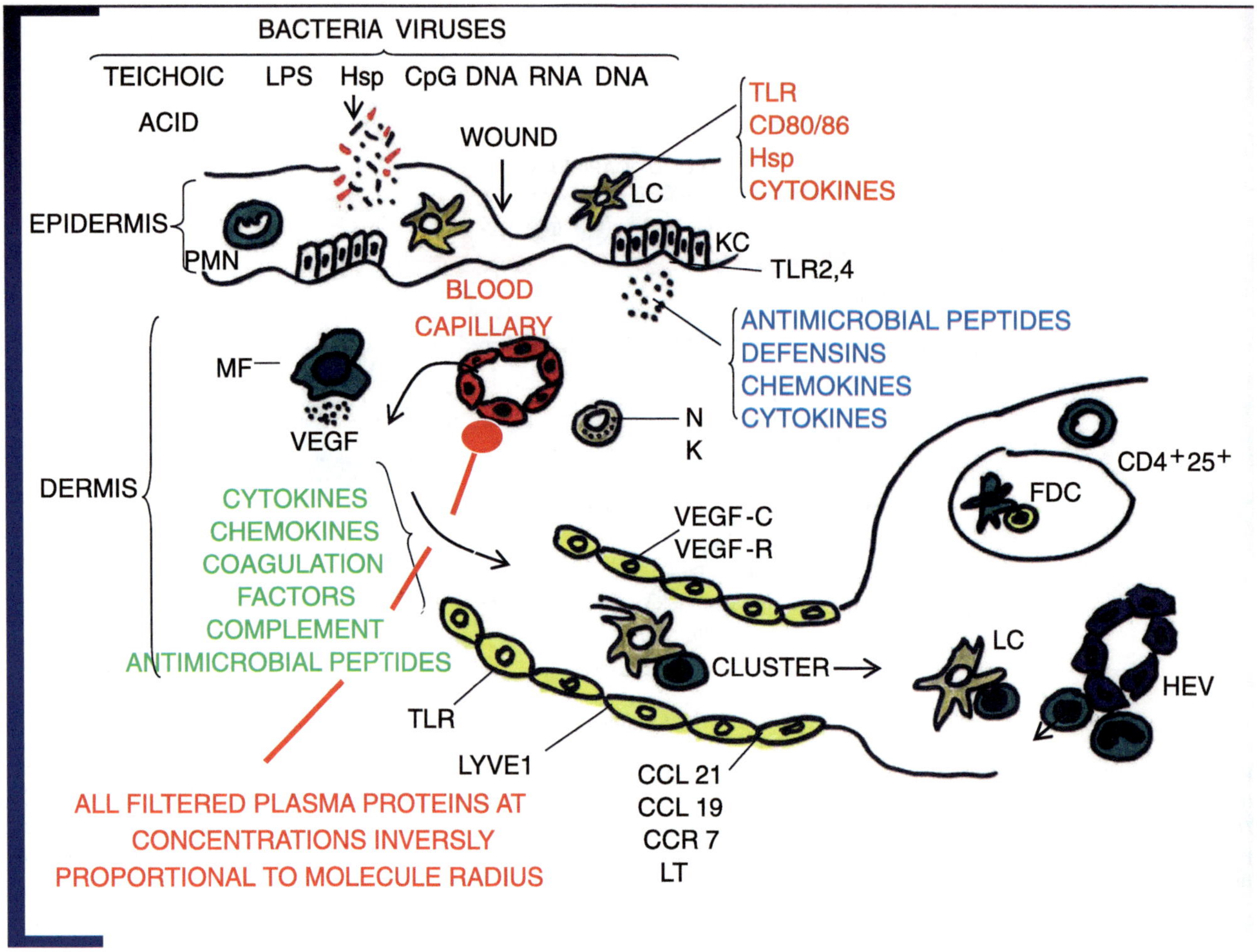

Fig. 1.4 Schematic presentation of the physiological events in the skin, draining lymphatics and nodes. The intercellular space with ground matrix and chemical molecules filtered from the blood and synthetized by resident and immigrating cells. Tissue fluid forms a hydrous environment for cells. It is continuously delivered from blood and transported to the initial lymphatics. Immune events are mediated by migrating lymphocytes and macrophages. A continuous process of elimination of penetrating microorganisms and own senescent cells debris is taking place. Microorganisms and mechanical injury of the epidermis impair the perfunctory stratum of keratinocytes. Langerhans' cells instantly identify bacteria antigens and fragments of damaged own cells. This initiates a series of immune events involving various cellular and humoral factors. "Yellow colored cells line out afferent lymphatics. *LPS* lipopolysaccharide, *hsp* heat-shock protein, *CpG DNA* bacterial DNA fragment, RNA, and DNA viral particles, *LC* Langerhans' cell, *KC* keratinocytes, *TLR* toll-like receptor, *MF* macrophage, *NK* natural killer cell, *VEGF* vascular endothelial growth factor (R-receptor), *LYVE 1* hyaluronate receptor specific for lymphatic endothelial cells, *CCL* lymphocyte chemo-attracting cytokine, *LT* lymphocytotoxin attracting lymphocytes, *FDC* follicular dendritic cells in B-cell follicles, *HEV* high endothelial venules—sites of extravasation of blood lymphocytes, *CD4+25+* regulatory lymphocytes." (Olszewski WL Pathology and biochemistry in BB Lee et al (eds) Lymphedema Springer 2018, p. 127) [3]

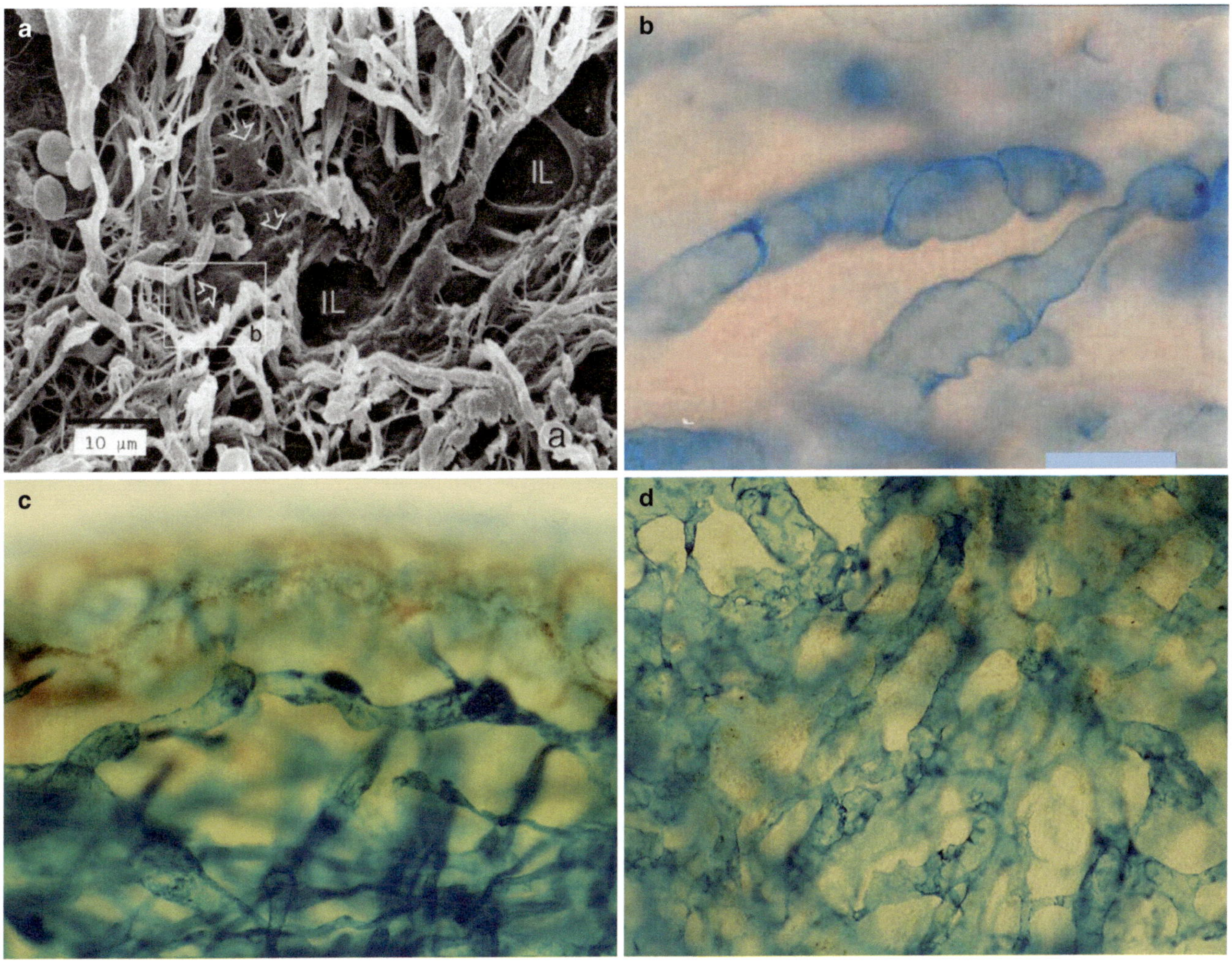

Fig. 1.5 Structure of the interstitial space where lymph is formed and initial and minor lymphatics conducting lymph. (**a**) Electron-microscopic picture of the skin interstitial space with entrance to the initial lymphatics (IL), (**b**) subepidermal and dermal lymphatics collecting tissue fluid from the skin (Paris Blue staining, ×40), (**c**) lymphatic collectors with valves (Paris Blue staining, ×40), and (**d**) intra-lymph node sinusoidal lymphatics, where the penetrating bacterial and viral antigens and own senescent cell debris are captured, and subsequently the immune reaction takes place

References

1. Olszewski WL. Peripheral lymph – formation and function. Boca Raton, FL: CRC Press; 1985.
2. Levick JR, Michel CC. Microvascular fluid exchange and the revised Starling principle. Cardiovasc Res. 2010;87(2):198–210.
3. Olszewski WL. Pathology and biochemistry. In: Lee BB, et al., editors. Lymphedema. Springer; 2018. p. 125–38.

Anatomy of Lymphatic System

2

Wei-Ren Pan, Zhi-An Liu, Chuan-Xiang Ma, and Fan-Qiang Zeng

Abstract

This chapter provides actual anatomical results of the human lymphatic system in regions of the head, neck, chest, and extremities. Most of the content was revealed and recorded for the first time. Presentation of photographs and radiographs combined with some schematic drawings enable readers to understand the detailed structure and distribution of the human lymphatic system in these regions. Content includes the lymph capillary plexus, precollecting and collecting lymph vessels, lymphatic trunk, lymphatic duct, and lymph node. In addition, details of the microanatomical morphology, unsymmetrical distribution pattern, and pathways of lymphatics, as well as the connection between lymph vessels and lymph nodes, have been presented and described. Furthermore, the latest findings of the lymphatic ampulla and diverticulum, transparent and degenerating lymph nodes, are explained in detail. This information upgrades the knowledge of the lymphatic anatomy, and results will be assisted for the clinical management of lymphoedema, cancer metastasis, and other lymphatic-related diseases.

Keywords

Lymphatic system · Lymph vessel · Lymph node · Head and neck · Chest · Limb

As a part of the vascular system, the lymphatic system is a broad network of tiny colorless vessels distributed over the body, which assists the removal of intracellular metabolic products and provides protection from disease. It is also the main route of cancer metastasis. Up to date, the knowledge of the lymphatic anatomy still remains the least described in the literature. The basic knowledge of the lymphatic system in the textbook is mostly based on Sappey's work that was done in the nineteenth century [1]. This knowledge is frequently discordant with clinical findings. In addition, it does not clarify clinical anomalies seen with breast cancer and melanoma patients using recent techniques such as lymphoscintigraphy, CT, MRI, and sentinel node biopsy for early-stage cancer management. It is well known that cancers can appear at distant sites without involving local lymph nodes. It has been suggested that disseminating cancer cells can access the circulation in the absence of local lymph node involvement [2].

Over the years, there have been attempts to accurately record actual regional lymphatic pathways but with varying success. A radiological study of the lymphatic system in cadavers has never been attempted until recently when elusive lymphatic pathways were radiologically marked by using the microvascular dissection and injection technique [3].

In this chapter, the superficial lymphatic system of the body is re-evaluated. There are still many regions where our knowledge is deficient and further studies are required.

2.1 Components of the Lymphatic System

The lymphatic system includes lymphatic channels, organs, and tissues, they are the lymph capillary plexus, precollecting and collecting lymph vessels including lymphatic ampullae and diverticulum, lymph nodes, lymphatic trunks and ducts, spleen and Peyer's patch, etc. (Figs. 2.1 and 2.2).

2.1.1 Lymph Capillary Plexus

Lymph capillary plexus exist in most organs and tissues of the body except the epithelials, cartilage and cornea, etc.

W.-R. Pan (✉) · Z.-A. Liu · C.-X. Ma · F.-Q. Zeng
Department of Anatomy, School of Biomedical Sciences, XuZhou Medical University, Xuzhou, Jiangsu, P.R. China

N. Liu (ed.), *Peripheral Lymphedema*, https://doi.org/10.1007/978-981-16-3484-0_2

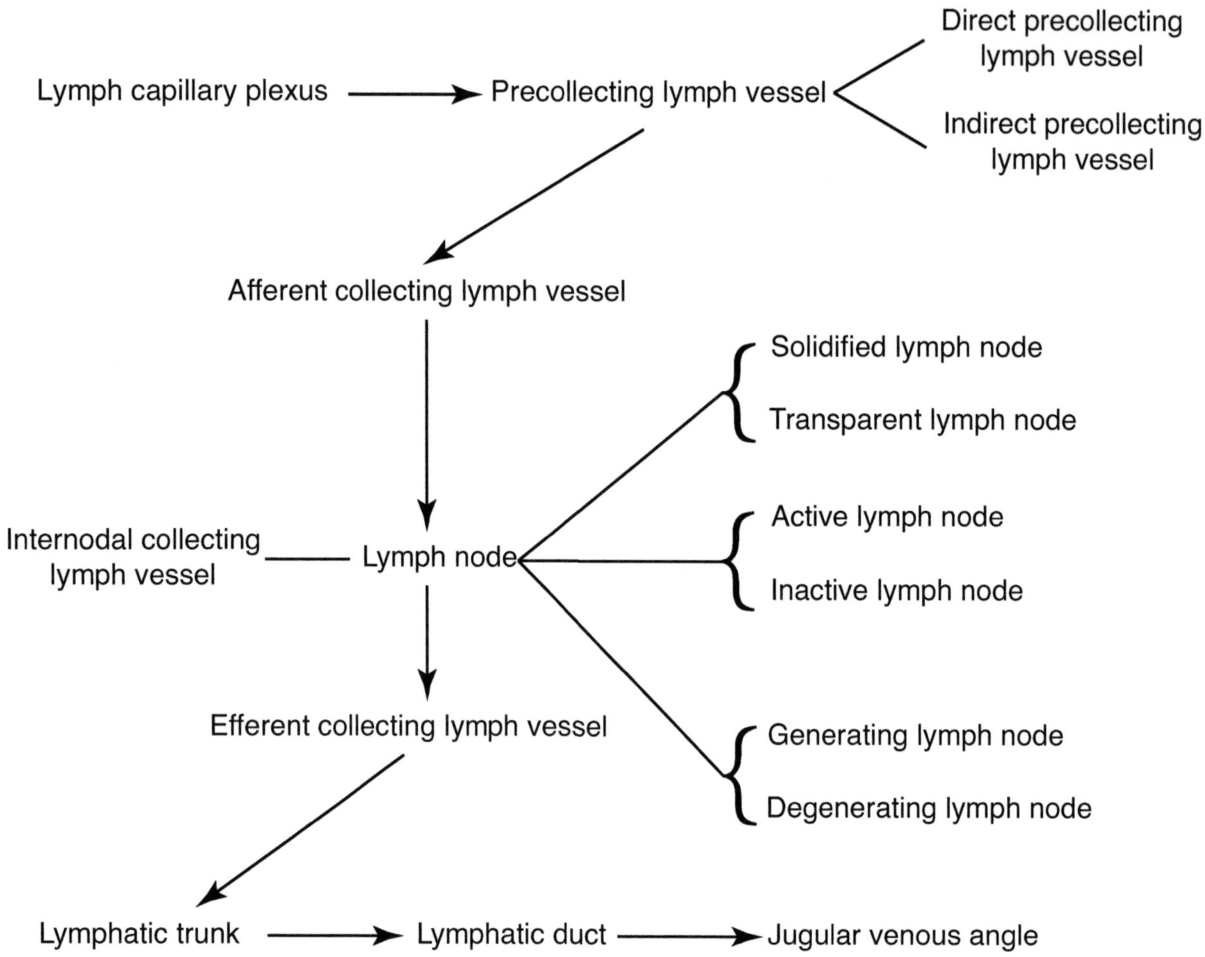

Fig. 2.1 Diagram of the lymphatic drainage

Originating from the dermis and the mucosa, lymph capillary plexus plays an important role in the immune defense mechanism, which has been well described in literatures (Hudack et al. 1933; Drinker 1941; Cowdry 1950). Those found in the galea layer have also been considered to have a similar function to those in the skin [4].

In the dermis (Fig. 2.2) and mucosa (Fig. 2.3), two layers of lymph capillary are visible—one is superficial and one deeper. They connect to each other, forming a three-dimensional (3D) network—lymph capillary plexus. The diameter of those vessels differs, tiny in the superficial layer (less than 0.02 mm) and slightly larger in the deeper. Sometimes, vessels with a diameter greater than 0.2 mm could be seen in the mucosa and the galea layer (Fig. 2.3b).

The wall of the lymph capillary plexus is thin and fragile. They are sometimes constricted and, at other times, dilated. They branch abundantly and anastomose freely to form a rich avalvular plexus. The microscopic morphology of these vessels is different in regions.

2.1.2 Precollecting Lymph Vessel

Containing sparse valves in the lumen, precollecting lymph vessel connects the lymph capillary plexus and collecting lymph vessels. The vessel arises from the dermis, mucosa, and the galeal layer, etc. From the superficial to deeper layers of the subcutaneous, it travels in an ascending, descending, horizontal, or looping manner and then drains into the collecting lymph vessels (Figs. 2.1 and 2.4).

Two types of precollecting lymph vessels, "Direct" and "Indirect (or bridge)", are presented in the scalp (Fig. 2.4). It has been shown that the former vessel arises from the lymph capillary plexus in the galea or dermis and drains directly to the collecting lymph vessel in the subcutaneous. The latter arises from the lymph capillary plexus in the dermis and crosses over the subcutaneous where bypassing the collecting vessel. Then It reaches the galeal layer where merging with the other precollecting lymph vessels, and travels within the subcutaneous again to link the collecting lymph vessel. Therefore the indirect precollecting lymph vessel connects the lymphatic drainage between the dermis and galeal layer in the scalp.

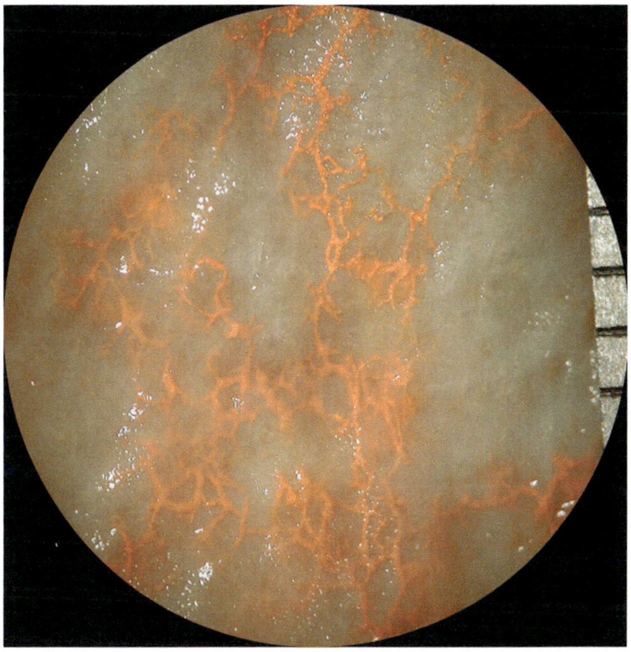

Fig. 2.2 The lymph capillary is filled with lead oxide compound in the dermis of the scalp

2.1.3 Collecting Lymph Vessel

Containing numerous valves in the lumen, the collecting lymph vessel links the precollecting lymph vessel and lymphatic trunk. It travels tortuously in the submucosa and subcutaneous (Figs. 2.1 and 2.5). According to the relationship between the vessel and lymph node, it can be named as the afferent collecting lymph vessel (ACLV), internodal collecting lymph vessel (ICLV), and efferent collecting lymph vessel (ECLV). ACLV carries lymph into the lymph node. ECLV drains lymph away from the lymph node. ICLV is either the efferent lymph vessel for the distal lymph node or the afferent vessel for the proximal node (Fig. 2.5).

2.1.4 Lymphatic Trunks and Ducts

Nine lymphatic trunks and two lymphatic ducts have been well described in related literatures (Standring et al. 2018; Moore et al. 2018). With numerous valves in the lumen, lymphatic trunks (the jugular, subclavian, bronchomediastinal, and lumbar trunks, each of which presented in pairs, and a single intestinal trunk) derived distally from the union of collecting lymph vessels, merged proximally to lymphatic ducts (the right lymphatic duct and the thoracic duct), the latter

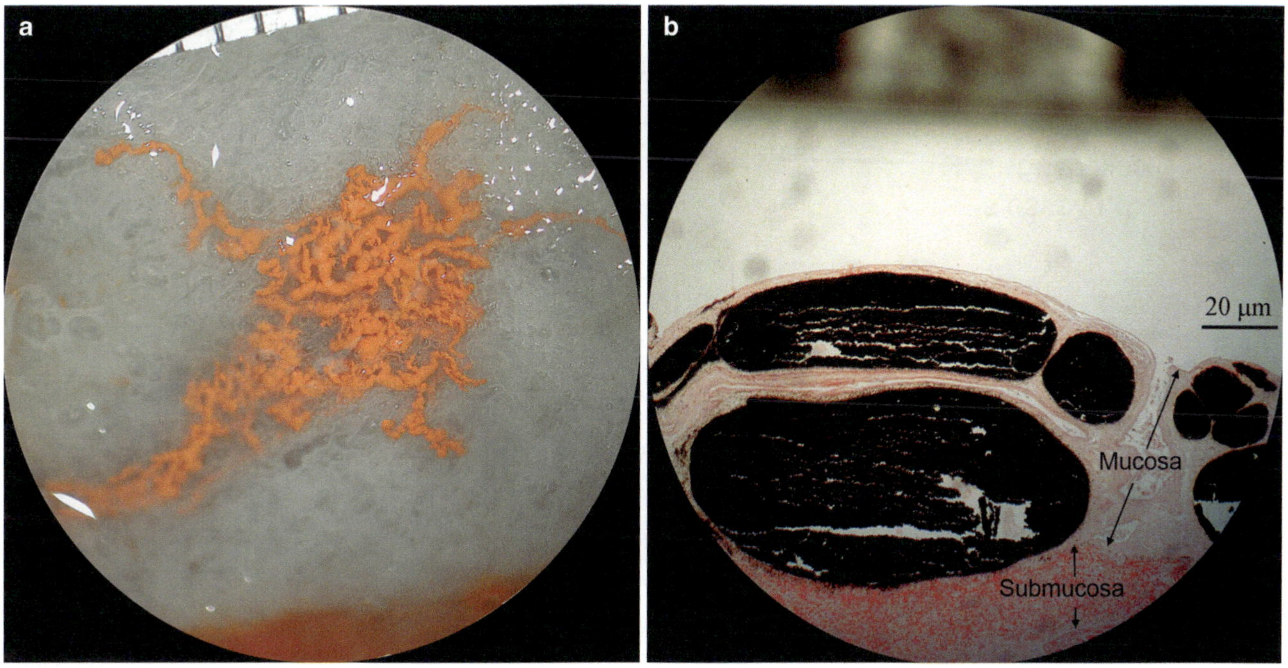

Fig. 2.3 (**a**) The "coral-like" lymph capillary is filled with lead oxide compound in the mucosa of the esophagus. (**b**) Various calibers of lymph vessels are noticed in different depths of the esophageal mucosa in the histological section

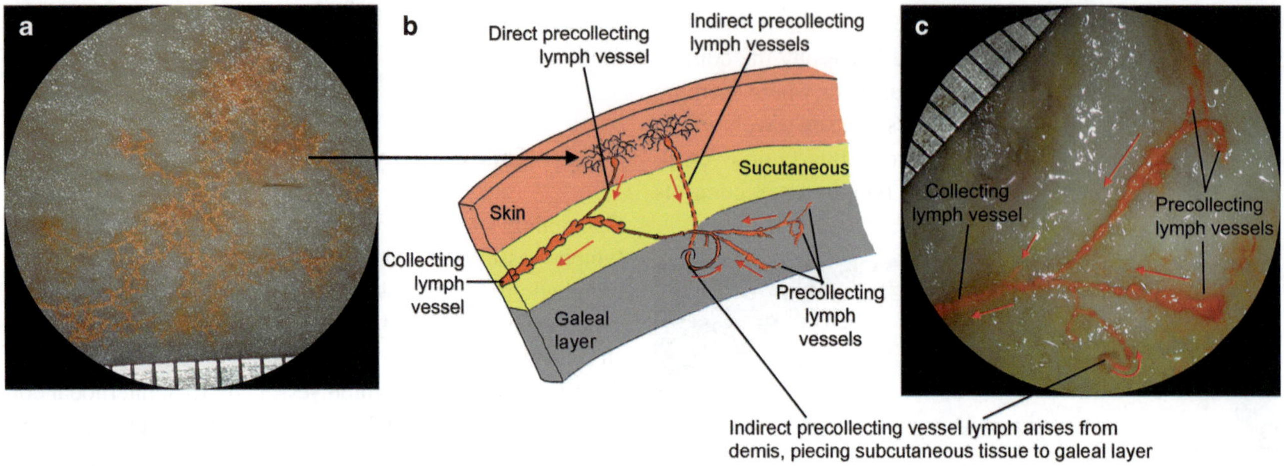

Fig. 2.4 Direct and indirect precollecting lymph vessels in the scalp. (**a**) The lymph capillary plexus filled with lead oxide mixture in the dermis of the scalp. (**b**) A sketch shows the distribution of the precollecting ("direct" and "indirect") and collecting lymph vessels in the scalp. (**c**) Lymphatic vessels in the galeal layer. Red arrows show the direction of the lymph flow

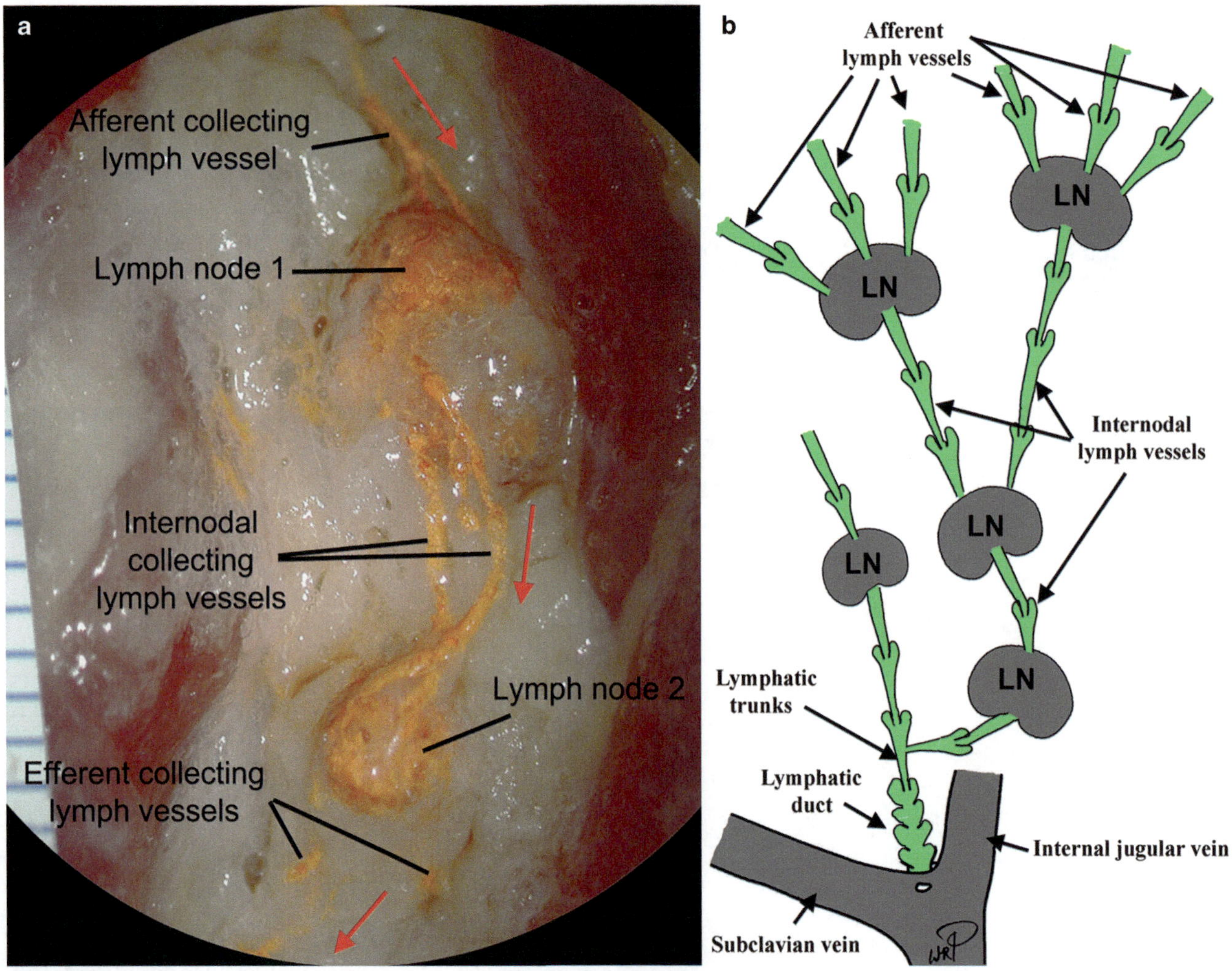

Fig. 2.5 (**a**) The relationship of ACLV, ICLV, EVLV, and lymph nodes in the preauricular region. ICLVs are ECLVs to the lymph node 1 and ACLVs to the lymph node 2. (**b**) A diagram of the relationship between collecting lymphatic vessels and the lymph nodes

then merged to large veins in corners of bilateral sides of the jugular and subclavian veins (Figs. 2.1 and 2.6).

2.1.5 Lymph Node

The details of the anatomy, function, and degeneration state of the lymph node have been described in literatures, which mostly based on studies of the solidified lymph node (Delamère et al. 1913, Rouvière 1938, Földi et al. 2003, Junqueira et al. 2003, Rubin et al. 2005, Guyton et al. 2006, Standring et al. 2018) [2, 5–12]. As early as the nineteenth century, it has been noticed that the lymph node had fully developed in regions of the neck, axilla, groin, and root of the mesentery in fetal life [5]. Soon after, Sabin [13] presented a detailed developmental process of lymph nodes in pig embryos, starting with the lymphatic heart (sac). In 1909, Lewis also found that lymph glands (nodes) could appear in early human embryos. In embryological study, Moore et al. [14] discovered and reported that the lymph sacs were converted into groups of the lymph node during the early fetal period. However, all these studies were based on solidified

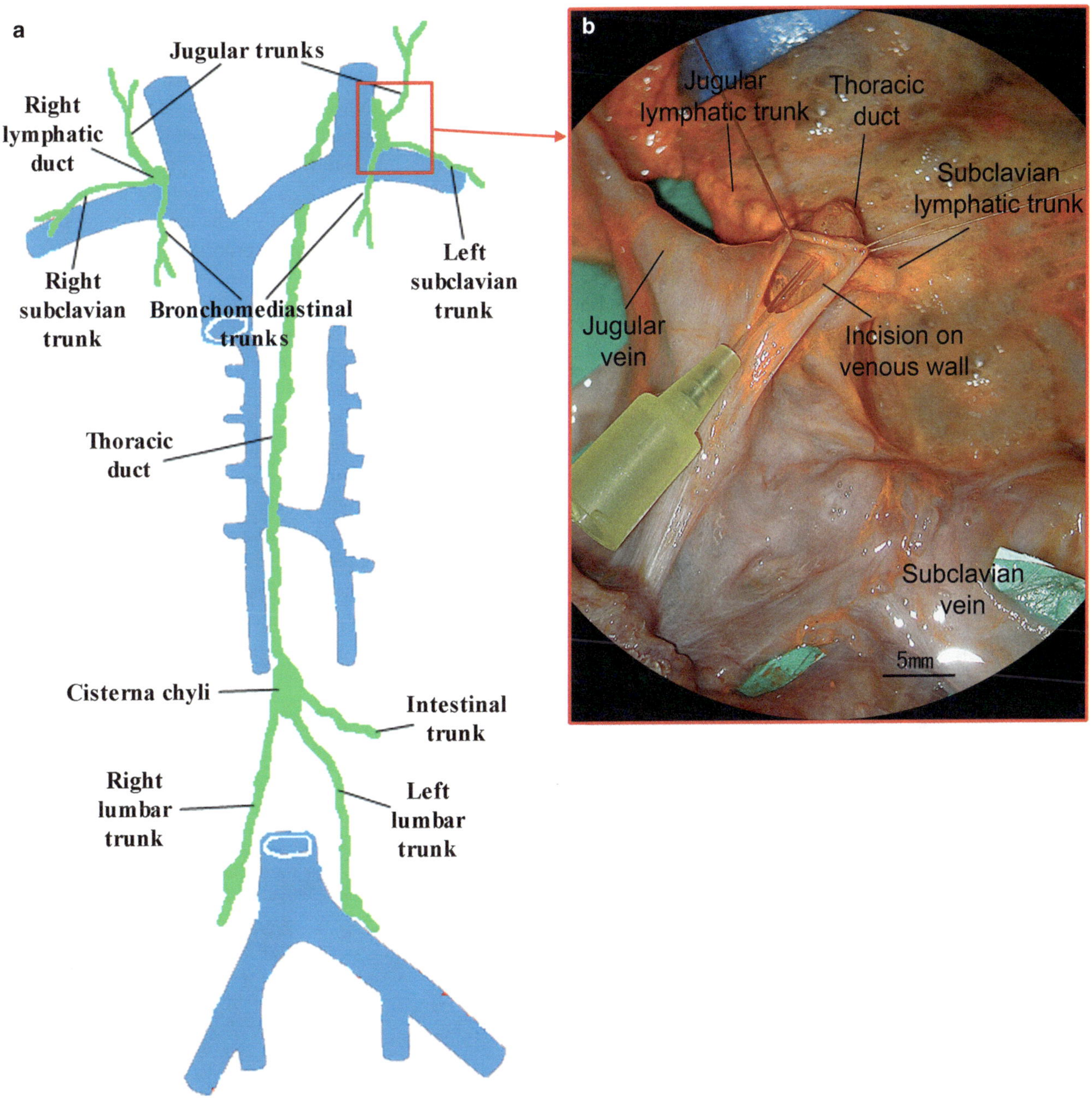

Fig. 2.6 (**a**) A diagram of the lymphatic trunks and ducts. (**b**) The left lymphatic trunks and duct drain to the corner of the subclavian and jugular veins in the left neck

lymph nodes. While Denz [6] concluded, after studying more than 300 lymph nodes, that the development of lymph nodes reached their maximum stage in childhood and decreased gradually in size after puberty. He also found that the cortical parenchyma decreased gradually and constituted an island surrounded by the medullary tissue in the node of the elderly. In some extremely old age, it could be seen that the extremely degenerated lymph nodes were similar to the undeveloped lymph node in the fetus. After studying 362 lymph nodes collected from the head and neck regions in 22 elderly cadavers, Pan et al. [4] proposed a new concept—transparent (inactive) lymph nodes. Figure 2.7 represents the concept of the generation and degeneration circle of lymph nodes combining previous knowledge with more recent findings.

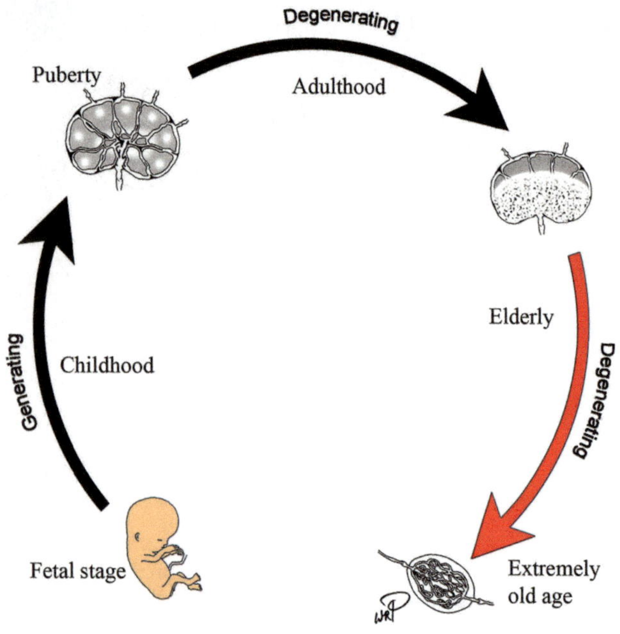

Fig. 2.7 A diagram of the generation and degeneration process cycle of the lymph node

It has been described that the medulla was predominantly affected during senile involution of the lymph node, while the cortex has remained unaffected. Report has shown that the degenerative process of the lymph node was changed qualitatively and gradually from solid to transparency [4]. Senile degeneration affected both the cortex and medulla of the lymph node. The medulla was involved in the early stage of the degenerative process. As the quantity of the lymphatic tissue was reduced, the lymph node was gradually become transparent (Fig. 2.8). The degenerative process continued until the transparent lymph node became an inactive lymph node that contained the lymphatic tubular coil, fibrous, and connective tissue rather than the lymphoid tissue. The histological section showed that the node contained neither cortex nor medulla. The result differed from previous reports that senile involution affected only the medulla predominately and that the cortex remained unaffected. It seems that the later stage of the degenerating process in the node was not observed in earlier studies.

Lymph nodes have been classified into five types according to the relationship between nodes and surrounding lymph vessels [15, 16]. However, since the lymphoscintigraphy has been applied clinically, the lymph node was described as the sentinel, interval (in transit), or regional nodes (Gould et al. 1960, Morton et al. 1992, Martini et al. 1994, Cascinelli et al. 1998, Krag 1998, Thompson et al. 1995, 2005) [2, 9, 17, 18]. With more recent findings, they could be classified as the transparent or solidified nodes based on their semblance; the active or inactive (degenerated) nodes according to histological structures; the generating or degenerating nodes based on their phases in the generation and degeneration cycle (Fig. 2.9) [4].

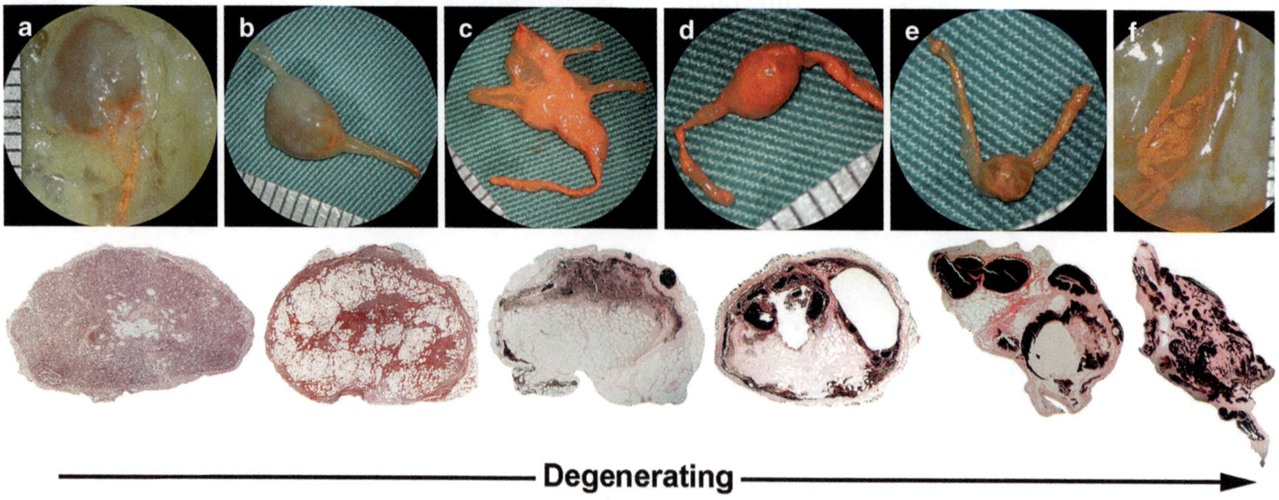

Fig. 2.8 The degenerative procedure of the lymph node. (Top row) The appearance of lymph nodes in different stages of degeneration (from **a** to **f**). (Bottom row) Histological sections show that the lymphoid tissue of lymph nodes is reduced gradually

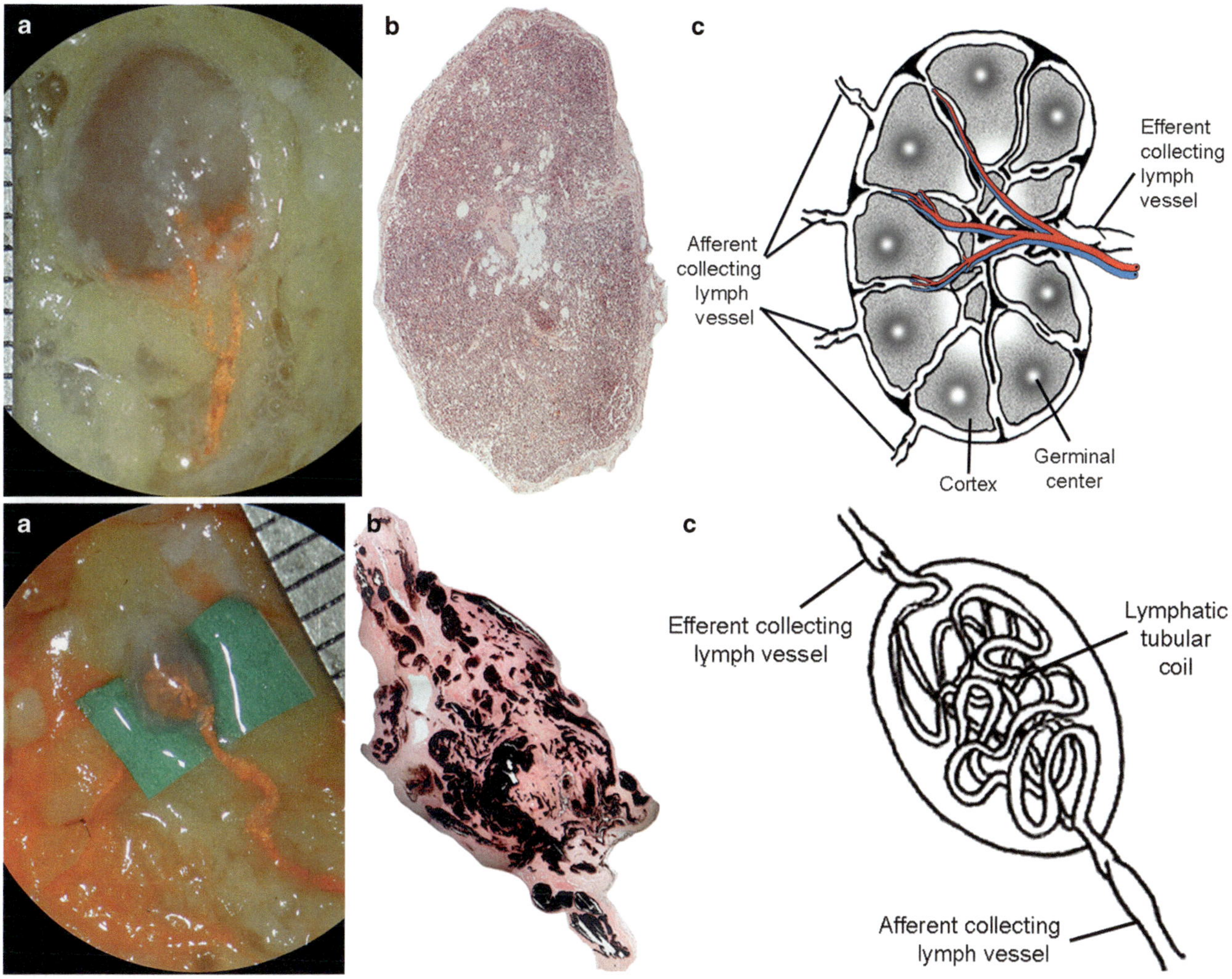

Fig. 2.9 Comparison figure of the solidified (top row) and transparent (bottom row) lymph nodes. (**a**) Semblance of lymph nodes; (**b**) Histological findings (HE); (**c**) A diagram of the solidified and transparent lymph nodes

2.2 Superficial Lymphatics of Head and Neck

Arising from the dermis, galea layer, and subcutaneous around the canthi, para-nasal area, mouth corners and neck, lymphatic vessels track radially towards the first-tier (sentinel) lymph nodes. Along their courses, vessels give branches or converge together. Sometimes, vessels are seen either crossing over or anastomosing with adjacent vessels (Fig. 2.10).

Different patterns of the lymphatic distribution are seen from person to person (Fig. 2.10). It is important that the lymph vessel in the head and neck do not always enter the first-tier lymph node, sometimes bypassed it (Figs. 2.10 and 2.11). In the head and neck section, it can be divided into three lymphatic territories—the scalp, face, and neck.

2.2.1 Scalp Region

Arising about 2 cm from the midline, collecting lymph vessels travel, in a tortuously fashion, inferiorly and posteriorly to reach the relevant first-tier (sentinel) lymph nodes in the subcutaneous (Figs. 2.10 and 2.11). They can be divided into the frontal, parietal, and occipital groups.

1. **Frontal Group**

Between the coronal suture and the upper edge of the eyebrow, three to six collecting lymph vessels can be found (average four vessels). They travel radially in the deep part of the subcutaneous and drain into the parotid and/or preauricular lymph nodes (Figs. 2.10 and 2.11); the nasolabial, parotid, and retroauricular lymph nodes (Figs. 2.10, 2.11, and 2.12a); the preauricular and retroauricular lymph nodes (Fig. 2.12b);

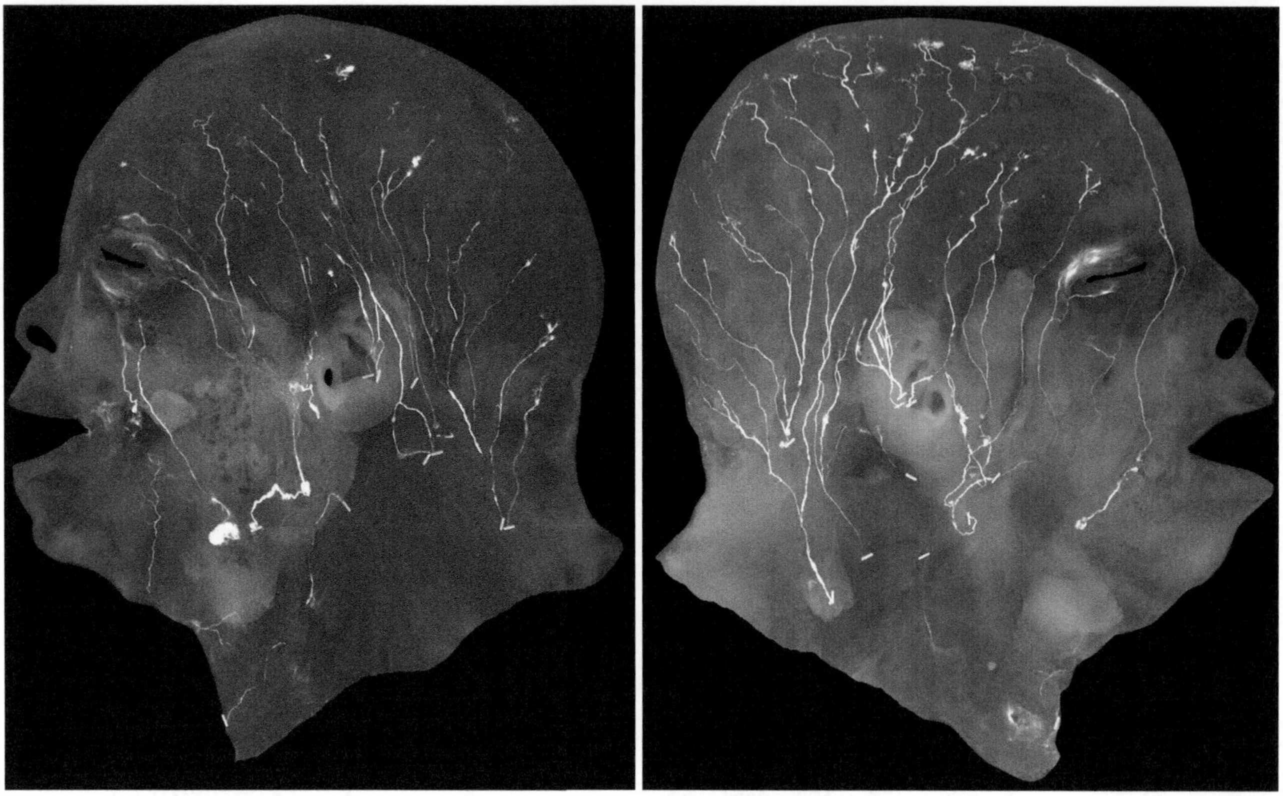

Fig. 2.10 After the lead oxide injection, radiographs of the integument on either side of the head and neck in the same body showing the asymmetrical distribution patterns of lymphatic vessels and nodes

the buccinators, preauricular, retroauricular and deep parotid lymph nodes (Fig. 2.12c).

2. **Parietal Group**

Between the coronal and the lambdoid sutures, 4–12 collecting lymph vessels can be found (average six vessels). They travel radially in the deep part of the subcutaneous and drain into single or multiple groups of the related lymph nodes (Figs. 2.10, 2.11, and 2.13).

3. **Occipital Group**

Between the lambdoid suture and the posterior hairline, four to nine collecting lymph vessels (average six vessels) are presented. They run radially in the deep part of the subcutaneous in the occipital section and drain into single or multiple groups of the related lymph nodes (Figs. 2.10, 2.11, and 2.14).

4. **Lymphaticovenous Shunt**

The phenomenon of non-iatrogenic lymphaticovenous anastomoses (LVA) is rare in the human body. A site of LVA is presented in the occipital region. The superficial occipital lymph node gives off the efferent lymph vessel that forms a lymphatic network at the junction of the occiput and neck. From there, two small lymphatic vessels arise and then connect to a superficial occipital vein in the subcutaneous (Fig. 2.15). This phenomenon confirms the clinical findings reported by Wallace et al. [19]. It should be recognized that this phenomenon can provide a systemic approach to metastatic disease.

2.2.2 Facial Region

Between the eyebrow and the inferior border of the mandible, lymphatic vessels distribute sparsely. Three to five main

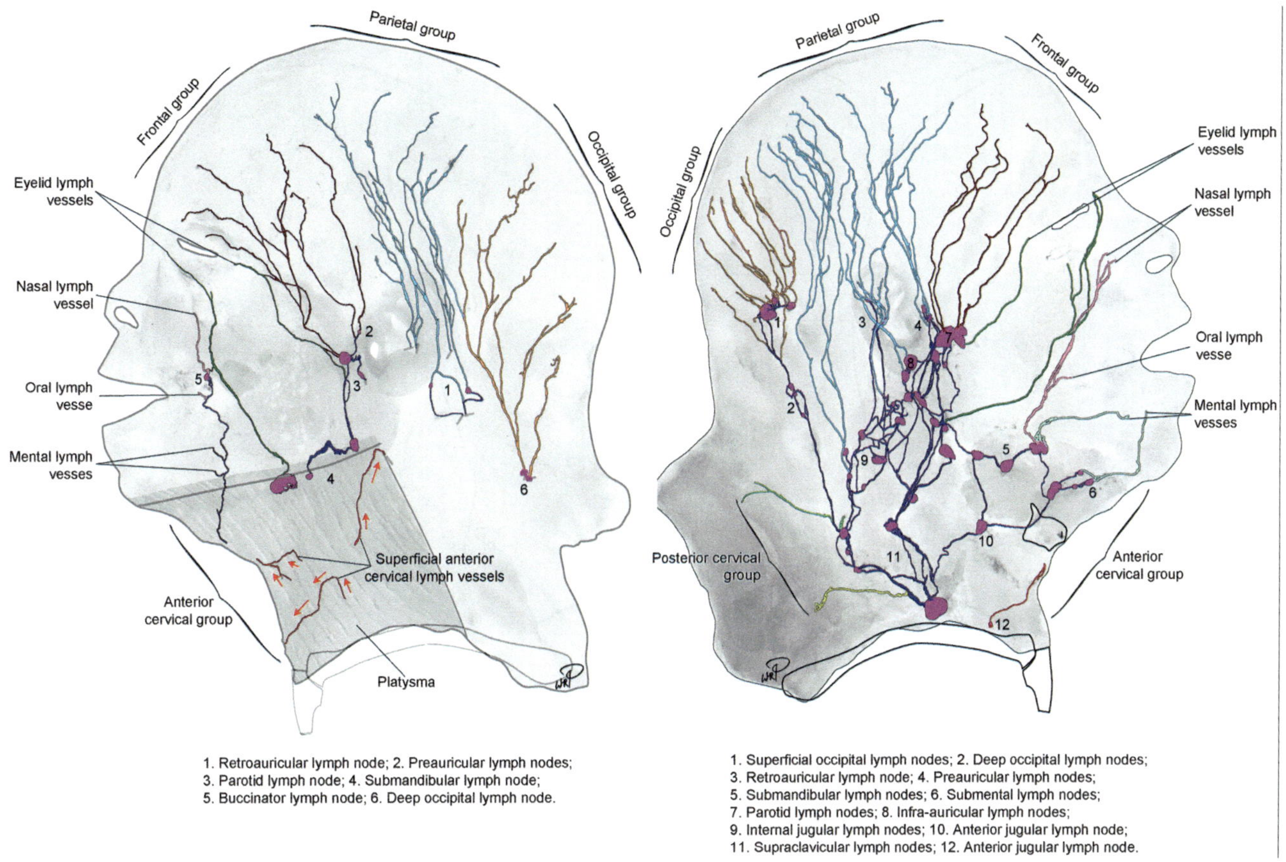

Fig. 2.11 The lymphatic distribution of the integument in the head and neck. (Left) Lymphatic vessels travel above the platysma in the neck. (Right) Vessels run under the platysma. Different groups of lymphatic vessels and nodes are highlighted in different colors

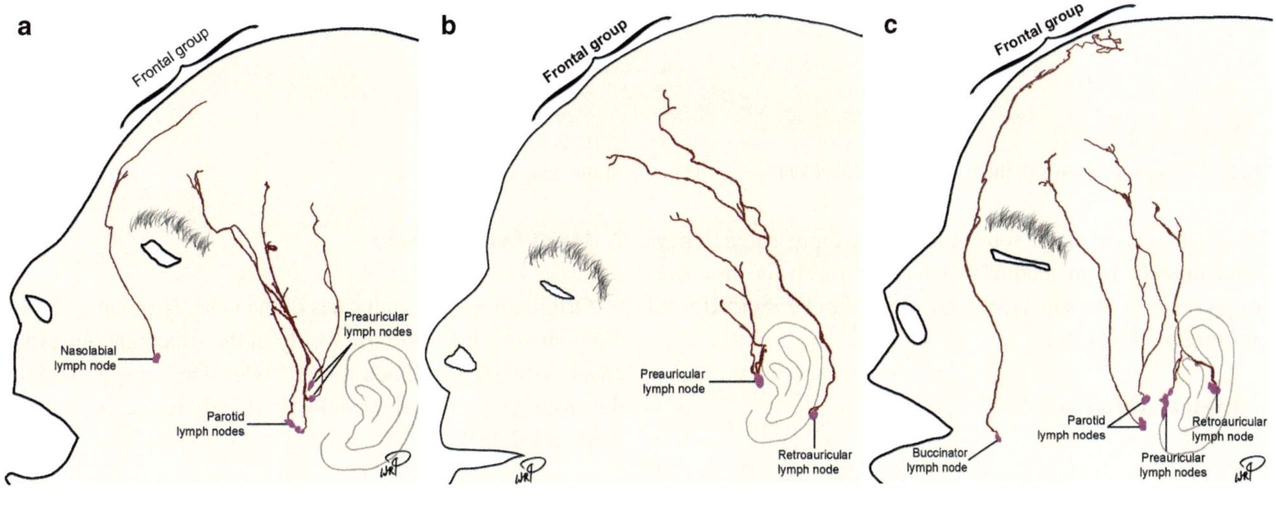

Fig. 2.12 Various patterns of the lymphatic drainage in the frontal group of the scalp region (**a** to **c**)

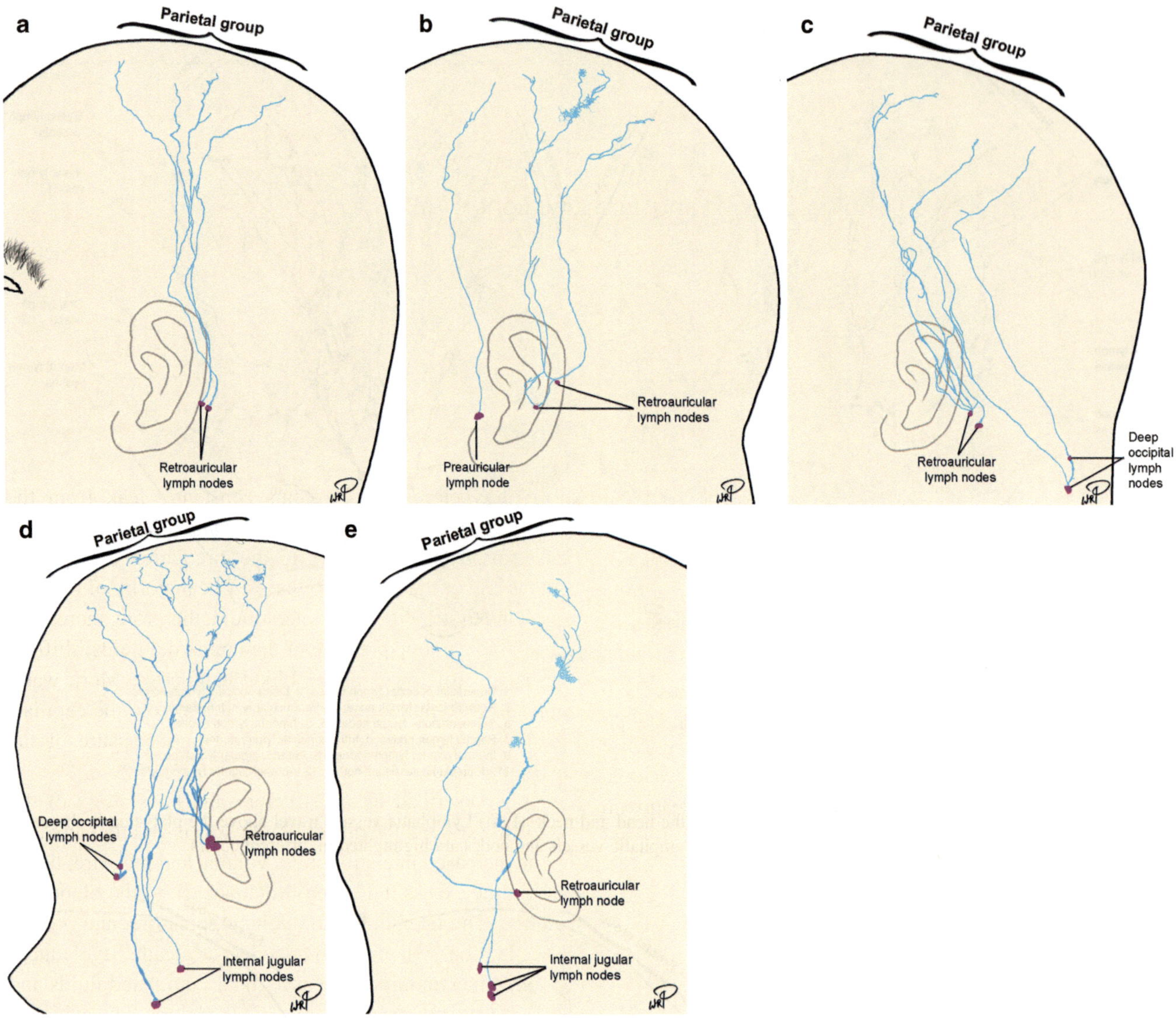

Fig. 2.13 Various patterns of the lymphatic drainage in the parietal group of the scalp region (**a** to **e**)

lymph vessels (average four vessels) were presented. They travel radially from medial to lateral to reach the first-tier lymph node in the subcutaneous, which can be divided into four groups of vessels.

1. **Eyelid Lymph Vessel**

Plexuses of the lymphatic capillary arise in the dermis of both superior and inferior eyelids. They form the outer and inner canthus lymph vessels at the outer and inner canthus. An inferior eyelid lymph vessel is presented at the middle-inferior area of the inferior eyelid (Fig. 2.16). The lymphatic drainage patterns of the eyelid are deferent in individuals (Figs. 2.11, 2.16, and 2.17).

2. **Nasal Lymph Vessel**

Originating from both sides of the nose, lymphatic vessels travel downwardly and outwardly in the subcutaneous of the cheek to reach the related lymph nodes. Drainage patterns of the nasal lymph vessel are deferent in individuals (Figs. 2.11, 2.12, and 2.18).

3. **Oral Lymph Vessel**

Originating from both corners of the mouth, oral lymph vessels traveled laterally and downwardly in the subcutaneous of the cheek and drained to related nodes. Drainage pat-

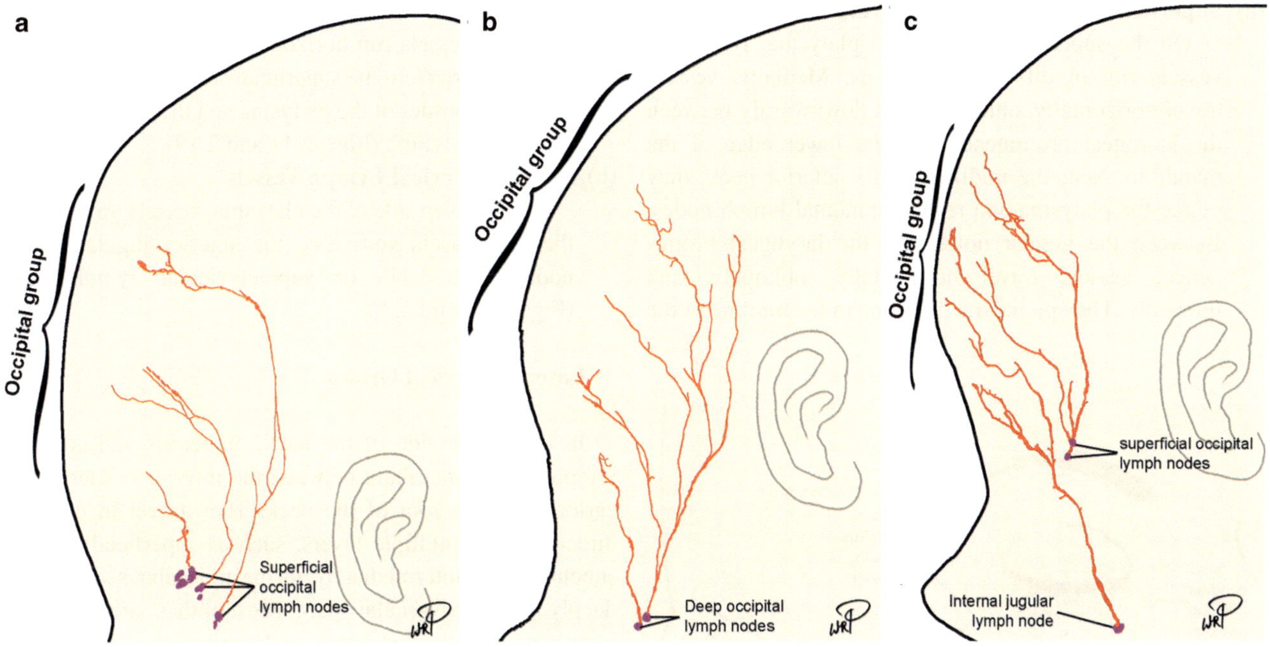

Fig. 2.14 Various patterns of the lymphatic drainage in the occipital group in the scalp region (**a** to **c**)

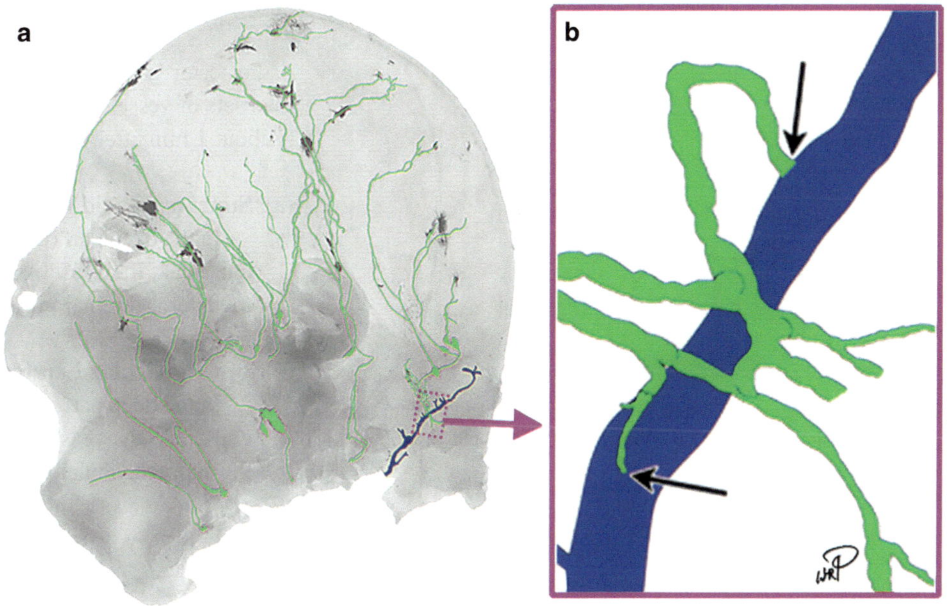

Fig. 2.15 LVA site in the junction of the occiput and neck. (**a**) A image shows LVA in the occipital area. (**b**) A Schematic diagram from the purple boxed area in (**a**) shows LVA site (black arrows). Blue = vein; Green = lymphatic vessels

terns of the oral lymph vessel are deferent in individuals (Figs. 2.11 and 2.18).

4. **Mental Lymph Vessel**

Originating from the deep aspect of the subcutaneous of the chin, mental lymph vessels were travel downward and drained to related nodes. Drainage patterns of the oral lymph vessel are deferent in individuals (Figs. 2.11 and 2.18).

2.2.3 Cervical Region

There are three groups of lymph vessels in the cervical region.

1. **Anterior Cervical Group**

There are two layers of lymphatic vessels in the anterior superficial tissue of the neck.

(a) **Superficial Anterior Cervical Lymph Vessels**
On the superficial side of the platysma, lymphatic vessels run in different directions. Medially, vessels travel horizontally, obliquely, and downwardly between the laryngeal prominence and the lower edge of the mandible. Near the midline of the anterior neck, they pierce the platysma and reach submental lymph nodes. Between the jugular notch and the laryngeal prominence, vessels travel horizontally, obliquely, and upwardly. They pierce the platysma in the midline of the anterior neck and reach the supraclavicular lymph node. Laterally vessels run horizontally, obliquely, upwardly, and then turn from the superficial side to the deep side at the lateral border of the platysma and then reach the submandibular lymph (Figs. 2.11 and 2.19).

(b) **Anterior Cervical Lymph Vessels**
On the deep side of the platysma, vessels travel above the deep fascia and reach the anterior jugular lymph node (Fig. 2.11) or supraclavicular lymph node (Figs. 2.19 and 2.20).

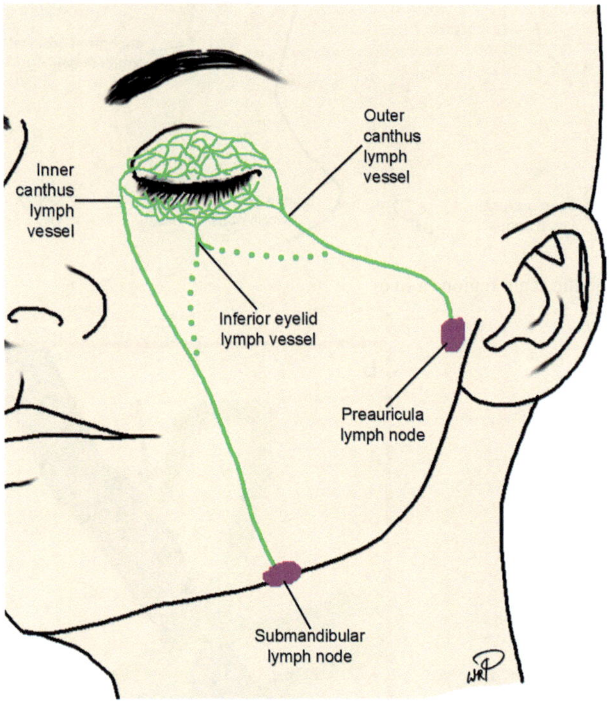

Fig. 2.16 A diagram of lymphatic drainage of eyelids. Dotted lines indicate that the inferior eyelid lymph vessel merges either the inner or outer canthus lymph vessels

2. **Lateral Cervical Group**

In the lateral side of the neck, numerous and complex lymph vessels distribute between the inferior border of the earlobe and the root of the neck. They travel in different directions and multiple layers, such as superficially in the subcutaneous, intermediately in the muscular septum, and deeply in the perivascular space. Most of them are internodal lymph vessels located between lymph nodes (Figs. 2.11, 2.19, and 2.20, lymph vessels are highlighted in blue).

3. **Posterior Cervical Group**

Posterior lymph vessels in the cervical region are sparse. Two sets of vessels are presented. The diameter of the vessel is about 1 mm after perfusion.

(a) **Supratrapezoid Lymph Vessels**
In the deep part of the subcutaneous of the posterolateral neck, the vessel travels anteromedially and reaches the lateral internal jugular and/or supraclavicular lymph nodes (Fig. 2.20).

(b) **Supraclavicular Lymph Vessels**
In the deep part of the subcutaneous of the posterolateral neck, the vessel travels anteromedially and reaches the supraclavicular lymph node (Fig. 2.20).

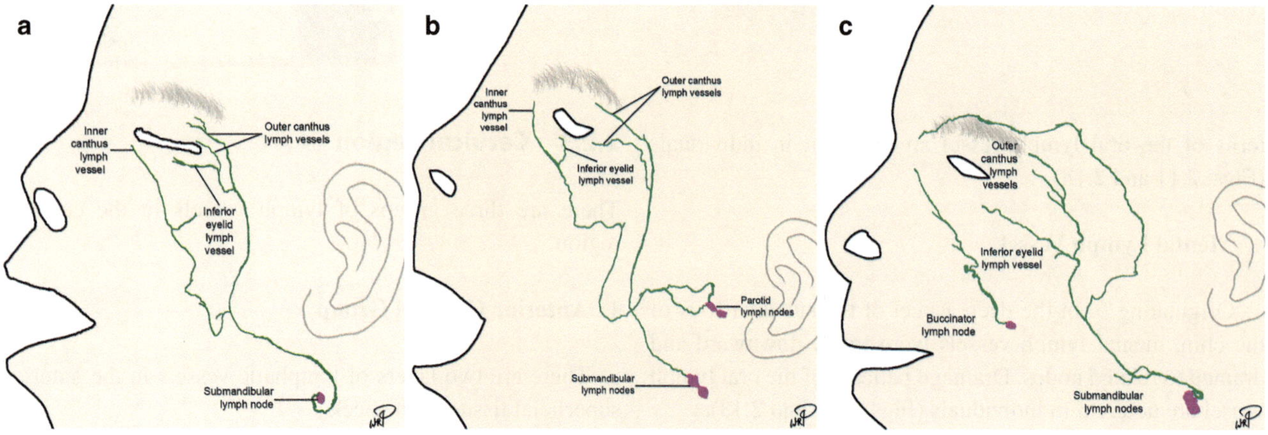

Fig. 2.17 Various drainage patterns of eyelids lymph vessels (**a** to **c**)

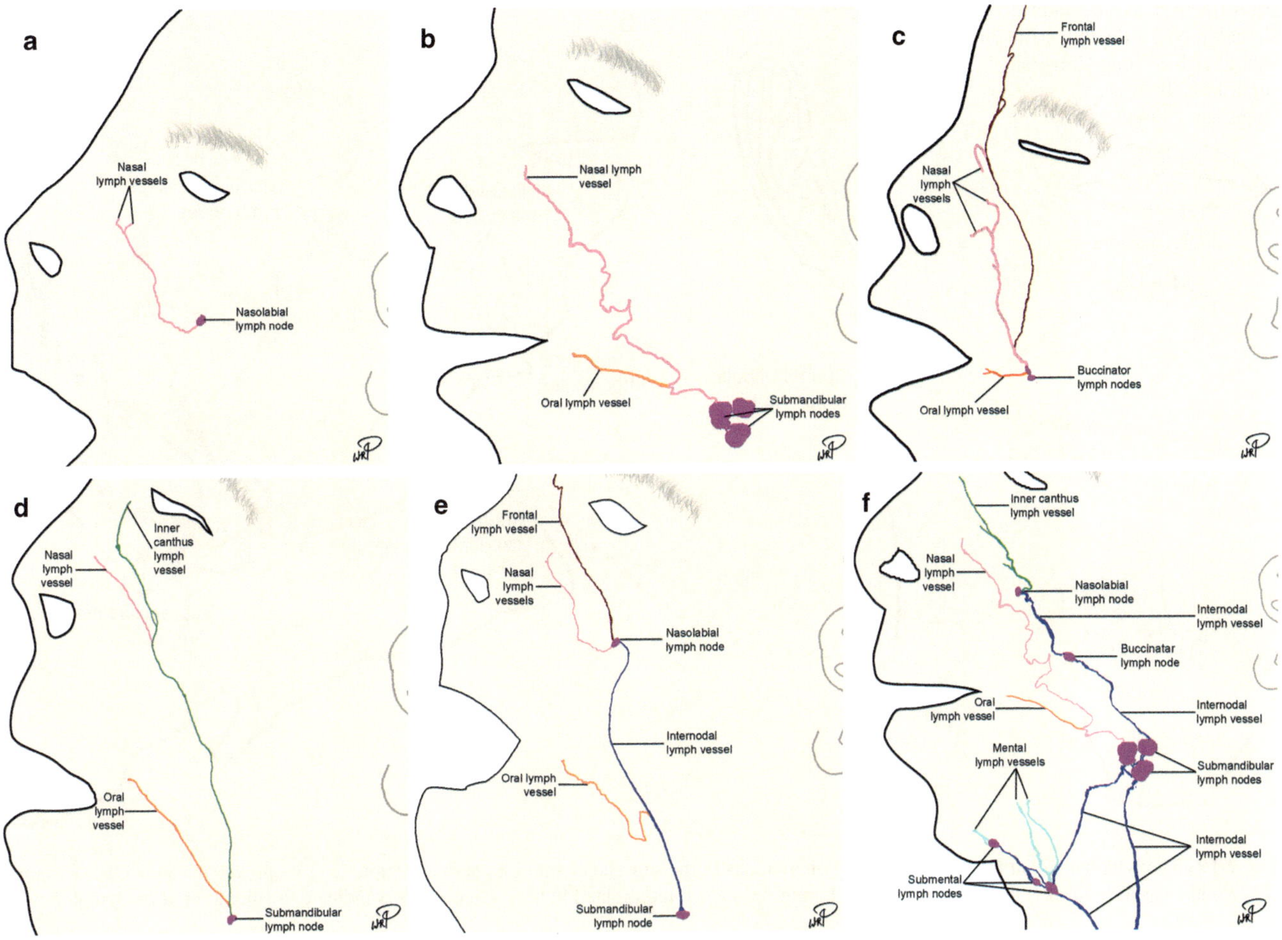

Fig. 2.18 Various drainage patterns of nasal, oral, and Metal lymph vessels. (**a**) The nasal lymph vessel (pink) drains to the nasolabial lymph node. (**b**) The nasal lymph vessel (pink) converges with the oral lymph vessel (light orange) and drains to the submandibular lymph node. (**c**) The nasal lymph vessel converges (pink) with a lymph vessel of the frontal group (brown) and drains to the buccinator lymph node. The oral vessel drains to the buccinator lymph node directly. (**d**) Both the nasal and oral lymph vessels merge to the inner canthus lymph vessels and drain to the submandibular lymph node. (**e**) The nasal lymph vessel drains to the nasolabial lymph node, the oral vessel merges to the internodal lymph vessel and then to the submandibular node. (**f**) The nasal and oral lymph vessels converged and drain to the submandibular lymph node, while mental lymph vessels drain to submental lymph nodes

2.2.4 Auricular Region

There are four groups of lymph vessels in the auricle (Fig. 2.21).

1. **Preauricular Lymph Vessel**

Arising from the lymph capillary plexus in the anterior aspect of the auricle, the preauricular lymph vessel travel *anteroinferiorly* in the subcutaneous of the crus of the helix and drain to the preauricular lymph node (Fig. 2.21 vessels highlighted in green).

2. **Supraauricular Lymph Vessel**

Arising from the superior part of the helix, supraauricular lymph vessels (ranged from 2 to 4) travel in the subcutaneous of the posterior aspect of the auricle. Then they converge together, run in the subcutaneous of the upper lateral part of the neck, and drain to the infraauricular and/or substernocleidomastoid lymph nodes (Fig. 2.21 vessels highlighted in orange).

3. **Midauricular Lymph Vessel**

Originating from the scaphoid fossa, mid auricular lymph vessels travel downwards, turn over at the middle of the auricular rim, and then run obliquely in the subcutaneous of the posterior aspect of the auricle. The mid auricular lymph vessel reaches to the infraauricular lymph node (Fig. 2.21 vessels highlighted in yellow).

4. **Infraauricular (Lobule) Lymph Vessels**

Originating from the lobule of the auricle, lymph vessels travel obliquely in the subcutaneous. Then they converge together and reach the infraauricular node (Fig. 2.21 vessels highlighted in blue).

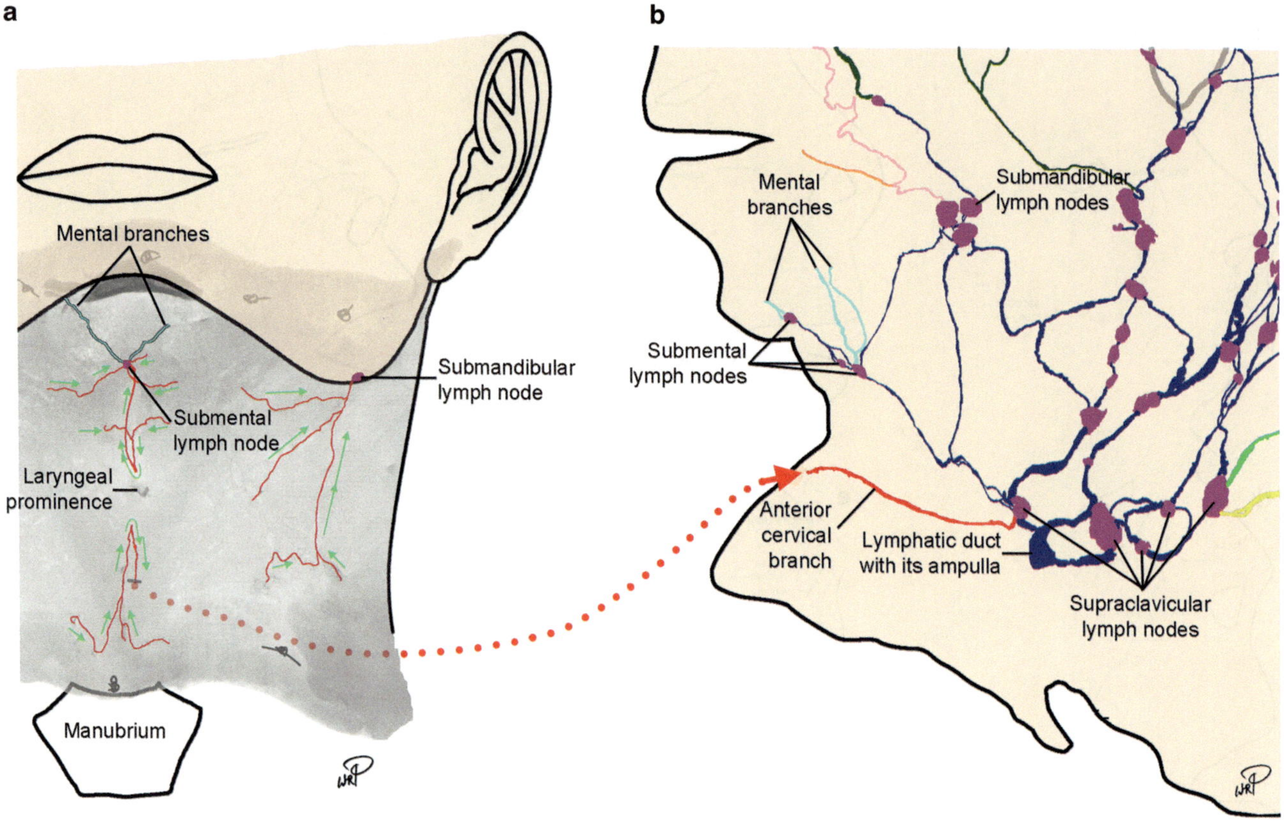

Fig. 2.19 The lymphatic distribution and related lymph nodes in the superficial anterior cervical region. (**a**) Lymph vessels above the platysma. (**b**) Lymph vessels below the platysma. Internodal lymph vessels are highlighted in blue. Green arrows indicate the direction of the lymph flow

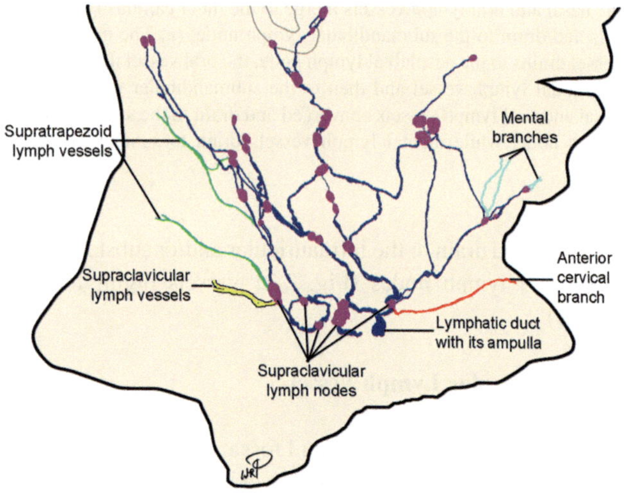

Fig. 2.20 The lymphatic distribution of the cervical region

2.3 Chest and Female Breasts

In the chest, numerous collecting lymph vessels distribute in the subcutaneous. The distribution pattern of lymphatics varies from person to person, and even an asymmetrical pattern can be seen on each side of the same body (Fig. 2.22). Vessels run in two layers (the superficial and deep). Three groups of the lymph vessel are presented in the region, two groups of them run in the integument of the chest and one the deep side (Fig. 2.22).

2.3.1 Paraareola Group

Originating from the lymph capillary plexus in the dermis of the areola, precollecting lymph vessels converge to collecting vessels (average two vessels) under the dermis around the areola. They travel superolaterally in the subcutaneous of the chest and converge with some lymph vessels of the superficial anterior group, and then enter one lymph node in the axilla (Fig. 2.22).

2.3.2 Superoanterior Group

Originating from the subcutaneous along the costal margin and the lateral side of the sternum, collecting lymph vessels travel radially to reach the axillary lymph node(s). During the process, most of them merge to form larger vessels, and then some divide into branches before entering nodes (Fig. 2.22).

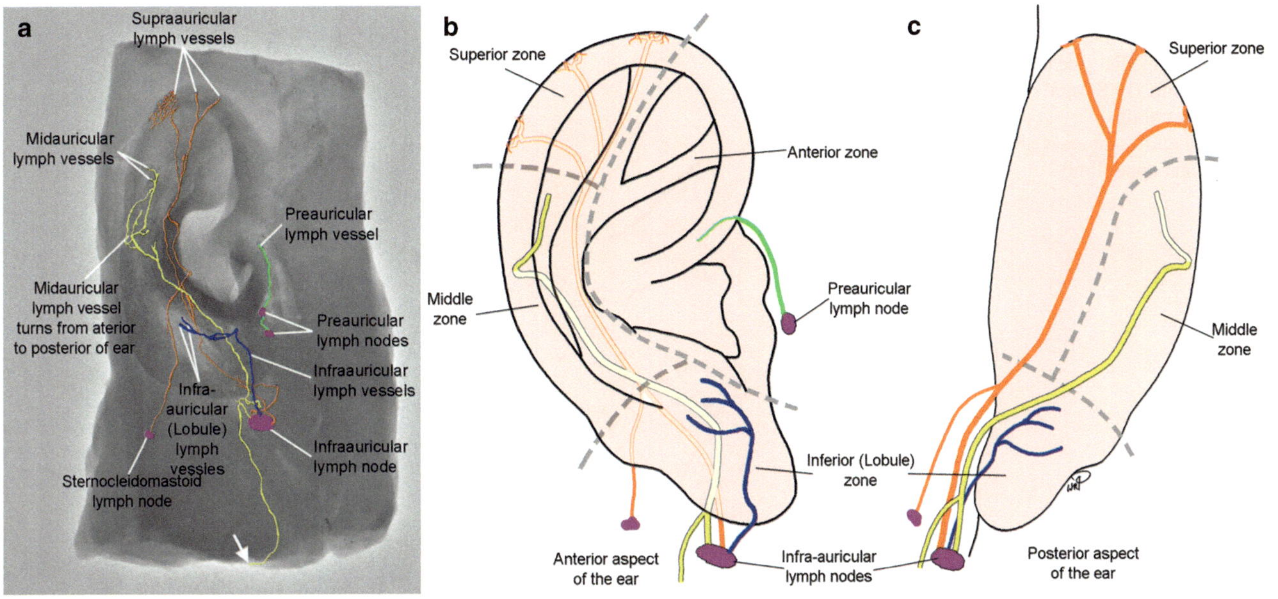

Fig. 2.21 The lymphatic distribution of the auricle. (**a**) Lymphangiogram of the lymphatic distribution of the auricle. (**b**) A diagram of the lymphatic distribution in the anterior aspect of the auricle. (**c**) A diagram of the lymphatic distribution in the posterior aspect of the auricle. Four lymphatic drainage zones are divided by the gray dashed lines

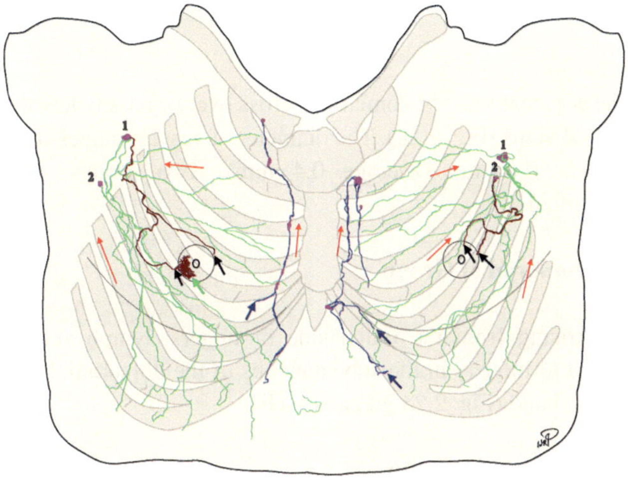

Fig. 2.22 The distribution of lymphatics in the chest. An asymmetrical pattern of lymphatic drainage is presented in the same specimen. Three groups of lymphatic vessels are highlighted by deferent colors. Brown = paraareola group (black arrows); Green = superoanterior group; Blue = parasternal-intercostal group; Purple = lymph nodes. The green arrow indicates the lymphatic capillary plexus in the dermis of the areola. Blue arrows indicate intercostal lymph vessels. Red arrows indicate the direction of the lymph flow. 1 and 2 = Axillary lymph nodes

2.3.3 Parasternal-Intercostal Group

In the internal side of the chest wall, one or two parasternal lymph vessels arise underneath the parietal pleura of the subcostal angle on each side of the chest. Along with the intrathoracic vascular bundle, lymph vessels ascend and pass through several parasternal lymph nodes and then merge to vessels in the supraclavicular region (Fig. 2.22).

Originating from the intercostals spaces, intercostal lymph vessels travel horizontally and obliquely to merge parasternal vessels or enter the relevant parasternal lymph nodes at different levels (Fig. 2.22).

2.3.4 Lymphatic Drainage Patterns in the Section of the Chest, Upper Limb, and Axilla

Axillary mph nodes receive lymph from both the chest and upper limb, but the drainage pattern varies from person to person, and even an asymmetrical pattern can be seen on each side of the same body (Figs. 2.22 and 2.23).

2.4 Superficial Lymphatics of Upper Extremity

Abundant collecting lymph vessels are presented in the subcutaneous of the upper extremity (Fig. 2.24). Originating beneath the dermis on bilateral sides of the finger, the wrist flexion crease, and the lateral area of the upper arm, lymph vessels travel centripetally and meander their way in the subcutaneous of different depths to reach lymph nodes in the axilla. One or two vessels pass through the cubital lymph node in the anteromedial elbow (Fig. 2.25). During the

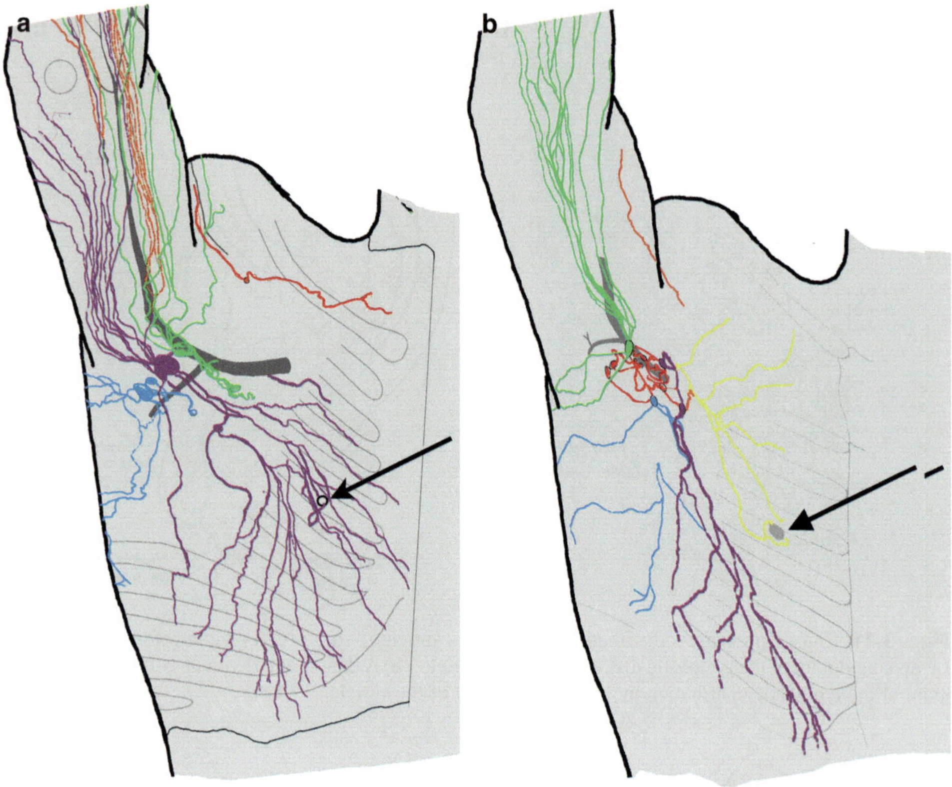

Fig. 2.23 (**a**) A lymph node in the axilla drains the most chest and the medial side of the upper limb. (**b**) Several lymph nodes drain respectively different areas of the chest and upper limb

process, vessels diverge and converge to each other, sometimes crossed over or pass through below the neighboring vessel. Most of them unite to form larger vessels, while some divide into smaller ones before entering axillary lymph nodes. The diameter of vessels ranges from 0.2 to 1.2 mm.

2.4.1 Finger

Initiating beneath the dermis on bilateral sides of the finger, digital lymph vessels (one or two vessels) travel meanderly in the subcutaneous along the central axis of the finger. They travel parallelly with digital arteries, veins, and nerves. Neighboring digital vessels merge together in the web spaces of the dorsal hand except those on the lateral edge of the thumb and the medial edge of the little finger that travel tortuously to unite with lymph vessels of the dorsal hand (Figs. 2.24 and 2.26). The diameter of vessels ranges from 0.2 to 0.5 mm (average 0.4 mm).

2.4.2 Hand

In the dorsal hand, 14–18 (average 6) collecting lymph vessels are presented (Fig. 2.24). During the process, vessels travel tortuously in the subcutaneous of the dorsal hand. They sometimes divide into branches or merge together with the adjacent vessels, sometimes cross over or pass below the dorsal veins (Fig. 2.24). The diameter of vessels ranges from 0.2 to 0.6 mm (average 0.4 mm). Two groups were identified.

1. **Dorsoradial Group**

Arising from the radial side of fingers, lymph vessels travel tortuously in the subcutaneous of the dorsoradial part of the hand (Fig. 2.24 green vessels).

2. **Dorsoulnar Group**

Arising from the ulnar side of fingers, vessels travel tortuously in the subcutaneous of the dorsoulnar part of the hand (Fig. 2.24 blue vessels).

2.4.3 Forearm

In the forearm, a range of 22–34 (average 26) collecting lymph vessels are presented (Fig. 2.24). Arising from the dorsal hand and the skin crease area of the ventral wrist, they meander in the subcutaneous of the forearm and travel parallelly with the basilic and cephalic venous systems. The diameter of vessels ranges from 0.3 to 0.6 mm (average 0.5 mm). Three groups of them are presented.

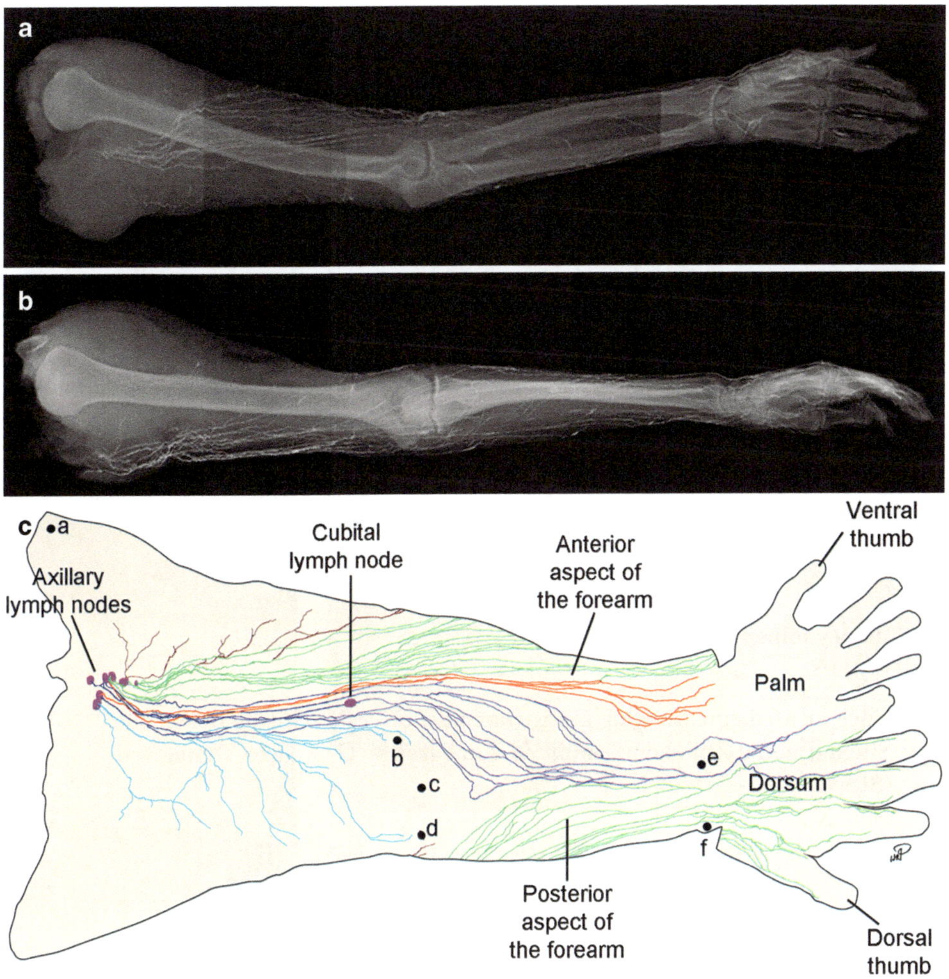

Fig. 2.24 The distribution of the superficial lymphatic in the upper left limb after a lead oxide mixture perfution. (**a**) Anteroposterial view. (**b**) Lateral view. (**c**) The lymphatic distribution in the subcutaneous of the upper extremity. a = Acromion of the scapula; b = Medial epicondyle of the humerus; c = Olecranon; d = Lateral epicondyle of the humerus; e = Styloid process of the ulna; f = Styloid process of the radius

1. **Radial Group**

They are continuation lymph vessels arising from the dorsoradial group of the hand. Vessels travel centripetally in the subcutaneous and cross the radial edge of the forearm from the dorsal wrist to the radial part of the cubital fossa (Fig. 2.24 green vessels).

2. **Ulnar Group**

They are continuation lymph vessels arising from the dorsoulnar group of the hand. Vessels travel centripetally in the subcutaneous and cross the ulnar margin of the forearm from the ulnar part of the wrist to the medial aspect of the cubital fossa (Fig. 2.24 blue vessels).

3. **Anterior Group**

Originating from the skin crease area of the ventral wrist, lymph vessels travel centripetally in the subcutaneous towards the cubital fossa (Fig. 2.24 Orange vessels).

2.4.4 Upper Arm

In the upper arm, a range of 17–21 (average 19) collecting lymph vessels are presented (Fig. 2.24). Traveling centripetally towards axillary lymph nodes in the subcutaneous of the upper arm, collecting lymph vessels distribute sparsely in the lateral and densely in the medial regions. The diameter of vessels ranges from 0.3 to 1.2 mm (average 0.6 mm). They are thinner in the lateral and larger on the medial sides. Three groups of collecting lymph vessels are presented in the upper arm.

1. **Anterolateral Group**

Originating from the lateral side of the upper arm, the anterolateral group of lymph vessels travels horizontally or obliquely in the subcutaneous of the anterior part of the upper arm to converge with the medial group of lymph vessels in levels and then drain to axillary lymph nodes (Fig. 2.24 brown vessels).

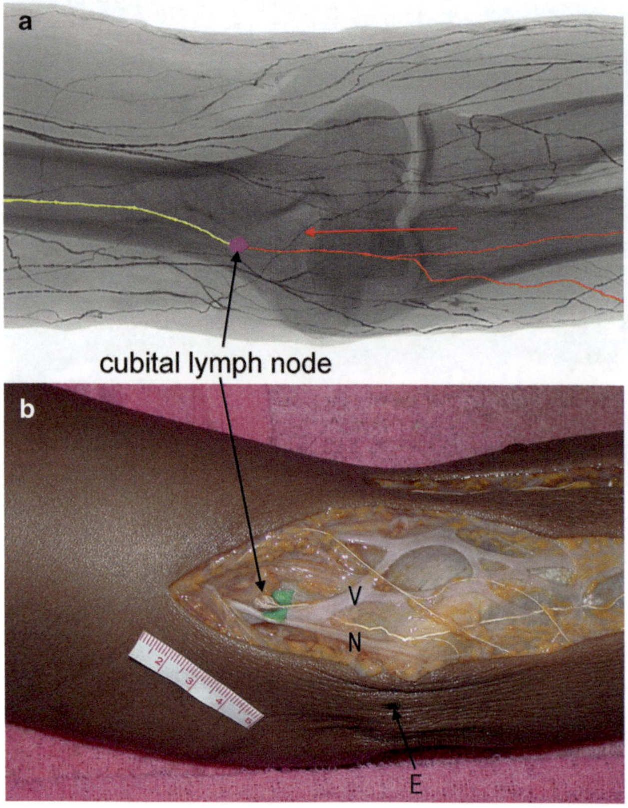

Fig. 2.25 The relationship between the cubital lymph node and lymph vessels in the left elbow. (**a**) Inverted radiograph. (**b**) Photograph

2. **Medial Group**

This group of lymph vessels, formed by three groups of collecting lymph vessels extending from the forearm in the elbow joint, travel in the subcutaneous of the medial part of the upper arm (Fig. 2.24 green, orange, and blue vessels). Vessels merge to unite larger caliber vessels and then reach axillary lymph nodes. During the course, some of them travel along with the medial cutaneous nerve and basilic vein, pierce the deep fascia and then run below the deep fascia before inflowing axillary lymph nodes (Fig. 2.27).

3. **Posterolateral Group**

The posterolateral group of lymph vessels arises from the lateral part of the upper arm. They travel horizontally or obliquely in the subcutaneous of the dorsal part of the upper arm towards the medial group of lymph vessels, where they unite together and then drain to lymph nodes in the axilla (Fig. 2.24 sky-blue vessels).

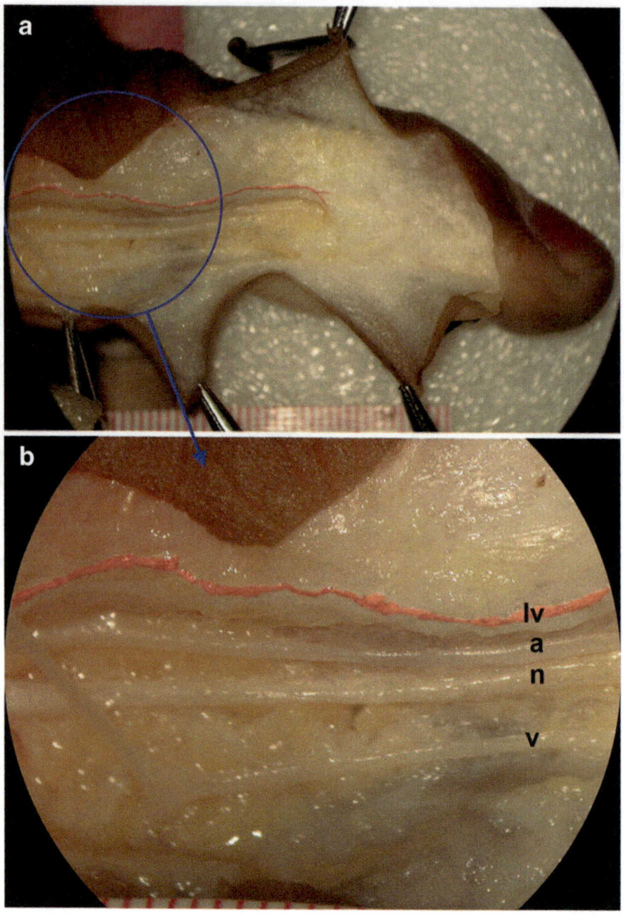

Fig. 2.26 The digital lymph vessel (lv) travels along with the digital artery (a), vein (v) and nerve (n), the image **b** is an enlarged view of the blue circled area in the image **a**

2.5 Superficial Lymphatics of Lower Extremity

Abundant collecting lymph vessels are presented in the subcutaneous of the lower extremity. Arising below the dermis on bilateral sides of the toe, the foot and the lateral area of the thigh, lymph vessels travel centripetally and meander their way in the subcutaneous of different levels to reach lymph nodes in the popliteal fossa and inguinal area. During the process, they diverge and converge to each other, sometimes crossed over or pass through below the neighboring vessel. Most of them unite to form larger vessels, while some divide into smaller ones before entering lymph nodes (Fig. 2.28).

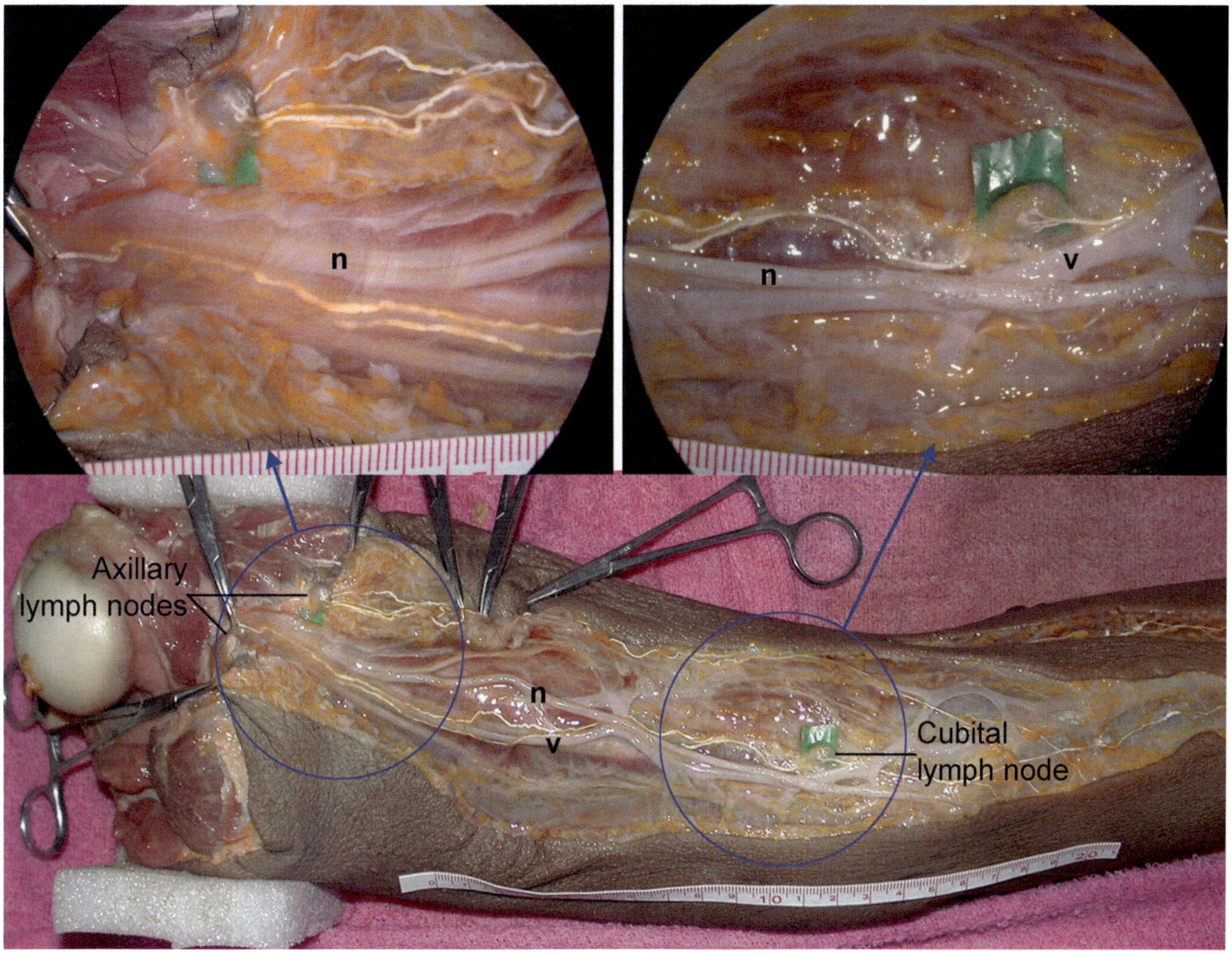

Fig. 2.27 Medial group of vessels travel along with the basilic vein (v) and medial cutaneous nerve (n)

2.5.1 Toes

Originated under the dermis on each side of toes, collecting lymph vessels travel tortuously along the mid-axial lines of the toe in the subcutaneous. They converge with neighboring vessels in the web spaces except those on the lateral side of the great toe and the medial side of the little toe. They then travel centripetally to unite with lymph vessels in the dorsal foot (Fig. 2.28 blue vessels). The diameter of vessels ranges from 0.2 to 0.8 mm (average 0.5 mm).

2.5.2 Foot

Situating in the subcutaneous of the dorsal foot, 9–19 (average of 14) collecting lymph vessels are presented. They travel centripetally, converge with or crossed over adjacent vessels. The diameter of vessels ranges from 0.2 to 1.2 mm (average 0.6 mm). Three groups are noticed (Fig. 2.28).

1. **Anterior Group**

Arising from toes, lymph vessels travel centripetally to unite the front and center portions of the network on the dorsal foot (Fig. 2.28 blue vessels).

2. **Medial Group**

Arising from the medial side of the foot, lymph vessels travel centripetally to unite the medial portion of the network on the dorsal foot (Fig. 2.28 sky-blue vessels).

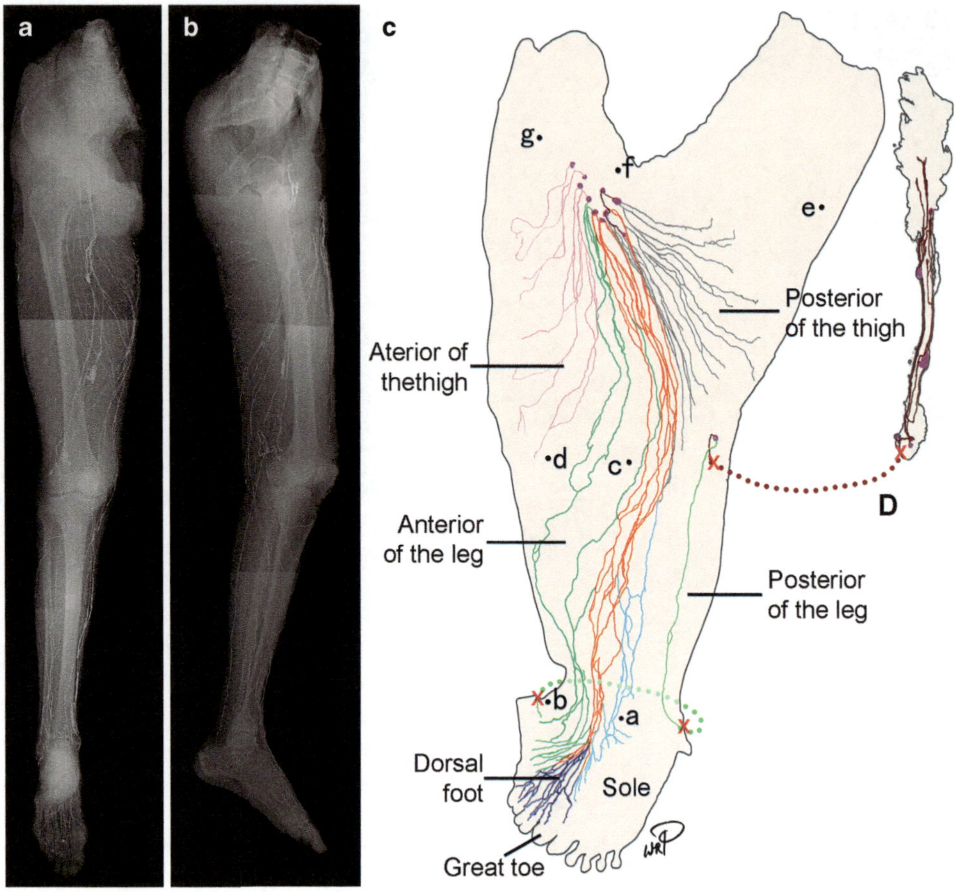

Fig. 2.28 The distribution of the superficial lymphatic in the lower limb after a lead oxide mixture perfusion. (**a**) Anteroposterial view of the radiograph. (**b**) Lateral view of the radiograph. (**c**) Lymphatic distribution in the subcutaneous of the lower extremity. (**d**) Lymphatic distribution in the femoral vascular bundle. a = Medial malleolus; b = Lateral melleolus; c = Medial epicondyle; d = Lateral epicondyle; e = Ischial tuberosity; f = Pubic tubercle; g = Anterosuperior iliac spine. Red crosses indicate points of divided vessels. The inguinal, popliteal, and femoral lymph nodes are colored in purple

3. **Lateral Group**

Arising from the lateral side of the foot, lymph vessels travel centripetally to unite the lateral portion of the network on the dorsal foot (Fig. 2.28 green vessels).

2.5.3 Leg

A range of 12–16 (average 13) collecting lymph vessels is presented in the subcutaneous of the leg. They are dense in the anteriomedial aspect and sparse in the lateral and posterior aspects. The diameter of vessels ranges from 0.2 to 1.8 mm (average 1.0 mm). Three groups are noticed (Fig. 2.28).

1. **Anteromedial Group**

Originating from the medial-dorsal foot, lymph vessels travel centripetally with the great saphenous vein (GSV) and its tributaries in the subcutaneous of the anteromedial side of the leg (Fig. 2.28 orange and sky-blue vessels and Fig. 2.29).

2. **Anterolateral Group**

Arising from the lateral-dorsal foot, lymph vessels travel centripetally in the subcutaneous of the anterolateral side of the leg (Fig. 2.28 green vessels).

3. **Posterior Group**

Arising from the lateral side of the heel, one or two lymph vessels travel centripetally with the small saphenous vein (SSV) in the subcutaneous of the posterior side of the leg. They enter the superficial popliteal lymph node (Fig. 2.28 light green vessels and Fig. 2.30). The diameter of vessels ranges from 0.7 to 1.4 mm (average 1.0 mm).

2.5.4 Thigh

A range of 27–31 (average 29) of collecting lymph vessels are presented in in the subcutaneous of the thigh. They distribute densely in the medial portion and sparsely in the lateral part. The diameter of vessels ranges from 0.3 to 1.7 mm (average 0.8 mm). Three groups of lymph vessel are noticed in the subcutaneous of the thigh (Fig. 2.28).

1. **Anterior Group**

Originating from the anterolateral portion of the thigh, collecting lymph vessels run centripetally in the subcutaneous of the thigh. They then drain to the lateral group of lymph nodes in subcutaneous of the inguinal region (Fig. 2.28 pink vessels).

2. **Medial Group**

The group of lymph vessels, extending from the anterior and medial groups of the leg, forms the medial group running in the medial portion of the thigh. They ascend centripetally in the subcutaneous next to the GSV and tributaries and then drain to the center group of lymph nodes in the subcutaneous of the inguinal region (Fig. 2.28 orange and green vessels and Fig. 2.31).

3. **Posterior Group**

Originating from the posterolateral portion of the thigh, collecting lymph vessels run centripetally in the subcutaneous of the posterior part of the thigh. They then drain to the medial group of lymph nodes in the subcutaneous of the inguinal region (Fig. 2.28 gray vessels).

2.5.5 Alternative Pathways from the Popliteal to Inguinal Lymph Nodes

Four lymphatic pathways are presented from the superficial popliteal to the inguinal lymph nodes in the lower limb.

1. **Superficial Pathway**

The lymph vessel arises from the superficial lymph node in the popliteal fossa and travels obliquely in the subcutaneous from the posterior part of the knee to the anteromedial side of the thigh via the medial side of the thigh. It converges with the medial group of lymph vessels and then drains to the superficial lymph node in the inguinal region (Fig. 2.32).

2. **Femoral Pathway**

The lymph vessel arises from the deep popliteal lymph node and travels in the femoral vascular bundle, and drains to the deep inguinal lymph node (Fig. 2.33).

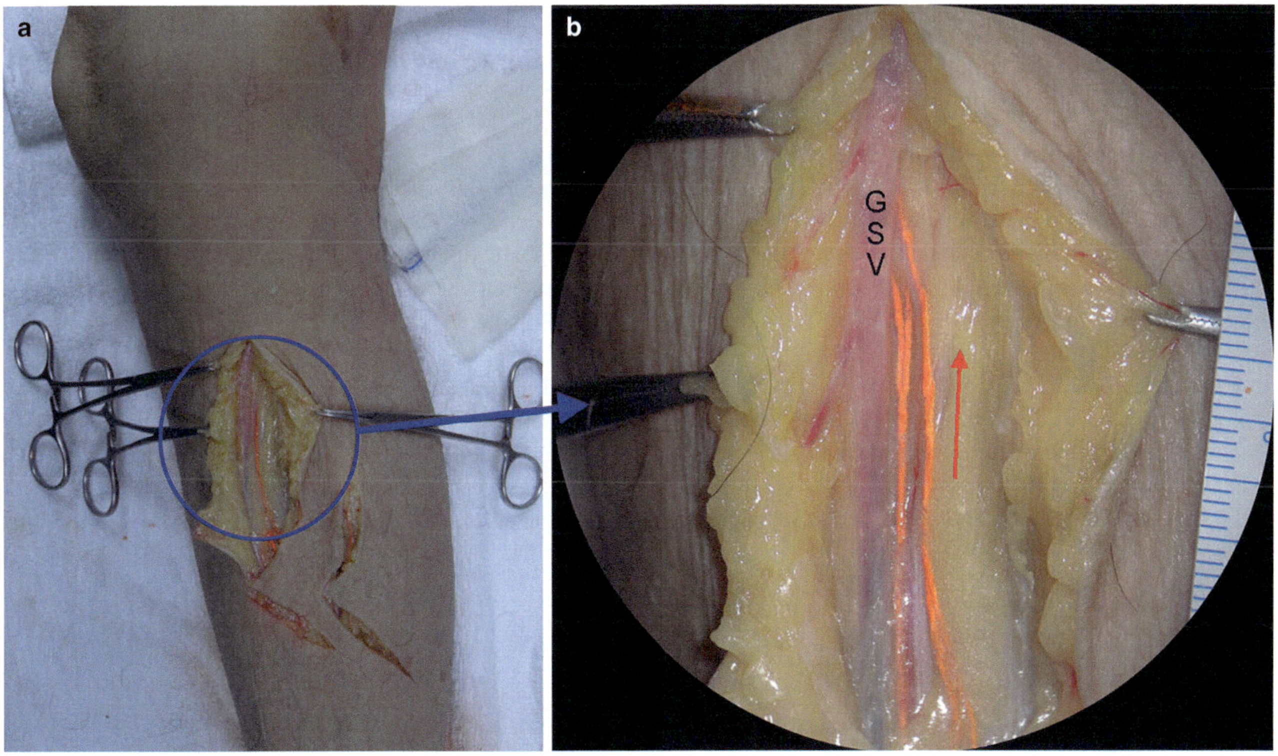

Fig. 2.29 Lymph vessels run with GSV in the anteromedial leg, image **b** is an enlarged view of the blue circle area in the image **a**

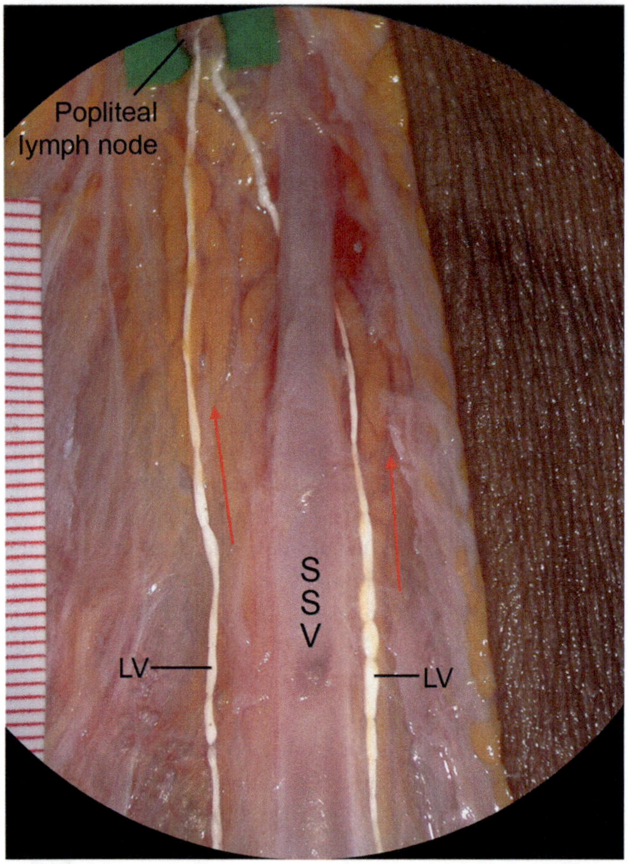

Fig. 2.30 Lymph vessels run with SSV in the posterior leg

3. **Profunda Pathway**

The lymph vessel arises from the deep popliteal lymph node, travels in the anterior aspect of the tibial nerve at the superior part of the popliteal fossa. It then runs along the profunda vascular bundle and drains either to the deep inguinal lymph node or the external iliac lymph node by passing through the obturator foramen (Fig. 2.33).

4. **Parasciatic Pathway**

This pathway has been described by Viamonte et al. [12]. Arising from the deep popliteal lymph node, the lymphatic vessel travels with the sciatic nerve and drains to the inferior gluteal lymph node (Fig. 2.34).

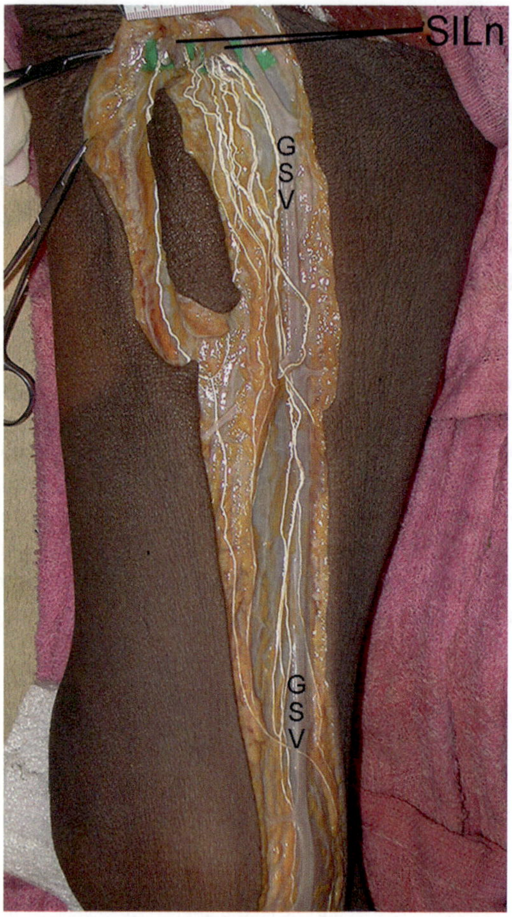

Fig. 2.31 Lymph vessels run along the GSV in the medial part of the thigh and enter lymph nodes in the subcutaneous of the inguinal region. *SILn* superficial inguinal lymph node

Therefore this anatomical feature could help to explain some patients who have not suffered from lymphedema after the lymphatic dissection in the groin, but on the other hand, it might be an alternative pathway for lymphatic metastases in cancer patients.

Acknowledgments Authors would like to pay tribute to body donors who contributed their bodies for this study and thank their families for assistance. Many thanks to the National Natural Science Foundation of China (No: 31671253), Xuzhou Medical University President special fund (No: 53051116), and the foreign experts' special fund from the Department of International Cooperation and Exchange (No: 537101) for supporting this study.

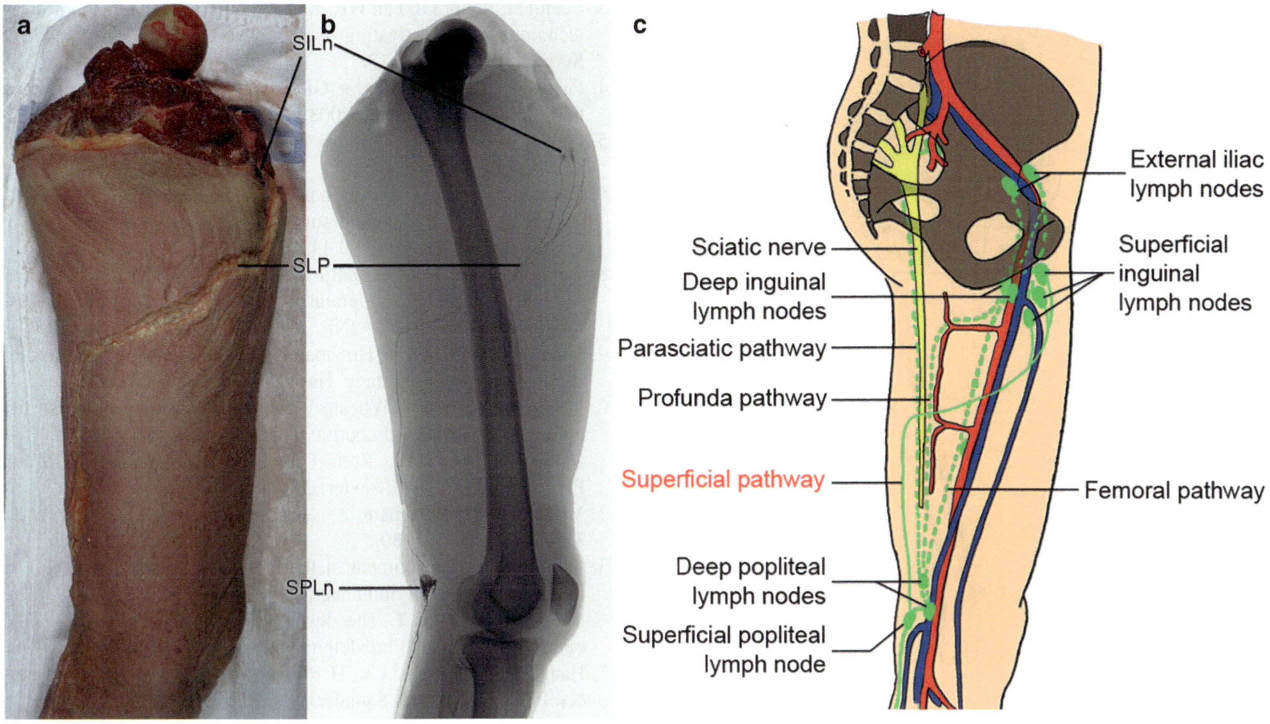

Fig. 2.32 The superficial lymphatic pathway of the thigh. *SILn* superficial inguinal lymph nodes; *SLP* superficial lymphatic pathway; *SPLn* superficial popliteal lymph node; (**a**) lateral view of the thigh; (**b**) lateral radiographic view of the thigh; (**c**) a sketch of lateral view of the pelvice and thigh

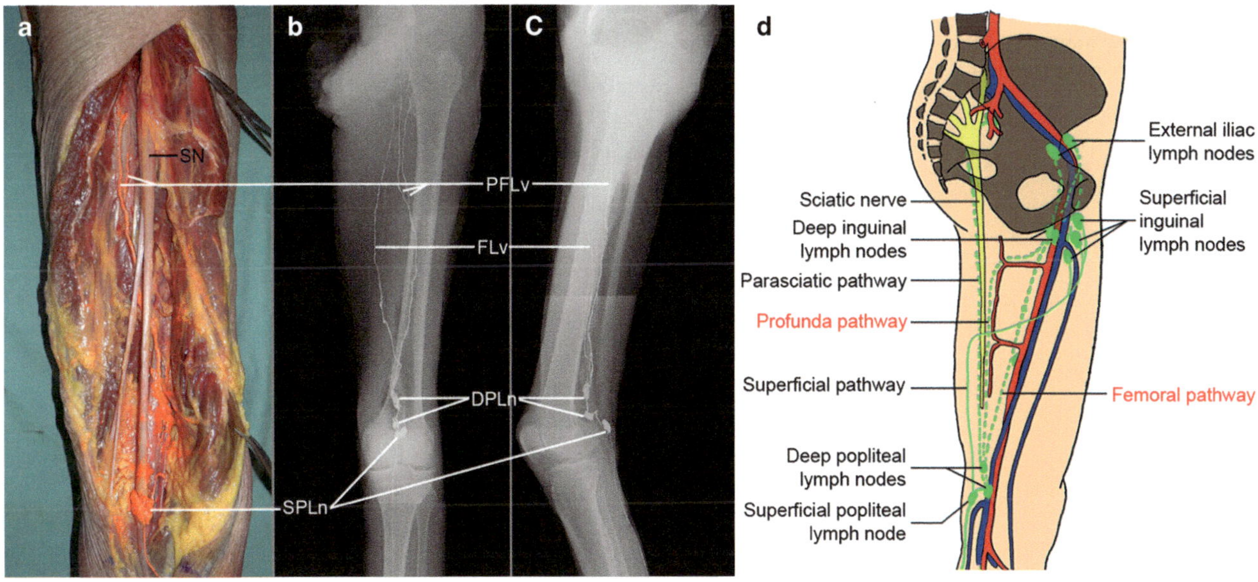

Fig. 2.33 Femoral and profunda lymphatic pathways in the thigh. *FLv* femoral lymph vessel; *PFLv* profunda lymph vessel; *SPLn* superficial politeal lymph node; *DPLn* deep popliteal lymph node; (**a**) dorsal view of the thigh; (**b**) anteroposterior radiographic view of the thigh; (**c**) lateral radiographic view of the thigh; (**d**) a sketch of lateral view of the pelvice and thigh

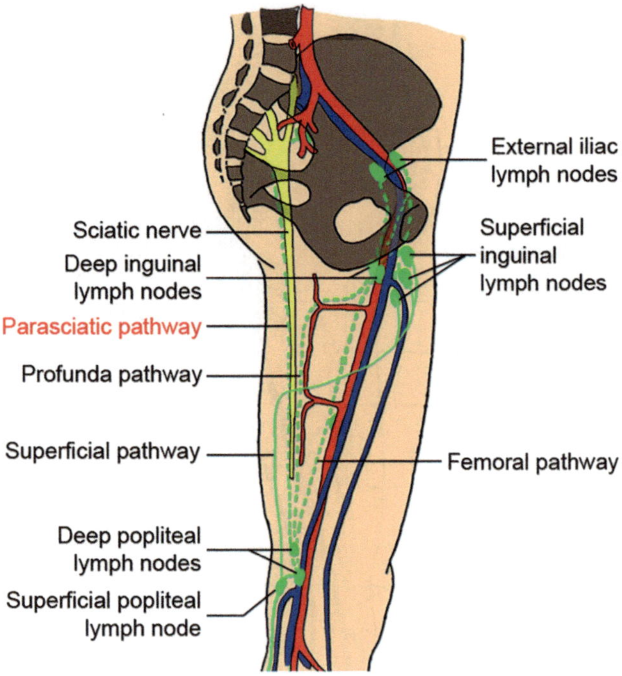

Fig. 2.34 Parasciatic lymphatic pathway in the thigh

References

1. Sappey PC. Anatomie, Physiologie, Pathologie des vaisseaux lymphatiques. Paris: Adrien Delahaye; 1874.
2. Thompson JF, Morton DL, Kroon BBR. Textbook of melanoma. London: Martin Dunitz; 2004.
3. Suami H, Taylor GI, Pan WR. A new radiographic cadaver injection technique for investigating the lymphatic system. Plast Reconstr Surg. 2005;115:2007–13.
4. Pan W-R, Suami H, Taylor GI. Senile changes in human lymph nodes. Lymphat Res Biol. 2008;6(2):77–83.
5. Gulland G. The development of lymphatic glands. J Path Bact. 1894;1:447–85.
6. Denz F. Age changes in lymph nodes. J Path Bact. 1947;59:575–91.
7. Furuta W. An experimental study of lymph node regeneration in rabbits. Am J Anat. 1947;80:437.
8. van den Brekel MW, Castelijns JA, Snow GB. The size of lymph nodes in the neck on sonograms as a radiologic criterion for metastasis: how reliable is it? AJNR. 1998;19:695–700.
9. Uren RF, Thompson JF, Howman-Giles RB. Lymphatic drainage of the skin and breast. Sydney: Harwood Academic; 1999.
10. Young B, Heath JW. Wheater's Functional histology; A text and colour atlas. 4th ed. Edinburgh: Churchill Livingstone; 2000.
11. Male D, Brostoff J, Roth DB, et al. Immunology. 7th ed. Philadelphia: Mosby Elsevier; 2006.
12. Viamonte MJ, Rüttimann A. Atlas of lymphography. New York: Thieme-Stuttgart; 1980.
13. Sabin F. The development of the lymphatic nodes in the pig and their relation to the lymph hearts. Am J Anat. 1905;4:355–89.
14. Moore K, Persaud T. The developing human-clinically oriented embryology. 6th ed. Philadelphia: WB Saunders; 1998.
15. Haagensen CD, Feind CR, Herter FP, et al. The lymphatics in cancer. Philadelphia: WB Saunders; 1972.
16. Ludwig V. Über Kurzschlußwege der Lymphbahnen und ihre Beziehungen zur lymphogenen Krebsmetastasierung. Path Microbiol. 1962;25:329–34.
17. Uren RF, Howman-Giles R, Thompson JF, et al. Interval nodes: the forgotten sentinel nodes in patients with melanoma. Arch Surg. 2000;135:1168–72.
18. Uren RF, Thompson JF, Howman-Giles R. Sentinel nodes. Interval nodes, lymphatic lakes, and accurate sentinel node identification. Clin Nucl Med. 2000;25:234–6.
19. Wallace S, Jackson L, Dodd GD, et al. Lymphatic dynamics in certain abnormal states. Am J Roentgenol Radium Ther Nucl Med. 1964;91:1187–206.

Formation and Transport of Lymph

3

Waldemar L. Olszewski and Marzanna T. Zaleska

Abstract

"Human limb soft tissues are composed of skin, subcutaneous tissue containing loose connective tissue structures as ground matrix, fibers and adipocytes, nerve fibers, blood and lymphatic vessels, muscular fascia and muscle fibers. All these solid elements bathe in tissue fluid." [Olszewski (Lymphedema. Complete medical and surgical management. CRC Press, 2016)]. Only part of tissue fluid is mobile, the rest is related to the matrix. In the normal condition, there is a balance between the volume of fluid inside the vessels and the volume of tissue fluid. Increased capillary filtration or obstruction or damage of the lymphatic system that impresses the outflow of fluid through lymphatic vessels into the blood circulation leads to an increase in the volume of tissue fluid in the interstitial space. This condition is diagnosed as tissue edema. The volume of extravascular extracellular tissue fluid may increase from 12% in physiological condition to 40–50% of total tissue volume in the lower limb in lymphedema (Fig. 3.1) [Olszewski (Lymphedema. Complete medical and surgical management. CRC Press, 2016)].

Keywords

Lymph · Tissue fluid · Lymphatics · Contractility Lymphedema

W. L. Olszewski (✉)
Department of Vascular Surgery, Central Clinical Hospital, Ministry of Internal Affairs, Warsaw, Poland

M. T. Zaleska
Department of Vascular Surgery, Central Clinical Hospital, Ministry of Internal Affairs, Warsaw, Poland

Department of Applied Physiology, Mossakowski Medical Research Institute, Polish Academy of Sciences, Warsaw, Poland

3.1 Clinical Aspects of the LS Function

3.1.1 Tissue Fluid and Lymph in Human Limbs in Normal Conditions and Obstructive Lymphedema (Fig. 3.1)

The knowledge of the site of surplus fluid accumulation and its pressure/flow mechanics becomes essential for the understanding of tissue fluid role in the metabolism of parenchymatous cells in physiological condition and in obstruction of flow called "lymphedema." It becomes indispensable for rational anti-edema therapy. The external force applied during compression therapy should depend on the sites of tissue fluid accumulation (under the epidermis, deep in the subcutaneous tissue, under the muscular fascia) and on tissue fluid hydraulic conductivity [1].

3.1.2 Where Do Tissue Fluid and Lymph Accumulate Under Normal Conditions and in Obstructive Lymphedema?

The ideal imaging method should show the shape and course of individual lymphatic vessels as well as the sites of fluid accumulation in the tissue space. The most common visualization method, lymphoscintigraphy, and lymphography, show the main vessels of the superficial and deep lymphatic system and lymph nodes. But they do not reveal the minor lymphatics of the subepidermal plexus. Direct lymphangiography with lipiodol indicates minor dermal lymphatics, but it is rarely used. Other methods like ultrasonography, computer tomography, and magnetic resonance show the structure of the tissue and sites of edema fluid retention. It remains difficult to imagine, the tissue fluid distributed in areas with obstructed lymphatics, find its way to the normal non-congested tissue regions and gets absorbed there. The best methods to show the network of the smallest lymph vessels and the area of fluid accumulation in tissue still remain histological processing of biopsy material [2] (Fig. 3.2).

N. Liu (ed.), *Peripheral Lymphedema*, https://doi.org/10.1007/978-981-16-3484-0_3

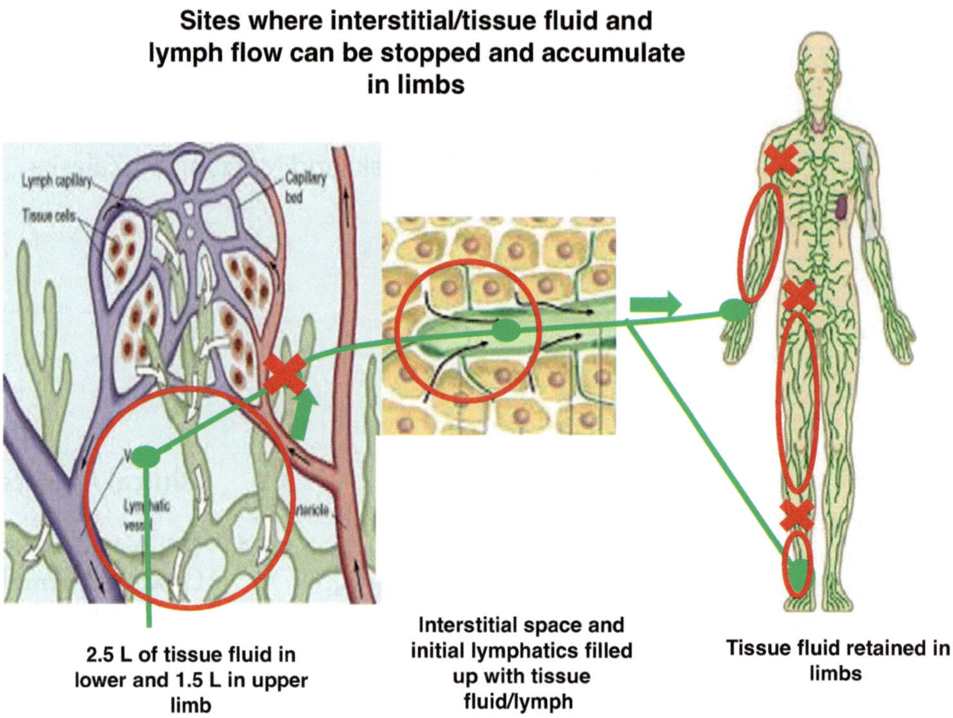

Fig. 3.1 This figure shows where the interstitial/tissue fluid and lymph flow is stopped and accumulates in limbs. Follow the green line and the red circles pointing to the pathological fluid reservoirs and tissue deformation

Important is also to know the topographical regions where most edema fluid is accumulating (Fig. 3.3). This is useful for compression therapy of lymphedema.

3.1.3 How Does the Tissue Fluid and Lymph Flow?

Schematic representation of tissue fluid and lymph flow in human legs is shown in Fig. 3.4. Under normal conditions, the volume of mobile tissue fluid in skin and subcutaneous tissue is negligible. However, it is continuously flowing toward the lymphatics.

3.1.4 Subcutaneous Tissue Fluid Pressures

Pressures in a normal limb. As we previously described, lower limb subcutaneous tissue fluid pressure measured at rest range between −1.8 to +3.0 mmHg (mean 0.8 ± 1.2 SD) [3, 4]. In animal studies also shown that it is insignificantly negative. The calf muscle contractions reduce the volume of tissue fluid in the interstitial space, which may lead to a slight, clinically insignificant drop in pressure.

Pressure in lymphedema. Tissue fluid pressure under the skin in the lymphedematous calf in rest ranged between −1.5 and +10 mmHg (mean 2.5 ± 3.0 SD) (Fig. 3.5). The pressure values were similar at different stages of lymphedema. Only in some advance cases pressure were insignificantly above average value. Change the position from horizontal to upright did not cause significant altered pressure. The relatively low tissue fluid pressure in lymphedema can be explained by the high pliability of the skin, especially in the initial stage of edema. This leads to the growth of subcutaneous tissue where fluid accumulates that cannot be drained through the lymph vessels. Water which is osmotically absorbed by matrix, dilates and stretches the skin, and a big space in the subcutaneous tissue is formed.

3.1.5 Lymph Pressure and Flow

The issues related to the hydromechanics of lymph and tissue fluid in normal and lymphedematous limbs have been investigated so far only in a few centers [6–11]. In a normal subcutaneous tissue, there is no detectable (with contemporary means) flow at rest and during walking or massage [3].

The hydromechanics of lymph and mobile tissue fluid (normal and stagnant-edema) differ considerably. Tissue fluid is located in the interstitial space restricted by solid elements of tissue (cells and fibers). Lymph is located, under physiological conditions, in lymph vessels, which contract spontaneously and rhythmically, causing pressure gradient. Any damage consisting in obstruction of lymph outflow through lymph vessels changes the hydraulic conditions.

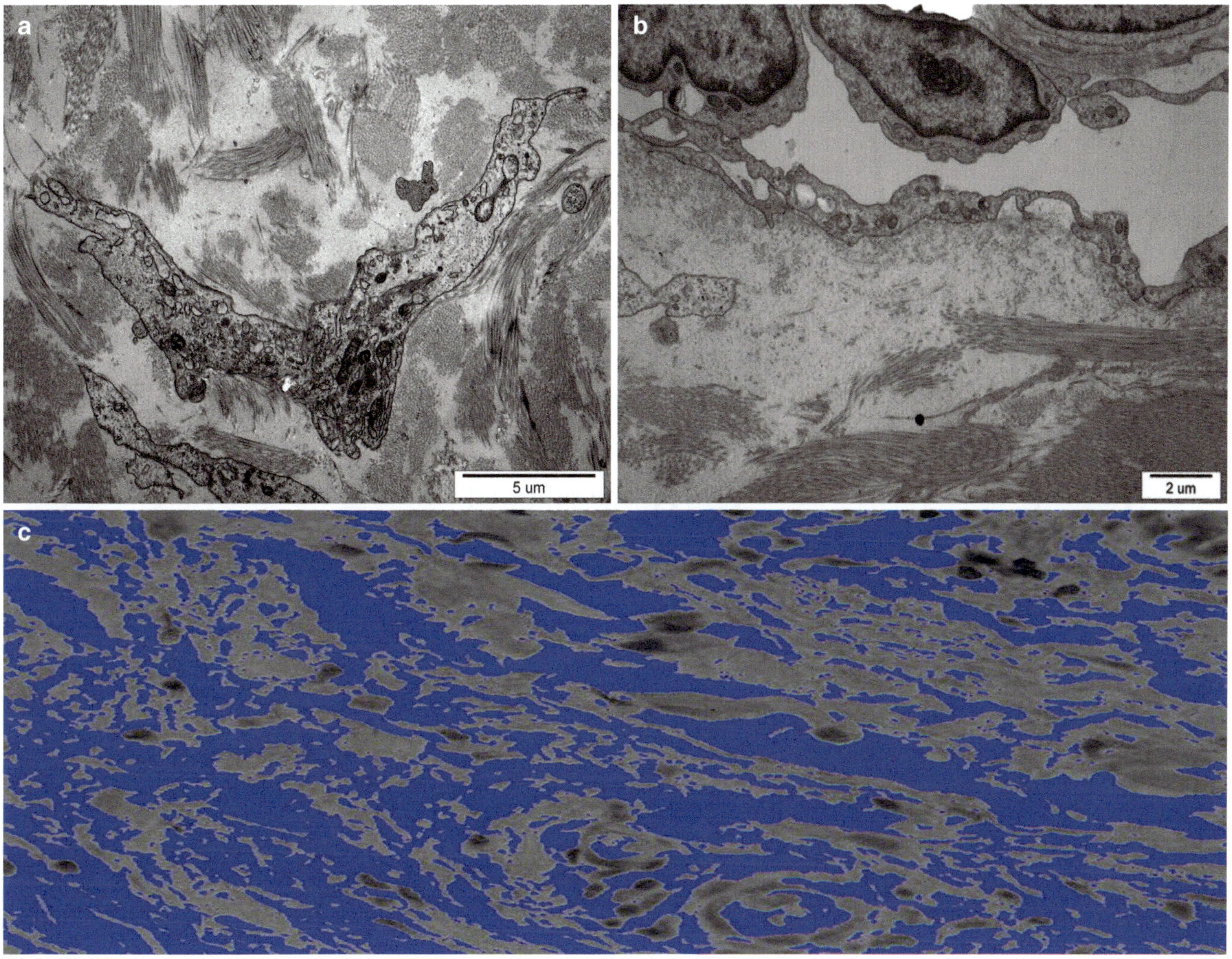

Fig. 3.2 Microscopical pictures of the lymphedema-deformed tissue with accumulated tissue fluid. (**a**) EM image of fluid between fibroblasts and collagen fibers, (**b**) EM image of a dilated initial lymphatic, (**c**) MicroImage (Olympus) picture of tissue spaces filled up with fluid (blue) (magn. ×40). Depending on the type of edema in its early stages, up to 50% of the entire skin and subcutaneous tissue specimen volume can be occupied by the lymphatic space. In advanced cases, fluid accumulates mainly in the artificially created interstitial "lakes" and less in the lymphatic space. Tissue fluid is also present in the perivascular spaces and even around the thickened fascia

3.1.6 Extrinsic Factors Propelling Lymph

Normal conditions. Neither active muscle contractions nor passive movement affects the lymph flow. The same lack of effect is observed with respiratory movements and pulsation of arterial vessels [6, 8, 10, 11]. Lymph vessels usually contain only a few microliters of lymph in some lymphangions. There is no hydrostatic pressure in normal leg lymphatics an in upright position [8, 11].

3.1.7 Intrinsic Factors Propelling Lymph

The flow of lymph in the lymphatic vessels is due to autoregulated rhythmic contractions of lymphangions [6, 11]. The tissue fluid flowing into the lymphangion stretches its wall, muscles of wall contract (according to the Starling's law for the heart muscle), and pushes the drop of lymph into the lymphangion above.

A drop of lymph contained in the big toe lymphatic will be transported to the collectors, cysterna chyli and thoracic duct, and finally subclavian-jugular venous angle by spontaneous rhythmic contractions of lymphangions (Fig. 3.6).

3.1.8 Lymph Pressures in Normal Limbs

"Human limb lymphatics contract rhythmically with a frequency depending on the volume of inflowing tissue fluid [8, 11] (Figs. 3.7 and 3.8). In area where capillary filtration and tissue fluid production is high the frequency of lymph vessel contraction is also high. The recorded pressures at

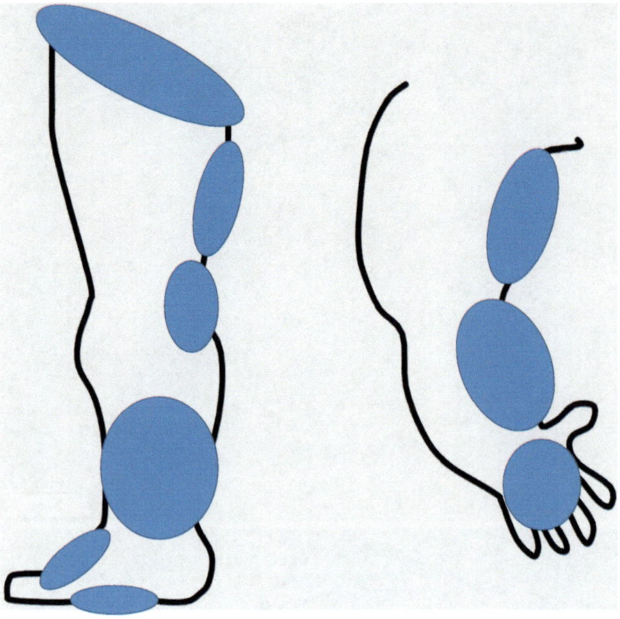

Fig. 3.3 Schematic presentation of sites with soft subcutaneous tissue with a predilection for edema fluid accumulation. Important for compression therapy

rest, irrespective whether in the lying or upright position, with free proximal flow (lateral pressure) range between 7 and 30 mmHg and during foot flexing between 10 and 30 mmHg. The pulse amplitude is 3–20 mmHg and 5–17 mmHg, respectively. The pulse frequency is 0.6 to 6/min and 2 to 8/min, respectively [8, 11]. The resting end pressures with obstructed flow (e.g., corresponding to lymphatic obstruction in postsurgical lymphedema) range between 15 and 55 mmHg, and during foot flexing 15 to 50 mmHg. The pulse amplitude is 3 to 35 mmHg and 3 to 14 mmHg, respectively. The pulse frequency is 2.5 to 10/min and 3 to 12/min, respectively." Massaging of foot, tapping of tissues containing lymphatics has no effect on lymph pressures. Heating of foot significantly increases pressure, amplitude, and frequency of lymphatic contractions" [8, 11]. There were no pressure changes during both massage and tapping the tissue. While heating the food significantly increased both the pressure and frequency of contraction of the lymphatic vessels [8, 11]. (All data are from our previous publication).

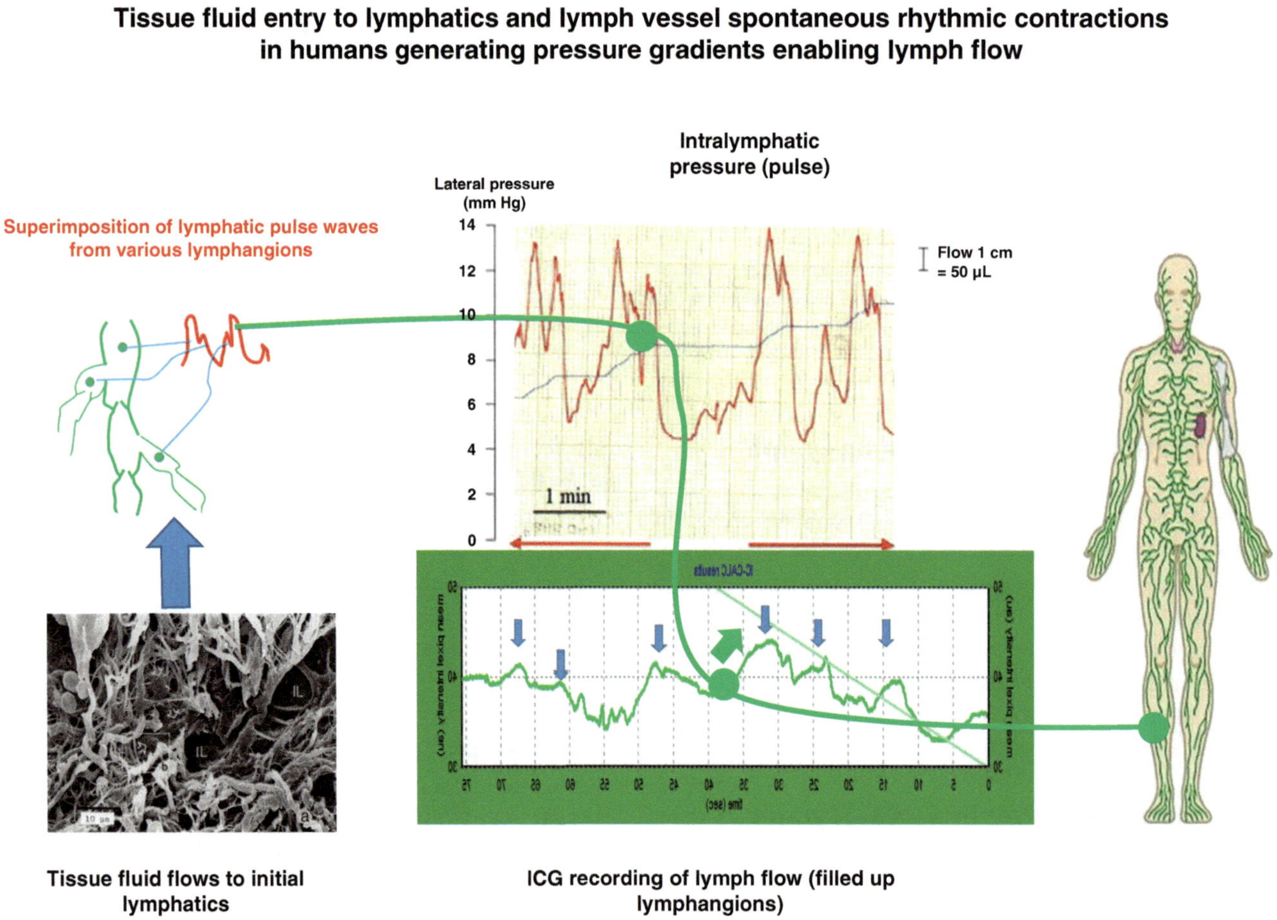

Fig. 3.4 Picture summary of the chapter. Left side—tissue fluid flows to the initial and collecting lymphatics; stretching of lymphangions evokes their contraction and generation of pressure gradient recorded as pulse curve (see scheme and dot on the green line); contraction of a distal lymphangion brings about filling of the proximal (dot on the green peak of the ICG lymphogram); right side—calf site where recordings were done

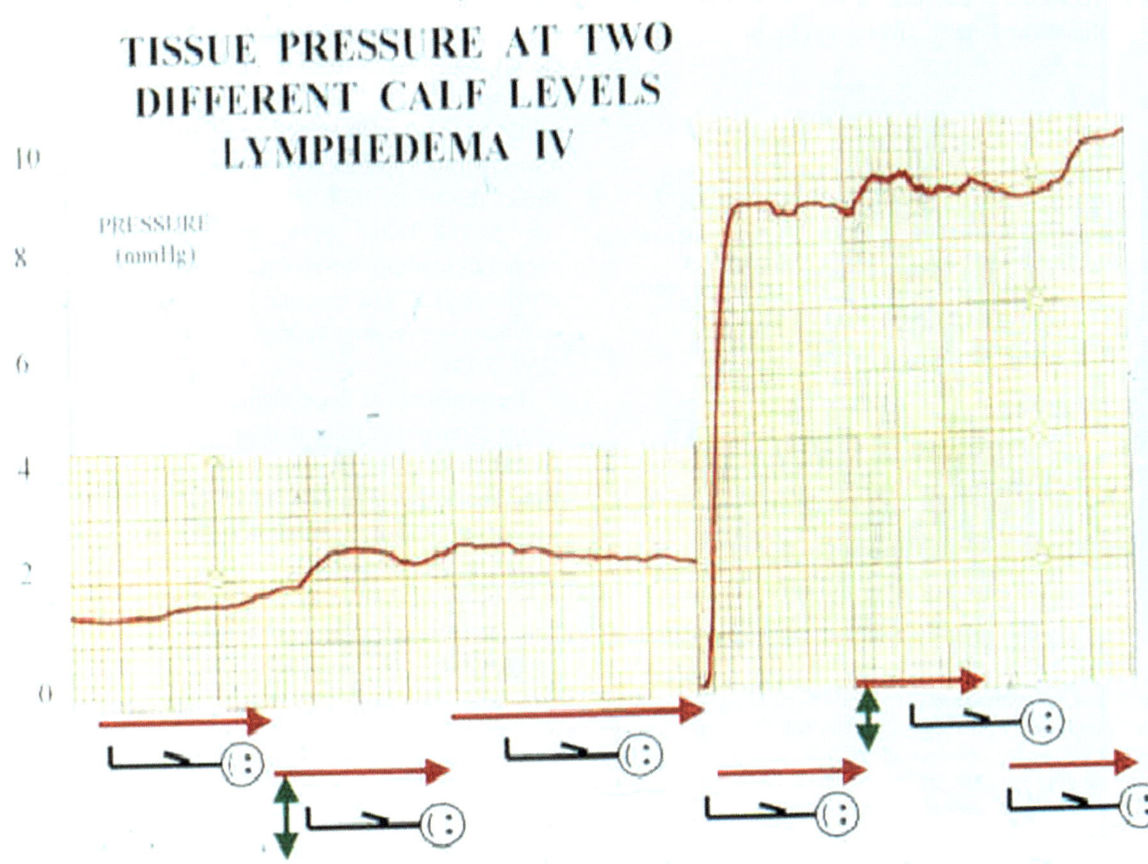

Fig. 3.5 Tissue fluid pressures in a normal and lymphedematous calf subcutaneous tissue in a horizontal position. Left panel—pressure around 2 mmHg. Right panel—pressure around 10 mmHg with minor oscillation during calf movements. Tissue fluid pressure remains low in advance stages of edema due to decompression by enhancement of subcutaneous space [5]

3.1.9 Lymph Flow in Normal Limbs

Flow occurs only during spontaneous contractions of lymphangions [8] (Fig. 3.9).

3.1.10 Lymph Pressure and Flow in Lymphatic Obstruction

General remarks. In the post inflammatory, postsurgical, and posttraumatic as well as in the so-called idiopathic (of unknown etiology) lymphedema, the intralymphatic pressures and flow are abnormal due to: (a) destruction of lymph vessel muscle cells, (b) destruction of valves, (c) partial or total obstruction of lumen. Tissue fluid finds its way to the non-swollen parts of the limb along the hydraulically created "tissue channels."

Lymph pressures in lymphedematous limbs. In obstructive lymphedema most of the lymph vessels are occluded. Those that remain open are filled with fluid. Tissue fluid pressure measured at rest ranges from 5 to 45 mmHg and depends on the ability of damaged or destructed lymph vessels to contract [4]. Pressure measured during movement of the lower limb is generally low and ranges from 10 to 25 mmHg, although tiptoeing may in some subjects generate end pressure of above 200 mmHg. Even this high pressure does not generate the fluid flow because the proximal lymph vessels are blocked (Figs. 3.10 and 3.11).

Lymph flow in lymphedematous limbs. Since most of the main lymphatics are completely or partially blocked, spontaneous flow can occur only in the remained fragments of patent lymphatic vessels at varies limb levels [3, 4]. Correlation of pressures and flow measurements reviled in most cases no effect of lymphangion's contractions (Fig. 3.12)

3.1.11 Lymph and Tissue Fluid Pressure and Flow During Various Types of Compression Procedures in Lymphedema

General remarks. Effective compression therapy requires knowledge about structure of tissue and changes occurring in them in the course of the lymphedema. Skin is relatively stiff, but as a result of hyperkeratosis and fibrosis, its stiffens increase (becomes less elastic). Subcutaneous tissue which contains collagen and elastic fibers, and fat is less stiff then

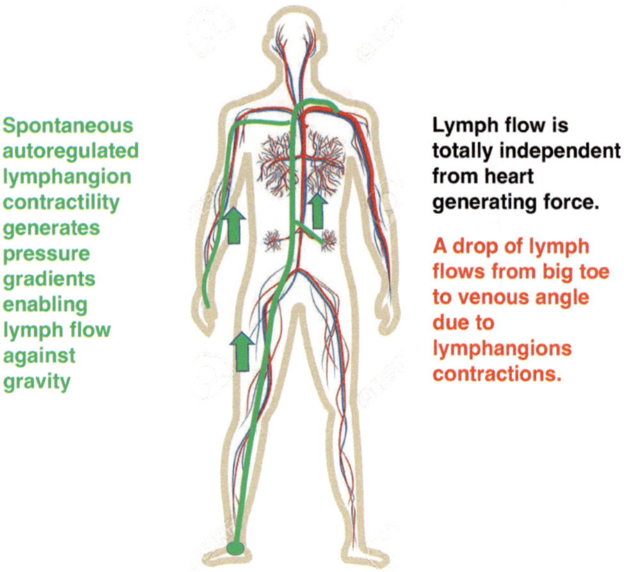

Fig. 3.6 Schematic presentation of plasma-filtrated capillary filtrate/tissue fluid/lymph flow from the big toe to the subclavian-jugular angle via lymphatics generated by autoregulated rhythmic lymphangion contractility generating pressure gradients enabling lymph flow against gravity. The role of lymphatics in maintaining cell fluid environment is crucial in all body regions, irrespective of position, movements, muscle contractions, respiration, and heart contraction force

skin. Because of the fibrosis, it becomes less elastic. Even the muscular facia become fibrotic (Fig. 3.13). As a result of these changes, the hydraulic conductivity was constantly decreasing. Therefore, higher external pressure to mobilized the edema fluid is necessary.

Edema tissue fluid accumulates in the spontaneously formed tissue spaces. Any type of external force is able to direct the tissue fluid into the lymphatic vessels as they are blocked. Using appropriate compression, we can only propel fluid along tissue spaces to the area where it can be absorbed [12]. The external force also works on skin, subcutaneous tissue, veins, lymphatics, and muscles (Fig. 3.14).

Deformation of these elements by external force brings about a transfer of force to the mobile issue fluid [5, 14–16]. Before the applied force increases the pressure of the tissue fluid and causes it to flow, much of it dissipates. Our study on edema fluid hydromechanics has shown that the minimum pressure of the tissue fluid that can cause its movement must be above 30 mmHg. To obtain such a tissue fluid pressure, an external pressure of 50–60 mmHg must be used in early stages of lymphedema, and up to 120 mmHg in advanced cases with hard skin.

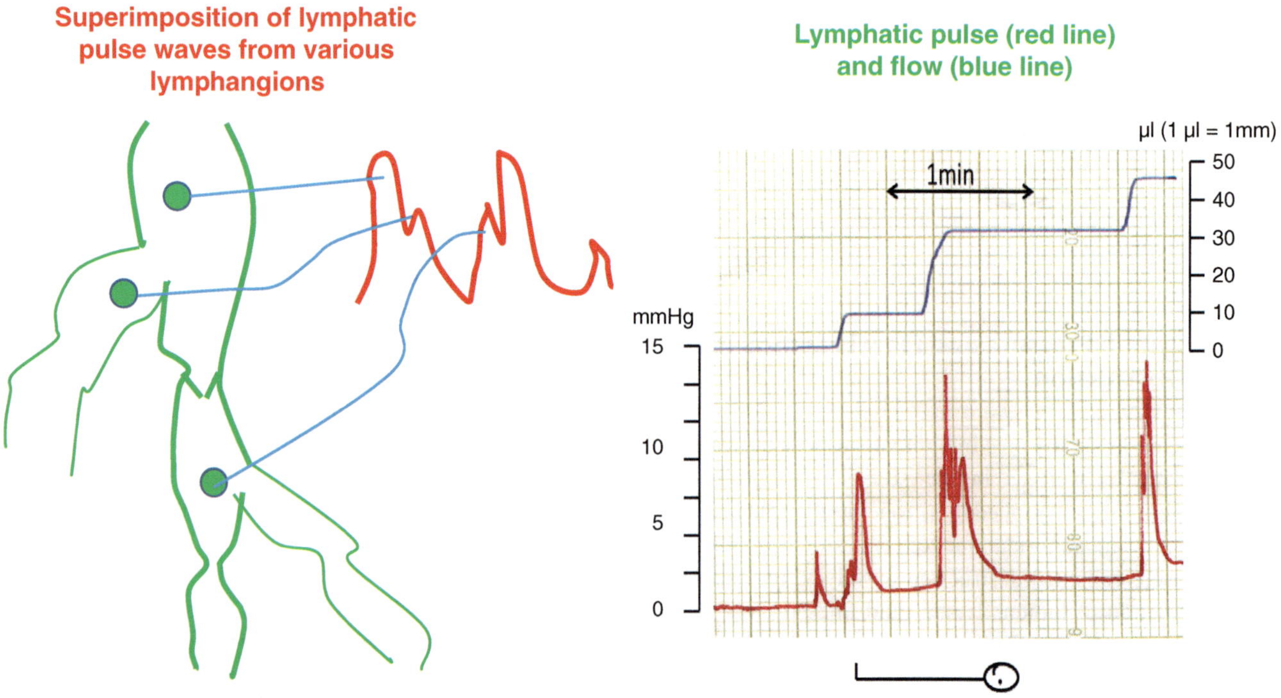

Fig. 3.7 Lymphatic pulse. Contractions of lymphangions generate pressures that can be recorded on high-sensitivity manometers. The recorded curves reflect forces created simultaneously by different lymphangions, expressed as separate peaks shown on the drawing. Recording in a calf collector shows various contours of pulse waves (red line). Normal pressures in a horizontal position remain around 10 mmHg. Note that lymph flow (blue line) occurs only during the rise in lymph pressure. The ejection fraction is from 1 to 10 μL per contraction

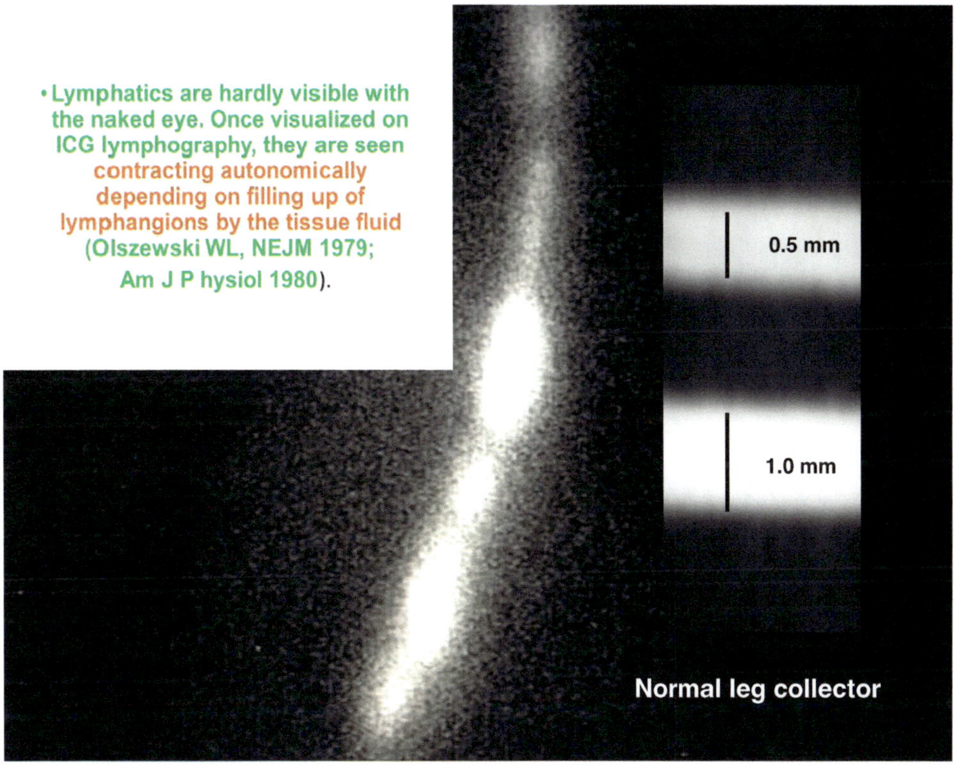

Fig. 3.8 The indocyanine green (ICG) near-infra-red fluorescent lymphography enables direct observation of lymph flow generated by spontaneous contractions of lymphangions. An ICG picture of a normal calf collector with filled up and proximal empty contracted lymphangions

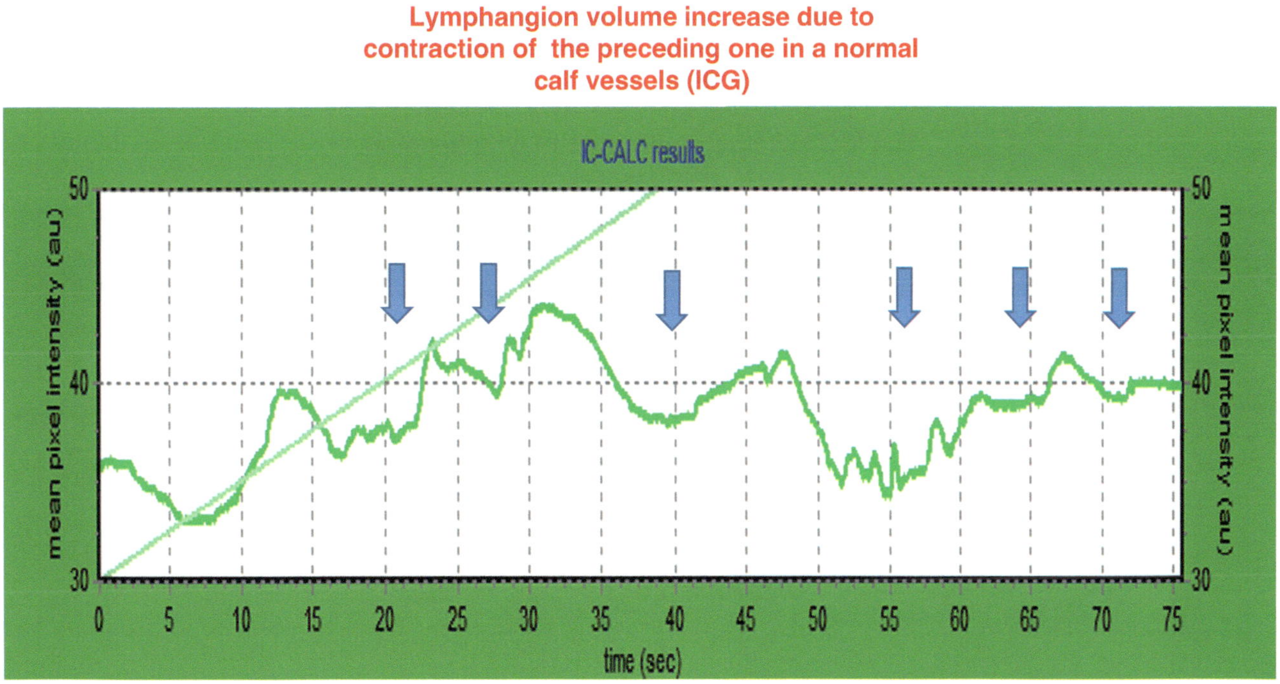

Fig. 3.9 The ICG fluorescence activity rate in a normal contracting calf collector. Blue arrows point to decrease of curve caused by contraction followed by rising due to filling of the proximal lymphangion

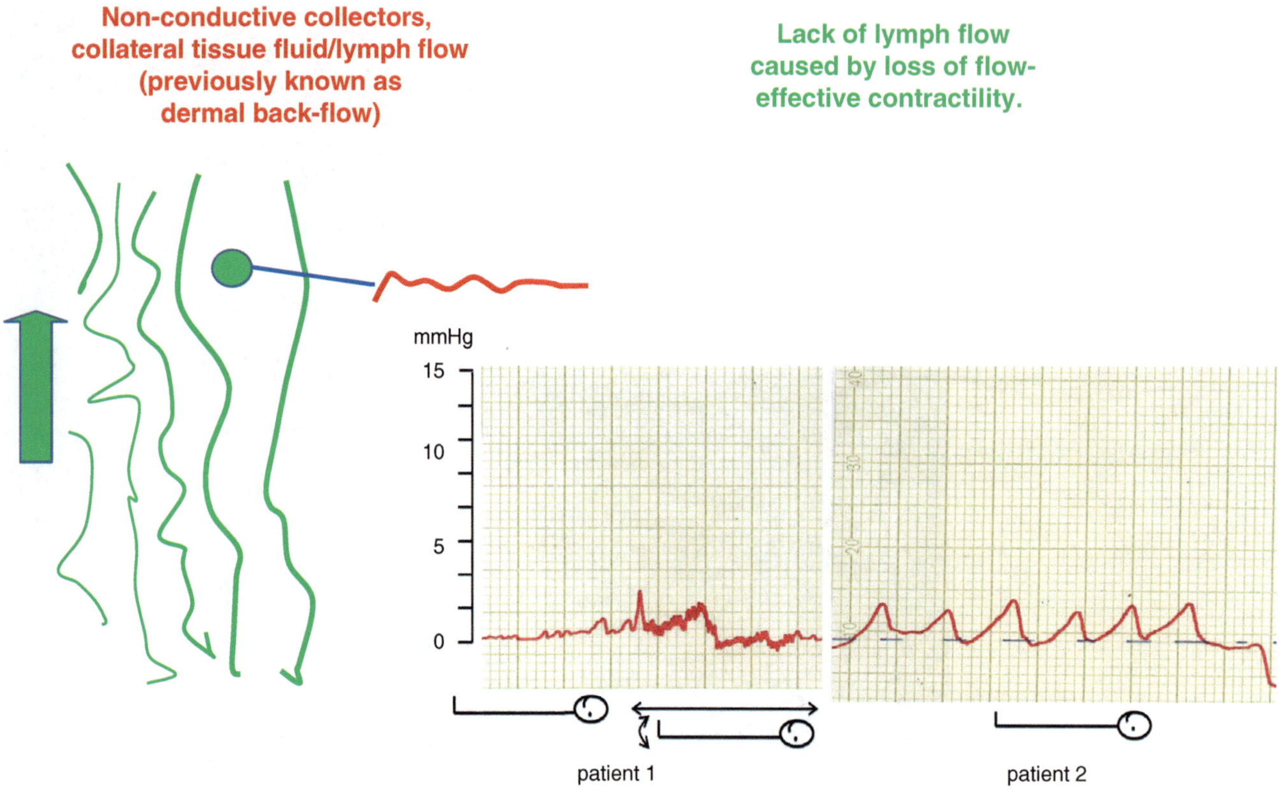

Fig. 3.10 Schematic presentation of the lymphatic pulse waves caused by damage to the lymphangion wall by inflammation or proximal obstruction. Lack of pulse—red line. Intralymphatic pressure in the calf collectors. Spurious non-effective contraction do not generate pressures high enough to propel lymph

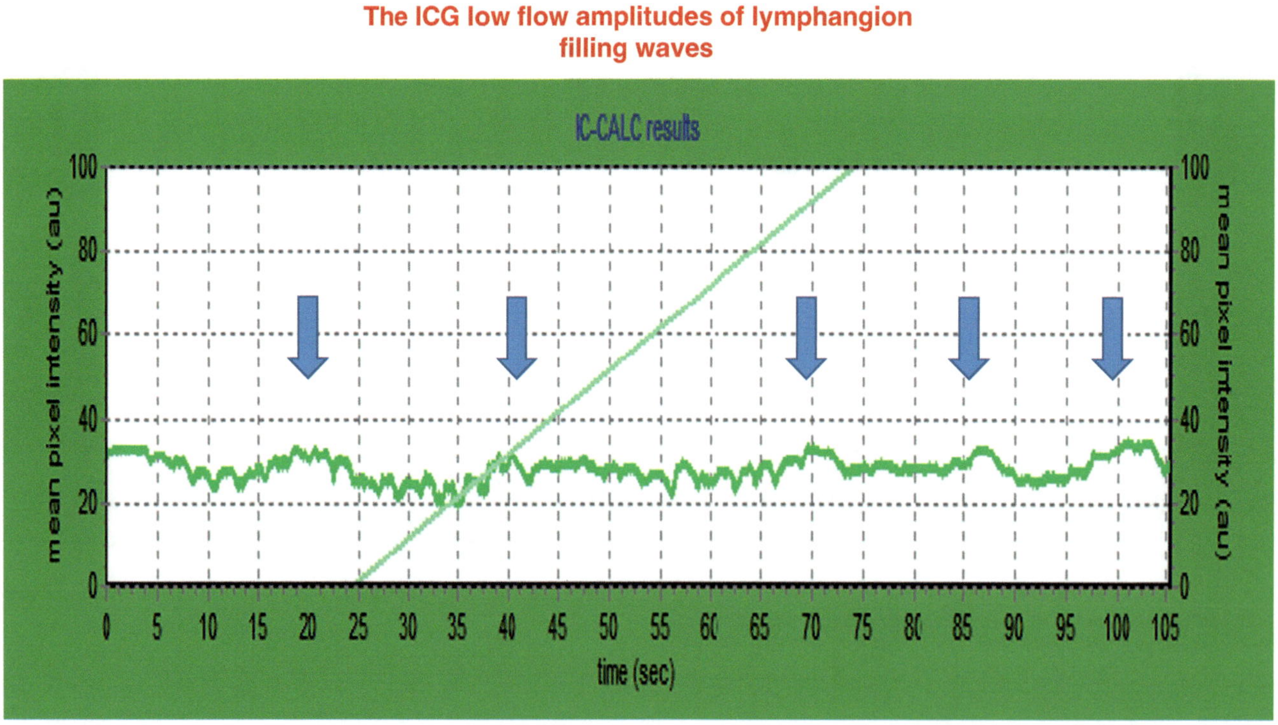

Fig. 3.11 The ICG fluorescence activity rate in a damaged non-contracting calf collector. Blue arrows point to the low amplitude of spuriously contracting lymphangions not generating effective flow pressures

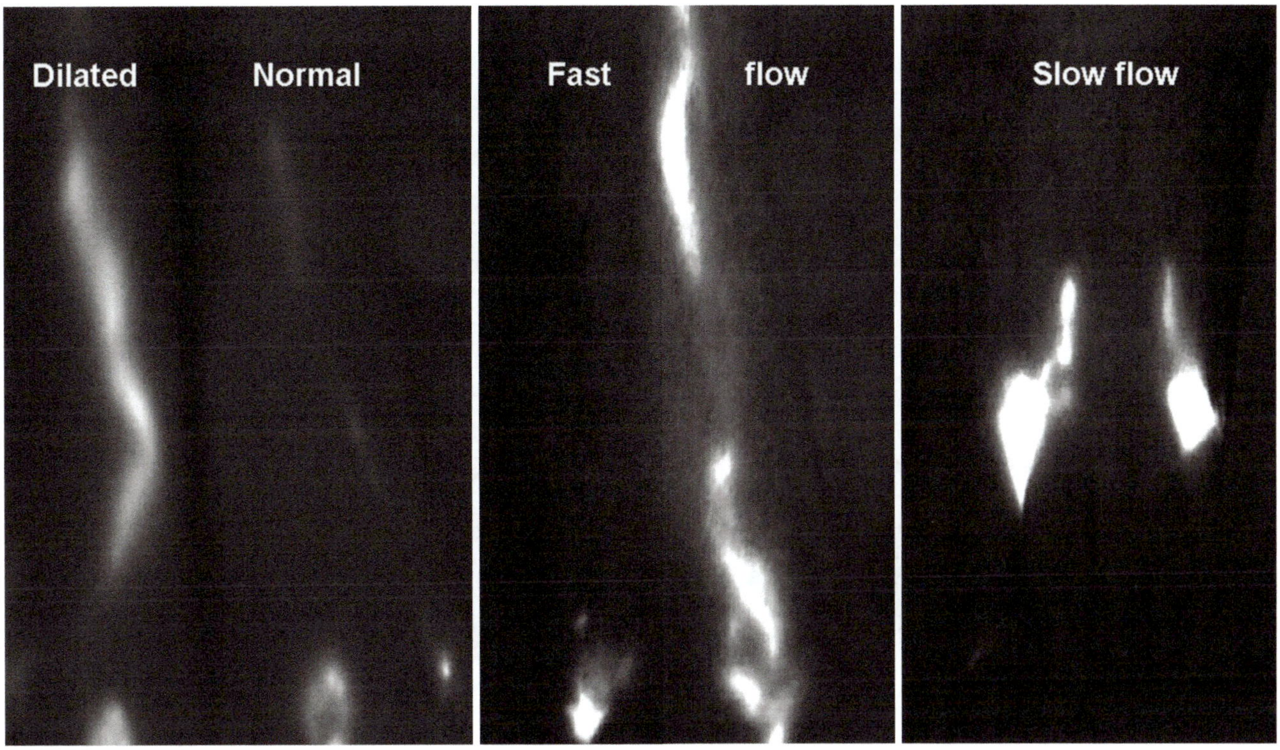

Fig. 3.12 The ICG images of leg lymphatics reflecting lymph flow. Dilated vs. normal calf collector. Fast dye flow in a normal lymphatic. Slow flow of dye from the foot. The ICG test is useful for early detection of lymph flow changes due to inflammation or obstruction

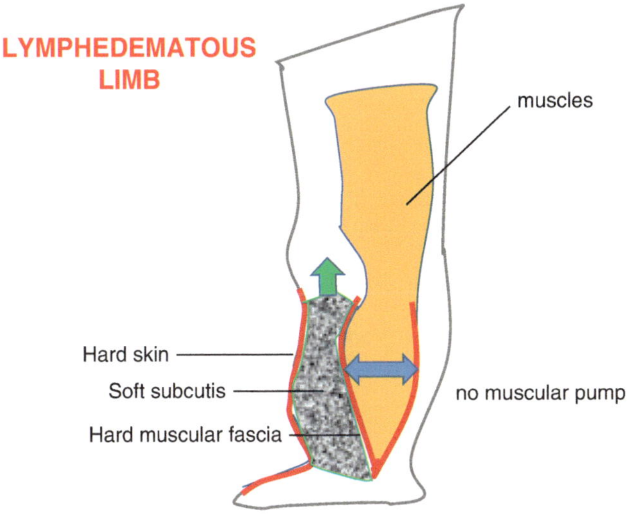

Fig. 3.13 Schematic presentation of tissue morphological changes in a lymphedematous lower limb. Hard skin, expanded subcutaneous tissue and fibrotic muscular fascia totally prevent muscle contractions to generate pressures propelling edema fluid. This requires the application of external massaging forces

3.1.12 How Much Force Is Lost During External Compression?

This can be estimated by measuring pressure at the therapist's hand, bandage, or pneumatic device—skin interface and that of the tissue fluid (Fig. 3.15).

Measuring the pressure on the skin surface and the pressure of the tissue fluid gives us information on how much force is dissipating on the solid elements of the tissue and how much is necessary to generate a fluid pressure gradient that will cause the flow (Fig. 3.16).

When planning compressor therapy, we should take into consideration that tissue fluid pressure will always be lower than that in the compression device and at the interface skin device (Figs. 3.17 and 3.18).

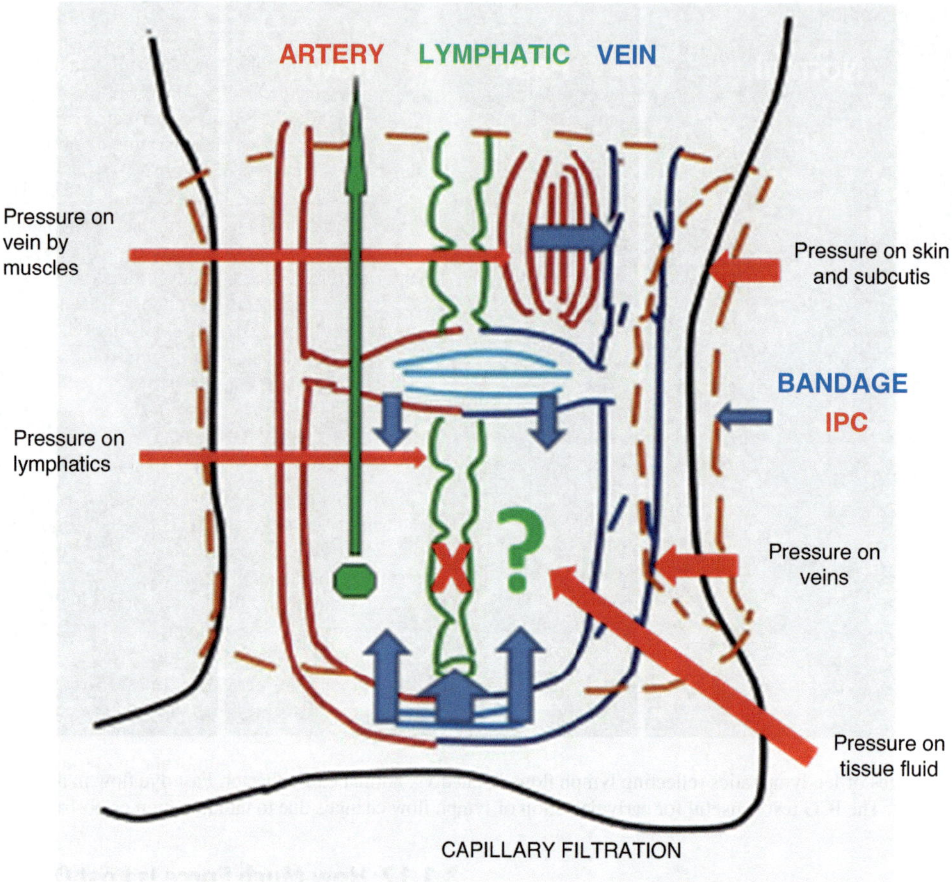

Fig. 3.14 Schematic presentation of anatomical structures and lymph and tissue fluid location in the foot and calf and forces acting upon tissues during manual compression or bandaging or intermittent pneumatic compression. Knowledge of which tissue structures are compressed before edema fluid can be mobilized during compression is necessary. The blue arrows indicate the area of the "exchange capillary vessels" where the process of capillary filtration occurs. Filtered fluid accumulates in the intercellular space (long red arrow pointing to green question mark ?). Lymphatic collectors are occluded (red X). External force must overcome skin, subcutaneous tissue, veins, lymphatics, and solid elements of tissue as fibers and ground matrix (red arrows) resistance before reaches the tissue fluid. The solid elements deform (long red oblique arrow) and transfer force to the tissue fluid. Some force (depending on the advancement of fibrous changes in skin and subcutaneous tissue) is dissipating before it reaches the tissue fluid, increases its pressure, and creates flow. The force applied should be high enough to cause fluid movement in the tissue (vertical green arrow), but not to obstruct blood flow in the arteries and veins. Interrupted circular and vertical lines point tissue calf deformation during compression procedures [13]

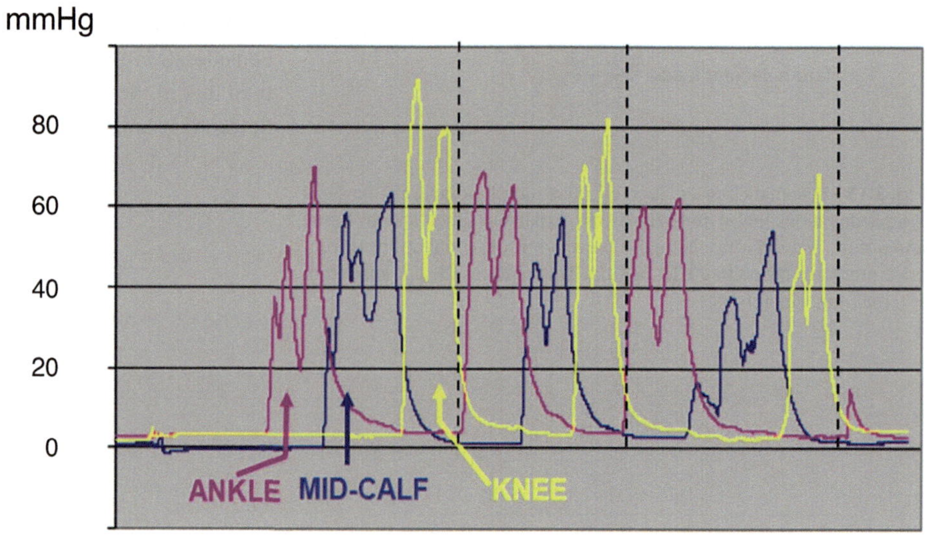

Fig. 3.15 The tissue (edema fluid) pressure bringing about flow is a product of external force against mechanical resistance of tissues. Pressure (force) distribution in the compressed leg tissues is different under the skin, in the subcutaneous tissue, and in the fluid

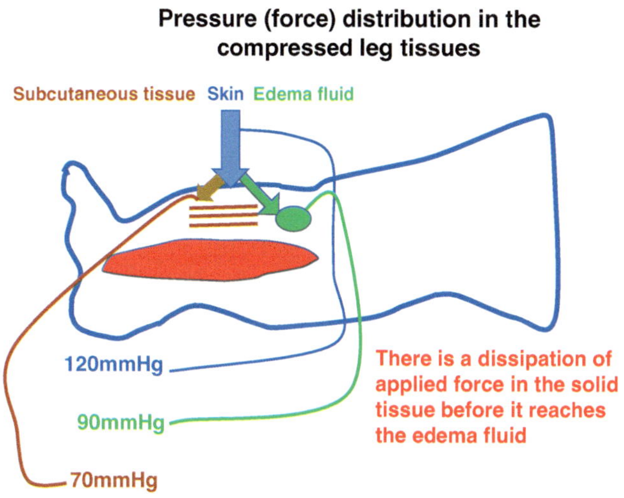

Fig. 3.16 Manual massage of the limb soft tissues generates tissue fluid pressures of some 60–80 mmHg. However, upon cessation of external pressure, the tissue fluid pressure drops to 1–5 mmHg, and flow stops. To reach an effective flow from the distal to proximal parts of the limb, sequential compression, as produced by a pneumatic sleeve, is needed

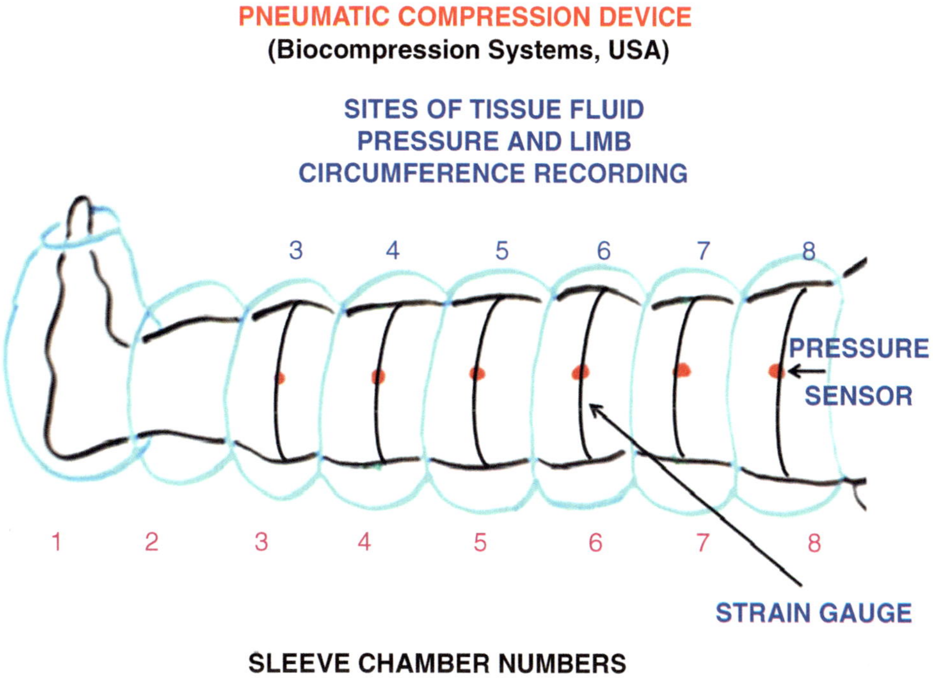

Fig. 3.17 Schematic presentation of a compression sleeve of eight chambers. Inflated from distal to proximal ones, without distal chambers deflation, each chamber inflated for 50 s. Sites of circumference and tissue pressure measurements. Recording of these parameters enables adjustment of adequate force at different limb levels

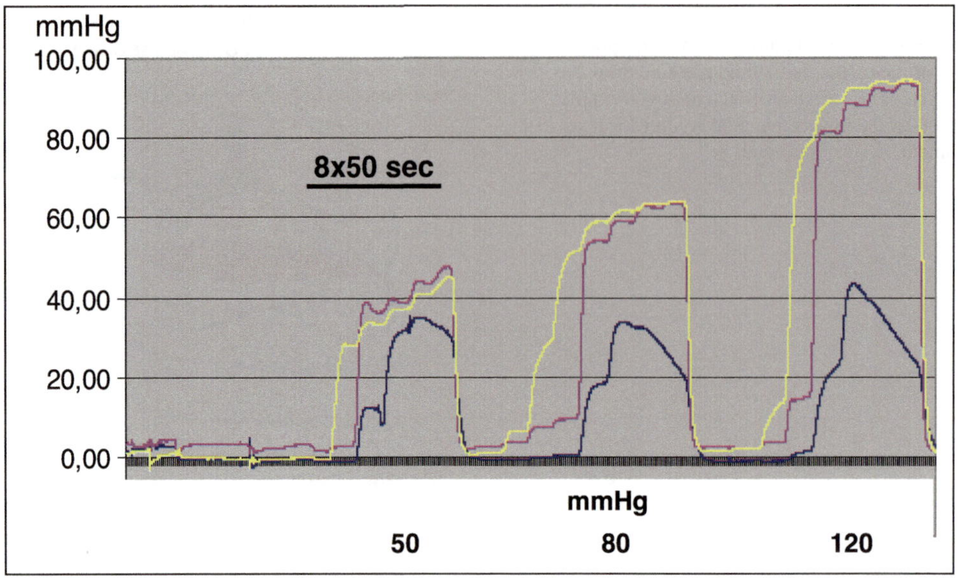

Fig. 3.18 Tissue fluid pressure recordings in the normal calf subcutaneous tissue during pneumatic compression of 50, 80, and 120 mmHg, 50 s/chamber. Pressures recorded at the chamber, level 3, above ankle (yellow curve), 4, mid-calf (rosy curve), and 5, below knee (blue curve). Inflation of sleeve to 50 mmHg produced tissue fluid pressure at ankle of 40 mmHg, to 80 mmHg reached 60 mmHg and to 120 mmHg rose to 90 mmHg. Note that pressures were lower in the mid-calf and below knee. This is the force dissipation effect caused by mechanical resistance of tissues [16]

References

1. Olszewski WL, Jain P, Ambujam G, Zaleska M, Cakala M. Topography of accumulation of stagnant lymph and tissue fluid in soft tissues of human lymphedematous lower limbs. Lymphat Res Biol. 2009;7(4):239–45.
2. Olszewski WL, Zaleska MT. Comments to Lymphatic medicine: paradoxically and unnecessarily ignored by Stanley G. Rockson LBR 15:315-316. Lymphat Res Biol. 2018;16(4):418–20.
3. Olszewski WL. Contractility patterns of normal and pathologically changed human lymphatics. Ann N Y Acad Sci. 2002;979:52–63.
4. Olszewski WL. Contractility patterns of human leg lymphatics in various stages of obstructive lymphedema. Ann N Y Acad Sci. 2008;1131:110–8.
5. Rockson Stanley G. Accruing evidence for a beneficial role of pneumatic biocompression in lymphedema. Lymphat Res Biol. 2010;8(4)
6. Olszewski WL, Engeset A. Intrinsic contractility of leg lymphatics in man. Preliminary communication. Lymphology. 1979;12:81–4.
7. Olszewski WL. Lymphatic contractions. N Engl J Med. 1979;8:300–16.
8. Olszewski WL, Engeset A. Intrinsic contractility of prenodal lymph vessels and lymph flow in human leg. Am J Physiol. 1980;239:H775–83.
9. Armenio S, Cetta F, Tanzini G, Guercia C. Spontaneous contractility in the human lymph vessels. Lymphology. 1981;14:173–8.
10. Sjöberg T, Norgren L, Steen S. Contractility of human leg lymphatics during exercise before and after indomethacin. Lymphology. 1989;22:186–93.
11. Olszewski WL. Lymph vessel contractility. In: Lymph stasis – pathomechanism, diagnosis and therapy. Boca Raton, FL: CRC Press; 1991. p. 115–54.
12. Olszewski WL, Cwikla J, Zaleska M, Domaszewska-Szostek A, Gradalski T, Szopinska S. Pathways of lymph and tissue fluid flow during intermittent pneumatic massage of lower limbs with obstructive lymphedema. Lymphology. 2011;44(2):54–64.
13. Olszewski WL. Hydromechanics of intercellular fluid and lymph. In: Neligan PC, et al., editors. Lymphedema. Complete medical and surgical management. CRC Press; 2016. p. 327–48.
14. Pilch U, Wozniewski M, Szuba A. Influence of compression cycle time and number of sleeve chambers on upper extremity lymphedema volume reduction during intermittent pneumatic compression. Lymphology. 2009;42:26–35.
15. Mayrovitz HN. Interface pressures produced by two different types of lymphedema therapy devices. Phys Therapy. 2007;87:1379–88.
16. Zaleska M, Olszewski WL, Jain P, Gogia S, Rekha A, Mishra S, Durlik M. Pressures and timing of intermittent pneumatic compression devices for efficient tissue fluid and lymph flow in limbs with lymphedema. Lymphat Res Biol. 2013;11(4):227–32.

4 Function of the Lymphatic System

Zhujun Li, Elan Yang, and Xiao Long

Abstract

The lymphatic system plays an important role in both the circulatory and immune systems. The main functions of the lymphatic system include maintenance of interstitial fluid homeostasis and prevention of edema, clearance of cellular debris and metabolic waste products, immune traffic, and lipid absorption from the intestines. Moreover, the lymphatic system is also observed to have a high regenerative capacity [Lee et al. (Lymphedema: a concise compendium of theory and practice. Springer London, 2011); Liu (Lymphedema—diagnosis and treatment. Science Press, 2014); Tammela and Alitalo (Cell 140:460–76, 2010)].

Keywords

Lymphatic system · Immune system · Lipid absorption
Self-renewal capacity

4.1 Maintenance of Interstitial Fluid Homeostasis

The plasma, interstitial fluid, and lymph are three compartments of extracellular fluid. Fluid flows continuously between the compartments and maintains a dynamic equilibrium in the steady state. One of the principal functions of the lymphatic system is to return excess fluid and proteins from the interstitial space back to the circulation as a supplement to the blood capillaries. It is estimated that lymph drains up to ~8 L/day, while the volume of human plasma is only ~3 L [1]. In fact, the lymphatic system is essential in controlling the volume, pressure, and protein concentration of the interstitial fluid.

In microcirculation, proteins constantly leak from the blood capillaries to the interstitium. Only a small amount of leaked protein returns back to the circulation through the venous end of the blood capillaries. The majority of the proteins tend to stack up in the interstitium, therefore, increasing the colloid osmotic pressure of the interstitial fluids, shifting the balance of forces at the blood capillaries. More water molecules are pulled into the interstitium from the capillaries, thus increasing both the volume and pressure of the interstitial fluid.

As is described in the structure and physiology of the lymphatic system, the rate of lymph flow is greatly increased by the increased interstitial fluid volume and pressure, transporting the excess fluids and proteins back to the blood circulation. The interstitial fluid volume, pressure, and protein concentration will be maintained at a steady level under homeostatic conditions, because the accumulated fluids and proteins cause an instant increase in the lymph flow, which is great enough to balance the rate of leakage into the interstitium.

Under pathophysiological conditions, that is, when some factors change the rate of leakage or interrupt lymph flow, the tissue could become swollen due to the accumulation of extra fluid and proteins, therefore causing lymphedema [2].

4.2 Clearance of Cellular Debris and Metabolic Waste Products

Since large molecules could not enter the blood capillaries, it is crucial to have an accessory passage for the clearance of cellular debris and metabolic waste products from the interstitial space. Lymphatic capillaries, due to their relatively loose intercellular conjunction, allow rather nonselective access into the lymphatic ducts. Take hyaluronic acid for an example, it is synthesized by fibroblastic cells and is a key constituent of the extracellular matrix (ECM). Unlike other ECM components, its degradation happens in lymph nodes and the liver. Therefore, it must be transported through the

Z. Li · E. Yang · X. Long (✉)
Division of Plastic and Reconstructive Surgery, Peking Union Medical College Hospital, Beijing, People's Republic of China

N. Liu (ed.), *Peripheral Lymphedema*, https://doi.org/10.1007/978-981-16-3484-0_4

lymphatic vasculatures to avoid accumulation in the interstitium. Lymphatic endothelial cells express hyaluronic acid receptor LYVE-1, which captures the molecules and transports them to lymph nodes and the liver. About one third of the total hyaluronic is transported and degraded. Obstruction of lymphatic ducts could result in impaired hyaluronic acid degradation, causing changes in interstitial fluid volume and composition [3].

4.3 Immune

Lymphatic vasculature is not a formal member of the immune system, yet it is indispensable in immunity. One of its principal tasks is to transport antigens and immune cells, providing a direct contact of the antigens with lymphoid organs. However, more and more studies have revealed that the lymphatic vessels play many other roles in immunity.

Plasma proteins constantly filtrate from the blood into the interstitial fluid. These proteins include complement, immunoglobulins, and many other proteins with active functions. The concentration of these functional molecules is lower in interstitial fluid than in plasma, because of the filtration barrier formed by capillary endothelial cells and their basal membrane. Vesicular transport, fenestrae, and numerous signals influencing capillary permeability to change the concentration of interstitial fluid protein, therefore regulating cells' accessibility to functional molecules. During tissue inflammation, proinflammatory mediators promote immunity by increasing the permeability of capillaries, allowing abundant effector molecules into the inflamed tissue. Since little protein could return to the blood circulation from the venous end of blood capillaries, their appearance in the plasma relies heavily on the lymphatic vessels. Moreover, the lymphatic system regulates the rate of interstitial fluid flow. A slow and steady flow of fluid ensures adequate contact between the functional molecules and tissue cells [4].

Lymphatic vessels and lymphoid tissue exist in all organs and tissues that contact directly with the external environment, for instance, the skin, the intestines, and the lungs. This distribution is crucial for the lymphatic system to fulfill its task, that is, to defend against foreign particles detrimental to our body [5]. The connection between lymphatic endothelial cells is rather loose compared to that of the vascular endothelial cells. Consequently, the lymphatic capillaries have gaps and flaps on their walls, making it easy for large molecules to enter rather non-selectively, yet difficult to flow back into the interstitium. Nevertheless, selective mechanisms may exist for some particles to enter the lymphatic capillaries. The migration of immune cells into the lymphatic capillaries is a step necessary for performing their functions. Since random interaction is inefficient and unreliable, chemotaxis to the lymphatic capillaries is essential for immune cells to locate and enter. For instance, the lymphatic endothelial cells express CCL21, a chemokine receptor that attracts dendritic cells, which have CCL21 receptor CCR7 on their surface.

Lymphatic capillaries converge into larger collecting vessels that are capable of contracting and pushing lymph forward due to the smooth muscle cells lining the outside of its wall.

Lymph, along with its contents, is transported further into lymph nodes. Lymph enters from the subscapular sinus along the border, filtrated by lymphoid tissue as it passes through, then leaves the lymph nodes from the efferent collecting lymphatic vessels in the center. Lymph nodes provide a specialized microenvironment for the migrating immune cells that come from two sources: the blood, where lymphocytes and DC precursors pass through the specialized high endothelial venules into lymph nodes, and the lymph, which drains from nearby tissues. The subscapular sinus of lymph nodes consists of two layers of lymphatic endothelial cells that form the floor and ceiling, respectively. The floor expresses LYVE-1 and CCL21 that attracts DCs. The ceiling, on the other hand, displays unique chemokines and receptors, such as CCL1, which scavenges CCL21, therefore, maintaining an effective CCL21 gradient from the floor to the ceiling, aiding the DCs' movement into the lymph nodes. The floor also functions as a sieve by the expression of plasma-lemma vesicle-associated protein (PLVAP), which constitutes endothelial fenestrae. The sieve limits access to the paracortex based on molecular size, with a cutoff value of about 70 kDa. In the medullary, lymphatic endothelial cells assist in T cell egress. They express sphingosine kinase 1 and sphingosine kinase 2, which are indispensable in T cell egress from the lymph nodes into efferent collecting lymphatic vessels. Moreover, a subgroup of lymphatic endothelial cells in the lymph node medulla mediates peripheral tolerance in coordination with other stromal cells through the expression of self-antigens like tyrosinase and immune-modulatory proteins like PD-L1. These PD-L1+ lymphatic endothelial cells have avid endocytosis of cellular debris and other materials in the lymph. They can mediate deletional tolerance by presenting these antigens directly to CD8+ T cells. Another way of presenting antigens is through the DCs. Lymphatic endothelial cells retain the engulfed particles for up to weeks. During late phases of the immune response, the lymph node begins to shrink, and excess lymphatic endothelial cells proliferated earlier must now undergo apoptosis. The dying endothelial cells, along with the engulfed antigens inside them, are devoured by DCs. In this way, the antigens are passed along to DCs, promoting CD8+ T cell memory response. Recent studies suggest that MHC II molecules found on lymphatic endothelial cells could also play a role in antigen presentation. Apart from its immune functions, the lymph nodes can also condense lymph. Lymph entering lymph nodes has a protein concentration less than half of the concentration in plasma, while it leaves with a concentration approximately equal to that of plasma. This concentration happens by means of water entering high endothelial venules and returning to the blood circulation [4].

4.4 Lipid Absorption

Dietary lipids are transported by the intestinal lymphatic system. The fact that the lymphatic vasculature plays a crucial role in lipid absorption and transportation was first discovered in 1662 by the Italian physician Gaspare Aselli. He observed the intestines of a well-fed dog and described the lacteal vessels, or chyliferous vessels, which are the lymphatic ducts of the guts. Historically, lipid transport through the lymphatic system was thought to be a passive process, which is simple and unregulated. Relatively modest attention was given to this subject until recent years, when specific markers of the lymphatic endothelial cells (LECs) and multiple imaging techniques developed, allowing us to get a deeper understanding of the lymphatic system under physiological and pathophysiological conditions. At present, we have discovered that the process of dietary lipid transport through the lymphatic system was never as simple as we initially presumed. Its metabolic implications and potential to become a target in the treatment of obesity are gaining it a rapid growth in interest.

Remember that the lymphatic system, unlike the blood-vascular network, is a unidirectional transport system whose principal function is to return fluid to the blood circulation. Fluid enters the blind-ended capillaries from the interstitium, then drains to the larger pre-collecting and collecting vessels. In the intestine, lymphatic capillaries, or lacteals, are found solely in intestinal villi, while collecting lymphatic vessels are located only in the mesentery. Lymph from the intestine funnels into the cisterna chyli then goes up to the thoracic duct, where it enters the blood circulation at the level of the subclavian vein.

Dietary lipids are digested and absorbed in the gastrointestinal tract following a series of steps. First, neutral lipids are disassembled into fatty acids and monoglycerides. These smaller molecules are able to pass through the apical membrane of mucosal cells, in which they are re-assembled into triglycerides (TGs). Second, different types of lipids, including TGs and cholesterol, are mixed together in the mucosal cell to form tiny lipid drops called chylomicrons (CMs), which are then released from the basal membrane of the mucosal cell. CMs will enter the intestinal lymphatic capillaries and travel through the lymphatic ducts till they reach the blood circulation.

In contrast with the notion of passive draining from the interstitial space, studies have shown that the process of CMs entering the lymphatic capillaries is an active process. Various molecular mechanisms have been proved to play a role in it. Pleomorphic adenoma gene-like 2 (*PlagL2*) null mice can secrete CMs, but the CMs do not appear in their lymphatic capillaries, indicating that the transcription factor *PlagL2* plays an important part in the regulation of CM uptake by lymphatic capillaries. VEGF-A signaling is also proved to be able to regulate CM uptake through the modulation of cell junctions.

Lymphatic ducts contract spontaneously to help pumping lymph forward. As we know, valves distribute at regular intervals along the ducts, forming one-way passages that prevent the backflow of lymph. Adjacent valves separate the duct into lymphangion, the functional unit of a lymphatic vessel. Lymph is propelled forward in the lymphangion by pressure changes from body movement like respiration and the pressure caused by lymphatic duct contraction. This contraction is controlled by the autonomic nervous system and is essential in the transport of dietary lipids. It is regulated by various factors. Increase in intraluminal pressure and wall shear stress would cause a differential release of prostaglandins, NO, and histamine, which would speed up the contraction frequency.

Apart from transporting dietary lipids, the lymphatic system also helps remove cholesterol from peripheral tissues. Links between impaired lymph drainage and chronic inflammatory disease are emerging, but there is still much to figure out [6].

4.5 Self-Renewal Capacity of the Lymphatic System

The lymphatic system has the power of self-renewal. The peripheral lymphatic system regenerates rather rapidly after injuries. Growth of a web of small lymphatic vasculatures follows any mechanical interruption of a lymphatic duct as an attempt to join the severed ends. Similarly, under a certain level of lymphatic duct obstruction, generation of a network of small lymphatics would ensue should the obstruction continue to exist. These small lymphatics can be observed under lymphangiography as dermal backflow [7].

Due to the discovery of specific markers of lymphatic endothelial cells, the field of lymphatic regeneration is experiencing a boost over the decades. Multiple molecules have been proved to play a part in lymphatic duct development and regeneration, including vascular endothelial growth factor receptor-3 (VEGFR-3), hyaluronic acid receptor LYVE-1, podoplanin, homeobox gene Prox-1, and so forth. Multiple researches have reported that VEGF-C gene therapy could promote regeneration of lymphatic vasculature and reduce lymphedema. More researches on the self-renewal capacity of the lymphatic system shall enhance our understanding and treatment efficacy of lymphedema [3, 7–9].

References

1. Levick JR, Michel CC. Microvascular fluid exchange and the revised Starling principle. Cardiovasc Res. 2010;87(2):198–210.
2. Hall JE, Guyton AC. Guyton and Hall textbook of medical physiology. 13th ed. Elsevier; 2016.
3. Liu N. Lymphedema – diagnosis and treatment. 1st ed. Beijing: Science Press; 2014. p. 191.
4. Randolph GJ, et al. The lymphatic system: integral roles in immunity. Annu Rev Immunol. 2017;35:31–52.
5. Lee B-B, Bergan J, Rockson SG. Lymphedema: a concise compendium of theory and practice. London: Springer London; 2011.
6. Cifarelli V, Eichmann A. The intestinal lymphatic system: functions and metabolic implications. Cell Mol Gastroenterol Hepatol. 2018.
7. Olszewski WL. The lymphatic system in body homeostasis: physiological conditions. Lymphat Res Biol. 2003;1(1):11–21. discussion 21–4
8. Tammela T, Alitalo K. Lymphangiogenesis: molecular mechanisms and future promise. Cell. 2010;140(4):460–76.
9. Alitalo K, Carmeliet P. Molecular mechanisms of lymphangiogenesis in health and disease. Cancer Cell. 2002;1(3):219–27.

Part II

Lymphedema

5 Introduction

Ningfei Liu

Lymphedema is a progressive and highly disabling disease that affects an estimated 200–300 million people worldwide [1]. Lymphedema can be either primary (hereditary) or secondary (acquired) and develops as tissue fluid retention and swelling. Primary lymphedema is caused by lymphatic system dysplasia or developmental dysfunction of unknown cause. The leading cause of secondary lymphedema worldwide is filariasis [2]. Tumor treatment is the main cause of secondary lymphedema in other regions. Peripheral lymphedema is the most common type and is caused by superficial lymphatic system disorders. Lymphedema may have serious consequences if it is neglected or not treated in time. Once lymphedema occurs, the edema fluid, which is rich in macromolecules, stays in the tissue, the fibrous tissue and fat continue to deposit, and the affected limb becomes deformity. Lymphedema is often accompanied by frequent attacks of erysipelas and cellulitis. Each infection exacerbates edema, creating a vicious circle. Currently, peripheral lymphedema is an incurable disease because the pathological changes in the affected tissue and the lymphatic system itself induced by lymphedema are generally irreversible. Secondly, the mechanisms underlying abnormal lymphatic system development and defective postnatal lymphatic regeneration remain largely unclear. This has led to a lack of effective and targeted treatments. To date, more than 20 underlying genes have been identified in lymphedema, and these are linked to different phenotypes of primary lymphedema [3], providing valuable insight into the molecular mechanisms that regulate the development and function of the lymphatic vasculature. Additionally, a new multi-modal imaging examination for the lymphatic system that was developed over the last decade is now available in many centers [4, 5]. Therefore, future studies into correlations between phenotype and genotype will help obtain a better understanding of this disease and explore new treatments.

References

1. Rockson SG, Rivera KK. Estimating the population burden of lymphedema. Ann N Y Acad Sci. 2008;1131:147–54. https://doi.org/10.1196/annals.1413.014.
2. International Society of Lymphology. The diagnosis and treatment of peripheral lymphedema: 2013 Consensus Document of the International Society of Lymphology. Lymphology. 2013;46(1):1–11.
3. Michelini S, Paolacci S, Manara E, Eretta C, Mattassi R, Lee BB, Bertelli M. Genetic tests in lymphatic vascular malformations and lymphedema. J Med Genet. 2018;55(4):222–32. https://doi.org/10.1136/jmedgenet-2017-105064.
4. Liu NF, Yan ZX, Wu XF. Classification of lymphatic-system malformations in primary lymphoedema based on MR lymphangiography. Eur J Vasc Endovasc Surg. 2012;44(3):345–9. https://doi.org/10.1016/j.ejvs.2012.06.019.
5. Yu ZY, Sun D, Wang L, Chen J, Han LH, Liu NF. Diagnosis of primary lymphedema with indocyanine green lymphography. Chin J Plast Surg. 2018;34(4):256–9.

N. Liu (✉)
Department of Plastic and Reconstructive Surgery, Shanghai Ninth People's Hospital, Shanghai Jiao Tong University School of Medicine, Shanghai, China

N. Liu (ed.), *Peripheral Lymphedema*, https://doi.org/10.1007/978-981-16-3484-0_5

Etiology of Primary Lymphedema

6

Ningfei Liu

Abstract

The clinical symptoms of primary lymphedema are diverse, and its pathogenesis is complicated. Previous studies have shown that primary lymphedema is a multi-gene-involved disease. More than 20 causative genes have been identified in patients. Newly developed imaging techniques can show morphological and functional anomalies of affected lymphatic systems. Study on the correlations between the phenotype and genotype of primary lymphedemas will uncover the complicated etiology of this disease.

Keywords

Primary lymphedema · Heterogeneous · Pathogenic Hereditary lymphedema · Sporadic lymphedema Genetic mutation · Extremity · Multi-segmental Phenotype · Genotype

Primary lymphedema refers to a class of lymphedema with heterogeneous symptoms and unknown causes [1, 2]. It is common in the limbs, especially the lower extremities, but also occurs in the external genitals, face, buttocks, and lower abdomen. In most cases, lymphedema occurs in a single limb, but may be multi-located and symmetrical or asymmetrical, such as those located in the upper left and lower right limbs. In most cases, lymphedema results from a superficial lymphatic anomaly, and less frequency are both the superficial and deep lymphatic systems involved. The diversity of clinical signs of primary lymphedema indicates a complicated underlying disease pathology. The etiology of primary lymphedema described here is based on our very limited current understanding of the disease [3].

N. Liu (✉)
Department of Plastic and Reconstructive Surgery, Shanghai Ninth People's Hospital, Shanghai Jiao Tong University School of Medicine, Shanghai, China

Classifications of primary lymphedema are simply made according to the onset of the disease as congenital (e.g., Milroy's disease), in which the disease occurs at birth or months after birth, or late-onset (praecox, tarda; e.g., lymphedema distichiasis syndrome [LDS]). The different mechanisms underlying early- and late-onset lymphedema are also poorly understood because of differences in the pathological anomalies of the lymphatic system between each type.

6.1 Hereditary Lymphedema

Inherited primary lymphedemas are classified according to their underlying genetic mutation as one of the following types.

1. Hereditary lymphedema type 1A (OMIM: 136352). The lymphatic system malformations associated with this type are lymphatic vessel dysplasia, aplasia, or dysfunction. Heterozygous mutations in *FLT4* (OMIM: 136352, *VEGFR3*) are strongly associated with lymphatic vessel development, and *FLT4* mutations show an autosomal dominant inheritance, with incomplete penetrance of 85–90% [4]. The *FLT4* mutations result in amino acid substitutions that increase the binding of the receptor to its ligand, VEGF-C/VEGF-D, producing abnormal signaling that affects the function of lymphatic endothelial cells [5]. However, not all Milroy's disease cases have identifiable variants of *FLT4*. It is generally believed that only the following symptoms suggested by Milroy can be diagnosed: having a family history (chromosome inheritance), congenital disease, nonprogressive development, and lower limb disease [6]. The features of Milroy's edema make the skin "woody," and secondary clinical changes include deep folds of the toe skin, papilloma-nourishing skin lesions, and a prominent great saphenous vein, which contribute to the diagnosis, as other congeni-

N. Liu (ed.), *Peripheral Lymphedema*, https://doi.org/10.1007/978-981-16-3484-0_6

tal lymphedemas do not present this phenomenon [7]. Different lymphatic imaging methods such as magnetic resonance lymphangiography (MRL), indocyanine green (ICG) lymphography, and lymphoscintigraphy (LSG) have been used to show impaired lymph backflow in the affected limb. These are classified as: no enhanced lymph collector in MRL or ICG [8] (Fig. 6.1), partial or delayed enhancement of collecting lymphatic vessels in the dorsum of the foot (ICG; Fig. 6.2), little uptake of contrast agent, and poor visualization of inguinal lymph nodes (LSG). Biopsies have shown various anomalies in capillary lymphatic vessels in the skin tissue of Milroy's disease patients, which are classified as: (1) aplasia—no initial lymphatics in the epidermis and dermis [9] (Fig. 6.3); (2) hypoplasia—a decrease in the number compared with the contralateral non-edema skin [8] (Fig. 6.1); and (3) not abnormal—which suggests that genetic variation affects lymphatic function rather than lymphatic formation.

2. Hereditary lymphedema type 1C (OMIM: 613480), which has an autosomal dominant inheritance, and the causative gene is *GJC2* (OMIM: 608803). The onset may be at birth or in youth or adulthood, and edema may be mild or severe and affect either lower or upper limbs. The impairment of lymph drainage may be due to lymphatic hypoplasia in the great saphenous vein [10, 11].
3. Hereditary lymphedema type 1D (OMIM: 615907), which has an autosomal dominant inheritance, and the causative gene is *VEGFC* (OMIM: 601528) with a loss-of-function mutation. The disease occurs at birth or as an adult. The lymphatic anomalies include tortuous vessels with reduced transportation [10, 11].

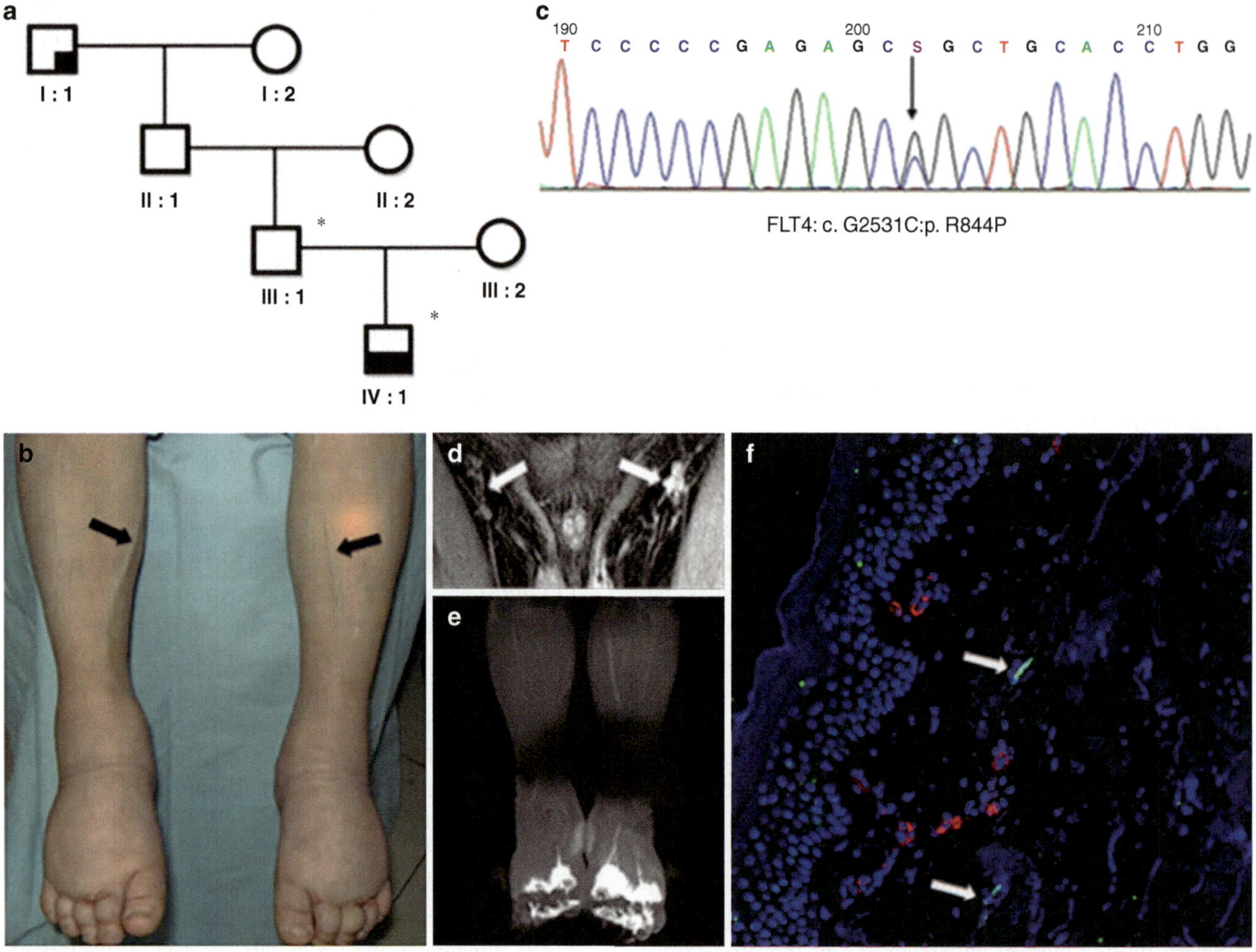

Fig. 6.1 Phenotype and genotype of *FLT4* mutation in an MD family. (**a**) Pedigree of the family, the half-filled shape indicates affected individuals with bilateral lower extremity lymphedema, a quarter-filled shape indicates unilateral (left) lower extremity lymphedema; * indicates mutation carrier; (**b**) Bilateral lymphedema of the lower extremity with prominent great saphenous veins (arrows) of IV:1; (**c**) DNA sequencing analysis shows a missense mutation of c.2531G>C in one allele of *FLT4* identified in III:1 and IV:1; (**d**) MRL imaging shows inguinal lymph nodes (arrows) in IV:1; (**e**) No lymph collector was visualized in the affected lower limbs on MRL imaging; (**f**) Dermal initial lymphatic vessels (arrows) stained with podoplanin of IV:1

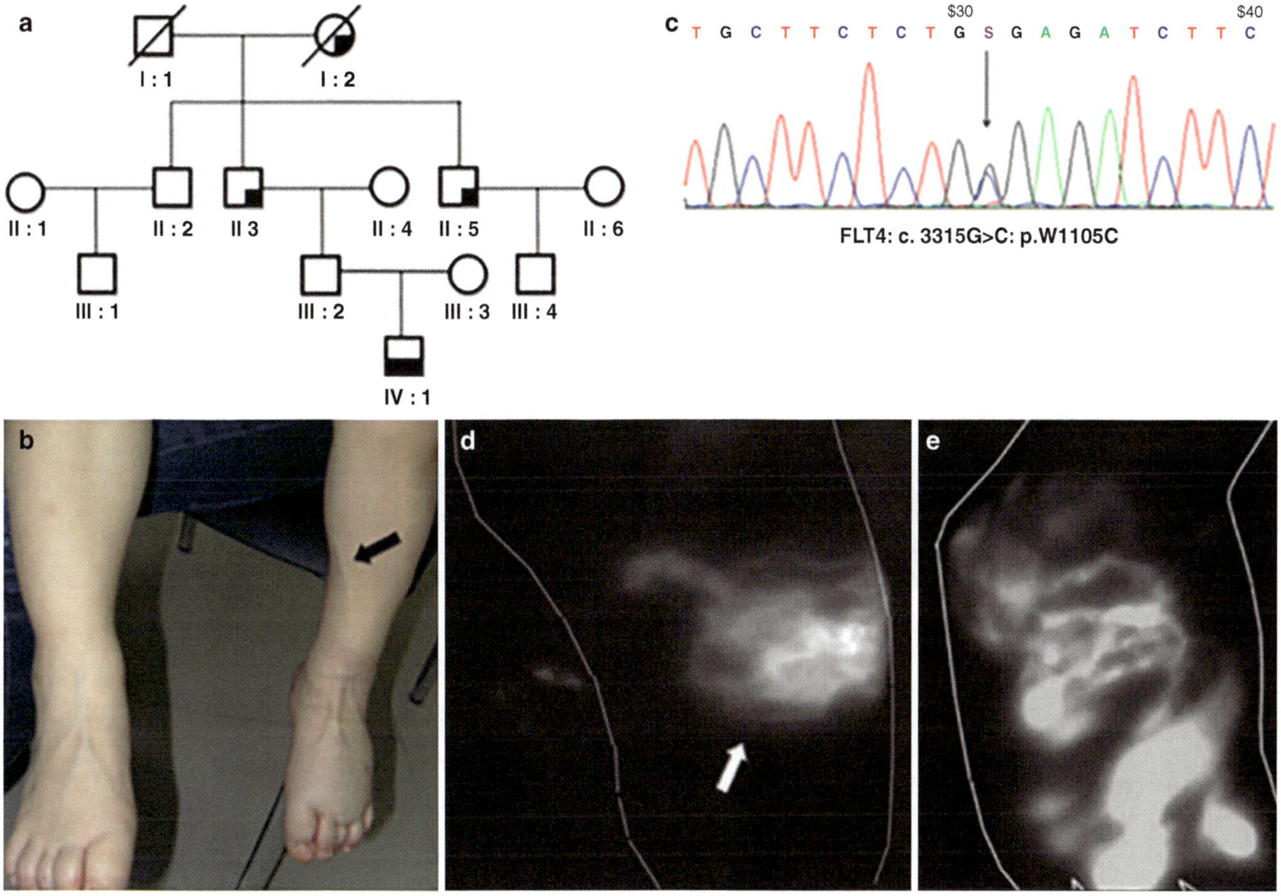

Fig. 6.2 Phenotype and genotype of *FLT4* mutation in an MD family. (**a**) Pedigree of the family, the half-filled shape indicates affected individuals with bilateral lower extremity lymphedema, a quarter-filled shape indicates unilateral (left) lower extremity lymphedema; (**b**) Bilateral lymphedema of the lower extremity of VI:1. The arrow points to prominent great saphenous veins; (**c**) DNA sequencing results: a missense mutation of c.3315G>C in one allele of *FLT4* identified in III:1 and IV:1; (**d**) ICG lymphogram shows few enhanced collecting lymph vessels at the bottom of left foot (arrow), and (**e**) shows tortuous lymph collectors in the dorsum of the right foot of IV:1

4. Hereditary lymphedema type 2, also known as Meige's syndrome (MIM 153200), which was first reported in 1898. Meige's syndrome is the most common hereditary lymphedema, accounting for approximately 65–80% of all hereditary cases. Hereditary lymphedema type 2, which shows chromosomal dominant inheritance and is characterized by puberty onset (ages 20–59). Both lower limbs can be involved. Edema is commonly seen in the ankle and anterior tibial region but also can also occur in the upper limbs and face. The disease is often accompanied by erysipelas and cellulitis. Other abnormalities include malformations in the cardiovascular system, cleft palate, deafness, pleural lymphatic leakage, varicose veins, double-row eyelashes, and spinal deformities. MR lymphangiography and direct lymphography have found that the number of lymphatic vessels was in the normal range or decreased and that vessels were dilated. Lymphoscintigraphy showed underdeveloped lymph nodes and lymphatic vessels. The molecular basis for the pathogenesis of heritable lymphedema type 2 is not well studied. Genetic variants in the transcription factor *FOXC2* (16q24.3) have been found in multiple families [12]. LDS (lymphedema distichiasis syndrome LDS) is one of the subtypes of heritable lymphedema type 2. Variations in *FOXC2* are also seen in hereditary cases such as lymphedema–yellow nail syndrome [13].

LDS is an inherited or sporadic primary lymphedema that is characterized by bilateral or unilateral lower limb lymphedema that presents after the onset of puberty. Affected individuals also usually have an abnormal second row of eyelashes. *FOXC2* is a fork-head box transcription factor and the only gene known to be involved in LDS [12]. *FOXC2* plays a central role in lymphatic vessel development and lymphatic valve formation [14]. Reflux of failed lymph and lymphatic valves has been suspected in the lower limbs of individuals with *FOXC2* mutations based on the low uptake of isotopic tracer in the ilioinguinal nodes during lymphoscintigram. Lymphatic dilatation and disruption with lymph leakage were visualized by MR lymphangiography [8]

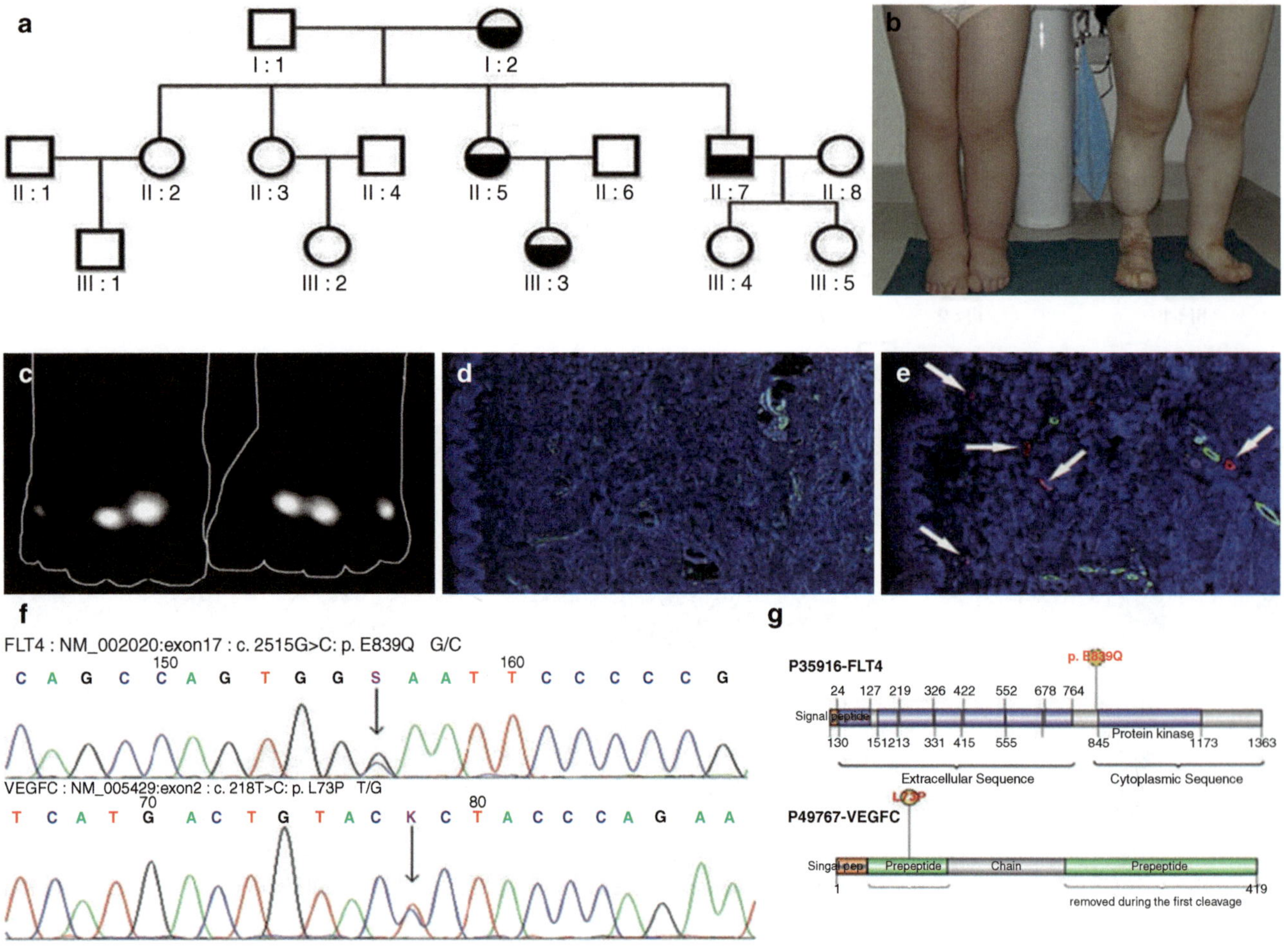

h

Table 1 Population frequency and disease prediction for the two variants

Gene	Ref Allele	Alt Allele	Chrs	Position	Mutation	dbSNP*	1000g‡	ExAC03†	Control 300‡	SIFT Score	SIFT Score Pred	POLYPhen V2 Score	POLYPhen V2 ScorePred	Mutation Taster	Mutation Taster Pred	Cadd Raw	Cadd Phred	Dann
FLT4	C	G	5	180047200	NM_002020:exon17: c.2515G>C:p.E839Q	-	0	0	0	0	D	1	D	0.999972	D	5.947646	27.6	0.999
VEGFC	A	G	4	177650830	NM_005429:exon2: c.218T>C:p.L73P	-	0	0	0	0.07	D	0.998	D	1	D	5.721332	26.9	0.999

*, NCBI dbSNP version 151. ‡, Frequency of the two variants in the 1000 genome database (https://www.ncbi.nlm.nih.gov/variation/tools/1000genomes/). †, Frequency of the two variants in the database of ~60,000 samples (http://exac.broadinstitute.org/). ‡, Frequencies of the two variante in 300 population-matched healthy controls.

Fig. 6.3 Phenotype and genotype of *VEGFR3/FLT4* and *VEGFC* co-mutations in a family with MD. (**a**) Pedigree of the family, the half-filled shape indicates bilateral lower extremity lymphedema; * indicates mutation carrier. (**b**) Bilateral lymphedema of lower extremity of III:3 (left) andII:5 (right). (**c**) DNA sequencing analysis: the top panel shows one missense mutation c.2515G>C (p.E839Q) in exon 17 of *VEGFR-3/FLT4,* and the bottom panel shows one missense mutation c.218T>C (p.L73P in exon 2 of *VEGFC.* (**d**) Locations of detected *FLT4* (top) and *VEGFC* (bottom) mutations in this study. (**e**) ICG lymphogram shows the stagnation of contrast in the injection sites of the dorsum of bilateral feet of III:3, and no enhanced lymphatic was visualized. (**f**) No podoplanin positive lymphatics were identified in the dorsum skin of subject III:3. (**g**) Dermal lymphatic vessels (arrows) stained with podoplanin the skin of control skin tissue

(Fig. 6.4). However, the pathological mechanisms underlying lymphatic valve defects in cases with *FOXC2* mutations remain unclear. In families with *FOXC2* mutations, there appears to be no clear genotype-phenotype correlation, and the severity of the disease varies widely, even within families [12]. It has been speculated that intra- and inter-familial variation results from stochastic effects or interactions with other genes in the *FOXC2* pathway [12].

The other genetic mutations associated with inherited lymphedema include homozygous or compound heterozygous mutations in *PIEZO1* (OMIM: 611184), which shows autosomal recessive inheritance with neonatal to prepuberty

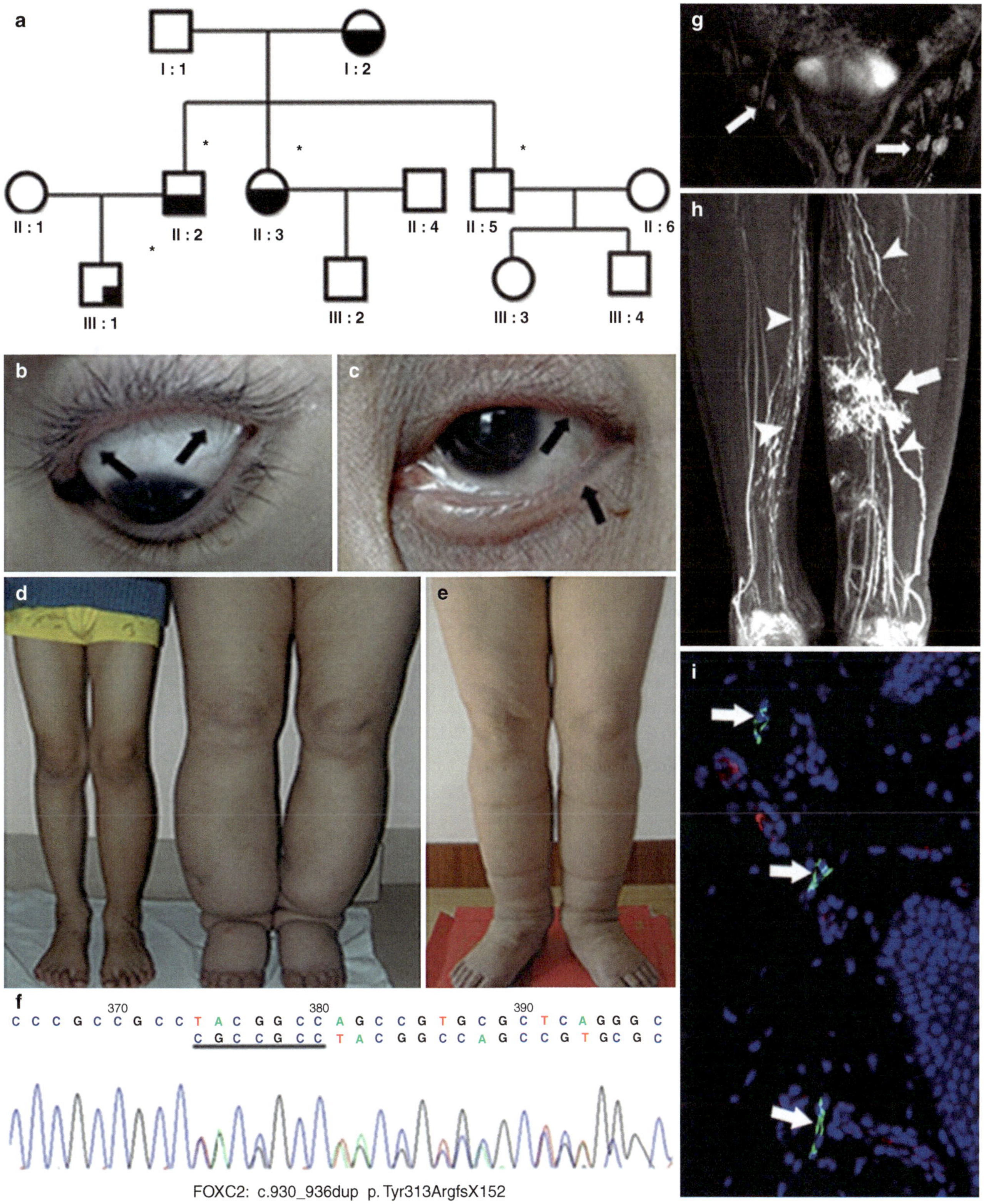

Fig. 6.4 Phenotype and genotype of *FOXC2* mutation in an LDS family. (**a**) Pedigree of the family, the half-filled shape indicates affected individuals with bilateral lower extremity lymphedema, and a quarter-filled shape indicates unilateral lower extremity lymphedema; (**b**, **c**) Aberrant eyelashes–distichiasis (arrows) in III: 1 and II:3; (**d**, **e**) lymphedema of the legs in III:1 and II:3 and II:2; (**f**) DNA sequencing analysis shows a 7-bp duplication, c.930_936dup of *FOXC2* identified in II:2, II:3, and III:1; (**g**) Inguinal lymph nodes (arrows) on MRL imaging; (**h**) Dilated collecting lymphatics (arrowheads) and lymphatic disrupture, and lymph leakage (arrow) in affected left leg (arrow) of III:1; (**i**) Slightly dilated dermal initial lymphatics in the skin of III:1 (arrows)

onset. The edema has been reported to be generalized in all segments of the body, with intestinal and pulmonary lymphangiectasia and chylothorax or pericardial effusion [15, 16]. Inherited lymphedema is also associated with missense mutations in lymphatic vessel endothelial hyaluronan receptor-1 (*LYVE-1*), which is one of the most specific lymphatic vessel markers in the skin and is specifically expressed by lymphatic endothelial cells. ICG lymphography showed a delayed and faint enhancement of tortuous lymphatics in the affected foot of one of these cases [17] (Figs. 6.5 and 6.6).

Primary lymphedema likely has multiple genetic causes despite its apparent transmission as a "single-gene" autosomal dominant disease. *FOXC2* mutations occur in both non-syndromic and syndromic lymphedema as well as in inherited and non-inherited cases [12]. Therefore, lymphatic abnormalities may be caused by several genes, similar to other disorders. A recent study showed co-mutation of *FLT4* and *VEGF-C* in a Milroy's disease family [9]. In this family, one missense mutation, c.2515G>C (p.E839Q), was identified in exon 17 of *VEGFR-3/FLT4* by whole-exome sequencing of blood samples from the proband and her mother (Fig. 6.3f). Another missense mutation, c.218T>C (p.L73P), was identified in exon 2 of *VEGF-C* (Fig. 6.3f) and is located within the N-terminal propeptide (Fig. 6.3g). No lymphatic vessels were seen during the ICG lymphography of the patient (Fig. 6.3c). Moreover, no initial lymphatics were identified in the superficial and deep dermis or the subcutaneous tissue of a biopsy from the dorsum of the patient's affected foot (Fig. 6.3d), which indicates a structural (maybe

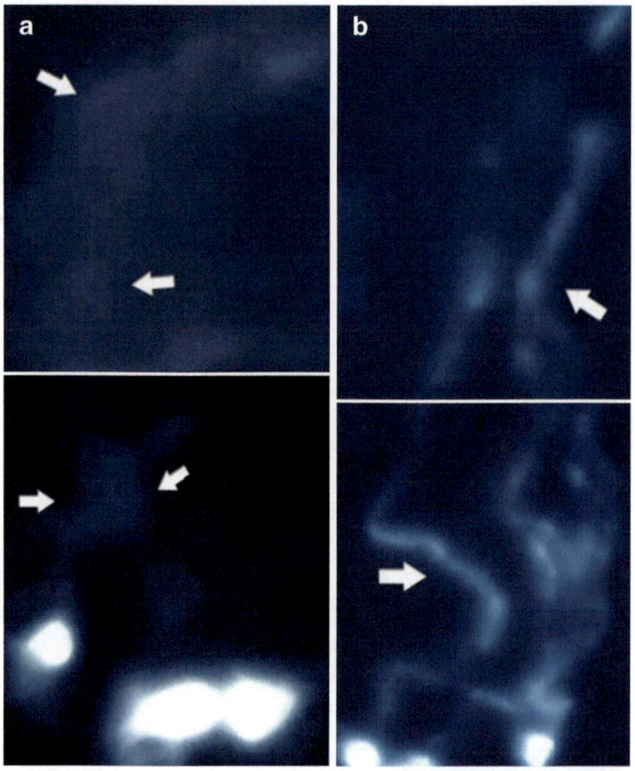

Fig. 6.6 Imaging results of ICG lymphography of subject II:7. (**a**) ICG lymphogram shows faintly enhanced tortuous lymphatics (arrows) with undefined shape in the lymphedematous right foot (bottom) and ankle (top) regions. (**b**) ICG lymphogram shows strongly enhanced lymph collectors (arrows) with clear shape in the dorsum (bottom) and ankle (top) regions of the non-edematous left foot

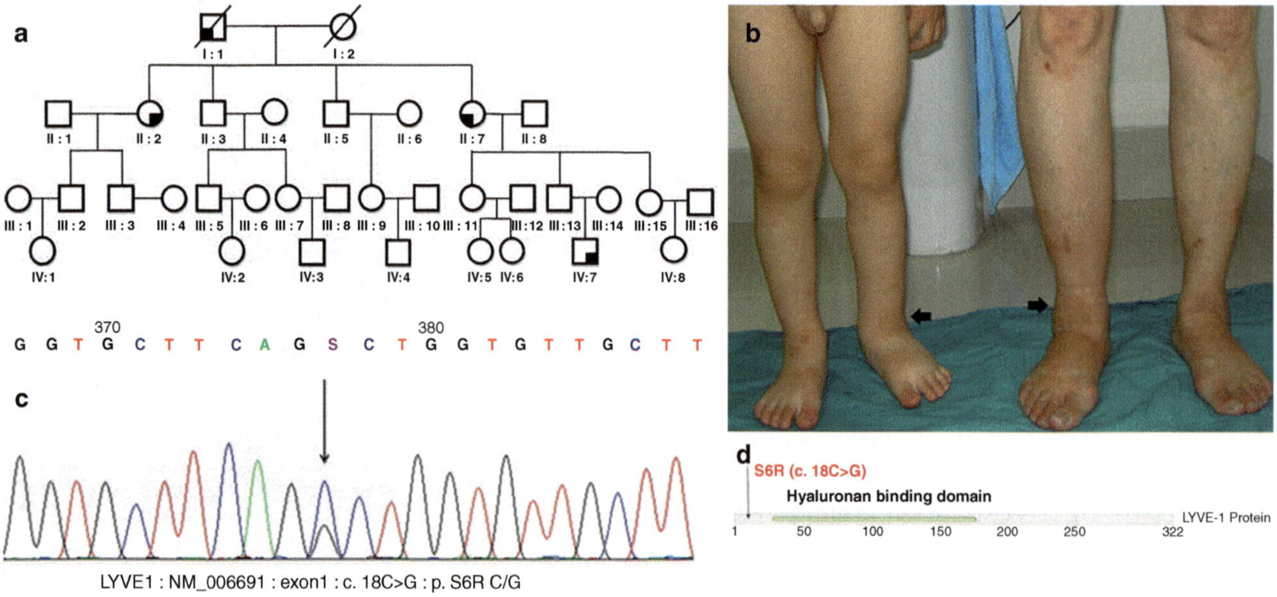

Fig. 6.5 Phenotype and genotype of *LYVE-1/CRSBP-1* mutations in a family with primary lymphedema. (**a**) Pedigree of the family, a quarter-filled shape indicates unilateral (right or left) lower extremity lymphedema; * indicates mutation carrier. (**b**) Unilateral lymphedema of the lower extremity (arrows) of IV:7 (left) and II:7 III:13 (right). (**c**) DNA sequencing analysis: the panel shows a missense mutation of c.18C>G (p.S6R) in exon 1 of *LYVE-1/CRSBP-1* changing amino acid 6 from serine to arginine in three generations of the family. (**d**) Locations of detected *LYVE-1/CRSBP-1* mutation in this family

also a functional) aplasia of the initial lymphatics. This study showed that primary lymphedema is likely to have multiple genetic causes despite its apparent transmission as a "single-gene" autosomal dominant disease. The individual reported mutations in *VEGFR-3* and *VEGF-C* in Milroy's disease or Milroy's disease-like primary lymphedema to reveal that these primarily affected lymphatic function or partially interfered with cutaneous lymphangiogenesis. However, when this receptor and ligand pair were simultaneously mutated, the development of dermal lymphatics may be seriously inhibited. Therefore, similar to other disorders, primary lymphedemas are most likely caused by several genes. The multiple phenotypes that arise in individuals with Milroy's disease are the cumulative result of multiple genetic and environmental influences.

6.2 Sporadic Lymphedema

Non-familial hereditary primary lymphedema accounts for approximately 90% of the total incidence of primary lymphedema. Patients who are <35 years old are generally referred to as early onset, while those >35 years old are referred to as late-onset. Early onset disease is more common in women, often between the ages of 10 and 20. This may be due to increased estrogen levels in the body, which result in water and sodium retention and increased capillary permeability, and reduced lymphatic contractility. Edema first appears in the dorsal foot and ankle, and 70% of cases are unilateral, with spreading to the entire leg after months or years, less to the thigh. On ICG lymphography, the lymphatic collector can be visualized in the dorsum of the feet, and the transportation of lymph flow is slow. Enhanced lymphatic vessel rarely goes above the ankle level. A minor injury such as a sprain may be a predisposing factor, compression, or displacement of the ankle lymphatic vessels may reduce the delivery of lymphatic vessels, and acute inflammation caused by the injury may aggravate the lymphatic load. Lymphedema persists after acute inflammation of tissue subsides. The slow development of edema because of the compensatory action of lymphatic vessels in youth is often not easy to detect. Delayed edema is aggravated in old age because the transporting function of the lymphatic vessels is gradually reduced. The pre-edema stage is clinically referred to as the edema incubation period, although lymphatic vessel development is abnormal and the number is reduced, it can sometimes still support the normal lymphatic transport. The genes identified in these families with heredity lymphedema were also found in isolated lymphedema cases, including *FIT4, FOXC2, HGF*, and *GATA2*. Among them, *FIT4* mutations are the most common (unpublished data). The sporadic LD cases exhibited similar clinical signs with inherited type, and the imaging of MRL demonstrated numerous tortuous lymph collectors with lymph reflux [8] (Fig. 6.7).

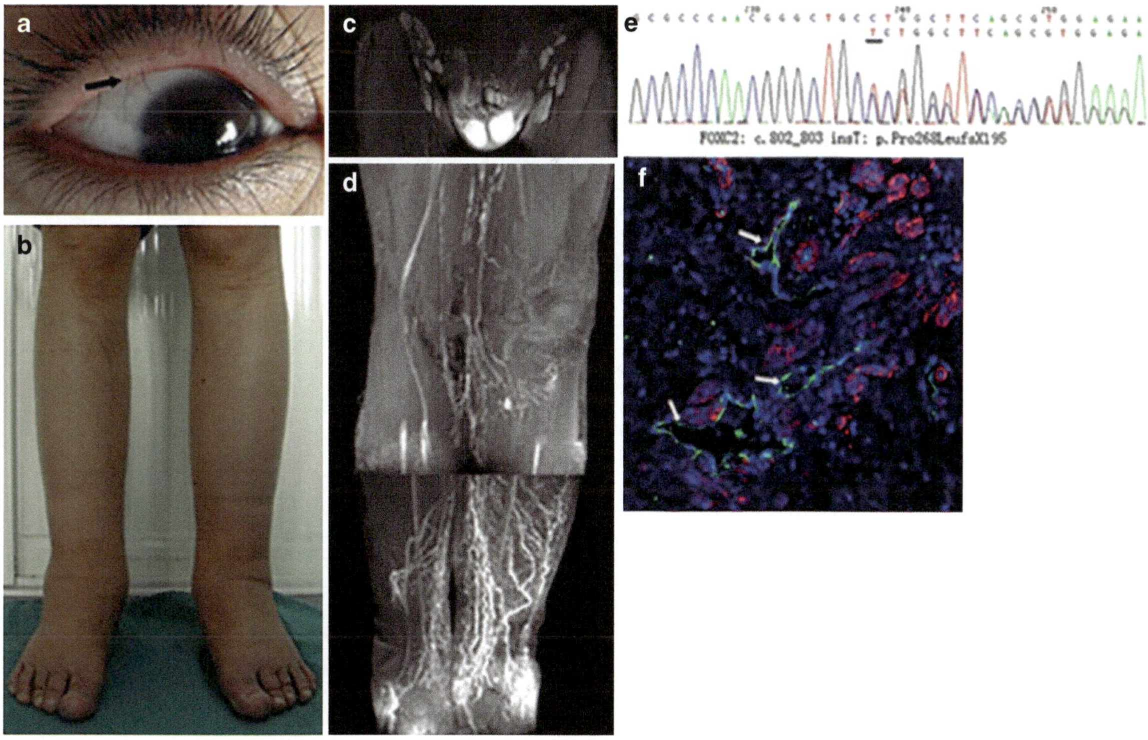

Fig. 6.7 Phenotype and genotype of *FOXC2* mutations in the isolated LDS case. (**a**) Double eyelashes (arrow); (**b**) Bilateral lower leg lymphedema; (**c**) Inguinal lymph node with normal structure and slightly increase in size; (**d**) Numerous, bead-like and tortuous lymphatics in the bilateral lower limbs with more severe pathology in the left lymphedematous limb; (**e**) DNA sequencing analysis shows 1-bp insertion mutation (c.802_803insT) of *FOXC2*; (**f**) Obviously dilated dermal lymphatics were found in the skin

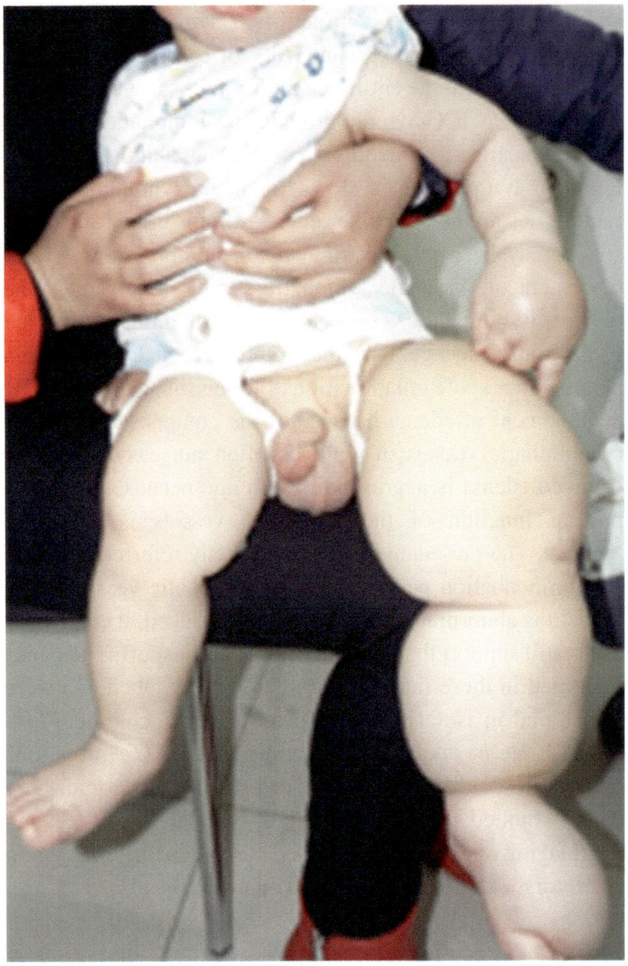

Fig. 6.8 Multi-segmental lymphedemas (left upper and lower limbs and extragenital) in a child

6.3 Multi-Segmental Lymphedema

Multi-location or multi-segmental lymphedema is rare. It is congenital and usually occurs without a family history. It can be general or affect more than two body parts and may locate asymmetrically in unilateral upper and lower limbs (Fig. 6.8). It may be associated with edema of the extra-genital, semi-face, and at a very low frequency with visceral involvement. The pathogenesis of multi-segmental lymphedema remains poorly understood because of the lack of a big data study. A cohort of nine children with multi-segmental lymphedema and their parents underwent DNA sequencing. A *GJL2* mutation was identified in one child with general lymphedema, and a *CELSR1* mutation was found in three cases (unpublished data). No parents had the same mutation as their child. No lymphatics or lymph nodes were visualized by lymphoscintigraphic imaging. In patients with external genitalia lymphedema, inguinal node anomalies were found. Lymphatic vessels were not detected in patients with affected upper extremity with LSG inspection (Fig. 6.9).

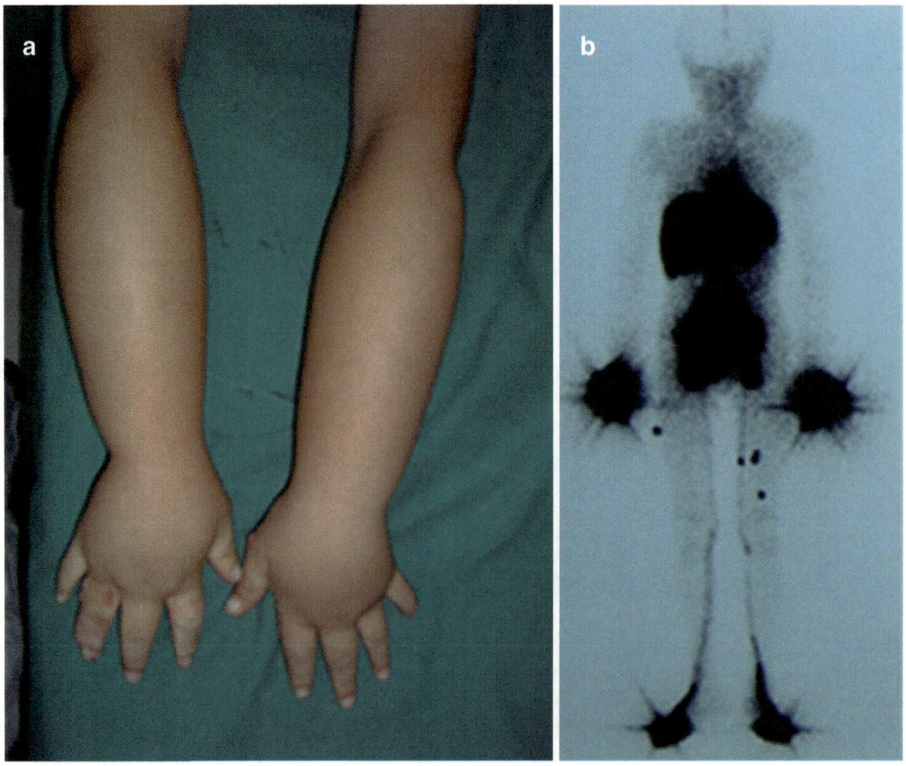

Fig. 6.9 (a) Bilateral upper limb lymphedema; (b) No lymphatic was identified on lymphoscintigram

References

1. Grada AA, Phillips TJ. Lymphedema: pathophysiology and clinical manifestations. J Am Acad Dermatol. 2017;77(6):1009–20. https://doi.org/10.1016/j.jaad.2017.03.022.
2. Lee BB, Laredo J. Pathophysiology of primary lymphedema. In: Neligan PC, Masia J, Piller NB, editors. Lymphedema: complete medical and surgical management. CRC Press, Taylor & Francis Group; 2015. p. 177–87.
3. Ferrell RE, Levinson KL, Esman JH, Kimak MA, Lawrence EC, Barmada MM, Finegold DN. Hereditary lymphedema: evidence for linkage and genetic heterogeneity. Hum Mol Genet. 1998;7(13):2073–8.
4. Gordon K, Spiden SL, Connell FC, Brice G, Cottrell S, Short J, Taylor R, Jeffery S, Mortimer PS, Mansour S, Ostergaard P. FLT4/VEGFR3 and milroy disease: novel mutations, a review of published variants and database update. Hum Mutat. 2013;34(1):23–31. https://doi.org/10.1002/humu.22223.
5. Karkkainen MJ, Ferrell RE, Lawrence EC, Kimak MA, Levinson KL, McTigue MA, Alitalo K, Finegold DN. Missense mutations interfere with VEGFR-3 signalling in primary lymphoedema. Nat Genet. 2000;25(2):153–9.
6. Milroy WF. An undescribed variety of hereditary edema. N Y Med J. 1892;56:505–8.
7. Brice G, Child AH, Evans A, Bell R, Mansour S, Burnand K, Sarfarazi M, Jeffery S, Mortimer P. Milroy disease and the VEGFR-3 mutation phenotype. J Med Genet. 2005;42(2):98–102.
8. Liu NF, Yu ZY, Sun D, Lou Y. Rare variants in LAMA5 gene associated with FLT4 and FOXC2 mutations in primary lymphedema may contribute to severity. Lymphology. 2016;49(4):192–204.
9. Liu NF, Yu ZY, Lou Y, Sun D. A Milroy case with FLT4/VEGFR3 mutation and an unusual skin biopsy. Br J Dermatol. 2019;180(1):223–4. https://doi.org/10.1111/bjd.17120.
10. Michelini S, Paolacci S, Manara E, Eretta C, Mattassi R, Lee BB, Bertelli M. Genetic tests in lymphatic vascular malformations and lymphedema. J Med Genet. 2018;55(4):222–32. https://doi.org/10.1136/jmedgenet-2017-105064.
11. Brouillard P, Boon L, Vikkula M. Genetics of lymphatic anomalies. J Clin Invest. 2014;124(3):898–904. https://doi.org/10.1172/JCI71614.
12. Brice G, Mansour S, Bell R, Collin JR, Child AH, Brady AF, Sarfarazi M, Burnand KG, Jeffery S, Mortimer P, Murday VA. Analysis of the phenotypic abnormalities in lymphoedema-distichiasis syndrome in 74 patients with FOXC2 mutations or linkage to 16q24. J Med Genet. 2002;39(7):478–83.
13. Finegold DN, Kimak MA, Lawrence EC, Levinson KL, Cherniske EM, Pober BR, Dunlap JW, Ferrell RE. Truncating mutations in *FOXC2* cause multiple lymphedema syndromes. Hum Mol Genet. 2001;10(11):1185–9.
14. Petrova TV, Karpanen T, Norrmén C, Mellor R, Tamakoshi T, Finegold D, Ferrell R, Kerjaschki D, Mortimer P, Ylä-Herttuala S, Miura N, Alitalo K. Defective valves and abnormal mural cell recruitment underlie lymphatic vascular failure in lymphedema distichiasis. Nat Med. 2004;10(9):974–81.
15. Lukacs V, Mathur J, Mao R, Bayrak-Toydemir P, Procter M, Cahalan SM, Kim HJ, Bandell M, Longo N, Day RW, Stevenson DA, Patapoutian A, Krock BL. Impaired PIEZO1 function in patients with a novel autosomal recessive congenital lymphatic-dysplasia. Nat Commun. 2015;21(6):8329. https://doi.org/10.1038/ncomms9329.
16. Andolfo I, De Rosa G, Errichiello E, Manna F, Rosato BE, Gambale A, Vetro A, Calcaterra V, Pelizzo G, De Franceschi L, Zuffardi O, Russo R, Iolascon A. PIEZO1 hypomorphic variants in congenital lymphatic dysplasia cause shape and hydration alterations of red blood cells. Front Physiol. 2019;15(10):258. https://doi.org/10.3389/fphys.2019.00258.
17. Liu NF, Yu Z, Luo Y, Sun D. A LYVE-1/CRSBP-1 mutation in inherited primary lymphedema. Lymphology. 2017;50(1):9–15.

Secondary Lymphedema of Different Types

7

Ningfei Liu

Filarial lymphedema is the most common type of secondary lymphedema worldwide [1]. Globally, 68 million people are infected with lymphatic filariasis, 17 million of whom have lymphedema [2]. Filarial lymphedema can be treated and prevented with an anti-filariasis drug, for which China is an example. Filariasis infections have been common in China for thousands of years. There were 330 million people at risk of filariasis and 30.94 million filariasis patients in the early 1950s. However, the disease was successfully eliminated after a decades long countrywide anti-filariasis treatment with Diethylcarbamazine Citrate [3, 4]. With approval from the World Health Organization in May 2007, China has taken the lead in eliminating filariasis in 83 countries and regions around the world. Currently, tumor-associated lymphedema has become more and more common with the increased survival rate of cancer patients. Thus, this situation will not change in the short term. This chapter focuses on tumor-related secondary lymphedema, the most common types of which are breast cancer-related lymphedema and gynecologic oncology-related lymphedema.

7.1 Breast Cancer-Related Lymphedema

Abstract
Breast cancer-related lymphedema accounts for the majority of the secondary lymphedema cases worldwide. Surgery, chemotherapy, and radiotherapy are the primary causes of lymph circulation failure, and improper use of the limbs, infection and injury are second hits to the overloaded lymphatic system. Early diagnosis and treatment may achieve better outcomes. For patients with stage II or III lymphedema, treatment is still challenging due to the irreversible pathological changes in the lymphedematous tissue.

Keywords
Secondary lymphedema, Breast cancer-related lymphedema (BCRL), Mastectomy, Axillary lymph node dissection, Radiation therapy, Chemotherapy

Breast cancer-related lymphedema (BCRL) is diagnosed in 15–30% of breast cancer survivors, making it the most common type of secondary edema in western countries. It is also one of the most common secondary lymphedemas in China. As in most other countries, breast cancer is now the most common cancer type in Chinese women; cases in China account for 12.2% of all newly diagnosed breast cancers and 9.6% of all breast cancer-related deaths worldwide. China's proportional contribution to the global breast cancer rate is increasing rapidly because of the population's rising socioeconomic status and unique reproductive patterns [5]. The total number of BCRL cases has increased along with the breast cancer incidence rate. The estimated number of new BCRL cases is 3–5 million per year. Axillary surgery contributes considerably to the incidence of BCRL, with the incidence and severity of swelling related to the number of lymph nodes removed [5]. It is generally believed that adjuvant radiotherapy to the breast or lymph nodes increases the risk of lymphedema in 9–40% of patients [6]. However, the risk of lymphedema is substantially decreased with newer sentinel lymph node sampling procedures. Selective modified surgery and selective radiotherapy may be important to prevent and reduce subsequent lymphedema in breast cancer treatment. Chemotherapy drugs may also trigger lymphatic reflux disorders. It has been noticed that taxane chemotherapy after or before surgery increases the risk of secondary lymphedema [7]. Patients developed transient systemic edema during chemotherapy with paclitaxel, and the edema gradually subsided in other parts of the body after chemotherapy but persisted in the affected upper limb. The lymphedema caused by chemotherapy can be diagnosed at early stages by signs such as non-pitting, tissue hardness, stiffness of the wrist and finger joints, and limited movement (Fig. 7.1).

N. Liu (✉)
Department of Plastic and Reconstructive Surgery, Shanghai Ninth People's Hospital, Shanghai Jiao Tong University School of Medicine, Shanghai, China

N. Liu (ed.), *Peripheral Lymphedema*, https://doi.org/10.1007/978-981-16-3484-0_7

Lymphatic regeneration failure after surgery can result in scar tissue, after which radiation can be a second hit to the fragile lymphatics that can lead to intensive tissue fibrosis that can further destroy the newly generated lymphatic capillaries. Some patients have transient edema after surgery, but most will subside on their own. Persistent edema occurs in months, years, or even decades after radical lymph node surgery. In a considerable number of patients, failure of the overload lymph flow occurs upon a trigger, including improper or overworking of the upper limb, acute infection, and venipuncture skin injury (e.g., mosquito bite or cut). Improper or overworking of the upper limb is the most common reason. A study proposed that the first abnormality during the development of BCRL is not lymphatic obstruction, but high fluid filtration, which overwhelms vulnerable lymphatics [8]. A recent magnetic resonance lymphangiogram imaging study showed that the collecting lymphatics underwent dilatation, disruption, and regeneration in BCRL limbs [9]. The number of lymph collectors increased along with the duration of the disease, indicating a self-compensatory mechanism of opening functional lymphatic vessels to deal with the edema. It is, therefore, the case that self-prevention of lymphedema will be a lifelong task for breast cancer patients. Early-stage edema is more common in the dorsum of the hand and will spread to the forearm and upper arm with time. Some edema is confined to the upper arm (Fig. 7.2). Early complete decongestion therapy can achieve good results and even cures. Long-lasting BCRL may turn into angiosarcoma or Stewart–Treves syndrome (Fig. 7.3). There has been an increased number of the report of angiosarcoma after breast-conserving surgery followed by radiation therapy over the past few years [10].

Recent association studies support the hypothesis that genetic susceptibility could be an important risk factor for developing secondary lymphedema [11–13]. The predisposing genes for secondary lymphedema are *HGF/MET, GJC2, VEGFR2, VEGFR3,* and *RORC*, which regulate lymphangiogenesis. Studies have also reported associations with *IL-4, IL-1,* and *NFKB2*, which are involved in inflammatory responses.

7.2 Gynecologic Oncology-Related Lymphedema

Abstract
Lower body lymphedema is a chronic condition and a significant cause of morbidity following treatment for gynecologic cancers, including cervical cancer, endometrial cancer, and ovarian cancer. Most studies on secondary lymphedema have investigated breast cancer-related lymphedema; thus, much less known about lower body lymphedema after treatment for gynecologic malignancies. The reported incidence of such cases was 0–50%, which suggests a need for standardizing evaluation and treatment.

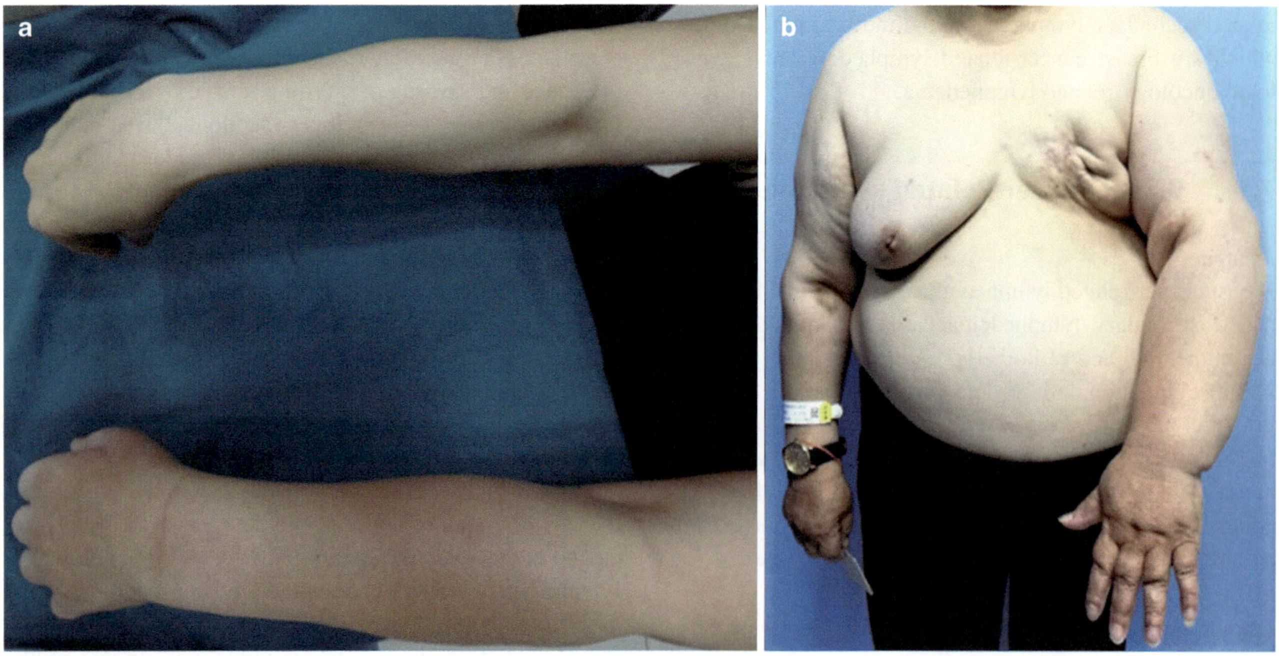

Fig. 7.1 (**a**) BCRL after chemotherapy of the left upper extremity at early stage (2 months). (**b**) BCRL of the left arm after chemotherapy at a later stage (6 years)

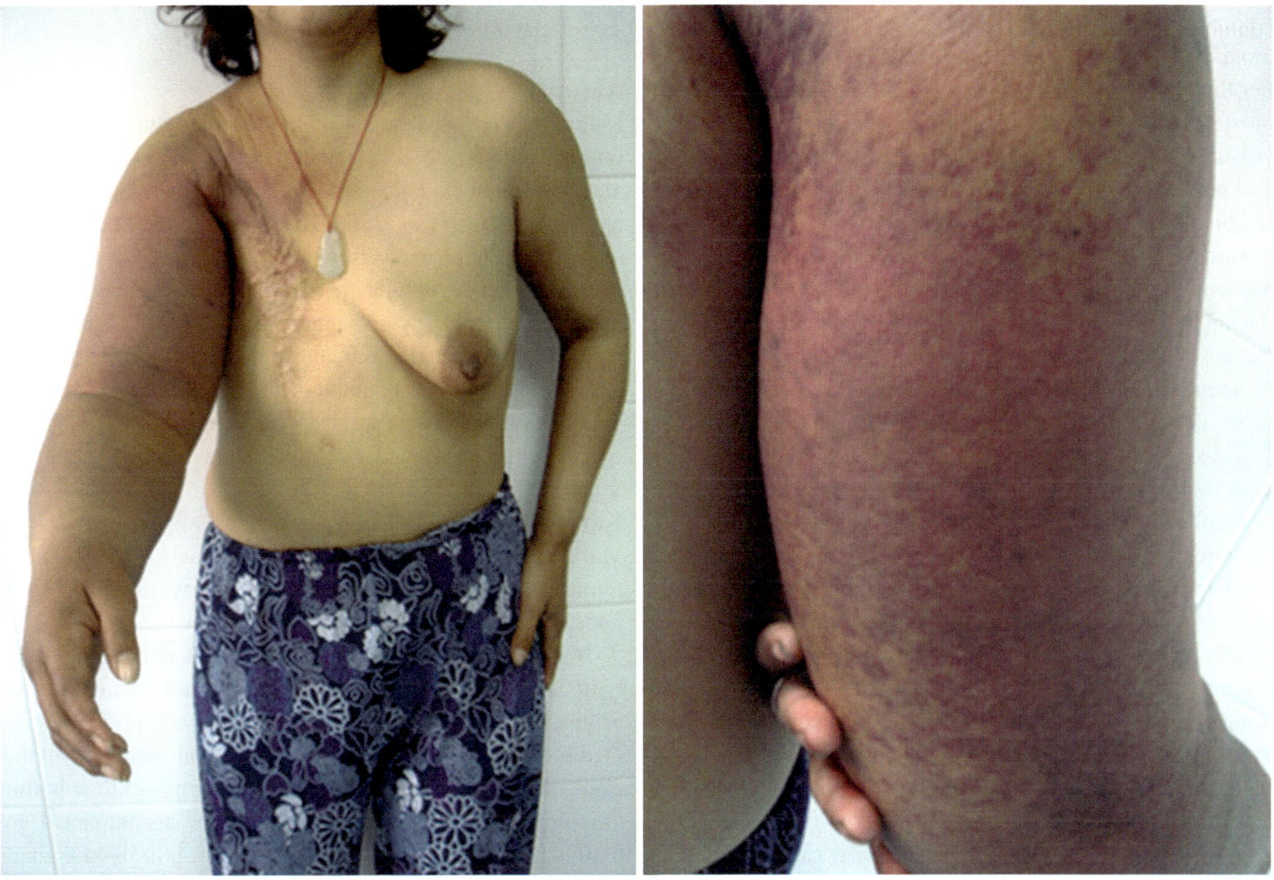

Fig. 7.2 A 45-year-old woman with BCRL and angiosarcoma in the right upper limb

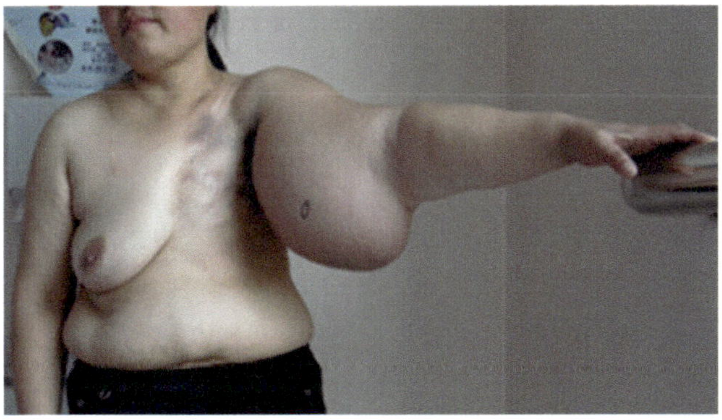

Fig. 7.3 A woman with BCRL in the left upper arm

Keywords
Gynecologic oncology-related lymphedema (GORL), Secondary lymphedema, Cervical cancer, Endometrial cancer, Ovarian cancer, Lower body, Pelvic lymph node dissection, Para-aortic lymphadenectomy, Radiation therapy, Lower extremity

Lower body lymphedema is a chronic condition and a significant cause of morbidity following treatment for gynecologic cancers, including cervical cancer, endometrial cancer, and ovarian cancer. This diagnosis is also called gynecologic oncology-related lymphedema (GORL). Most studies of secondary lymphedema have focused on breast cancer-related lymphedema treatment, so much less is known about lower body lymphedema after gynecologic malignancies. The reported incidence of GORL has been dramatically different among previous studies [14]. Endometrial cancer is the most common gynecologic malignancy in developed countries, and the GORL incidence following endometrial cancer varies from 1.2% to 47% [15]. Cervical cancer affects young women and is almost always diagnosed at an early stage due to the widespread availability of screening in developed countries. The GORL incidence in this population ranges from 0% to 55.9% [16, 17]. In China, cervical cancer ranks second among malignant tumors in women. There are approximately 150,000 new cases of cervical cancer in China every year. Ovarian cancer is the leading cause of death among gynecologic malignancies. The reported incidence of lymphedema among ovarian cancer patients ranges from 4.7% to 40.8% [18]. The potential risk factors for GORL include surgical aggressiveness, the number of removed nodes, the removal of specific nodes, the use of adjuvant radiotherapy, and patient characteristics that cause temporary and/or permanent impairment of lymph backflow [18, 19]. The introduction of sentinel node (SLN) biopsy for selected cases of endometrial, cervical, and vulvar cancer is promising as it minimizes the risk of lymphedema [20].

Approximately 75% of GORL cases presented within 12 months of surgery [19]. The onset of GORL is relatively earlier than in breast cancer-related lymphedema. Lymphedema most commonly occurs proximal in the thigh, mons pubis, vulvar, and inguinal regions, as it is due to para-aortic, bilateral pelvic, or inguinal lymph node dissection or irradiation. In some cases, edema begins at the thigh level and descends towards the calf and foot, which can remain unaffected. In particular for cervical cancer patients, lymphedema occurs in the ankle region and further extends to the whole lower limb. Because of the role of standing and gravity, the progression of secondary lymphedema in the lower limbs is relatively rapid, i.e., edema extends to tissue fibrosis, and it is common to see stage III or VI lymphedema patients with a short history, such as only 1–2 years. Damage to the pelvic lymphatic system can affect the inguinal lymph nodes and cause impaired lymph backflow through the inguinal lymph node. MRI can investigate soft tissue edema with good sensitivity and specificity. Magnetic resonance lymphangiography clearly shows anomalies in inguinal lymph nodes/collecting lymph vessels such as structural damage, atrophy, reduced number, disrupted transport, and lymph leakage in affected limbs (Fig. 7.4). Early complete decongestive therapy treatment can effectively decrease edema in the lower leg, but is less effective in cases with lymphedema in the thigh, lower abdomen, and vulva region. Complications such as frequent inflammation and vaginal and vulva lymphatic leakage can seriously reduce patients' quality of life. The treatment of lymphedema after pelvic surgery to remove a tumor remains a significant clinical challenge.

7.3 Malignant Lymphedema

Abstract
Malignant lymphedema differs from traditional chronic lymphedema in that it is characterized by rapid development and poor treatment outcomes. For patients with lower extremity lymphedema who do not have a history of treatment for malignant tumors or infections and whose lymphedema occurs over a short time with the fast development, it is necessary to exclude malignant lymphedema. Magnetic resonance lymphangiography can detect metastatic lesions in the inguinal or iliac lymph nodes and pathological changes of blocked lymphatic vessels for an early and accurate imaging-based diagnosis of obstructive secondary lymphedema.

Keywords
Malignant lymphedema, Tumor metastasis, Lymph node, Lymphatic vessel, Cancer, Lower extremity, Inguinal lymph node, Iliac lymph node

Malignant lymphedema is any lymphedema caused by lymphatic metastasis of a malignant tumor or tumors that originate in the lymph node as a lymphoma [21]. The spread of tumors to lymph nodes is an important means of tumor dissemination. Because of impaired lymph backflow within the tumor, inguinal metastasis is often accompanied by malignant lymphedema of the affected lower limb. Malignant lymphedema could be the first or the only physical sign of tumor metastasis through the lymph nodal pathway [22, 23] and is often confused with benign lymphedema. The latter occurs in the extremities because of congenital lymphatic

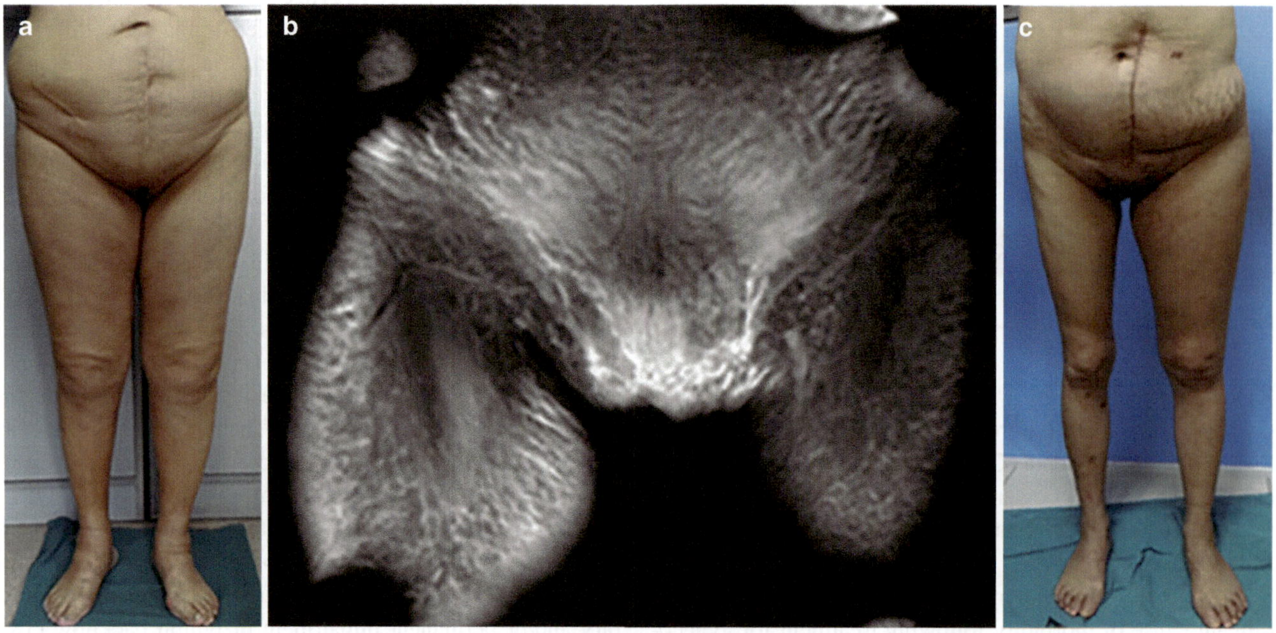

Fig. 7.4 (**a**) A woman with secondary lymphedema of the lower abdomen and bilateral lower limbs after cervical cancer surgical treatment and radiation therapy. (**b**) MRI showed extensive edema in the subcutaneous layer of the lower abdomen and inguinal region. (**c**) A woman with lymphedema of the lower abdomen and left thigh after endometrial cancer treatment

system dysplasia or acquired lymphatic damage caused by injury, infection, or surgery. Therefore, the differential diagnosis of benign and malignant lymphedema is of primary importance. Malignant tumor cells can penetrate the lymphatic wall and block lymphatic vessels, or the tumor itself may compress the lymphatic vessels to block lymphatic circulation. More commonly, tumor metastases to the inguinal or iliac lymph nodes block lymph circulation [21]. Different from benign lymphedema, malignant lymphedema has the characteristics of a short course and rapid development; it is also called acute lymphedema. Because the primary tumor may be undetected, the patient came to the hospital because of lower limb edema with an enlarged inguinal mass, which was actually the affected lymph node. The edema can spread rapidly over the whole limb, as well as to the lower abdomen, vulva, and buttocks (Fig. 7.5). Inguinal lymph node metastasis can be a manifestation of different tumor origins. Tumor cells that metastasize to the inguinal and/or iliac lymph node are either from a nearby tumor such as cervical cancer, ovarian cancer, or endometrial cancer in women, or prostate cancer, bladder cancer, penile cancer, or Paget's disease in men. The tumor cells could also come from distant tumors with more complex sources, including nasopharyngeal carcinoma, lung cancer, colon cancer, gastric cancer, liver cancer, or cancers of unknown origin in the digestive tract [24]. A sensitive and reliable imaging modality to detect the involved lymph node would help achieve earlier diagnoses. Magnetic resonance imaging (MRI) is superior to computed tomography for local staging of carcinomas [25–27]. Recently, high-resolution MRI with various contrast agents that are injected intravenously has emerged as a new diagnostic method in the clinic [28, 29]. This modality has much higher accuracy rates for detecting nodal metastasis than conventional MRI [21]. Because of the high quality of imaging soft tissues, including lymph nodes and lymphatics, patients with suspected malignant lymphedema should first undergo an MRL examination. On contrast, MRL imaging of malignant lymphedema, the lower extremity collecting lymphatic vessels were obviously dilated (the diameter could be up to 10-fold increased from 1 mm to 10 mm), and the vessel wall may rupture, which causes lymph leakage [30]. The most significant findings were enlargement of the inguinal lymph nodes and various spaces of occupying lesions with different manifestations of the filling defects in the lymph nodes, including totally non-filling, needle-like filling, and irregular lymph nodes. A study of 23 cases of malignant lymphedema in the lower extremities showed that only 5 had inguinal palpable lymph nodes, while there was no significant change in the lymph node volumes of the remaining cases (Figs. 7.6 and 7.7). MRL can be used as a preliminary screening, on the basis of which suspected subjects should be further examined for cancer-related antigens, computed tomography scans, and lymph node aspiration histology to detect distant primary lesions.

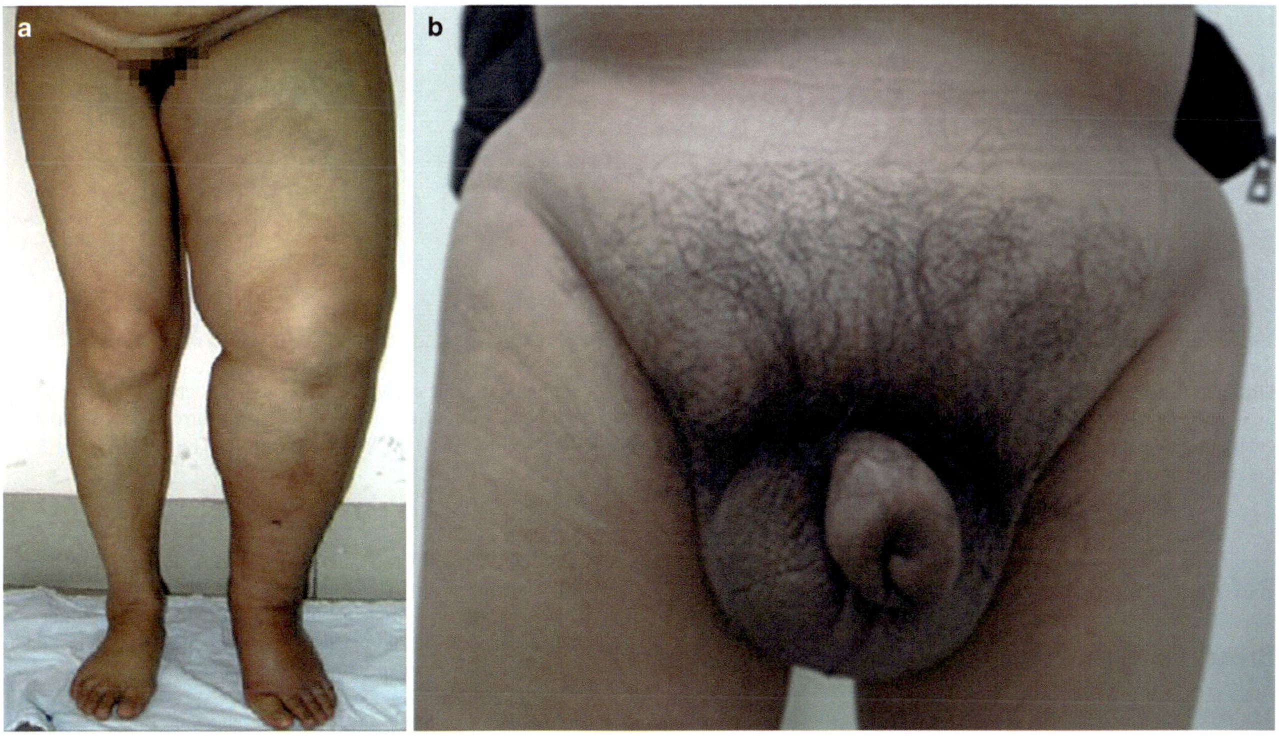

Fig. 7.5 (**a**) A 35-year-old woman with atypical fibrous histiocytoma with early metastasis to the left inguinal lymph nodes and developed acute lymphedema of the left lower limb. (**b**) A 70-year-old man exhibits its extensive selling in the lower abdomen and extra-genital region due to prostatic cancer metastasis of bilateral inguinal lymph nodes

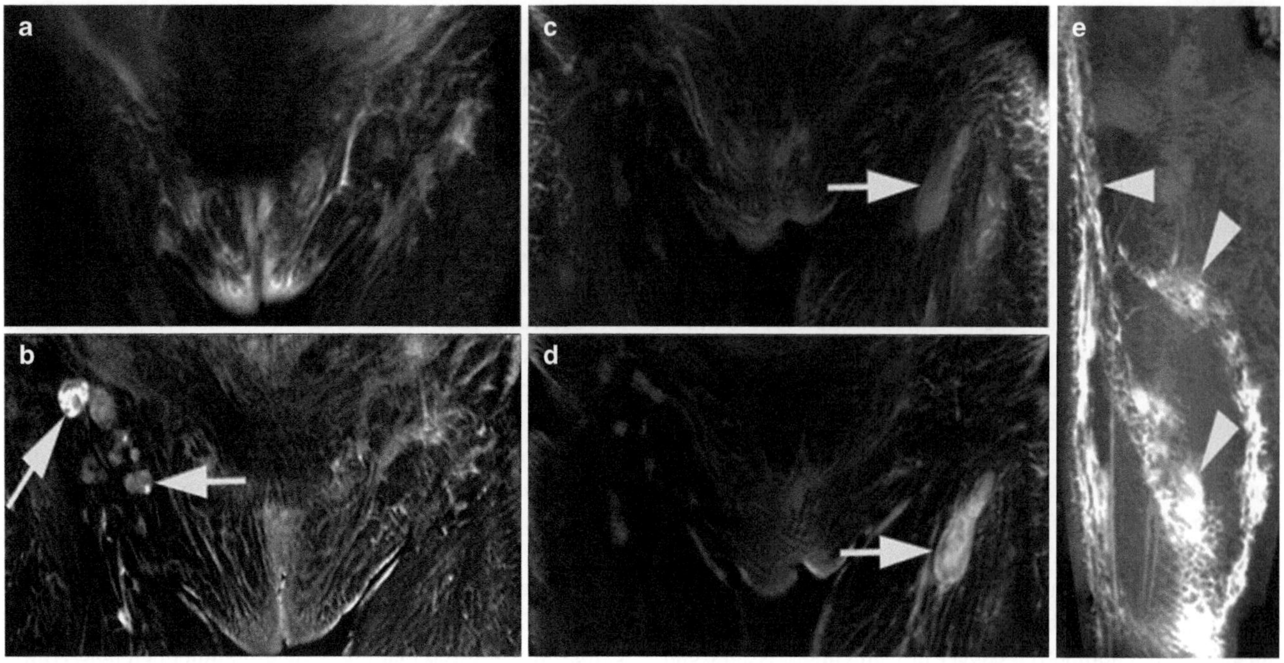

Fig. 7.6 (**a**) A 62-year-old woman with right inguinal lymph node metastasis of colon cancer, the inguinal lymph nodes could hardly identify on T2-weighted magnetic resonance (MR) image. (**b**) Post-contrast T1 MR lymphangiogram clearly displays enlarged superior and central lymph nodes (arrows) with partial contrast enhancement. (**c**) A 56-year-old woman with left inguinal lymph node metastasis o rectal cancer. Pre-contrast T2-weighted MR image shows enlarged inferior node without obvious structural change (arrow). (**d**) Post-contrast T1-weighted lymphangiogram shows heterogeneous structure with the partial enhancement of the enlarged node (arrow)

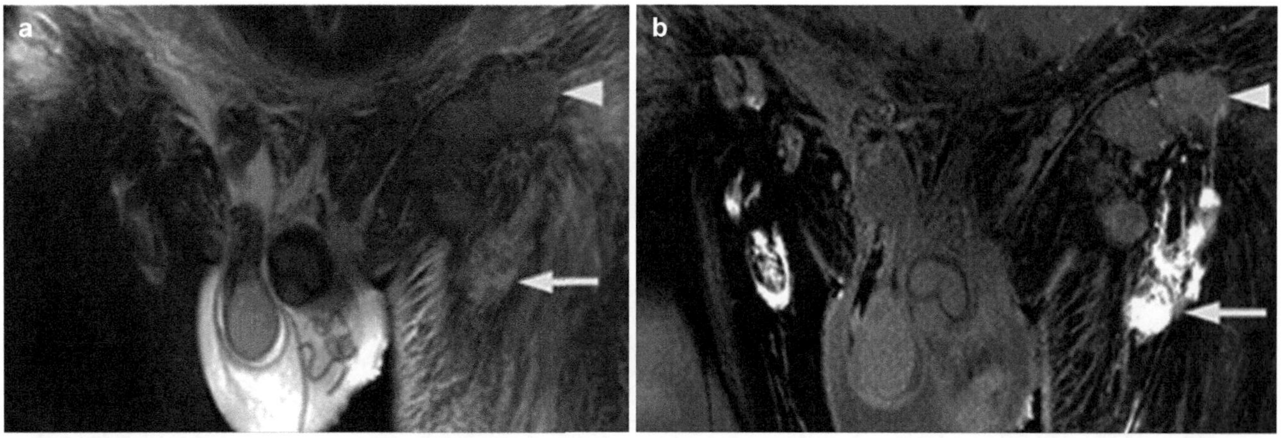

Fig. 7.7 (**a**) A 78-year-old man with non-Hodgkin lymphoma of left inguinal lymph nodes metastasis. T2-weighted MR image shows the enlarged superior (arrow head) and inferior lymph nodes (arrow) without evidence of architectural change. (**b**) Post-contrast T1-weighted MR lymphangiogram shows homogeneous structure of the enlarged superior node without contrast enhancement (arrowhead) in contrast with the inferior nodes that were fully enhanced (arrow)

References

Breast Cancer-Related Lymphedema

1. Executive Committee. The diagnosis and treatment of peripheral lymphedema: 2016 Consensus Document of the International Society of Lymphology. Lymphology. 2016;49(4):170–84.
2. Cassidy T, Worrell CM, Little K, Prakash A, Patra I, Rout J, Fox LM. Experiences of a community-based lymphedema management program for lymphatic filariasis in Odisha State, India: an analysis of focus group discussions with patients, families, community members and program volunteers. PLoS Negl Trop Dis. 2016;10(2):e0004424.
3. Shi ZJ, Sun DJ. Study on prevention and control of filariasis in China for 50 years. Chin J Parasitol Parasit Dis. 1999;17(5):267–70.
4. Sun DJ. The global significance of eliminating lymphatic filariasis in China. Chin J Parasitol Parasit Dis. 2005;23(5 Suppl):329–31.

5. Fan L, Strasser-Weippl K, Li JJ, St Louis J, Finkelstein DM, Yu KD, Chen WQ, Shao ZM, Goss PE. Breast cancer in China. Lancet Oncol. 2014;15(7):e279–89. https://doi.org/10.1016/S1470-2045(13)70567-9.
6. Morrell RM, Halyard MY, Schild SE, Ali MS, Gunderson LL, Pockaj BA. Breast cancer-related lymphedema. Mayo Clin Proc. 2005;80(11):1480–4.
7. Kilgore LJ, Korentager SS, Hangge AN, Amin AL, Balanoff CR, Larson KE, Mitchell MP, Chen JG, Burgen E, Khan QJ, Dea AP, Nye L, Sharma P, Wagner JL. Reducing breast cancer-related lymphedema (BCRL) through prospective surveillance monitoring using bioimpedance spectroscopy (BIS) and patient directed self-interventions. Ann Surg Oncol. 2018;25:2948–52.
8. Stanton AW, Modi S, Mellor RH, Levick JR, Mortimer PS. Recent advances in breast cancer-related lymphedema of the arm: lymphatic pump failure and predisposing factors. Lymphat Res Biol. 2009;7(1):29–45. https://doi.org/10.1089/lrb.2008.1026.
9. Ningfei L, Shun WB. Functional lymphatic collectors in breast cancer-related lymphedema arm. Lymphat Res Biol. 2014;12(4):232–7. https://doi.org/10.1089/lrb.2014.0021.
10. Goldust M, Giulini M, Weidenthaler-Barth B, Gupta M, Grabbe S, Schepler H. Increased risk of angiosarcoma secondary to cancer radiotherapy: case series and review of the treatment options. Dermatol Ther. 2020;29:e13234. https://doi.org/10.1111/dth.13234.
11. Finegold DN, Schacht V, Kimak MA, et al. HGF and MET mutations in primary and secondary lymphedema. Lymphat Res Biol. 2008;6:65–8.
12. Newman B, Lose F, Kedda MA, et al. Possible genetic predisposition to lymphedema after breast cancer. Lymphat Res Biol. 2012;10:2–13.
13. Newman B, Lose F, Kedda MA, Francois M, Ferguson K, Janda M, Yates P, Spurdle AB, Hayes SC. Possible genetic predisposition to lymphedema after breast cancer. Lymphat Res Biol. 2012;10(1):2–13. https://doi.org/10.1089/lrb.2011.0024.

Gynecologic Oncology-Related Lymphedema

14. Biglia N, Zanfagnin V, Daniele A, Robba E, Bounous VE. Lower Body Lymphedema In Patients With Gynecologic Cancer. Anticancer Res. 2017;37(8):4005–15.
15. Miller KD, Siegel RL, Lin CC, Mariotto AB, Kramer JL, Rowland JH, Stein KD, Alteri R, Jemal A. Cancer treatment and survivorship statistics, 2016. CA Cancer J Clin. 2016;66(4):271–89. https://doi.org/10.3322/caac.21349.
16. Biglia N, Librino A, Ottino MC, Panuccio E, Daniele A, Chahin A. Lower limb lymphedema and neurological complications after lymphadenectomy for gynecological cancer. Int J Gynecol Cancer. 2015;25(3):521–5. https://doi.org/10.1097/IGC.0000000000000341.
17. Abu-Rustum NR, Gemignani ML, Moore K, Sonoda Y, Venkatraman E, Brown C, Poynor E, Chi DS, Barakat RR. Total laparoscopic radical hysterectomy with pelvic lymphadenectomy using the argon-beamcoagulator: pilot data and comparison to laparotomy. Gynecol Oncol. 2003;91(2):402–9.
18. Beesley V, Janda M, Eakin E, Obermair A, Battistutta D. Lymphedema after gynecological cancer treatment: prevalence, correlates, and supportive care needs. Cancer. 2007;109(12):2607–14.
19. Hayes SC, Janda M, Ward LC, Reul-Hirche H, Steele ML, Carter J, Quinn M, Cornish B, Obermair A. Lymphedema following gynecological cancer: Results from a prospective, longitudinal cohort study on prevalence, incidence and risk factors. Gynecol Oncol. 2017;146(3):623–9. https://doi.org/10.1016/j.ygyno.2017.06.004.
20. Cibula D, Oonk MH, Abu-Rustum NR. Sentinel lymph node biopsy in the management of gynecologic cancer. Gynecol Oncol. 2015;136(1):54–9.

Malignant Lymphedema

21. Liu N, Yan Z, Lu Q, Wang C. Diagnosis of inguinal lymph node metastases using contrast enhanced high resolution MR lymphangiography. Acad Radiol. 2013;20(2):218–23. https://doi.org/10.1016/j.acra.2012.09.014.
22. Ali M, Vinay KM, Mujtaba H. Metastatic inguinal lymphadenopathy presenting as the only physical evidence of recurrent ovarian carcinoma. J Gynecol Surg. 2003;19(2):81–3.
23. Zhang Q, Yu JW, Yang WL, Liu XS, Yu JR. Gastrointestinal stromal tumor of stomach with inguinal lymph nodes metastasis: a case report. World J Gastroenterol. 2010;16(14):1808–10.
24. Tobler NE, Detmar M. Tumor and lymph node lymphangiogenesis—impact on cancer metastasis. J Leukocyte Biol. 2006;80(4):691–6.
25. Harisinghani MG, Barentsz J, Hahn PF, Deserno WM, Tabatabaei S, van de Kaa CH, de la Rosette J, Weissleder R. Noninvasive detection of clinically occult lymph-node metastases in prostate cancer. N Engl J Med. 2003;348(25):2491–9.
26. Jager GJ, Barentsz JO, Oosterhof GO, Witjes JA, Ruijs SJ. Pelvic adenopathy in prostatic and urinary bladder carcinoma: MR imaging with a three-dimensional T1-weighted magnetization-prepared-rapid gradient-echo sequence. AJR Am J Roentgenol. 1996;167(6):1503–7.
27. Weissleder R, Elizondo G, Josephson L, Compton CC, Fretz CJ, Stark DD, Ferrucci JT. Experimental lymph node metastases: enhanced detection with MR lymphography. Radiology. 1989;171(3):835–9.
28. Liu NF, Lu Q, Jiang ZH, Wang CG, Zhou JG. Anatomic and functional evaluation of the lymphatics and lymph nodes in diagnosis of lymphatic circulation disorders with contrast magnetic resonance lymphangiography. J Vasc Surg. 2009;49(4):980–7. https://doi.org/10.1016/j.jvs.2008.11.029.
29. Lu Q, Xu J, Liu N. Chronic lower extremity lymphedema: a comparative study of high-resolution interstitial MR lymphangiography and heavily T2-weighted MRI. Eur J Radiol. 2010;73(2):365–73. https://doi.org/10.1016/j.ejrad.2008.10.041.
30. Olszewski WL, Liu NF. Magnetic resonance lymphography (MRL): point and -point. Lymphology. 2013;46(4):202–7.

Stage of Lymphedema

8

Ningfei Liu

Abstract

The practical way of staging limb lymphedema is divided into stages I–IV. It is refer to the physical condition of the extremities.

Keywords

Stage of lymphedema · Pitting edema · Non-pitting edema · Skin fibrosis · Fat deposition · Elephantiasis

Staging lymphedema requires making a judgment of the pathological changes of the lymphedematous skin and subcutaneous tissue in the affected limb [1]. The practical way of staging limb lymphedema is divided into stages I–IV (Figs. 8.1 and 8.2). The definitions of these stages are as follows:

Stage I: The protein content of the edema fluid in the early tissue is relatively high (compared with "venous" edema), and the edema is pitting, can fade after limb elevation. Increased proliferation of various cell types may also occur.

Stage II: Edema does not recede after limb elevation. In more severe Stage II cases, there can be the formation of a large amount of subcutaneous fat and fibrosis, and edema no longer presents as a depression.

Stage III: Non-pitting edema, limb thickening and hardening, further deposition of subcutaneous fat, and fibrosis.

Stage IV: Also known as elephantiasis is advanced lymphedema, where there is diseased soft tissue hypertrophy, trophic skin changes such as acanthosis, alterations in skin character and thickness, further deposition of fat and fibrosis, and warty overgrowths have developed.

The above I–IV staging system is only refer to the physical condition of the extremities and does not include the pathogenic mechanisms and the anatomical and functional pathology of involved lymphatic vessels or lymph nodes under the condition of lymphatic stasis.

N. Liu (✉)
Department of Plastic and Reconstructive Surgery, Shanghai Ninth People's Hospital, Shanghai Jiao Tong University School of Medicine, Shanghai, China

N. Liu (ed.), *Peripheral Lymphedema*, https://doi.org/10.1007/978-981-16-3484-0_8

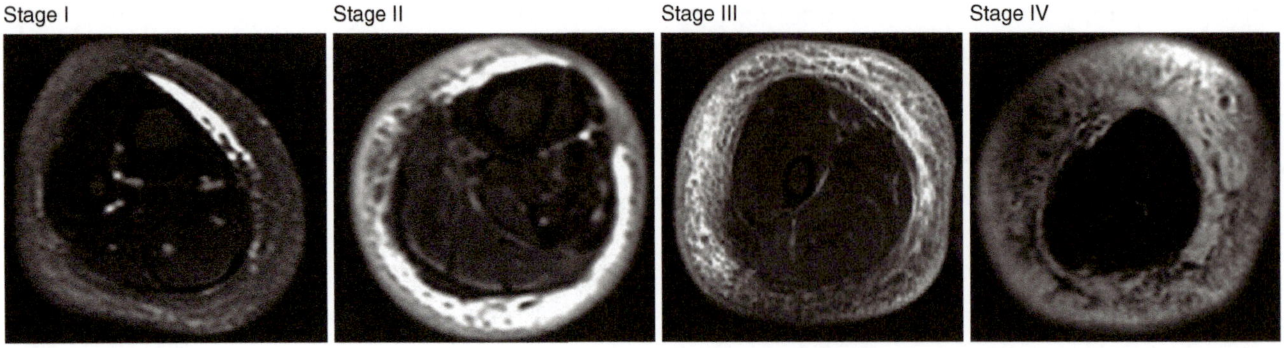

Fig. 8.1 Magnetic resonance cross-sectional image (MRI) showing edema fluid, fibrosis, and fat tissue in lymphedematous of the lower leg of I–IV stages

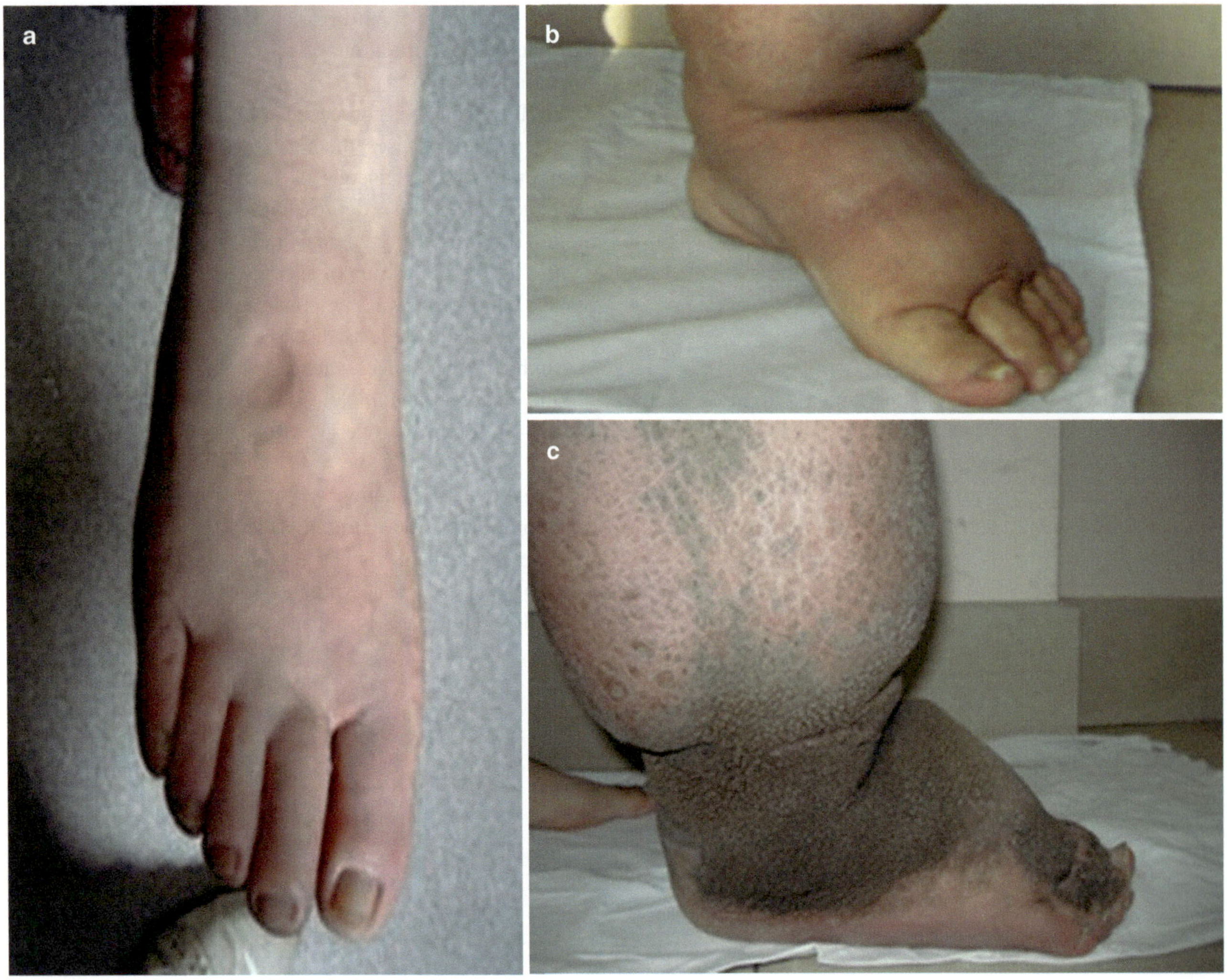

Fig. 8.2 Clinical signs of different stages of lymphedema of lower limbs. (**a**) Lymphedema stage I: pitting edema of the foot; (**b**) lymphedema stage III: edema with obvious skin fibrosis; (**c**) lymphedema stage IV: elephantiasis

Reference

1. Executive Committee. The Diagnosis and treatment of peripheral lymphedema: 2016 Consensus Document of the International Society of Lymphology. Lymphology. 2016;49(4):170–84.

Part III

Pathogenesis of Lymphatic System in Lymphedema

Changes in Lymphatic Vessels in Primary Lymphedema

9

Ningfei Liu

Abstract

The lymphatic anomalies in primary lymphedema can be morphological or functional or a combination of both. Lymphedema can occur at any level of the lymphatic system. The morphological changes of the lymphatic system in primary lymphedema can be clearly demonstrated with magnetic resonance lymphangiography (MRL) and are classified into three major subtypes. Dysfunction of lymph collectors, including valve deficiency and transporting delay, can be demonstrated by indocyanine green lymphography (ICG) in patients with lymphedema distichiasis syndrome (LDS) and Milroy's disease.

Keywords

Primary lymphedema · Lymphatic system · Lymphatic anomalies · Lymphatic dysfunction · Lymph node anomalies · MR lymphangiography · ICG lymphography Valve deficiency · Milroy's disease · Lymphedema distichiasis syndrome (LDS)

9.1 Morphological Changes of Lymph Vessel

Primary lymphedema is a heterogeneous condition with diverse clinical manifestations [1]. The anomalies of the lymphatic vessel in primary lymphedema include morphological and functional types though the two may coexist and interconnect. Changes of the lymphatic system in primary lymphedema can occur in the lymph vessels, the nodes, or both. A recent study that used magnetic resonance lymphangiography (MRL) in a group of 378 patients to define anomalies of the lymphatic system demonstrated morphological anomalies in collecting lymph vessels [2]. In this study, 63 (17%) patients exhibited defects in inguinal lymph nodes with mild or moderate dilatation of afferent lymph vessels. A total of 123 (32%) patients exhibited lymphatic anomalies, including lymphatic aplasia, hypoplasia, or hyperplasia, with no obvious defects in drainage lymph nodes. The involvement of both lymph vessel and node abnormalities in the affected limb was found in 192 (51%) patients. Primary lymphedema was classified as one of three major types as follows: (1) only lymph nodes affected; (2) lymph vessels affected (with three subtypes); and (3) both lymph vessels and lymph nodes affected (with subgroups). Lymphatic abnormalities were primarily determined on the basis of the number and shape of vessels. In cases of aplasia/hypoplasia, the peripheral vessels were either absent or severely hypoplastic in terms of number and size, only one or two deep lymph vessels were identified (Fig. 9.1b), or the enhanced vessels stopped in the distal part of the limb (above the ankle) (Fig. 9.1). In cases of hyperplasia, the varicose lymphatic vessels in the limb and trunk were numerous, tortuous, and dilated. Both the superficial and deep lymphatic systems were affected, which can be chylous reflux. No enhanced lymph vessels were visualized in most contralateral healthy limbs. The number of lymphatic vessels ranged from 0 to numerous, and the diameter ranged from 0.5 to 8 mm in lymphedematous limbs (Fig. 9.1). Based on these observations, the morphological malformations of lymphatic system anomalies in primary lymphedema can be classified as follows (Fig. 9.2):

N. Liu (✉)
Department of Plastic and Reconstructive Surgery, Shanghai Ninth People's Hospital, Shanghai Jiao Tong University, School of Medicine, Shanghai, China

N. Liu (ed.), *Peripheral Lymphedema*, https://doi.org/10.1007/978-981-16-3484-0_9

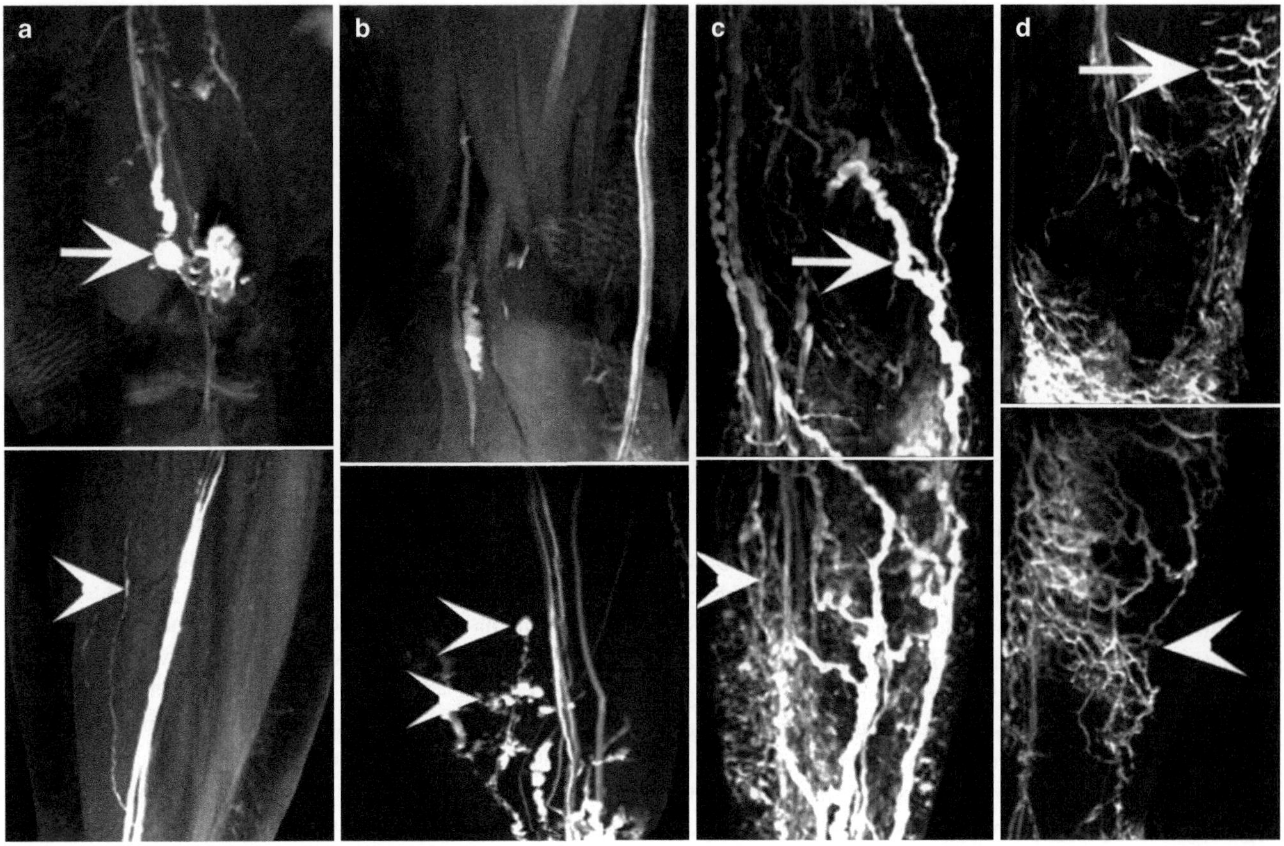

Fig. 9.1 Composition images of MR lymphangiogram show various lymphatic drainage pathways in primary lymphedematous limbs. (**a**) Enhanced deep lymphatic and popliteal lymph nodes (arrow) and single superficial lymphatic (arrowhead); (**b**) Enhanced lymph vessels with cystic dilatation (arrowhead) in the distal part of the leg. (**c**) Numerous aberrant tortuous vessels with a mixture of larger (arrow) and smaller vessels (arrowhead). (**d**) A crisscross network of hyperplastic vessels in the thigh (arrow) and the calf (arrowhead)

1. Lymph node anomalies: nodal changes can be clearly demonstrated with MRL, including:
   (a) Lymph node structural abnormalities: this was the most common type and causes secondary lymphatic dilatation (Fig. 9.3). The nodal pathology is unclear. The only known example is lymph nodal angiomyoma hamartoma.
   (b) Lymph node hyperplasia: This is commonly seen in hydrometric lymphatic malformations as Klippel–Trenaunay syndrome together with lymphatic and venous malformations.
   (c) Lymph node hypoplasia or lymph node aplasia: This type occurs in either primary lymphedema alone or can be associated with syndromic diseases.
2. Lymphatic anomalies: Collecting lymphatic malformations, including functional and morphological, which can be demonstrated by MRL and indocyanine green (ICG) lymphography, including:
   (a) Collecting lymphatic hyperplasia in the lower extremity (Fig. 9.4): unilateral or bilateral, the superficial system involved or together with deep lymphatics.

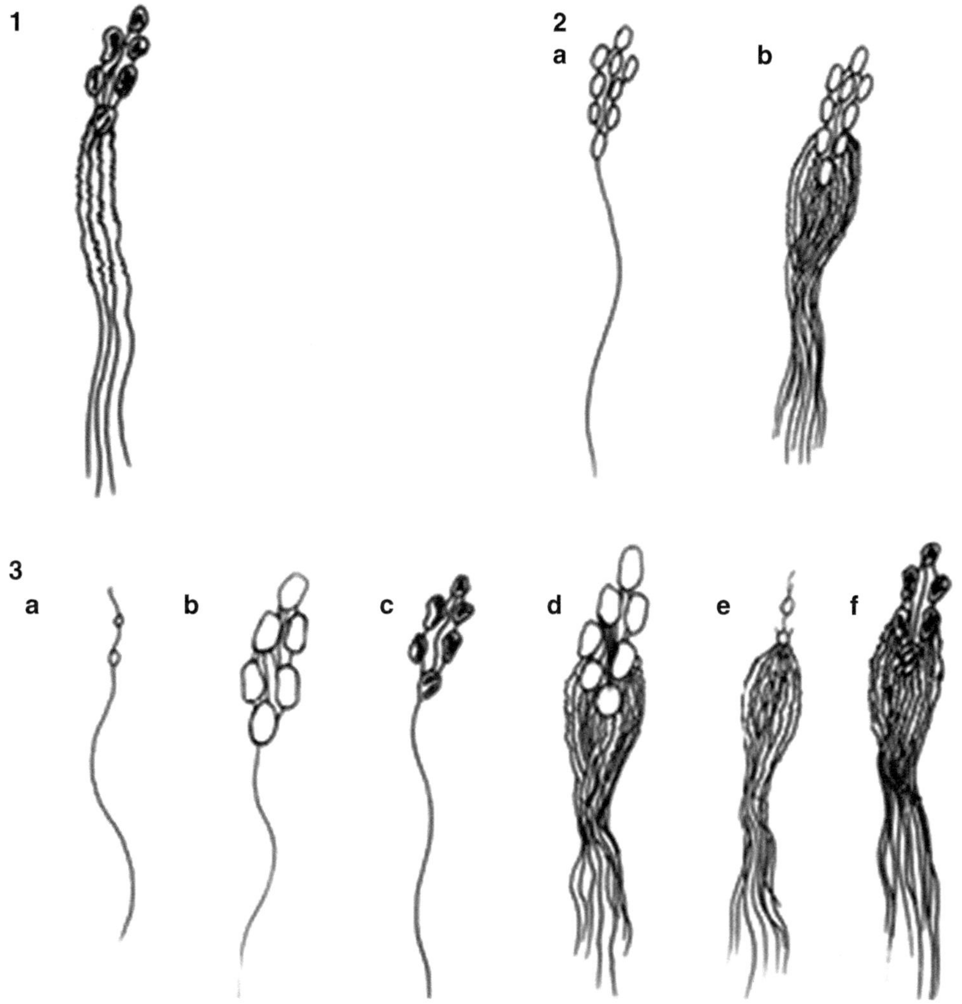

Fig. 9.2 Schematic drawing of classification of lymphatic system anomalies based on MRL. (1) lymph node affected only; (2) lymphatic affected only; (3) both lymphatic and lymph node affected with subtypes

(b) Collecting lymphatic hypoplasia in the lower extremity (Fig. 9.5): single superficial or deep lymph vessel or a few small lymph vessels in the distal region of the lower leg.
(c) Collecting lymphatic aplasia: this type is rare and may be confused with other lymphatic dysfunctions on the lymphoscintigraphy and MRL. This must be verified with ICG lymphography.
(d) Initial lymphatic hyperplasia: this phenomenon in initial lymph vessels is visualized together with lymph collector hyperplasia.
(e) Initial lymphatic hypoplasia and aplasia: this type of lymphatic abnormality is found in the skin of Milroy's disease patients with *FLT4* mutations.

3. Lymphatic and lymph node anomalies: Lymph vessels and nodes are affected together in some subtypes of this

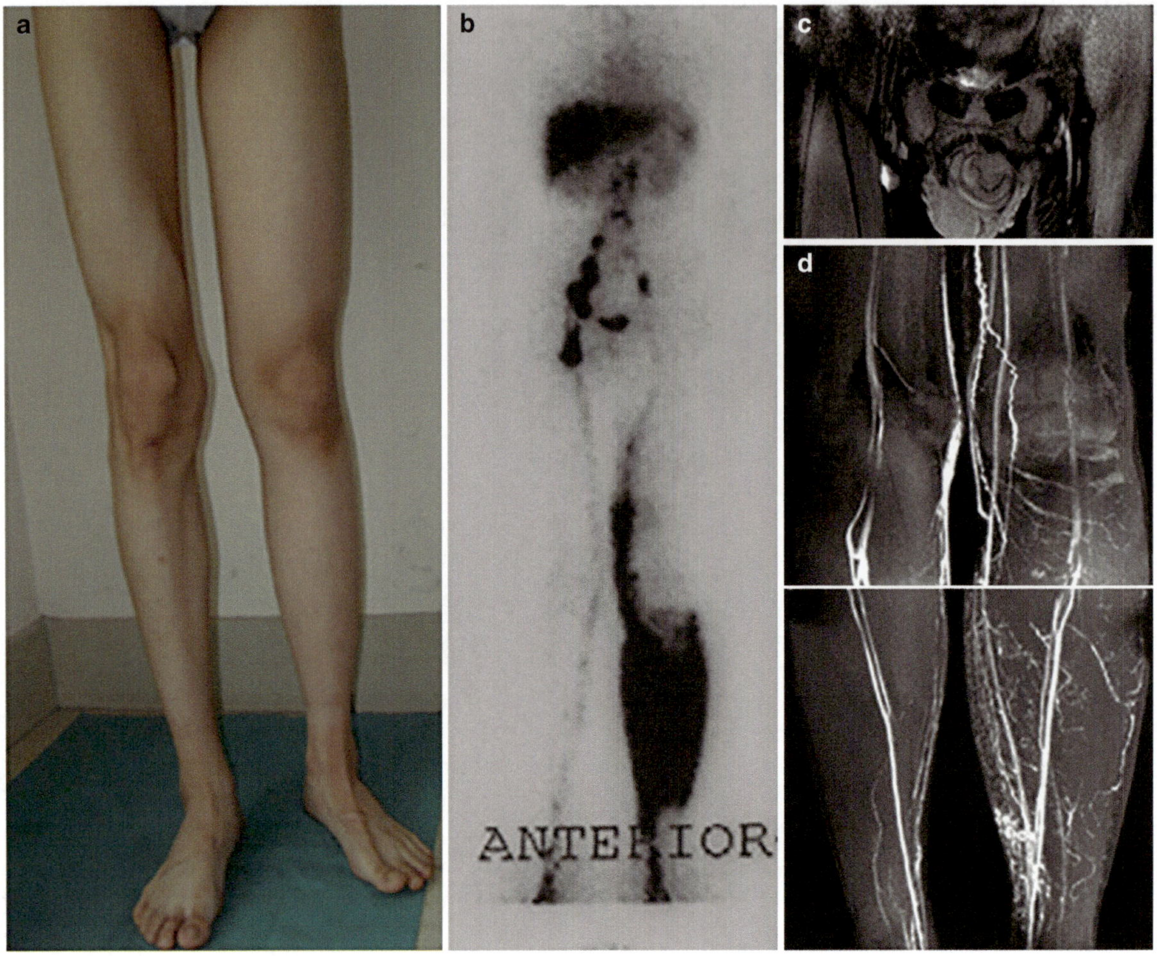

Fig. 9.3 Classification type 1: Lymph node abnormal with secondary lymphatic dilatation

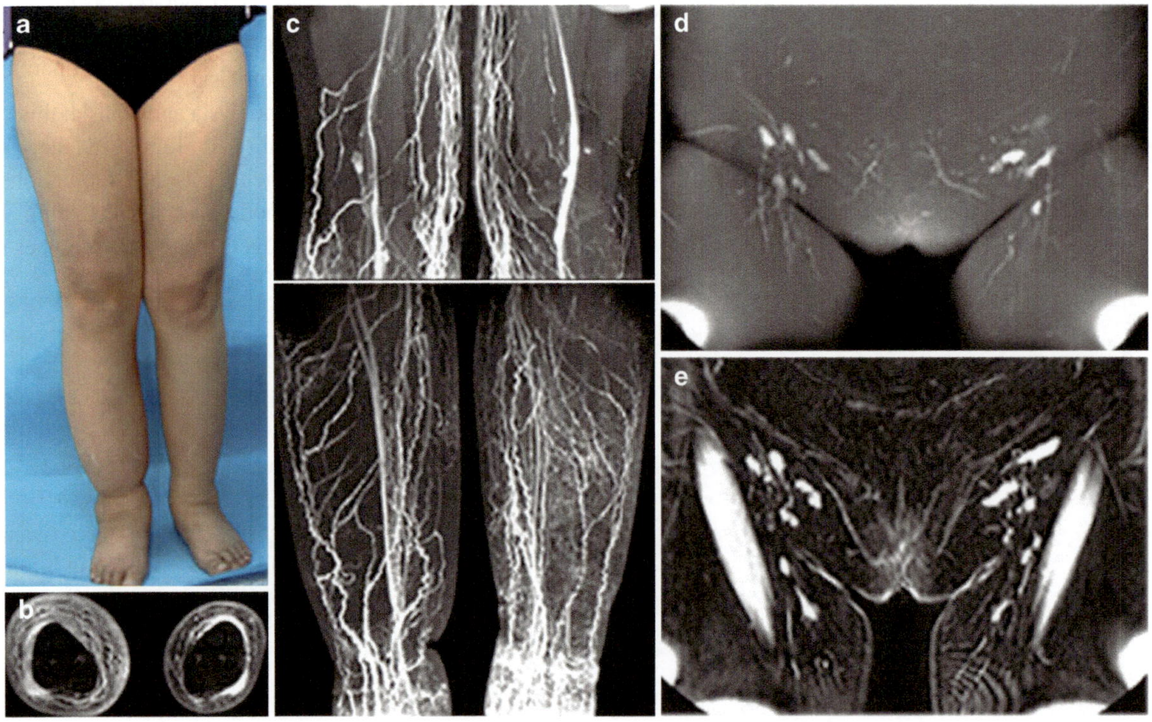

Fig. 9.4 Classification type 2: lymphatic anomalies—bilateral hyperplastic collecting lymph vessels with normal inguinal lymph nodes in a girl with lower extremity primary lymphedema

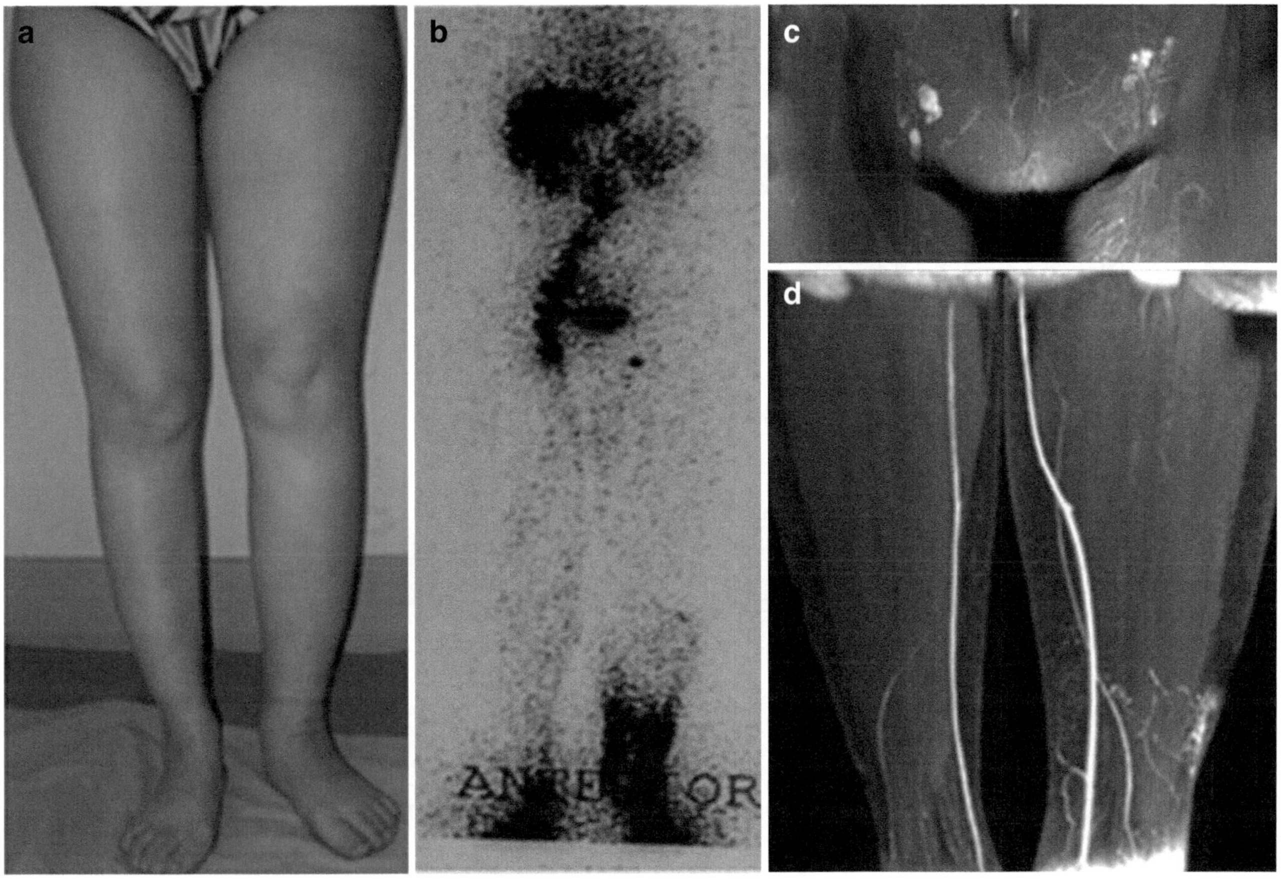

Fig. 9.5 Classification of type 2: lymphatic anomalies. (**a**) Agirl with primary lymphedema of the left lower limb. (**b**) Lymphoscintigram showed dermal-back flow in the distal region of the leg and no enhanced inguinal lymph node. C&D. MRL demonstrated small enhanced lymphatics in the ankle region and the left inguinal lymph nodes

group of mixed lymphatic system malformations as hyperplasia, hypoplasia, or aplasia of vessels and nodes. The malformations of the lymphatics can be concordant or not concordant with those of the lymph node in primary lymphedema (Figs. 9.6, 9.7, and 9.8).

This updated classification system clearly defines the location and pathological characteristics of these diseases to provide a clear and more useful definition. Therefore, the proposed system is likely to be more convenient and understandable for clinical workers and patients and could facilitate investigations into the respective etiologies of the pathological changes in the vessels and nodes in the different disease classifications.

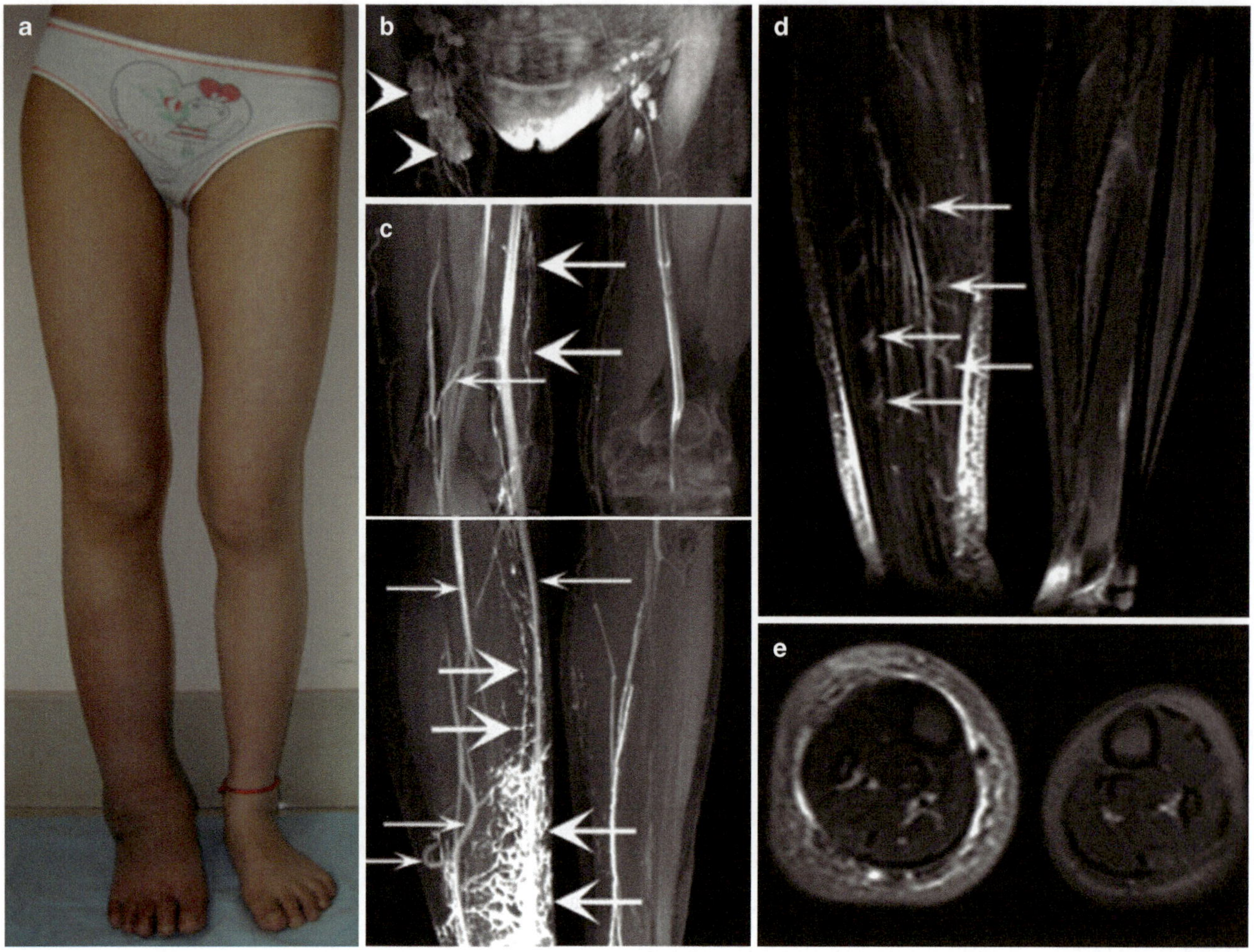

Fig. 9.6 Classification type 3: Lymphatic and lymph node anomalies—lymphatic and lymph node hyperplasia. (**a**) A 15-year-old girl with the enlarged and longer right lower extremity. (**b**) MRL shows enhanced inguinal lymph nodes (arrow head) with increased size and number on the right side. (**c**) MRL shows hyperplastic lymphatic vessels (large arrows) and enlarged superficial veins (small arrows) of the right lower extremity. (**d**) MR image shows increased intramuscular blood vessels (arrows) of the right lower limb. (**e**) MR image shows hypertrophy and edema of subcutaneous tissue

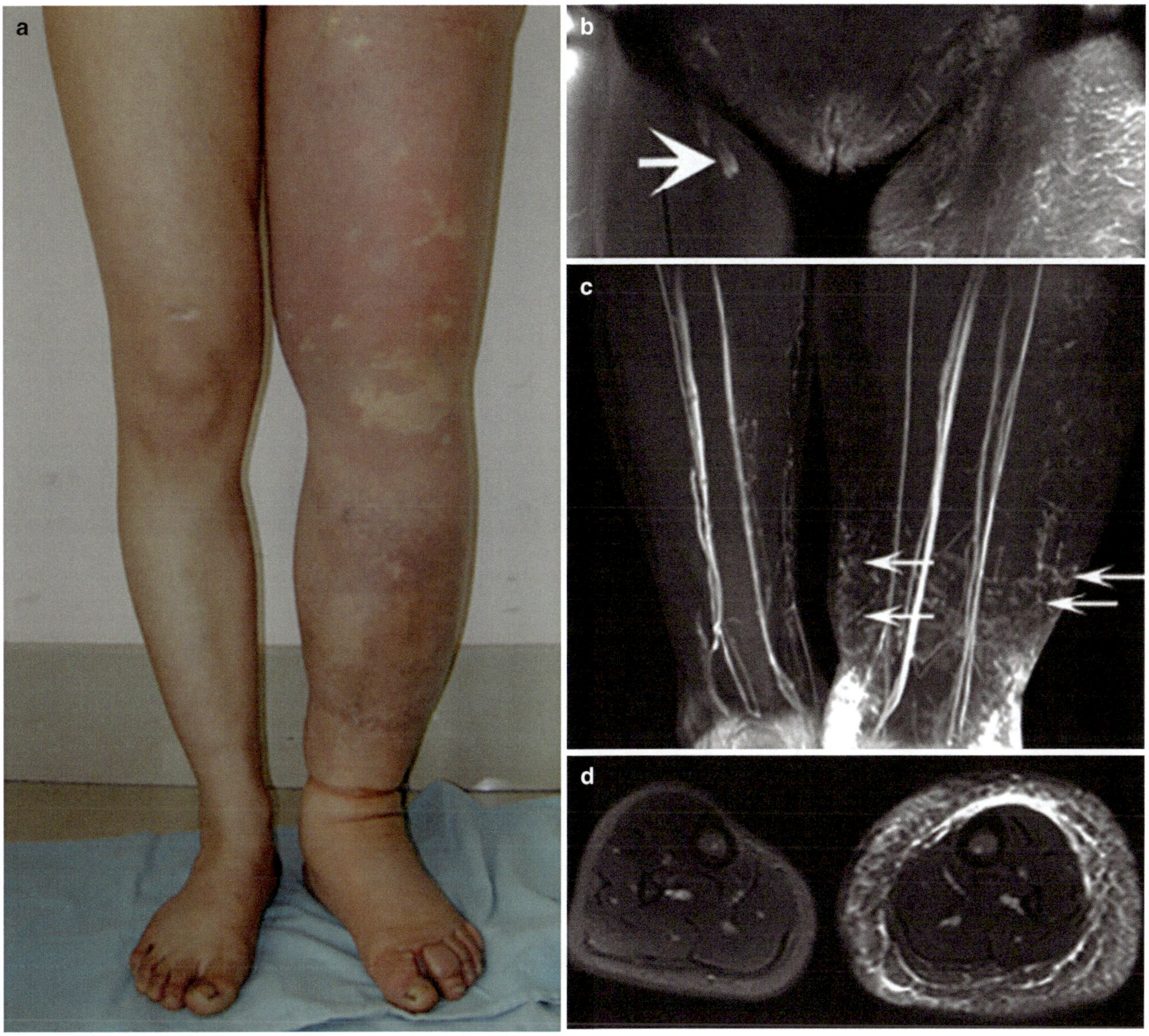

Fig. 9.7 Classification type 3: lymphatic and lymph node anomalies—lymphatic hyperplasia and lymph node aplasia. (**a**) A 27-year-old woman with extensive skin port-wine staining and enlarged left lower extremity. (**b**) No lymph node was identifiable in the inguinal region of the left side in contrast with clearly visualized lymph nodes (arrow) on the right side MRL images. (**c**) Fine lymphatic vessels (arrows) are found in the distal region of the lower leg. (**d**) MRI shows hypertrophy and edema in the subcutis of the left lower extremity

9.2 Functional Changes of Lymph Vessels

Valve deficiency is the most common cause of lymphatic dysfunctions in primary lymphedema and causes lymph reflux (xx). It has also been reported in patients with lymphedema distichiasis. *FOXC2* mutations are responsible for the failure in lymphatic valve development [3]. Lymphatic function can be examined using lymphatic imaging tests, including lymphoscintigraphy, magnetic resonance lymphography, and indocyanine green (ICG) lymphography; however, the results of these three modalities can be inconsistent. Because MRL scanning does not cover the feet, lymphatics in the distal region of the limb are missed. ICG lymphography is used as a supplemental test for patients in whom the diagnosis of lymphatic aplasia or hypoplasia was doubted. In this population, the functional status of collecting lymph vessels in the affected limbs should be investigated further. Recent studies have demonstrated that dysfunction of localized lymph collectors (and possibly pre-collecting vessels) is involved in primary lymphedema (unpublished data). This has also been found in the well-known congenital lymphedema, Milroy's disease with *VEGFR3* mutations, in which a severe transport delay of lymph fluid and tortuous dorsal lymphatic vessels were visualized in the affected feet by ICG lymphography [4]. A similar phenomenon was also found in sporadic cases of lower extremity lymphedema with or without *VEGFR3*

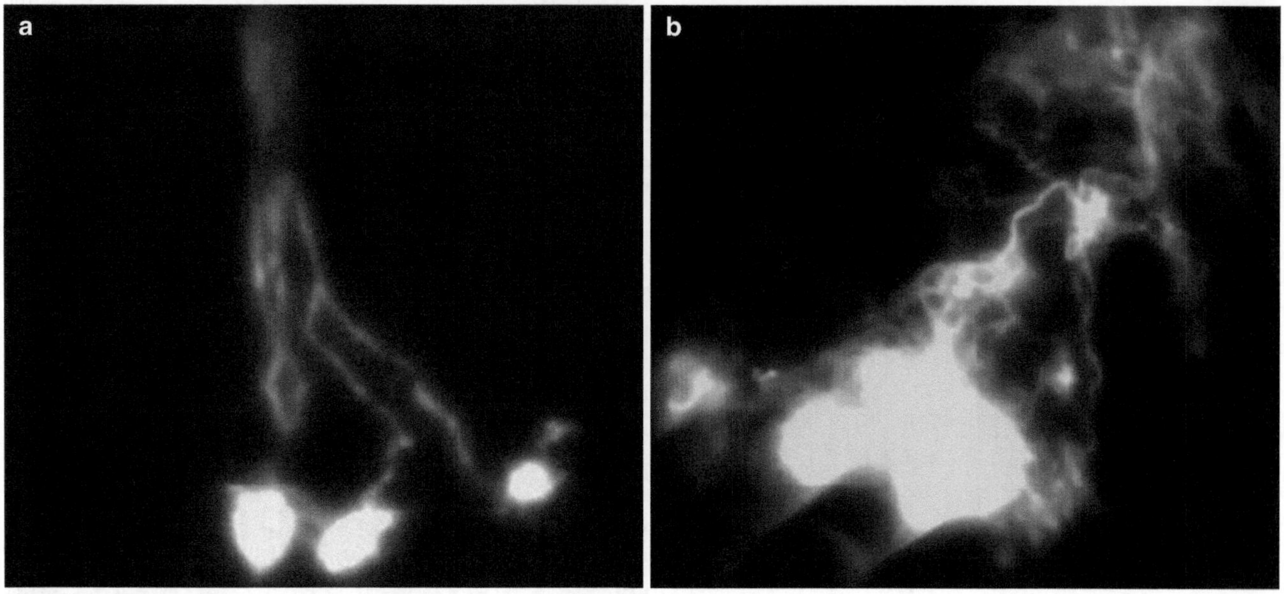

Fig. 9.8 ICG lymphography imaging tested on the dorsum of the foot. (**a**) Contrast-enhanced lymph collectors in the contralateral non-edema foot. (**b**) Tortuous and dilated lymphatics in the dorsum of the lymphedematous foot

mutations [5]. However, the pathophysiology that underlines such lymphatic malfunctions remains unclear.

References

1. Drada AA, Phillips TJ. Lymphedema: pathophysiology and clinical manifestations. J Am Acad Dermatol. 2017;77(6):1009–20.
2. Liu NF, Yan ZX, Wu XF. Classification of lymphatic-system malformations in primary Lymphoedema based on MR lymphangiography. Eur J Vasc Endovasc Surg. 2012;44(3):345–9. https://doi.org/10.1016/j.ejvs.2012.06.019.
3. Mellor RH, Brice G, Stanton AW, French J, Smith A, Jeffery S, Levick JR, Burnand KG, Mortimer PS. Mutations in FOXC2 are strongly associated with primary valve failure in veins of the lower limb. Circulation. 2007;115(14):1912–20.
4. Liu NF, Yu ZY, Sun D, Lou Y. Rare variants in LAMA5 gene associated with FLT4 and FOXC2 mutations in primary lymphedema may contribute to severity. Lymphology. 2016;49(4):192–204.
5. Yu ZY, Sun D, Wang L, Chen J, Han LH, Liu NF. Diagnosis of primary lymphedema with indocyanine green lymphography. Chin J Plast Surg. 2018;34(4):256–9.

10 Changes in Lymph Node in Primary Lymphedema

Ningfei Liu

Abstract

Lymph node malformations alone account for approximately 20% of primary lymphedema cases, and malformations are more common in inguinal nodes. Lymph node anomalies in primary lymphedema include hypertrophy, dysplasia, and aplasia. However, the pathology of lymph nodes is far from clear. Although rare, lymph node angioleiomyomatous hamartoma may be an anomaly in cases of primary lymphedema, for which the histological changes are clear.

Keywords

Primary lymphedema · Lymph node anomaly
Hypertrophy, dysplasia, aplasia · Angioleiomyomatous hamartoma

Lymph node anomalies are one of the main causes of primary lymphedema. Investigations into lymph node malformation are primarily performed using imaging tests and only very rarely with histological examination. A study involving magnetic resonance lymphangiography analysis of 378 patients with primary lymphedema of the lower limbs showed that lymph nodal dysplasia could be grouped into three categories: structural anomalies, hypoplasia/aplasia, and hyperplasia [1].

Detailed pathological characteristics of the affected lymph nodes were: marked enhancement or reduction of size and/or number (including absence), irregular shape, uneven structure, and partial contrast filling (Fig. 10.1).

Among all tested cases, 72% demonstrated anomalies of the inguinal and iliac lymph nodes. Furthermore, 45% had no history of cellulitis or erysipelas, while 23% showed severe nodal changes that extended beyond lymph vessels. Pathological changes in the lymphatic vessels were not always consistent with those of the corresponding lymph nodes [2].

Among patients with hypoplasia of the inguinal lymph nodes, 49% showed hyperplasia of efferent lymph vessels. Conversely, 29% of patients with lymph nodal hyperplasia also exhibited lymphatic hypoplasia. The co-existence of lymphatic and lymph node hyperplasia was present in 24% of tested cases, while the co-existence of lymphatic and lymph node hypoplasia was present in 50% of cases. Among patients with hyperplasia of the inguinal lymph nodes, 29% exhibited lymphatic hypoplasia. However, these lymph nodes anomalies are based on imaging findings and most lack a histological diagnosis.

Angioleiomyomatous hamartoma (AH) is a rare type of primary lymph node malformation [3–8] that only occurs in the inguinal node in single- and multi-node cases. The patients come to the hospital because of the enlargement of inguinal lymph nodes and are suspected as lymphadenitis. Lymphedema develops in the ipsilateral limb before or after the lymph node biopsy. No significant discomfort was described by most of these patients, but a few reported pain. AH is vascular benign disease of unknown etiology. Microscopically, most lymph node structures were replaced by pathological tissue. The hamartoma partially displayed the original lymph node architecture with stromal collagenization and the proliferation of blood/lymph vessels with thickened walls that were surrounded by irregular hyperplasia of smooth muscle bundles. Immunohistochemical staining revealed that smooth muscle cells were positive for SMA and desmin (Figs. 10.2 and 10.3). The positive staining with lymphatic endothelial antigen LYVE-1 and podoplanin in the vascular lesions of the affected nodes strongly point that AH are lymphatic origins (Figs. 10.2 and 10.3). The imaging diagnosis can only show a decreased number of inguinal lymph nodes and edema in the operated limb with limited information of structural changes [9].

N. Liu (✉)
Department of Plastic and Reconstructive Surgery, Shanghai Ninth People's Hospital, Shanghai Jiao Tong University School of Medicine, Shanghai, China

N. Liu (ed.), *Peripheral Lymphedema*, https://doi.org/10.1007/978-981-16-3484-0_10

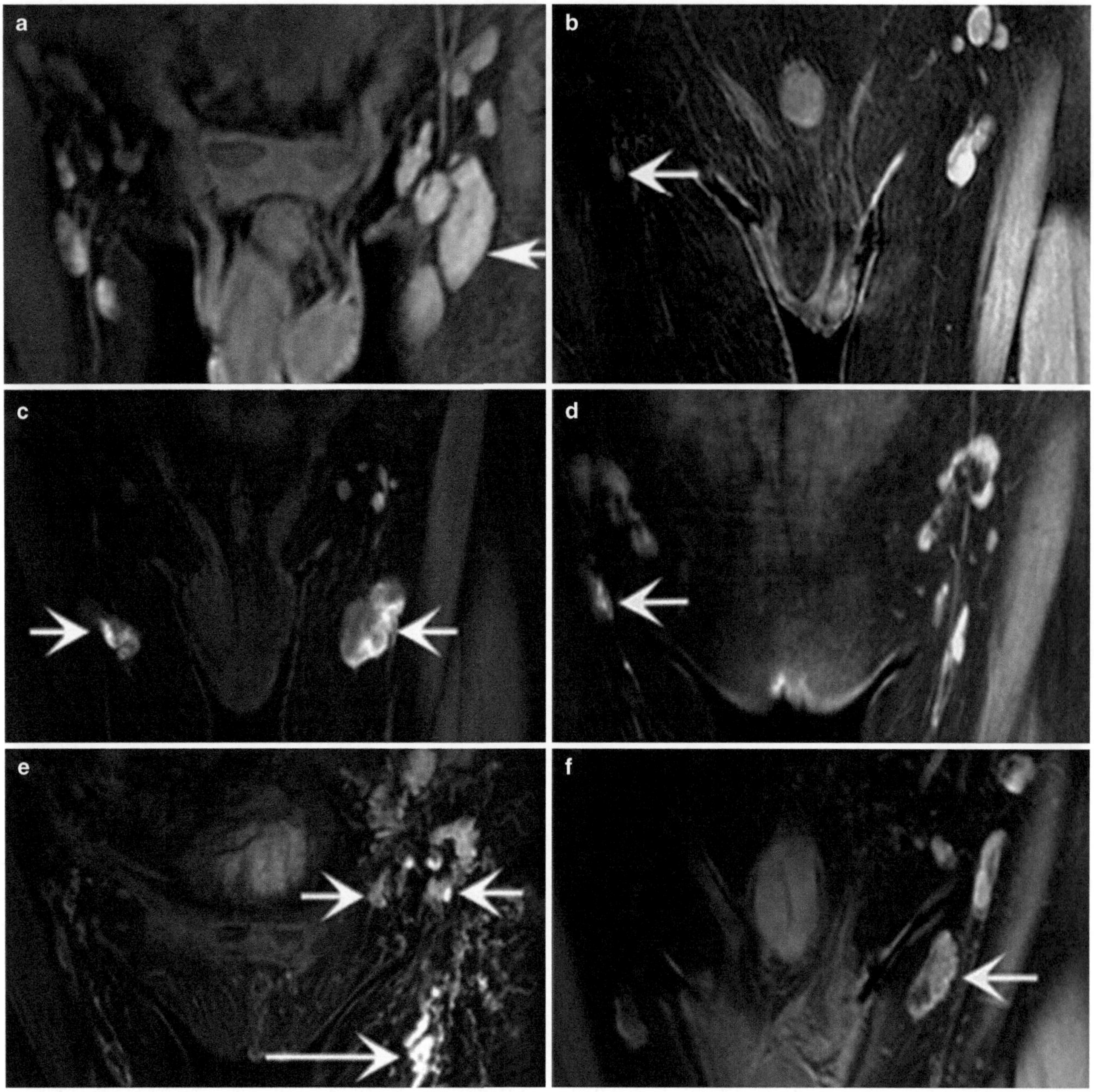

Fig. 10.1 Pathological changes in inguinal nodes of primary lymphedema lower limbs demonstrated on MR Lymphangiograms. (**a**) Enlarged inguinal lymph nodes (arrow) with homogeneous texture in the left affected limbin contrast with lymph nodes of normal size in non-lymphedema side. (**b**) Small node in a limb (arrow) with lymphatic hypoplasia and lymphedema is compared with lymph nodes in a non-lymphedema left limb. (**c**) Partially contrast-filling and enlarged size on the left inguinal lymph nodes. (**d**) Partially enhanced inferior inguinal node (arrow) compared with evenly enhanced contralateral healthy nodes. (**e**) Small nodes that are irregularly shaped (small arrow) in a limb with lymphangiectasia (large arrow). (**f**) Enlarged inguinal lymph nodes (arrow) with homogeneous texture in the left limb. Used with permission from [1]

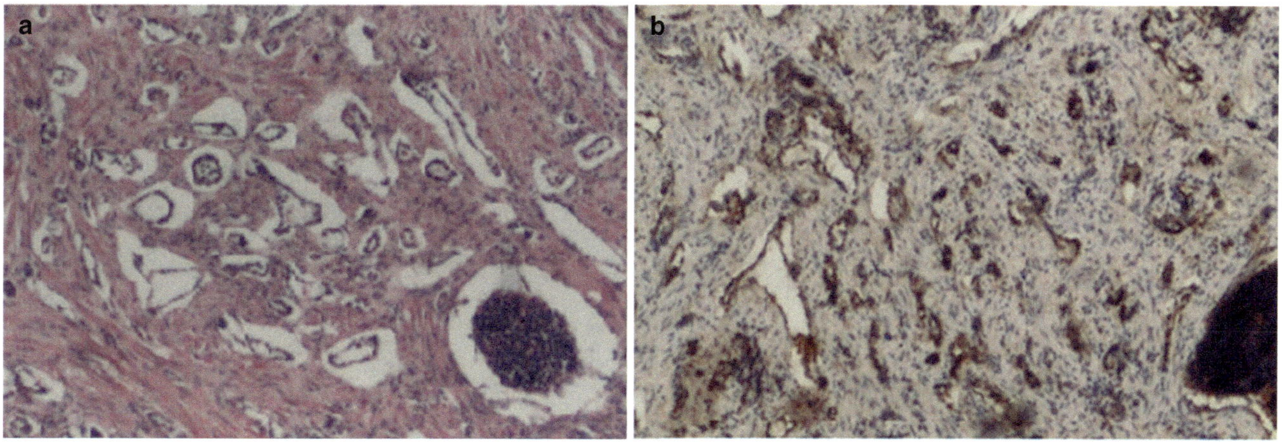

Fig. 10.2 A female, 6 years old, lower right lower abdomen and vulva primary lymphedema, right inguinal lymph node enlargement was removed and diagnosed as angioleiomyomatous hamartoma. (**a**) H.E staining showed the proliferation of blood/lymph vessels with thickened wall that were surrounded by hyperplastic smooth muscle bundles. (**b**) Anti-lymphatic endothelial cell-specific antigen LYVE-1 antibody staining showed that the hyperplastic vasculature in the lymph nodes was lymphatic vessel origin

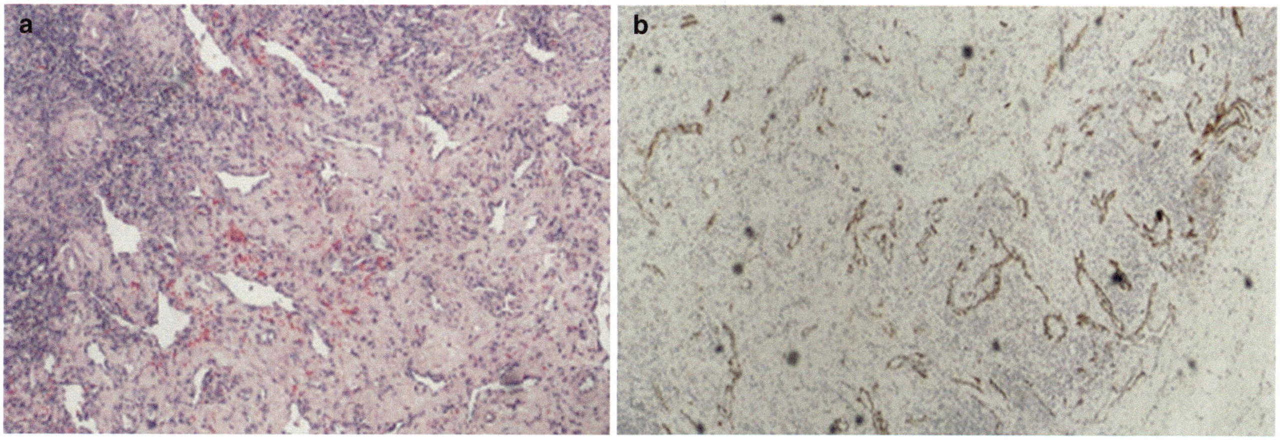

Fig. 10.3 Female, 8 years old, right groin mass surgery removal, pathology diagnosed as inguinal lymph node angioleiomyomatous hamartoma. (**a**) HE staining showed an increase in the intranode vasculature (arrow), fewer lymphoid tissue, and hyperplasia of smooth muscle cells. (**b**) lymphatic endothelial cell-specific antibody podoplanin staining revealed hyperplastic lymphatic vessels

References

1. Liu NF, Lu Q, Jiang ZH, et al. Anatomic and functional evaluation of the lymphatics and lymph nodes in diagnosis of lymphatic circulation disorders with contrast magnetic resonance lymphangiography. J Vasc Surg. 2009;49(4):980–7.
2. Liu NF, Lu Q, Yan ZX. Lymphatic malformation is a common component of Klippel-Trenaunay syndrome. J Vasc Surg. 52(6):1557–63. https://doi.org/10.1016/j.jvs.2010.06.166.
3. Rong OY, De Chun L, De Chen L, Qun X, Nong CZ. Angioleiomyomatous hamartoma of lymph nodes: a clinicopathological analysis of 10 cases. J Clin Exp Pathol. 2006;22(3):291–3.
4. Sullu Y, Gun S, Dabak N, Karagoz F. Angiomyomatous hamartoma in the inguinal lymph node: a case report. Turk J Pathol. 2006;22(1):42–4.
5. Lee CH, Chang TC, Ku JW. Angiomyomatous hamartoma in an inguinal lymph node with proliferating pericytes/smooth muscle cells, plexiform vessel tangles, and ectopic calcification. Indian J Pathol Microbiol. 2015;58(2):226–8. https://doi.org/10.4103/0377-4929.155325.
6. Sakurai Y, Shoji M, Matsubara T, Imazu H, Hasegawa S, Ochiai M, Funabiki T, Mizoguchi Y, Kuroda M, Kasahara M. Angiomyomatous hamartoma and associated stromal lesions in the right inguinal lymph node: a case report. Pathol Int. 2000;50(8):655–9.
7. Dzombeta T, Francina M, Matković K, Marković I, Jukić Z, Lez C, Kruslin B. Angiomyolipomatous hamartoma of the inguinal lymph node—report of two cases and literature review. In Vivo. 2012;26(3):459–62.
8. Piedimonte A, De Nictolis M, Lorenzini P, Sperti V, Bertani A. Angiomyomatous hamartoma of inguinal lymph nodes. Plast Reconstr Surg. 2006;117(2):714–6.
9. Bourgeois P, Dargent JL, Larsimont D, Munck D, Sales F, Boels M, De Valck C. Lymphoscintigraphy in angiomyomatous hamartomas and primary lower limb lymphedema. Clin Nucl Med. 2009;34(7):405–9. https://doi.org/10.1097/RLU.0b013e3181a7d013.

Pathology of Collecting Lymph Vessels in Secondary Lymphedema

11

Ningfei Liu

Abstract

Using the high-resolution imaging of magnetic resonance lymphangiography, pathological changes of lymph collectors in secondary (obstructive) lymphedema limbs, including dilatation, disruption, occlusion, and regeneration, can be clearly demonstrated. The morphological and functional information regarding lymph vessels in secondary lymphedema show the evolution of affected vessels in breast cancer-related lymphedema and pelvic malignancy-related lymphedema, which is helpful for choosing the proper treatment.

Keywords

Secondary lymphedema · Lymph collector · Lymphatic disruption · Breast cancer-related lymphedema · Upper limb · Pelvic malignant tumor · Lower limb

Lymph collectors play important roles in the onset and development of lymphedema. The damage and obstruction of lymphatic vessels in secondary lymphedema can be caused by surgery, radiation, injury, or inflammation. Failure of lymphatic regeneration impairs the lymph back flow, causing lymphedema in the drainage region. It is important to understand the pathological changes of lymph collecting vessels to ensure accurate diagnoses and choose proper treatments. Past studies have mainly focused on histological findings concerning lymph collectors [1, 2]. However, it is unclear what pathological changes occur in lymphatic vessels during secondary lymphedema, including whether these vessels are occluded after injury or obstruction of upstream pathways. Furthermore, the functional conditions of lymph collectors in secondary lymphedematous limbs are unknown. The current lack of understanding regarding lymphatic pathology in patients with lymphedema may be attributable to the lack of reliable research tools for the assessment of such vessels in the human body. Because of its insufficient resolution, the commonly used lymphoscintigraphy method cannot clearly display functional lymph vessels in limbs with secondary lymphedema, such as in arms with BCRL.

A study on the arms of a group of patients with breast cancer-related lymphedema (BCRL) tested by magnetic resonance lymphangiography [3] revealed the following findings involving collecting lymph vessels:

1. Lymph collectors were present in the affected arm in 85% of patients. The diameter of visualized vessels ranged from 0.5 to 5.0 mm (Fig. 11.1).
2. Morphological changes in the lymph collectors included dilatation, tortuosity, disruption, leakage, and formation of small lymph vessel networks between large collectors, which may have resulted from lymphatic regeneration (Fig. 11.1).
3. The number of contrast-enhanced lymph vessels increased with increasing disease duration (Fig. 11.2).
4. The number of lymph collectors in arms with BCRL was closely associated with the thickness of skin and the degree of subcutaneous edema (Fig. 11.2).

These results imply persistent collecting lymphatic function and lymph stasis in arms with BCRL. Magnetic resonance lymphangiography imaging is helpful for predicting patient prognosis and guiding therapy.

The processes that occur in the main lymphatic trunks during the evolution of obstructive lymphedema in the lower limbs are also poorly understood. The most common type of such lymphedema is gynecologic oncology-related lymphedema (GORL) following treatment for cervical cancer, endometrial cancer, and ovarian cancer. Compared with BCRL, the swelling in GORL occurs earlier and faster, is

N. Liu (✉)
Department of Plastic and Reconstructive Surgery, Shanghai Ninth People's Hospital, Shanghai Jiao Tong University School of Medicine, Shanghai, China

N. Liu (ed.), *Peripheral Lymphedema*, https://doi.org/10.1007/978-981-16-3484-0_11

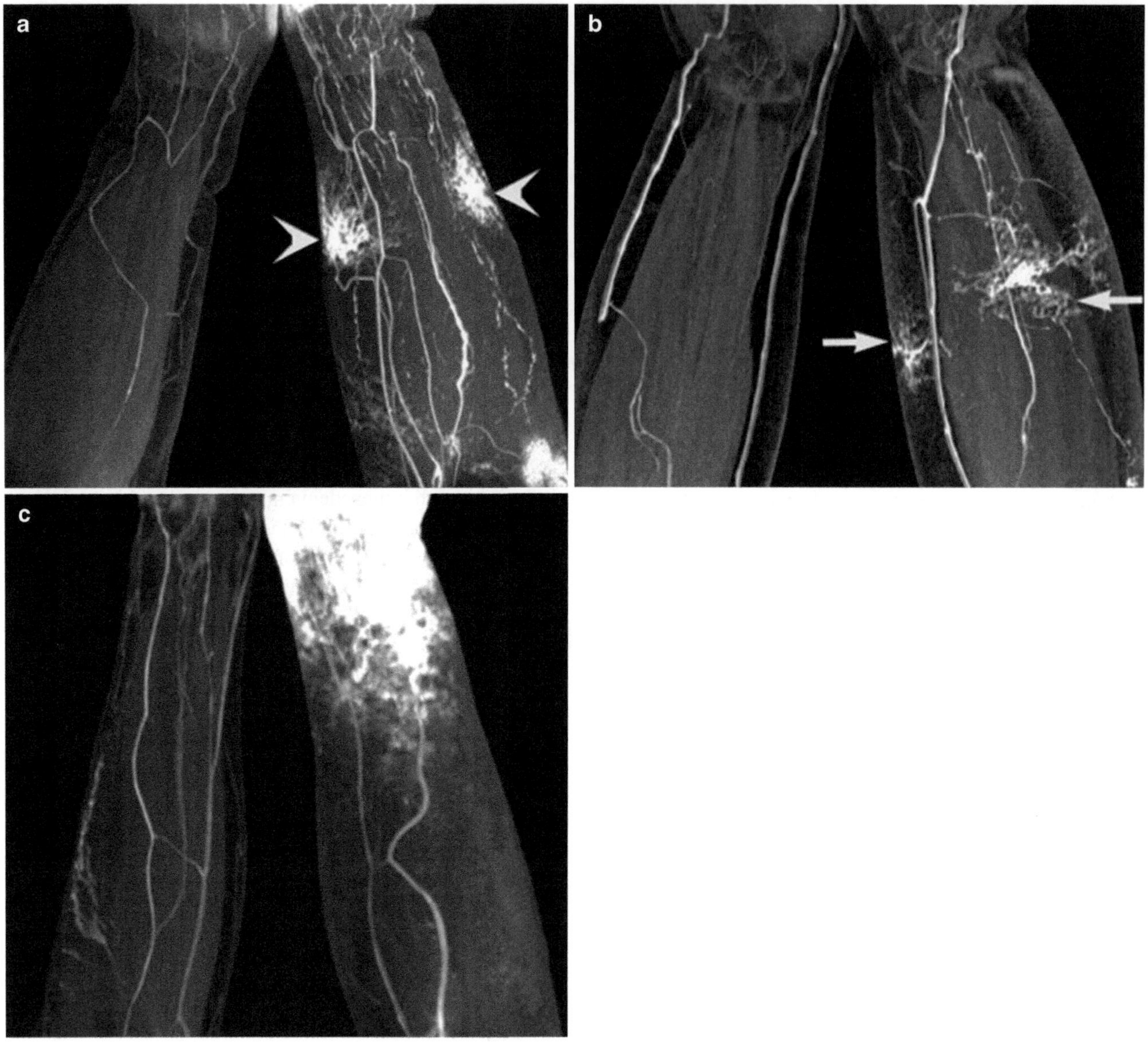

Fig. 11.1 MRL imaging shows lymphatic damage in the lymphedematous upper extremity after mastectomy. (**a**) Lymph collector disruption and lymphorrhea (arrowheads) in the forearm. (**b**) Lymphatic network regeneration (arrows) in the forearm. (**c**) The "dermal backflow" was seen as massive high signal intensity in the distal region of the arm

more severe, and more extensively affects regions of the body, including the lower abdomen, extra-genital region, and lower limbs. The pathological changes of the affected lymph collectors can be characterized as acute or chronic [4–8]. The acute changes can occur at very early stages of the disease (initial 2 months) (Fig. 11.3), with extreme dilatation of lymph vessels in the thigh and extensive "dermal backflow" in the calf, which suggest significantly increased intravascular pressure and massive damage to the lymphatics. The common chronic changes include: (1) lymphatic disruption in the anterior tibial area of the lower leg that involves the anterior tibial lymph vessel with leakage of contrast-enhanced lymph into the surrounding region (Fig. 11.1a). (2) In some patients, a segment of enhanced lymphatic network can be seen bridging the trunks of collecting vessels without lymph leakage in the tibial area, indicating regeneration of disrupted lymph vessels (Fig. 11.4). These results suggest that the anterior tibial lymph vessel is the weak point of the lymphatics in the lower extremities, and the imaging features of the vessels, such as disruption, lymphorrhea, and regeneration, reflect the evolution of both lymphatic damage and repair in obstructive lymphedema (Fig. 11.4) [9]. (3) Finally, the pathological changes are mild in patients without pelvic-iliac lymphadenectomy or radiation. In this population, the lymph vessels are persistently clear and dilated (Fig. 11.5).

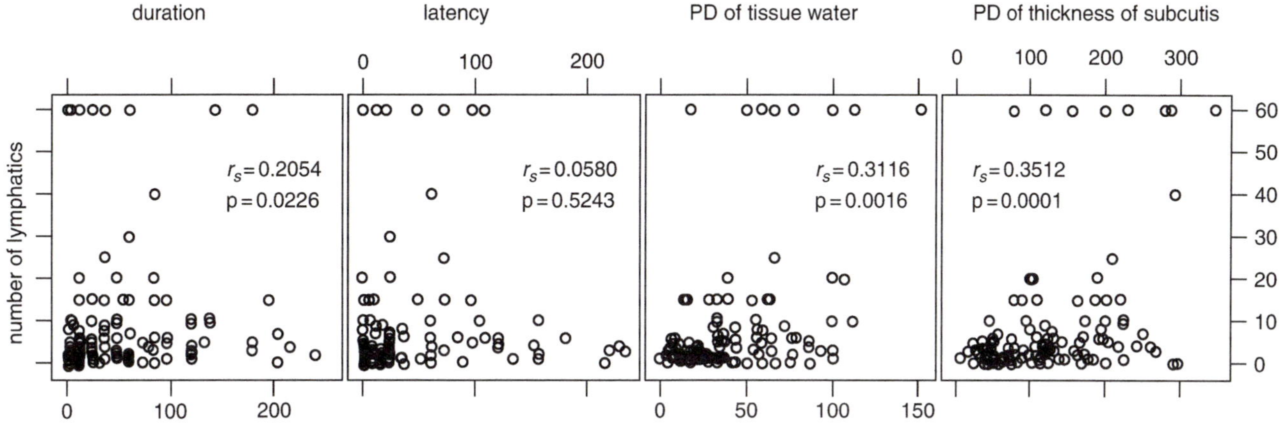

Fig. 11.2 Scatter plot of the number of lymphatics with respect to duration, latency of lymphedema, PD of tissue water, and PD of the thickness of subcutis. There are significant correlations between number of lymphatics and three clinical characteristics: duration of lymphedema, percentage difference of tissue water, and percentage difference of the thickness of subcutis. (*PD of tissue water: Percentage difference of tissue water between the edematous and nonedematous upper limbs (%); *PD of thickness of subcutis: Percentage difference of thickness of subcutis between the ipsilateral lymphedematous and contralateral nonedematous limbs (%).). Used with permission from [10]

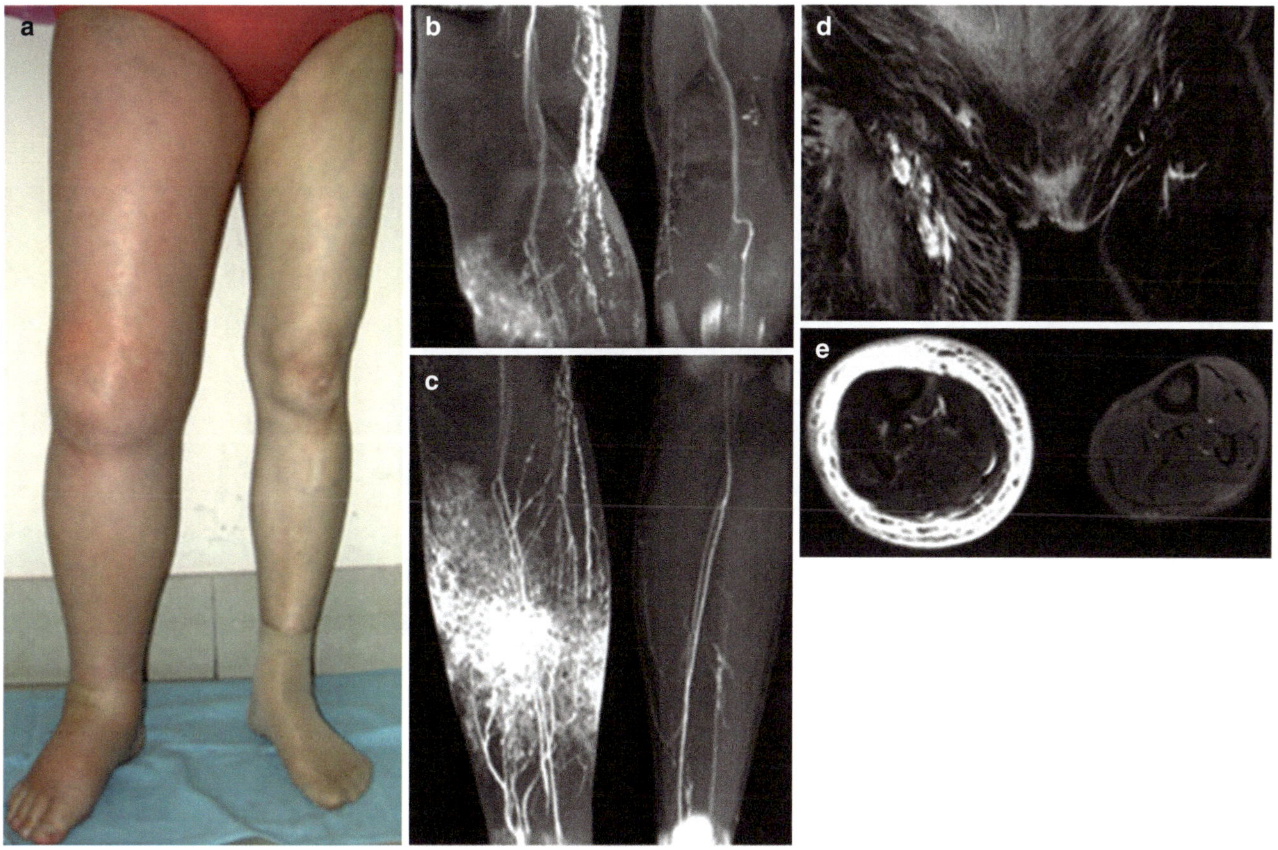

Fig. 11.3 (**a**) A woman received radiotherapy for cervical cancer 6 months ago and right lower limb lymphedema of 2 months. (**b**) Extremely dilated lymph collector in the thigh; (**c**) Massive dermal backflow in the calf; (**d**) Contrast-enhanced inguinal lymph nodes with irregular shape; (**e**) Intensive swelling in the subcutaneous layer of the calf

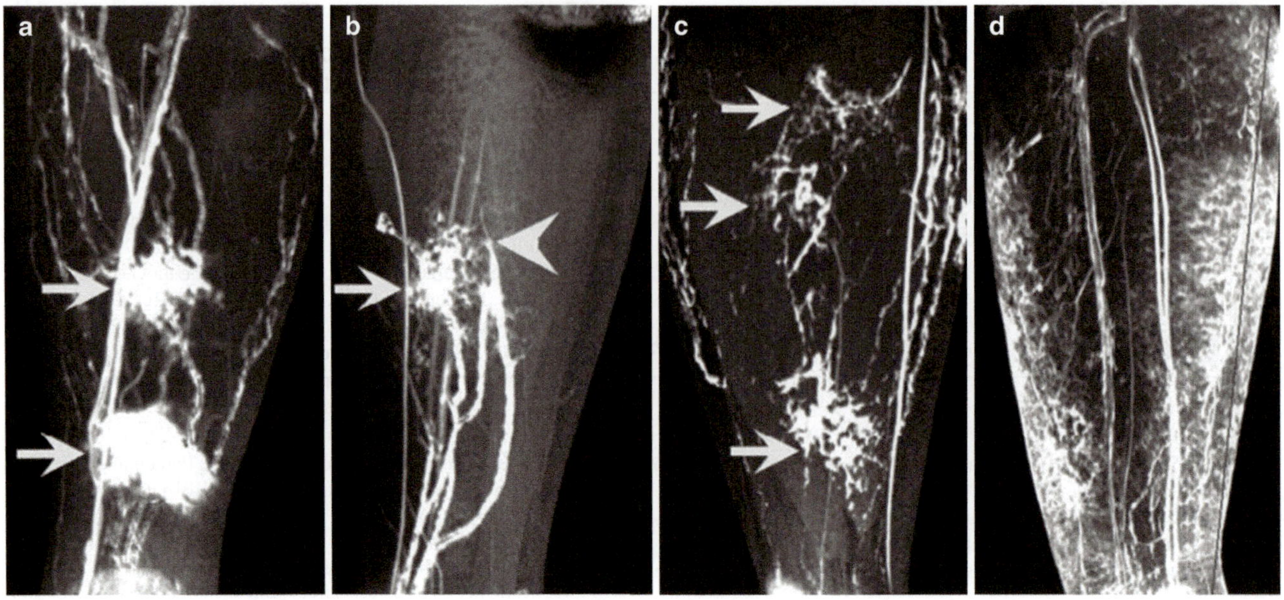

Fig. 11.4 Anterior tibial lymphatic damage on MR lymphangiogram. (**a**) Lymphatic rupture and lymphorrhea (arrows) in a left lower leg lymphedema. (**b**) Disruption of the collecting lymph vessels with lymph leakage (arrow) in a left lower leg. Only lymph collectors distal to the rupture point were enhanced (arrowhead). (**c**) Segments of the regenerated lymphatic network (arrows) displayed in a lymphedematous right leg. (**d**) "Dermal backflow" characterized by massive diffusion of high signal intensity in the skin of an affected right leg

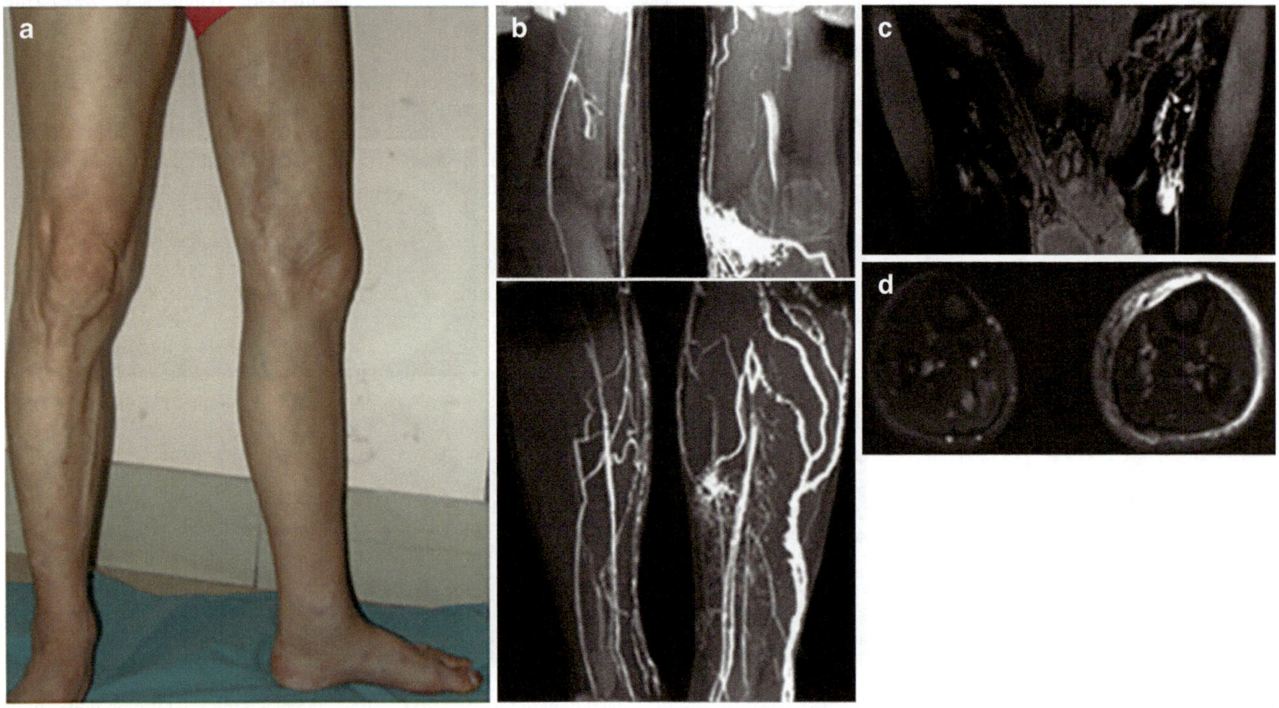

Fig. 11.5 (**a**) A 40 years old man with lymphedema of the left lower limb after surgical treatment of liposarcoma. (**b**) MRL showed significantly dilated lymphatic trunks, which was severed in the median of the left thigh. (**c**) Partial enhanced left inguinal nodes. (**d**) Edema in the subcutaneous layer of the left leg

References

1. Koshima I, Kawada S, Moriguchi T, Kajiwara Y. Ultrastructural observations of lymphatic vessels in lymphedema in human extremities. Plast Reconstr Surg. 1996;97(2):397–405.
2. Wu X, Li R, Liu N. Microscopic analysis of lymphatic vessels in primary lymphedematous skin. Phlebologie. 2012;41(1):13–7.
3. Liu NF, Wang BS. Functional lymphatic collectors in breast cancer-related lymphedema arm. Lymphat Res Biol. 2014;12(4):232–7. https://doi.org/10.1089/lrb.2014.0021.
4. Liu NF, Lu Q, Jiang ZH, et al. Anatomic and functional evaluation of the lymphatics and lymph nodes in diagnosis of lymphatic circulation disorders with contrast magnetic resonance lymphangiography. J Vasc Surg. 2009;49(4):980–7.
5. Lu Q, Bui D, Liu NF, Xu JR, Zhao XH, Zhang XF. Magnetic resonance lymphography at 3T: a promising noninvasive approach to characterise inguinal lymphatic vessel leakage. Eur J Vasc Endovasc Surg. 2012;43(1):106–11. https://doi.org/10.1016/j.ejvs.2011.09.007.
6. Liu N, Zhang Y. Magnetic resonance lymphangiography for the study of lymphatic system in lymphedema. J Reconstr Microsurg. 2016;32(1):66–71. https://doi.org/10.1055/s-0034-1384213.
7. Lu Q, Xu J, Liu N. Chronic lower extremity lymphedema: a comparative study of high-resolution interstitial MR lymphangiography and heavily T2-weighted MRI. Eur J Radiol. 2010;73(2):365–73. https://doi.org/10.1016/j.ejrad.2008.10.041.
8. Lu Q, Delproposto Z, Hu A, Tran C, Liu N, Li Y, Xu J, Bui D, Hu J. MR lymphography of lymphatic vessels in lower extremity with gynecologic oncology-related lymphedema. PLoS One. 2012;7(11):e50319. https://doi.org/10.1371/journal.pone.0050319.
9. Liu NF, Yan ZX, Wu XF, Luo Y. Magnetic resonance lymphography demonstrates spontaneous lymphatic disruption and regeneration in obstructive lymphedema. Lymphology. 2013;46(2):56–63.
10. Liu NF, Yan ZX, Wu XF. Classification of lymphatic-system malformations in primary lymphoedema based on MR lymphangiography. Eur J Vasc Endovasc Sur. 2012;44:345–9.

Pathology of the Initial Lymph Vessels in Lymphedematous Skin

12

Ningfei Liu

Abstract

Lymphedema is caused by lymphatic circulation disorders, which are caused by congenital lymphatic malfunctions and developmental disorders (primary) or acquired injury of lymphatic vessels and lymph nodes. Previous studies have focused more on the collecting lymph vessels than on the initial lymphatic vessels. The initial lymphatic vessels are responsible for both forming and transporting lymphatic fluid from tissues, but little is known about the role of these fragile vessels in the occurrence and development of lymphedema. This section comprehensively introduces the latest studies, including those investigating the histology, imaging, and genetics of capillary lymphatics in lymphedematous tissue. The results demonstrated significant pericyte coverage of the lymphatic capillaries in both primary and secondary lymphedema skin. The observed pathological changes of the initial lymph vessel may be a common phenomenon in lymphedematous tissues that need further investigation.

Keywords

Lymphedema · Initial lymphatic · Pericytes · Smooth muscle cell SMC · Lymphaticosclerosis · Lymphatic capillary · Lymphatic endothelial cell · ICG lymphography · Dermal backflow

Lymphatic circulation originates with the lymphatic capillaries, or initial lymph vessels, which perform the important functions of interstitial fluid absorption and lymph formation. Capillary endothelial cells have loosely overlapping junctions and are connected to the surrounding extracellular matrix by anchoring filaments. Unlike blood capillaries, lymphatic capillaries are devoid of pericytes and smooth muscle cells [1–3]. As initial lymphatic vessels play an important role in lymph formation and transportation, the morphological and functional abnormalities of dermal lymph vessels may play important roles in the occurrence and development of lymphedema. Studies that focus on lymphatic vessels in the affected skin revealed the importance of lymphatic vessels for the pathogenesis of primary lymphedema with the use microlymphography and indirect lymphography in the last decades [4, 5]. Recent histological studies on skin samples from primary and secondary lymphedema patients demonstrated that a large proportion of lymphatic capillaries in thickened lymphedematous skin were significantly dilated in contrast to healthy control skin samples [6–8] (Fig. 12.1). Additionally, the median luminal areas of the dermal lymphatics in patients with primary and secondary lymphedema were significantly higher than in controls (Fig. 12.2a). The most significant pathological change was significantly increased mural cell coverage of lymphatic capillaries, which were identified as α-SMA^{+} lymphatic vessels in 39 of 44 lymphedematous skin cases compared with 0% of control non-edema skin samples [8] (Figs. 12.2 and 12.3). Thus, this disease could be described as "lymphatic capillary sclerosis," similar to the previously described "lymphaticosclerosis" of collecting lymph vessels [9].

There are several potential explanations for this pathological mural cell coverage. One possibility is that long-term lymphostasis and distension of the vessel wall may induce compensatory proliferation and remodeling of the lymphatic muscle cells to withstand the high intraluminal pressure loading and to maintain lymph vessel tone. It is speculated that in lymphedema, lymphatic capillaries that originally absorb lymph might begin to transform into muscular conductive lymph vessels to increase lymph propulsion. A second explanation for the increase in mural cells is that it results from altered secretion of cytokines, chemokines, or growth factors by lymphatic endothelial cells in the chronic inflammatory microenvironment [10, 11].

N. Liu (✉)
Department of Plastic and Reconstructive Surgery, Shanghai Ninth People's Hospital, Shanghai Jiao Tong University School of Medicine, Shanghai, China

N. Liu (ed.), *Peripheral Lymphedema*, https://doi.org/10.1007/978-981-16-3484-0_12

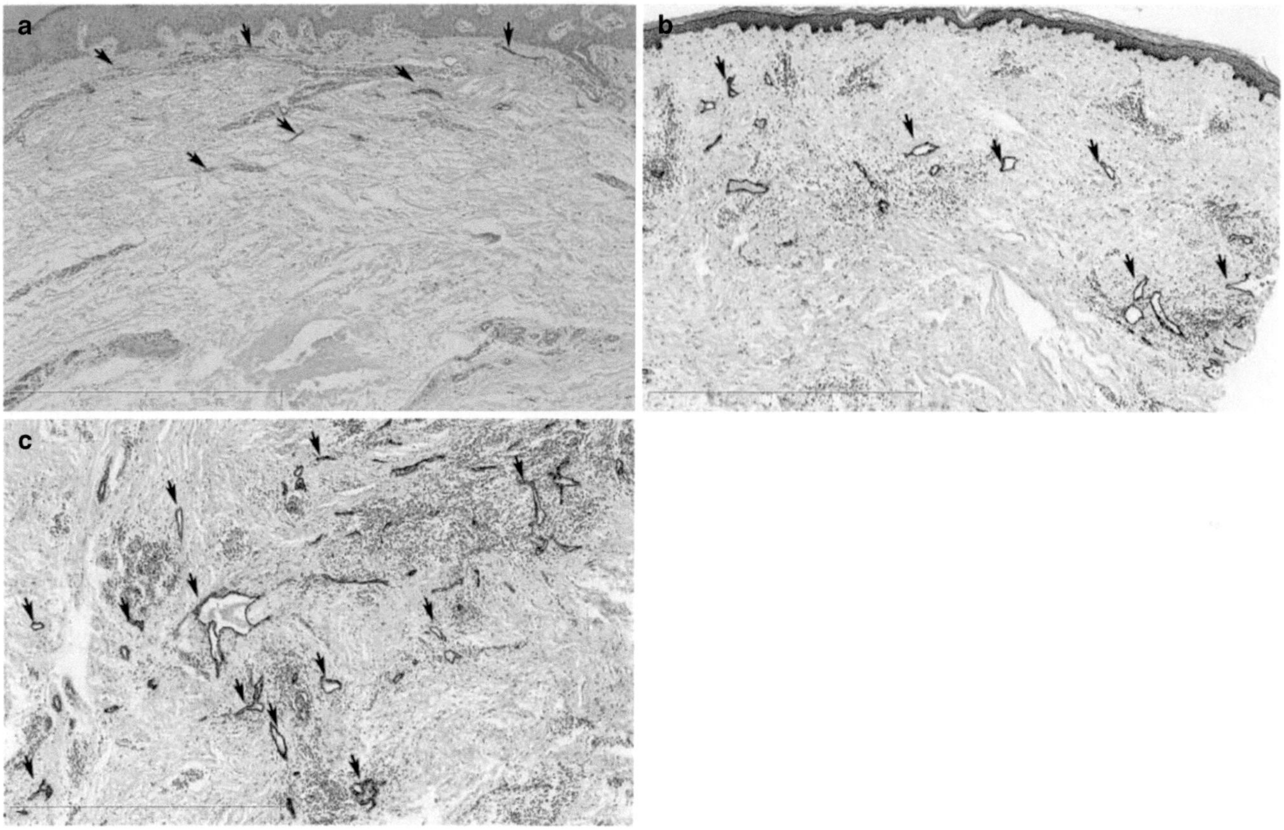

Fig. 12.1 Histological sections of skin stained with antibodies to podoplanin. (**a**) Control limb. (**b**) Primary lymphedema limb. (**c**) The deep part of affected skin of primary lymphedema foot. Lymphatic vessels, indicated by arrows, are positive for podoplanin (brown)

Subsequent thickening of the lymphatic vessel walls might lead to decreased permeability, thereby impairing the absorptive function of these vessels. Additionally, it is possible that the recruited pericytes/smooth muscle cells may interfere with the structure and/or function of the delicate anchoring filaments that control the opening and closing of lymphatic endothelial junctions, thus reducing lymph formation. The test of the functional impairment of skin lymph vessels by real-time indocyanine green imaging of the affected limbs revealed that, although the collecting lymph vessel in the lower leg could be observed immediately after contrast injection, they were not visible 30 min later, at which point dermal backflow and massive subcutaneous diffusion of contrast were seen [8] (Fig. 12.4). It is possible that the contrast agent was initially absorbed by the lymphatic capillaries and transported to the lymphatic collectors but subsequently flowed back toward the distal part of the lymphatics and interstitial spaces because of lymphatic blockage or dysfunction. These findings indicate that the lymph flows bidirectionally between the "hardened" lymphatic capillaries and the interstitial spaces (Fig. 12.5). The relationship between altered lymph flow and abnormal mural cell coverage of lymphatic capillaries is currently unknown, but the altered configuration and fluid dynamics

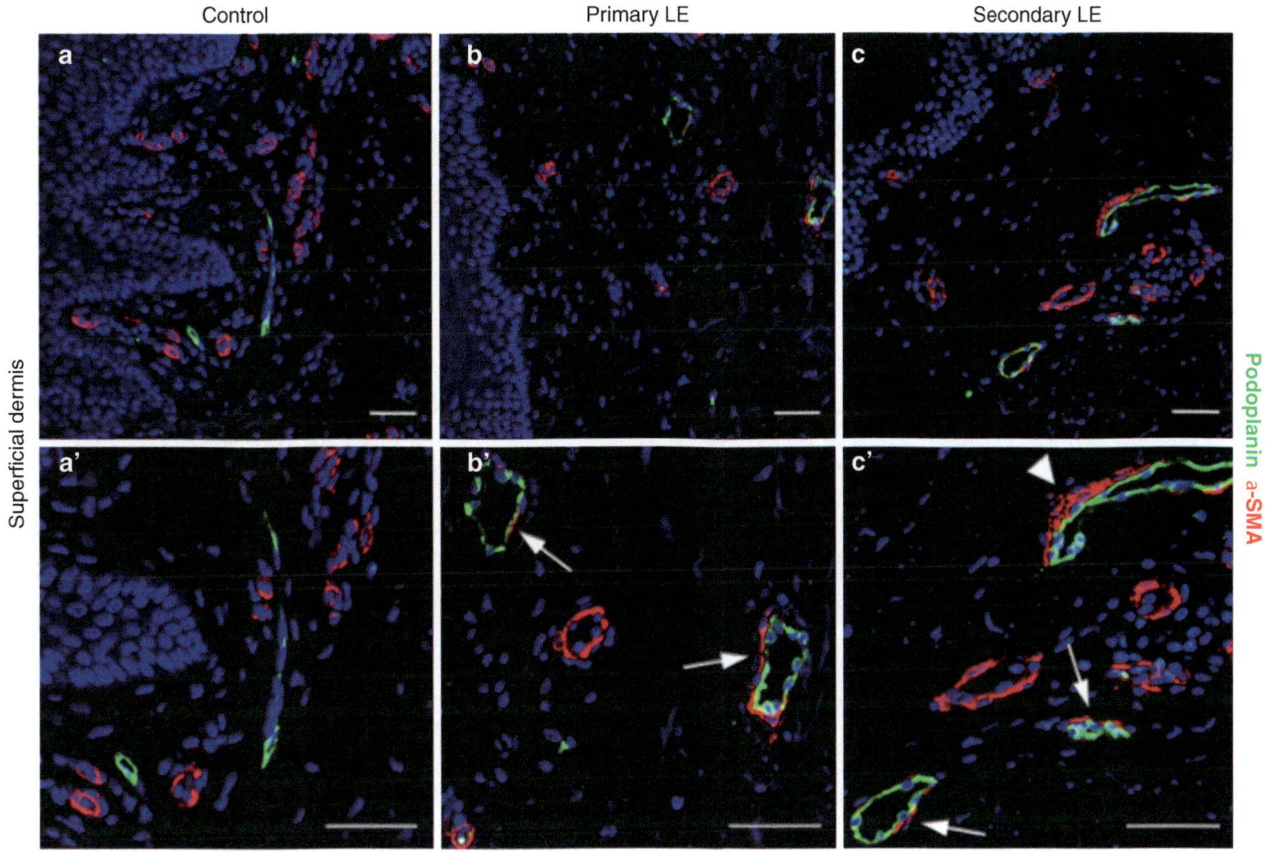

Fig. 12.2 Superficial dermis of skin sections from controls, patients with primary lymphedema, and patients with secondary lymphedema were immunofluorescently stained with podoplanin (green) and α-smooth muscle actin (red). In contrast to the lymph vessel in the control group which are devoid of smooth muscle cells and exhibit a "collapsed" morphology, the lymph vessel in lymphedema patients are dilated and encircled by scattered (**b** & **c**: arrow) or grouped (**c**: arrowhead) α- SMA + mural cells in primary and secondary lymphedema

in the dermal lymphatic vasculature suggest that the function of capillary lymph vessels is greatly impaired in patients with lymphedema. The increased SMC coverage of skin lymphatics was detected in primary lymphedema patients with and without *FOXC2* mutations [8]. Thus, rather than being an abnormal consequence of a specific gene defect [12], the pathological increase in SMCs appears to be a common feature of patients with either primary or secondary lymphedema. It is noteworthy that the changes may occur at a very early stage of the disease [8] and potentially result in fewer functioning skin initial lymph vessels, thus aggravating lymphatic circulation disorders by disrupting the absorptive function of these vessels. The observed pathological changes in dermal lymphatic vessels may help to explain the irreversibility of the disease, the current difficulties in treating patients with lymphedema and will help identify potential therapeutic targets.

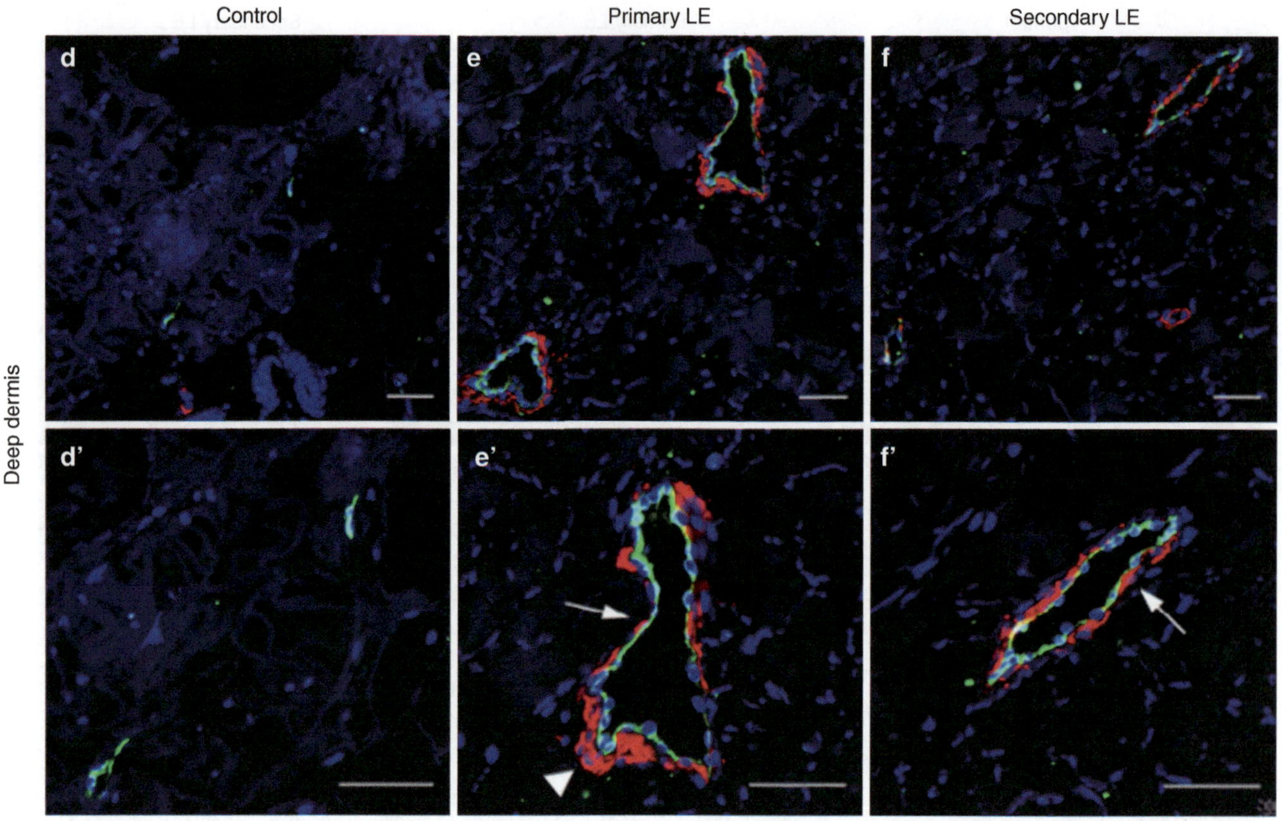

Fig. 12.3 Deep dermis of skin sections from controls, patients with primary lymphedema, and patients with secondary lymphedema were immunofluorescently stained with podoplanin (green) and α- smooth muscle actin (red). In contrast to the lymph vessel in the control group which are devoid of smooth muscle cells and exhibit a "collapsed" morphology, the lymph vessel in lymphedema patients are dilated and encircled by scattered (**e** & **f**: arrow) or grouped (**e**: arrowhead) α-SMA + mural cells in primary and secondary lymphedema

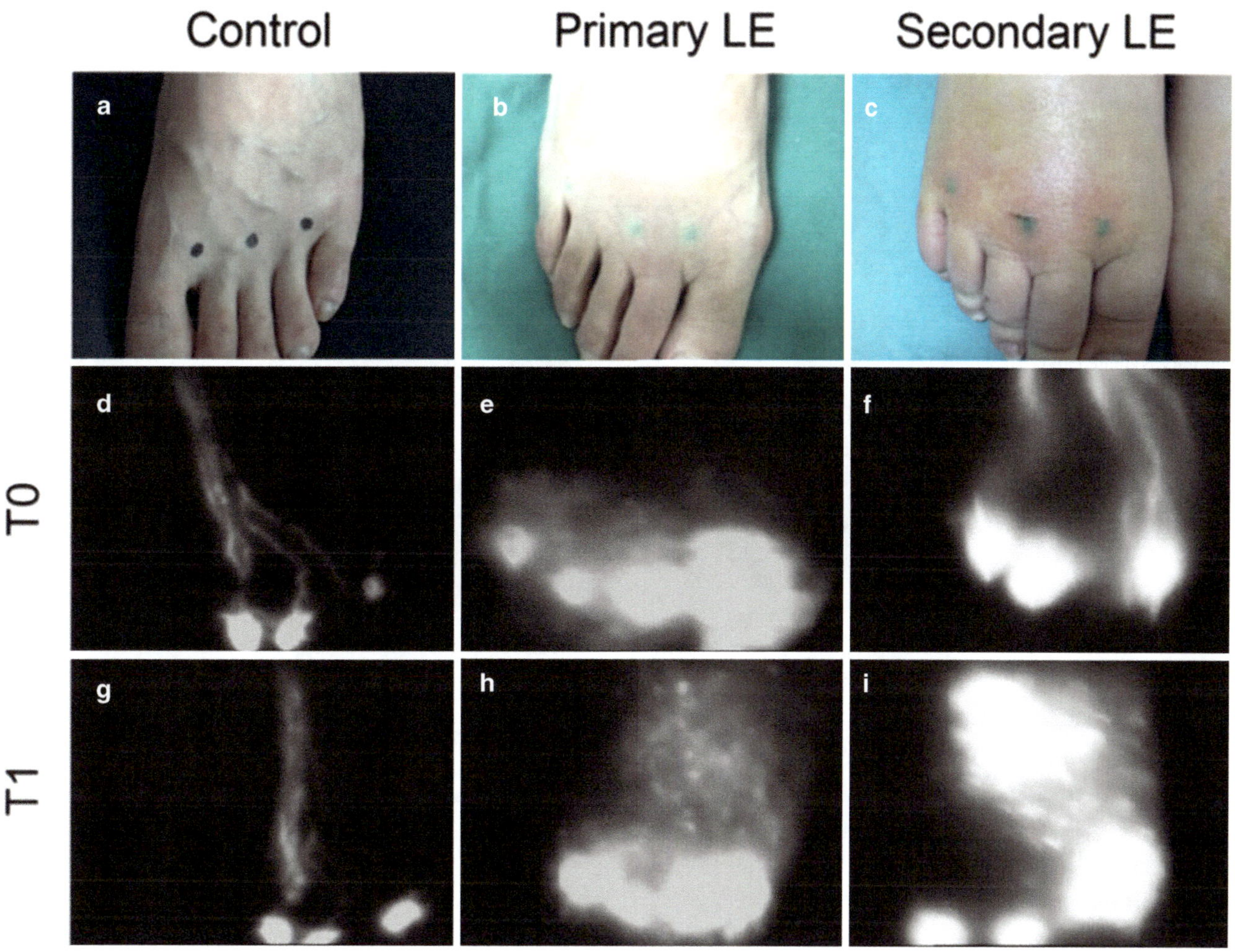

Fig. 12.4 ICG lymphographic image on the dorsum of the feet in controls and patients with lymphedema at T0 and T1. (**a**, **d**, **g**) Clear fluorescent image of the collecting lymph vessels could be visualized in controls at T0 and T1. (**b**, **e**, **h**) In primary lymphedema, lymph vessels could barely be identified at T0 (**e**), and dermal backflow with massive contrast diffusion on the dorsum of the feet was seen at T1 (**h**). (**c**, **f**, **i**) In secondary lymphedema, the contrast-enhanced lymph vessels were observed at T0 (**f**), and dermal backflow with massive subcutaneous contrast diffusion on the dorsum was visualized at T1 (**i**)

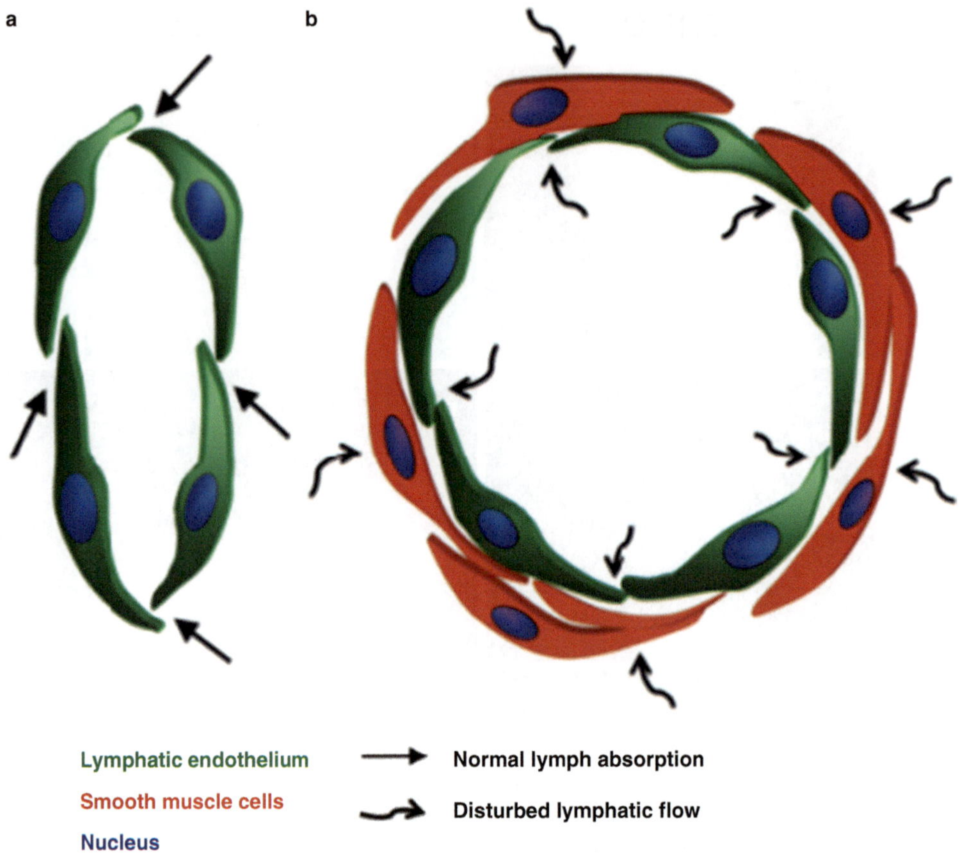

Fig. 12.5 Schematic diagram of skin lymphatic capillaries in normal and lymphedematous condition. (**a**) Normal lymphatic capillary consists only of a single layer of lymphatic endothelial cells and usually exhibits a "collapsed" morphology. Interstitial fluid is absorbed through cellular junctions. (**b**) In chronic lymphedema, lymphatic capillary is dilated and encircled by smooth muscle cells. Bidirectional flow of lymph is formed between the "hardened" lymphatic capillary and interstitial spaces

References

1. Alitalo K, Tammela T, Petrova TV. Lymphangiogenesis in development and human disease. Nature. 2005;438(7070):946–53.
2. Ryan TJ. Structure and function of lymphatics. J Invest Dermatol J Invest Dermatol. 1989;93(2 Suppl):18S–24S.
3. Schmid-Schonbein GW. Microlymphatics and lymph flow. Physiol Rev. 1990;70(4):987–1028.
4. Partsch H, Urbanek A, Wenzel-Hora B. The dermal lymphatics in lymphoedema visualized by indirect lymphography. Br J Dermatol. 1984;110(4):431–8.
5. Bollinger A, Amann-Vesti BR. Fluorescence microlymphography: diagnostic potential in lymphedema and basis for the measurement of lymphatic pressure and flow velocity. Lymphology. 2007;40(2):52–62.
6. Wu X, Yu Z, Liu N. Comparison of approaches for microscopic imaging of skin lymphatic vessels. Scanning. 2012;34(3):174–80. https://doi.org/10.1002/sca.20285.
7. Wu X, Li R, Liu N. Microscopic analysis of lymphatic vessels in primary lymphedematous skin. Phlebologie. 2012;41(1):13–7.
8. Yu ZY, Sun D, Luo Y, Liu NF. Abnormal mural cell recruitment in lymphatic capillaries: a common pathological feature in chronic lymphedematous skin? Microcirculation. 2016;23(7):495–502. https://doi.org/10.1111/micc.12299.
9. Mihara M, Hara H, Hayashi Y, Narushima M, Yamamoto T, Todokoro T, Iida T, Sawamoto N, Araki J, Kikuchi K, Murai N, Okitsu T, Kisu I, Koshima I. Pathological steps of cancer-related lymphedema: histological changes in the collecting lymphatic vessels after lymphadenectomy. PLoS One. 2012;7(7):e41126. https://doi.org/10.1371/journal.pone.0041126.
10. Abramsson A, Lindblom P, Betsholtz C. Endothelial and nonendothelial sources of PDGF- B regulate pericyte recruitment and influence vascular pattern formation in tumors. J Clin Investig. 2003;112(8):1142–51.
11. Armulik A, Abramsson A, Betsholtz C. Endothelial/pericyte interactions. Circ Res. 2005;97(6):512–23.
12. Petrova TV, Karpanen T, Norrmén C, Mellor R, Tamakoshi T, Finegold D, Ferrell R, Kerjaschki D, Mortimer P, Ylä-Herttuala S, Miura N, Alitalo K. Defective valves and abnormal mural cell recruitment underlie lymphatic vascular failure in lymphedema distichiasis. Nat Med. 2004;10(9):974–81.

Co-Existence of Lymphatic and Venous System Malformation

13

Ningfei Liu

Abstract

Lymphatic and venous malformations co-exist not uncommonly in patients with primary lymphedema. The clinical manifestations in the affected limb generally resemble the effects of lymphedema. Imaging of both lymphatic and blood vessels may assist in making an accurate diagnosis.

Keywords

Primary lymphedema · Lymphatic malformation
Lymphatic origin · Venous malformation
Co-malformations · Mixed edema · *FOXC2* mutation
VEGFR-3 mutation · Valve insufficiency

Co-existence of lymphatic and venous system malformation is not rare in primary lymphedema. Phlebolymphedema, which occurs in many older people with chronic swelling of their lower limbs, is the result of a combination of chronic venous insufficiency caused by venous circulatory disorders and lymphedema that is not associated with obvious malformations in the lymphatic system; this is a type of secondary lymphedema rather than a form of primary lymphedema.

Genuine mixed venous-lymphatic edema caused by malformations of lymphatic and blood circulatory systems is commonly seen in the lower extremity. It can be congenital or first become apparent in adolescence or middle age. The co-existence of venous and lymphatic system dysplasia suggests that they may interact with each other, worsening the already impaired venous and lymph circulation and aggravating swelling. Clinical manifestations of co-existing venous-lymphatic edema are similar to those of pure lymphedema and do not include skin sclerosis, hyperpigmentation, pain, or chronic ulcers in the affected limb. The absence of edema in the muscles of the affected limb suggests that the edema is mainly caused by lymphatic malfunction and is less attributable to venous malformation.

Mixed edema involving both lymphatic and venous circulatory systems is commonly seen in:

1. Syndrome-related lymphedema, which includes lymphedema associated with lymphedema–distichiasis (LD) syndrome (characterized by varicose veins and venous valve insufficiency/reflux) [1, 2] and that associated with Klippel–Trenaunay syndrome (characterized by aplasia and dysfunction of deep venous valves, malformation of veins in the skin, subcutaneous tissue, and muscles together with severe lymphatic malformations such as lymphatic and/or lymph node hyperplasia or hypoplasia [3] (Fig. 13.1).
2. Inherited lymphedema such as Milroy's disease, which is characterized by prominent great saphenous veins and hypoplasia, dysfunction, or aplasia of lymphatic vessels [4, 5] (Fig. 13.2).
3. Sporadic lymphedema, which is the commonest type of mixed edema. The venous malformations include deep venous valve aplasia or insufficiency and varicose veins, and the associated lymphatic anomalies are lymphatic hyperplasia or hypoplasia (Figs. 13.3 and 13.4).

The malformations can be accurately diagnosed by MR lymphangiography (MRL), Doppler ultrasound, and CT venography. It may be more difficult to treat venous/lymphedema than pure lymphedema. For patients with no surgical indications for varicosities and vascular malformation, lymphedema should be treated actively, based on the diagnosis established. Early diagnosis and proper treatment may effectively prevent or slow the course of lymphedema.

Co-malformations of the lymphatic and venous circulatory systems in patients with primary lymphedema may have developmental and molecular origins. The embryonic ori-

N. Liu (✉)
Department of Plastic and Reconstructive Surgery,
Shanghai Ninth People's Hospital, Shanghai Jiao Tong University
School of Medicine, Shanghai, China

N. Liu (ed.), *Peripheral Lymphedema*, https://doi.org/10.1007/978-981-16-3484-0_13

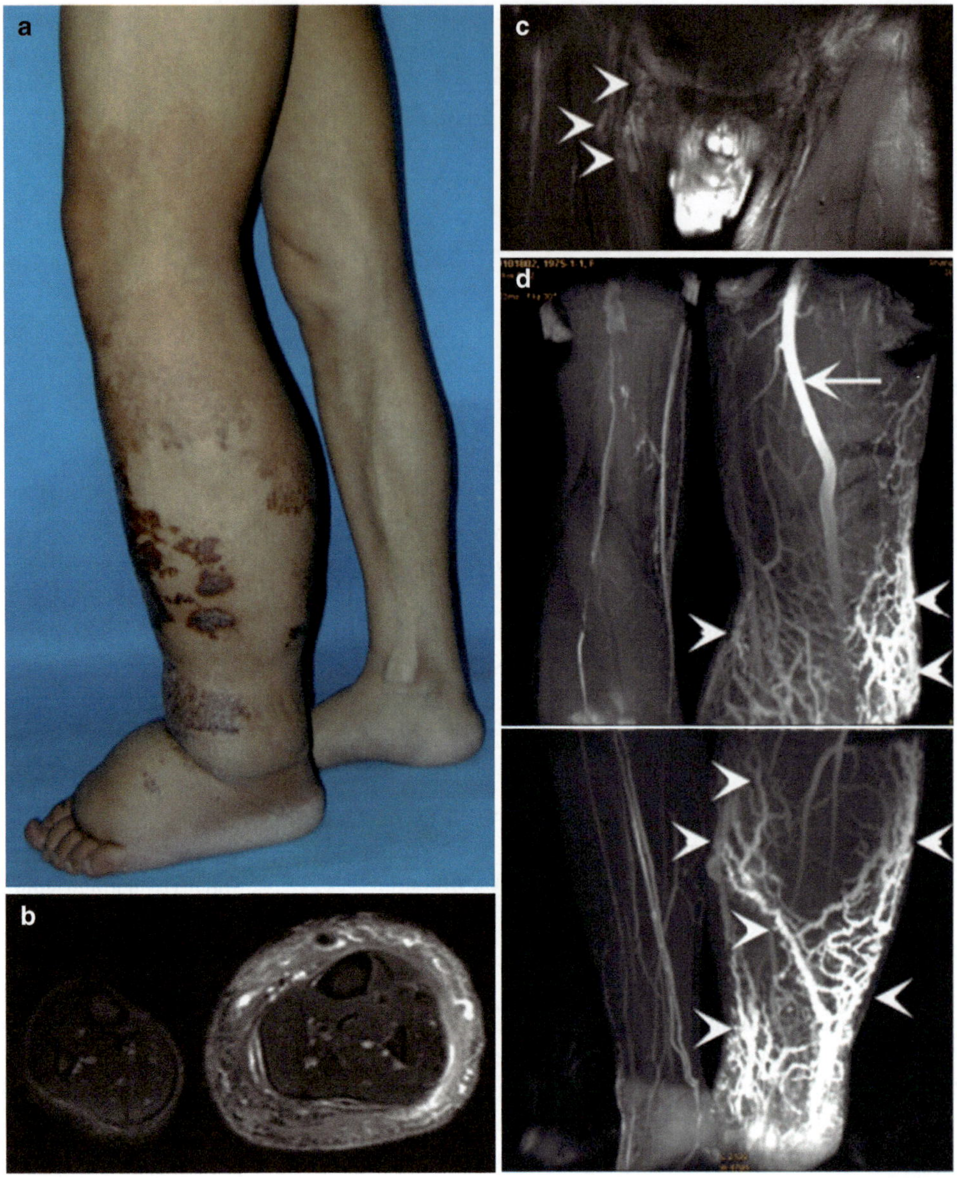

Fig.13.1 (**a**) A 34-year-old man with chief clinical features of KTS including skin port-wine stain and hypertrophy of left lower limb. (**b**) The axial section of T2-weighted MR image shows hypertrophy of subcutaneous tissue and edema (high signal intensity) in the whole subcutaneous layer. (**c**) No inguinal lymph nodes were visualized on the left side in contrast with lymph nodes (arrowheads) visualized on the contralateral side on the coronal T2-weighted MR image. (**d**) Composition image of MR lymphangiogram shows numerous hyperplastic lymphatic vessels (arrowheads) and an enlarged deep vein (arrow)

gins of lymphatic vessels were proposed a century ago, the predominant view being that the lymphatic endothelium has a venous origin [6, 7]. Recent studies on the molecular regulation of lymphatic and venous development have identified some genes that have important effects on both lymphatic and venous development and specification. For example, mutations in *FOXC2* have been identified as the cause of LD. The findings of studies in patients with LD and *Foxc2*-deficient mouse mutants indicate that the underlying cause of lymphatic failure in LD is abnormal valve morphogenesis [8]. Patients with LD and their relatives who carry *FOXC2* mutations but do not have clinical evidence of LD all have long saphenous vein reflux, which supports the role of FOXC2 in venous and lymphatic valve development [1, 2]. Mutations in *VEGFR3* cause lymphatic dysfunction in Milroy disease, the most common form of congenital lymphedema; most patients with Milroy disease also have reflux in the great saphenous vein [4]. These findings suggest that Foxc2-VEGFR3 signaling may regulate the development of valves in both lymphatic and venous vessels.

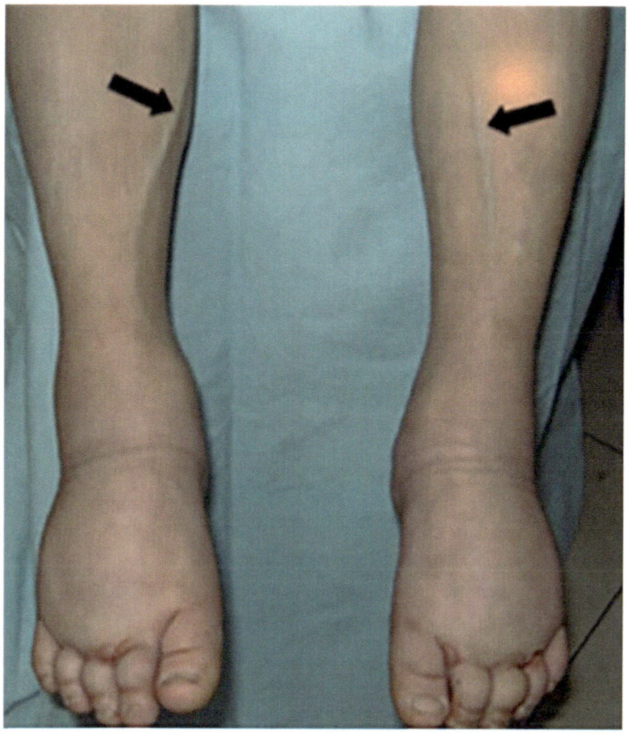

Fig. 13.2 Prominent great saphenous veins (arrows) in bilateral lower limbs of a child with Milroy's disease

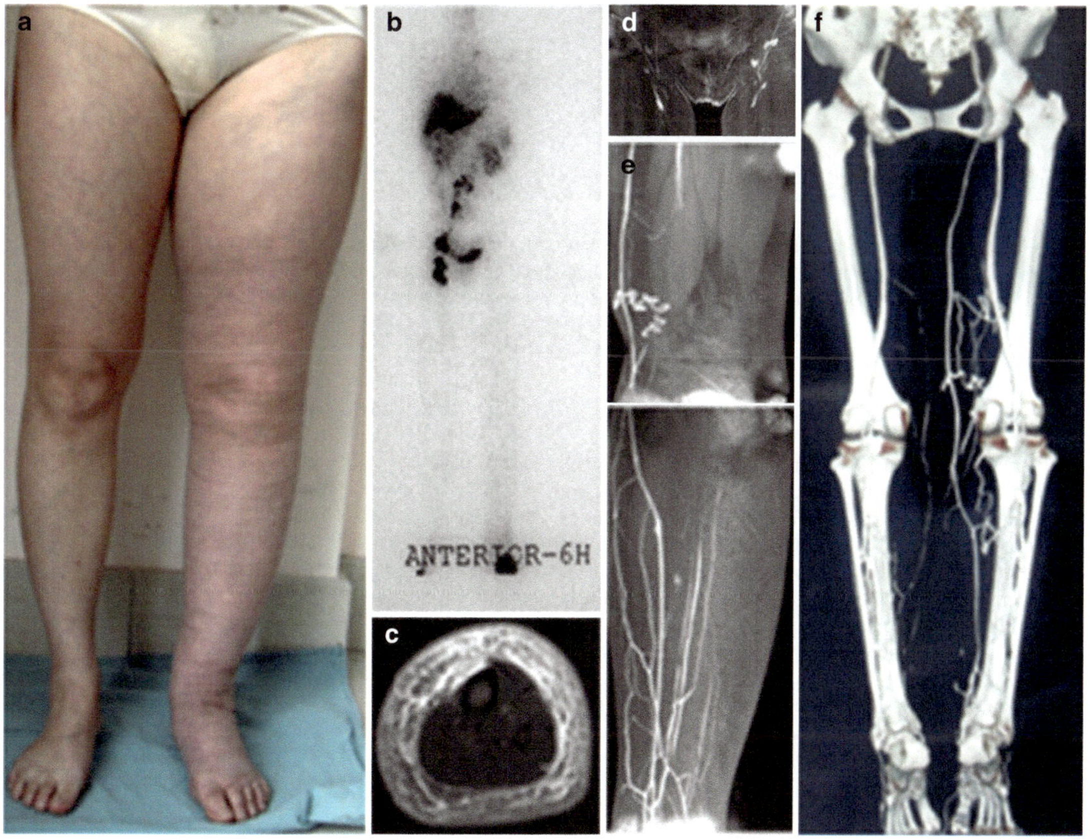

Fig. 13.3 (**a**) A 38 years old woman with congenital left lower extremity lymphedema. (**b**) No lymph node and lymphatic collector were visualized in the lymphoscintigram on the affected limb. (**c**) Axial section of T2-weighted MR image shows edema in the subcutaneous layer but not in the muscle. (**e**) MR lymphangiography showed normal inguinal lymph nodes and varicose venous but not the collecting vessels in the left lower extremity. (**f**) CT venography further confirmed venous malformation in the lymphedema limb

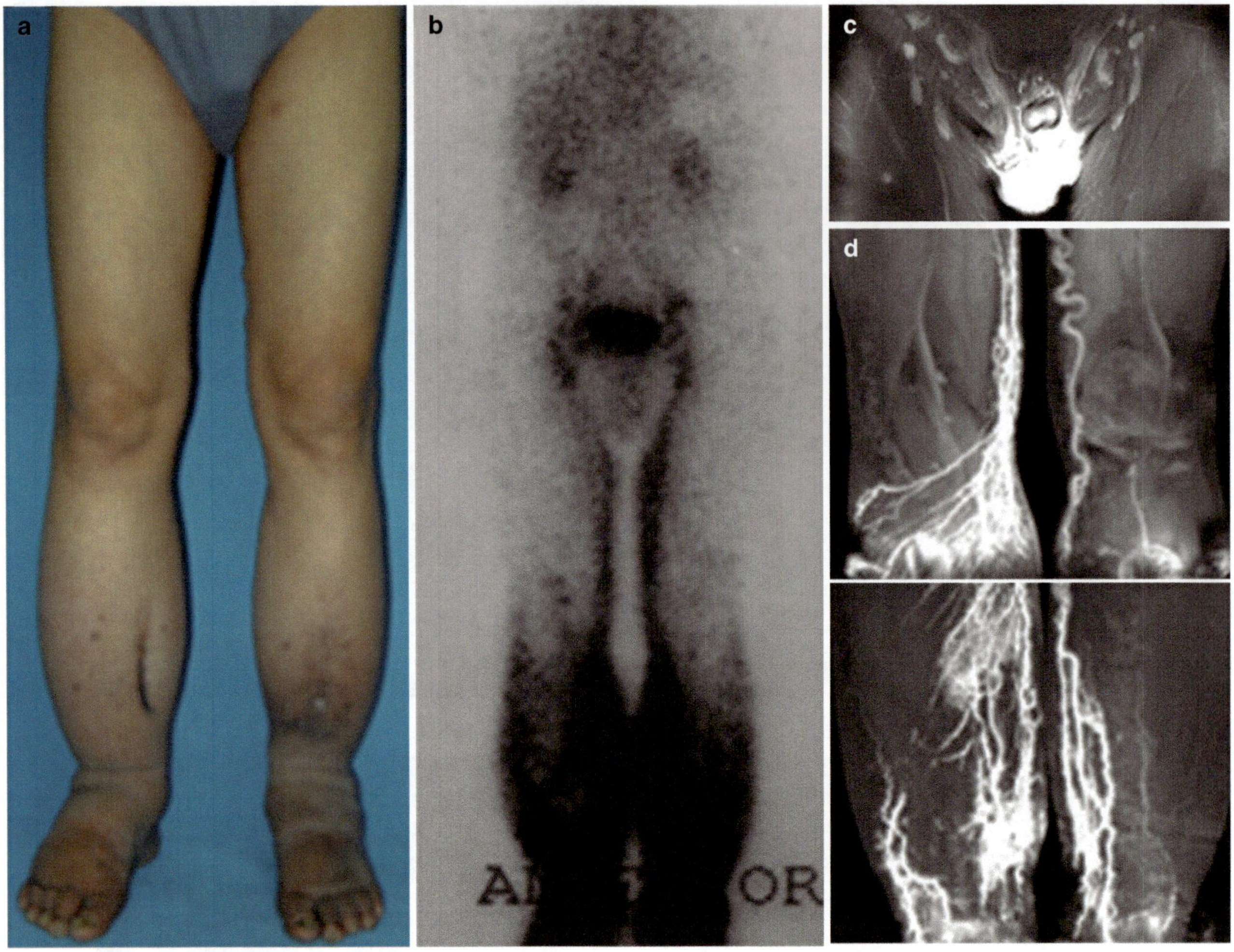

Fig. 13.4 (**a**) A 23 years old man with bilateral lower limb lymphedema of 11 years. (**b**) The lymphoscintigram showed unclear inguinal lymph nodes and lymphatic trunks in the thigh and isotopic concentrated in the calf. (**c**) MRL demonstrated inguinal lymph nodes. (**d**) Hyperplasia of bilateral tortuous lymph vessels with the varicose saphenous big vein on MRL imaging

References

1. Mellor RH, Brice G, Stanton AW, French J, Smith A, Jeffery S, Levick JR, Burnand KG, Mortimer PS. Mutations in FOXC2 are strongly associated with primary valve failure in veins of the lower limb. Circulation. 2007;115(14):1912–20.
2. Petrova TV, Karpanen T, Norrmén C, Mellor R, Tamakoshi T, Finegold D, Ferrell R, Kerjaschki D, Mortimer P, Ylä-Herttuala S, Miura N, Alitalo K. Defective valves and abnormal mural cell recruitment underlie lymphatic vascular failure in lymphedema distichiasis. Nat Med. 2004;10(9):974–81.
3. Liu NF, Lu Q, Yan ZX. Lymphatic malformation is a common component of Klippel-Trenaunay syndrome. J Vasc Surg. 52(6):1557–63. https://doi.org/10.1016/j.jvs.2010.06.166.
4. Gordon K, Spiden SL, Connell FC, Brice G, Cottrell S, Short J, Taylor R, Jeffery S, Mortimer PS, Mansour S, Ostergaard P. FLT4/VEGFR3 and Milroy disease: novel mutations, a review of published variants and database update. Hum Mutat. 2013;34(1):23–31. https://doi.org/10.1002/humu.22223.
5. Mellor RH, Hubert CE, Stanton AW, Tate N, Akhras V, Smith A, Burnand KG, Jeffery S, Mäkinen T, Levick JR, Mortimer PS. Lymphatic dysfunction, not aplasia, underlies Milroy disease. Microcirculation. 2010;17(4):281–96. https://doi.org/10.1111/j.1549-8719.2010.00030.x.
6. Sabin FR. On the origin of the lymphatic system from the veins and the development of the lymph heart and thoracic duct in the pig. Am J Anat. 1902;1:367–89.
7. Semo J, Nicenboim J, Yaniv K. Development of the lymphatic system: new questions and paradigms. Development. 2016;143(6):924–35. https://doi.org/10.1242/dev.132431.
8. Bazigou E, Lyons OT, Smith A, Venn GE, Cope C, Brown NA, Makinen T. Genes regulating lymphangiogenesis control venous valve formation and maintenance in mice. J Clin Invest. 2011;121(8):2984–92. https://doi.org/10.1172/JCI58050.

Part IV

Pathology of Lymphedematous Tissue

14 Lymphedema Fluid

Marzanna T. Zaleska and Waldemar L. Olszewski

Abstract

The mobile intercellular fluid flowing to and in the lymphatics contains filtered plasma products and substances synthetized and excreted by tissue cells. Among them are signaling proteins as cytokines, chemokines, enzymes, and growth factors. Lipids are transported to and from cells. They act locally in autocrine and paracrine systems regulating cell metabolism and proliferation and formation of the ground matrix. They play an immunoregulatory role in infections, wound healing, and tumor cell growth. They reflect what has been filtered from plasma and produced by local cells. This gives an insight into the tissue metabolic processes that cannot be detected by the study of plasma biochemistry with respect to the given tissue or organ. Lymph chemistry provides the most valuable information on cell metabolic events. Legs are exposed to infections and trauma, often resulting in the development of lymphedema. Our studies showed generally higher concentrations of cytokines, chemokines, enzymes, and growth factors in lymph than in serum. The total protein L/S ratio was 0.22, whereas that of various lymph signaling proteins ranged between 1 and 10. Reverse lipid flow from cells to tissue fluid adds to lipoprotein concentration. This indicates that in addition to proteins filtered from the blood, local cells contribute to lymph concentration by their own production, depending on the actual cell requirement. Moreover, there were major individual differences of lymph levels with simultaneous stable serum levels. This suggests the existence of a local autonomous regulatory humoral mechanism in tissues, not reflected in serum.

M. T. Zaleska
Department of Applied Physiology, Mossakowski Medical Research Institute, Polish Academy of Sciences, Warsaw, Poland

Department of Vascular Surgery, Central Clinical Hospital, Ministry of Internal Affairs, Warsaw, Poland

W. L. Olszewski (✉)
Department of Vascular Surgery, Central Clinical Hospital, Ministry of Internal Affairs, Warsaw, Poland

14.1 Proteins and Lipids in Peripheral Normal and Lymphedema Lymph

14.1.1 Lymph Proteins in Normal and Lymphedema Limbs

Lymph contains a number of proteins that are similar to blood plasma, as it is generally referred to as an ultrafiltrate of plasma. The components of human afferent lymph and how similar or different they are compared with plasma, remain largely undetermined. In the afferent lymph, we expect the presence not only of proteins and peptides derived from filtered plasma but also metabolic products of keratinocytes and connective tissue cells, cytokines, chemokines, growth factors, and antibacterial peptides originating from immune cells normally present in tissues (Fig. 14.1).

Signaling proteins are represented in the tissue fluid/lymph from soft tissues of normal human legs at concentrations different from serum (Fig. 14.2).

Tissue cell metabolic processes, proliferation, differentiation, senescence, and apoptosis are regulated by a plethora of low molecular proteins and peptides, among them cytokines, chemokines, growth factors, enzymes, and neurotransmitters. These signaling proteins are present in the tissue fluid [1–4]. They easily diffuse in the liquid environment and get access to individual cells. Here they are absorbed by cell multimerized specific receptors, subsequently activating the JAK/STAT signal transduction pathway. The concentration of signaling proteins in tissue fluid is not regulated solely by filtration from blood but also by local production by parenchymatous and immigrating immune cells. In skin and subcutaneous tissue, these are keratinocytes, blood and lymphatic endothelial cells, Langerhans' cells, fibroblasts, and recirculating lymphocytes. Tissue fluid flows into lymphatics, and since then, it

N. Liu (ed.), *Peripheral Lymphedema*, https://doi.org/10.1007/978-981-16-3484-0_14

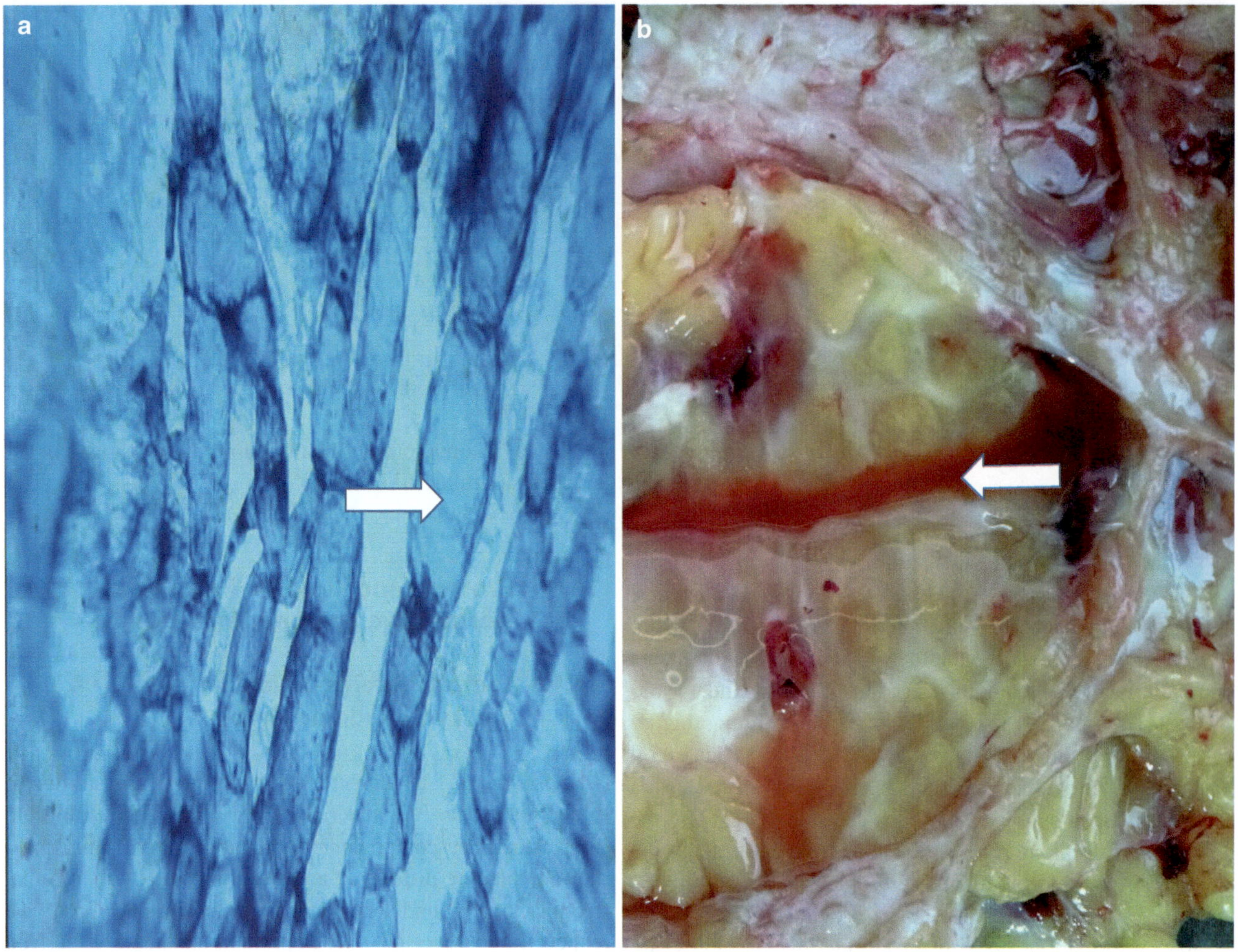

Fig. 14.1 Picture of peripheral lymphatics where lymph may be collected from, by cannulation of the vessel or from the surgical cut of tissue, where mobile tissue fluid accumulates in lymphedema. Biochemistry of tissue fluid/lymph provides most information on tissue function

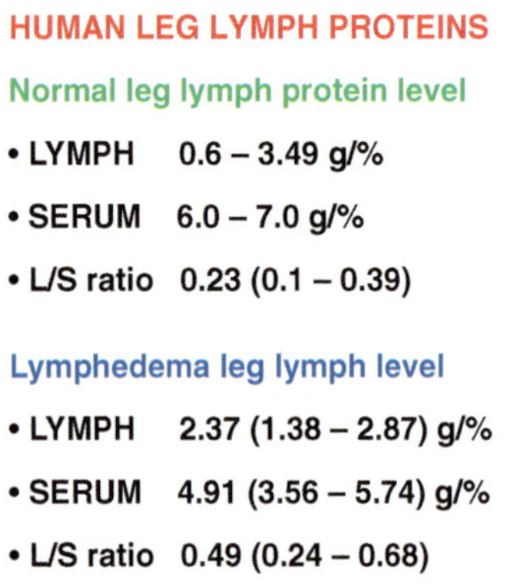

Fig. 14.2 Protein concentration in tissue fluid/lymph of normal legs and in obstructive lymphedema. Note that it is lower than in serum with the L/S ratio 0.1 to 0.6. There are no statistically significant differences between normal and lymphedema lymph protein levels. The L/S ratio cannot reach values close to that of serum as, according to the Starling's equation, the oncotic pressure of proteins attracts water bringing about protein dilution. Finally, the total protein mass in edema fluid is increased in parallel to the increased fluid volume; however, the concentration remains low

is called lymph. It is known from multiple studies that lymph composition changes continuously due to the influx of plasma components and consumption and production/secretion of various substances by the parenchymatous cells. Consequently, lymph flow rate and its composition change from minute to minute [5]. The venous hydrostatic pressure also has a major impact on the actual protein concentration (Fig. 14.3).

The knowledge of their concentration and activity can give insight into the cellular and interstitial processes of the studied tissue. Harvesting lymph from the cannulated lymphatic collectors provides volumes sufficient for biochemical studies [6]. Blood samples from the studied tissue do not provide data reflecting intercellular events to such an extent as lymph.

The literature on the chemical composition of lymph is scarce and provides only limited knowledge on the chemical processes in the intercellular space [7–10]. Lower limbs are exposed to infections and trauma, and the signaling proteins

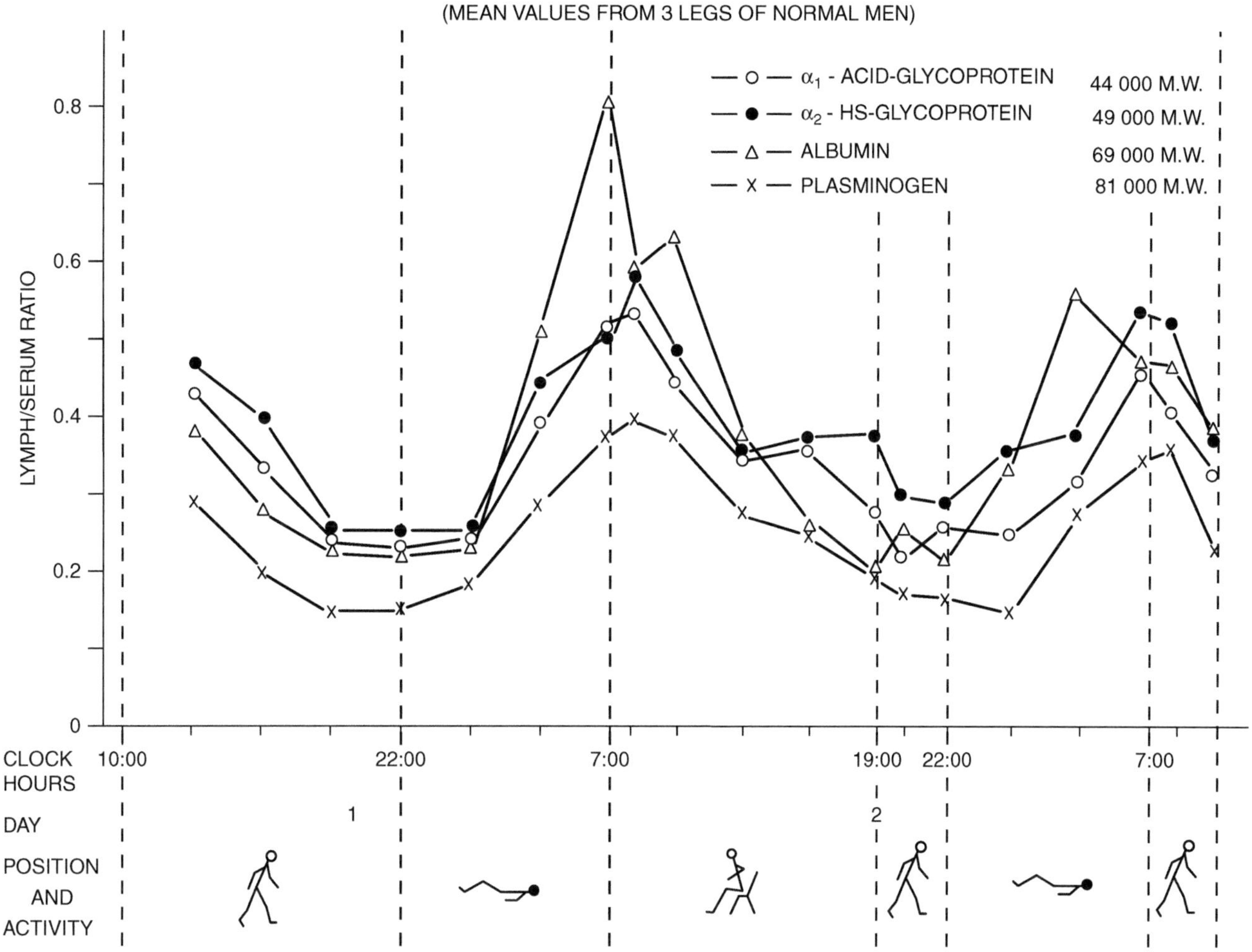

Fig. 14.3 The concentration of various lymph proteins in normal legs in different body positions. Tissue fluid/lymph protein concentration in leg tissues (and most likely other sites) changes depending on the capillary plasma filtration. This in turn depends on the body's horizontal or upright position depending on the changes of leg venous hydrostatic pressure. There is no stable lymph protein concentration as it is in plasma. The volume of filtered proteins depends on the capillary wall molecular sieve. The larger is the protein molecule, the less of it will penetrate through the capillary wall. E.g., note the difference between the acid-glycoprotein and plasminogen lymph levels

play here a dominant role in regulating the immune homeostasis.

14.1.1.1 Normal Leg Lymph and Serum Cytokines, Chemokines Enzymes, and Growth Factors

The investigated pro-inflammatory cytokines were interleukins IL1β, IL6, and TNFα (tumor necrosis factor), anti-inflammatory IL1Rα (anty-IL1-receptor). The chemokines were MIP1 α (macrophage inflammatory protein), CCL2/MCP1 (macrophage chemotactic protein), enzymes TIMP1, lymphocyte chemokine CCL21, and KGF (keratinocyte growth factor). Moreover, there were VEGF (vascular endothelial growth factor), VEGF-C, leptin, and adiponectin.

The concentrations of investigated cytokines, chemokines, enzymes, and growth factors in pg/ml and ng/ml have been presented on Fig. 14.4 [11]. The obtained data for total protein L/S ratio that was 0.22 ± 0.1 (concentration 1.66 ± 0.14 g/dl and 7.30 ± 0.1 g/dl, respectively). It was 1.39 for IL1β, 1.7 for IL6, 10.2 for IL1Ra (all $p < 0.05$), and 0.94 for TNFα.

The growth factor, tissue enzyme, and chemokine L/S were 6.0 for KGF, 2.5 for TIMP1, 2.5 for CCL2/MCP1, and 3.0 for CCL21. The angiogenic and adipocytogenic factor L/S was 1.0 for VEGF, 1.3 for VEGF C, and 2.6 for leptin (both $p < 0.05$). Together, there the lymph concentration was higher than in serum for all but TNFα and VEGF (Fig. 14.5).

14.1.1.2 Lymphedema Leg Lymph Cytokines, Chemokines Enzymes, and Growth Factors

The concentrations of investigated cytokines, chemokines, enzymes, and growth factors in pg/ml and ng/ml have been presented on (Figs. 14.6, 14.7 and 14.8).

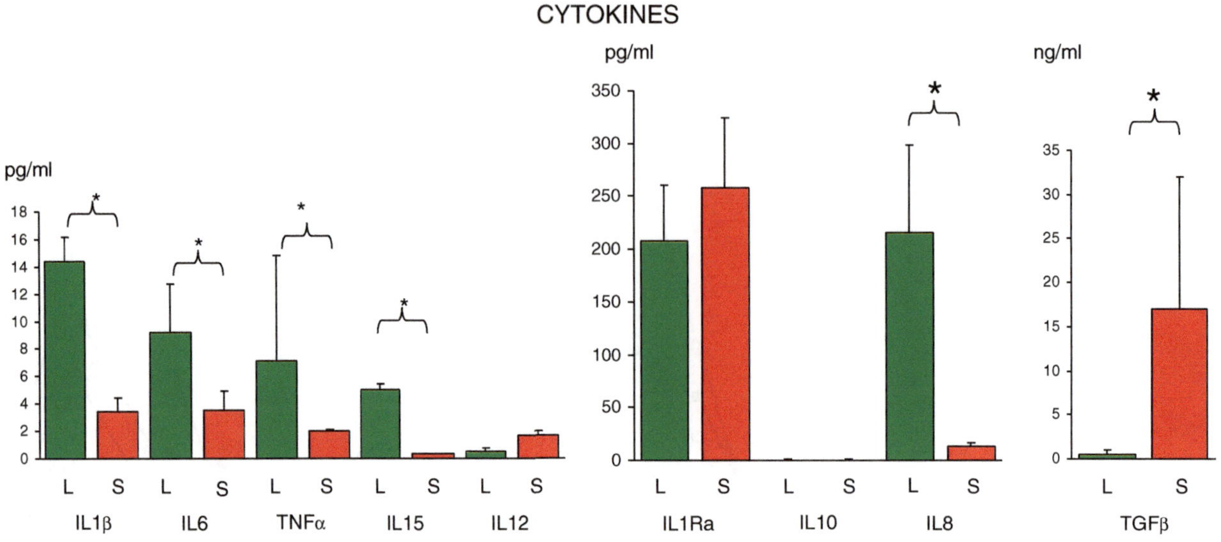

Fig. 14.4 Cytokine, chemokine, growth factors, and adipogenic hormones concentration in normal leg lymph (L) and serum (S). $N = 25$, mean ± sd, $*p < 0.05$. Note that the IL1Ra, keratinocyte growth factor (KGF), tissue metalloproteinase, chemokine CCL2, lymphocyte attracting chemokine CCL21, and leptin lymph levels are higher than in the tissue percolating serum

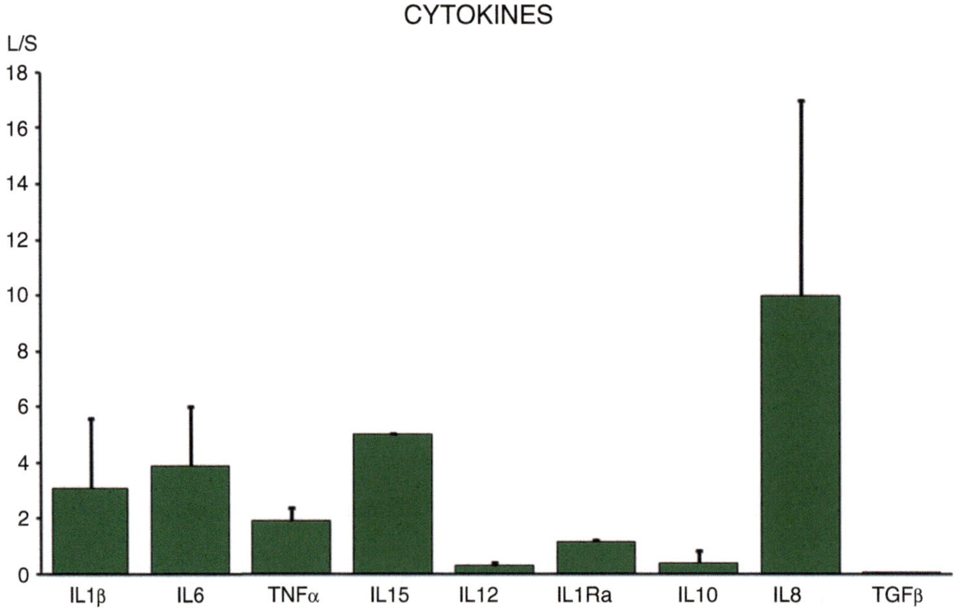

Fig. 14.5 The normal leg lymph to serum (L/S) ratio for cytokine, chemokine, growth factors, and adipogenic hormones. $N = 25$. 1-IL1β, 2-IL6,3-IL1Ra, 4-TNFα, 5-KGF, 6-TIMP1, 7-CCL2, 8-CCL21, 9-VEGF (vascular endothelial growth factor), 10-VEGF C, 11-leptin, and 12-adiponectin. The red line shows the L/S ratio 1.0. All values above 1.0 point to higher lymph than serum levels

The L/S ratio of lymphedema lymph to normal lymph was 0.73 vs. 1.4 for IL1β, 3.2 vs. 1.7 for IL6, 18.0 vs. 10.2 for IL1Ra ($p < 0.05$), 0.5 vs. 0.9 for TNFα, 10.7 vs. 6.0 for KGF ($p < 0.05$), 3.0 vs. 2.5 for TIMP1, 6.0 vs. 2.5 for CCL2/MCP1 ($p < 0.05$), 1.7 vs. 3.0 for CCL 21, 3.1 vs. 1.0 for VEGF ($p < 0.05$), 3.1 vs. 1.3 for VEGF C ($p < 0.05$), 7.6 vs. 2.6 for leptin (p, 0.01) and 0.13 vs. 0.34 for adiponectin (Fig. 14.9). Together, there was significantly more of IL1Ra, KGF, CCL2/MCP1, VEGF, VEGF C and leptin in the stagnant lymphedema lymph compared with the normally flowing leg lymph.

14.2 General Analysis

Our studies have shown generally higher concentrations of cytokines, and growth factors, and enzymes in lymph than in serum. This indicates that in addition to proteins filtered from the blood, local cells contribute to lymph concentration by their own production, depending on the actual cell requirement. Interestingly, the lymphedema lymph contains more of IL1Ra, KGF, CCL2/MCP1, VEGF, VEGF C, and leptin than normal leg lymph. These proteins may play a significant role

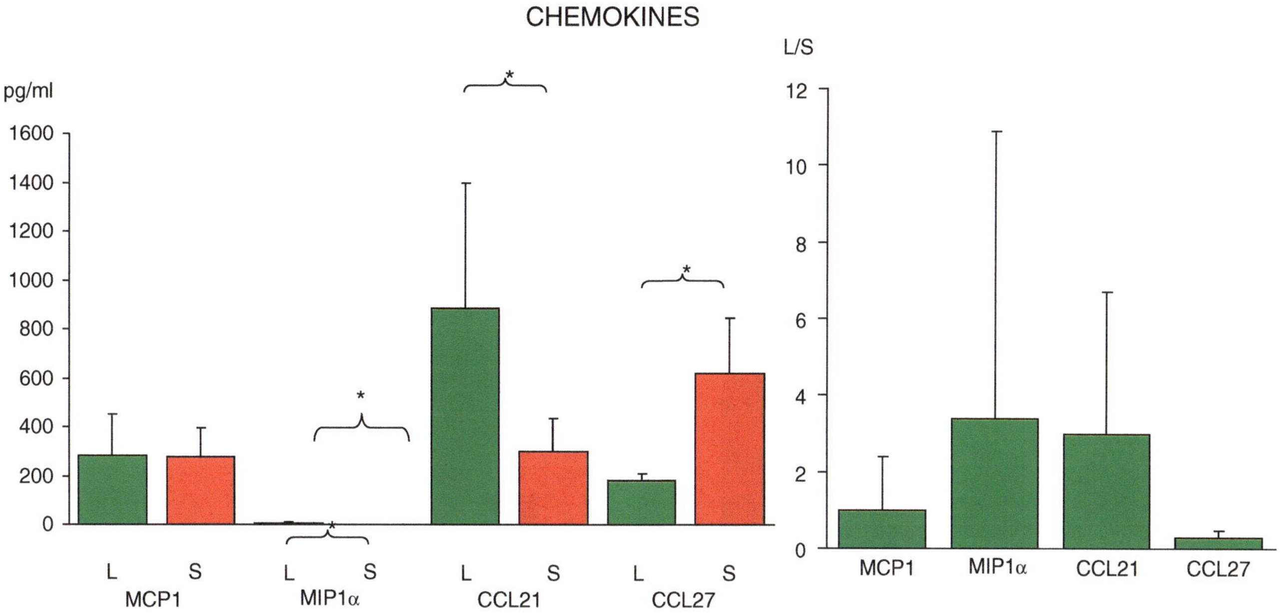

Fig. 14.6 The normal (N) and lymphedema leg (L) lymph cytokine concentration (mean, $n = 20$). Note more lymphedema than the normal level for IL1Ra

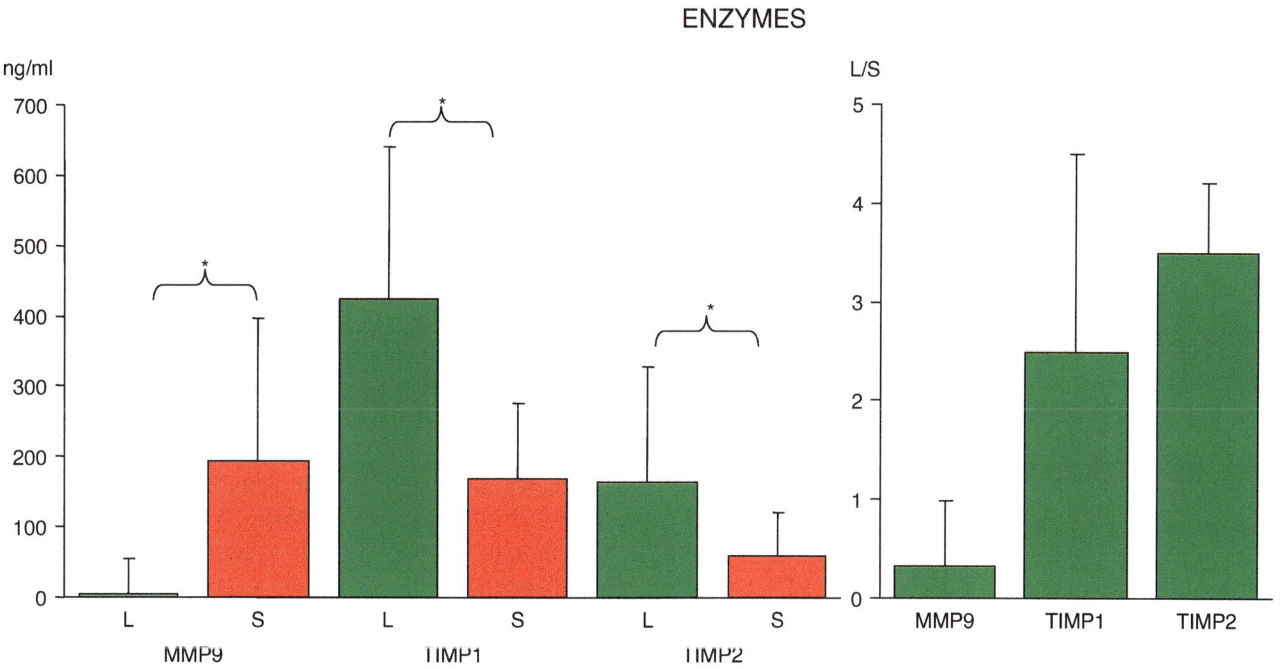

Fig. 14.7 The normal (N) and lymphedema leg (L) lymph enzyme and chemokine concentration (mean, $n = 20$). Higher values for lymphedema lymph for KGF and CCL2 compared with normal

in the inflammatory and fibrotic skin and subcutaneous tissue changes. Cytokines and chemokines can be classified as proteins, peptides, or glycoproteins. The original members of the IL-1 superfamily are IL-1α and IL-1β are produced by epithelial cells, macrophages, monocytes, fibroblasts, and dendritic cells. They form an important part of the inflammatory response of the body against infection. These cytokines increase the expression of adhesion factors on endothelial cells to enable the transmigration of leukocytes [12]. Interleukin-6 (IL-6) is an interleukin that acts as both a pro-

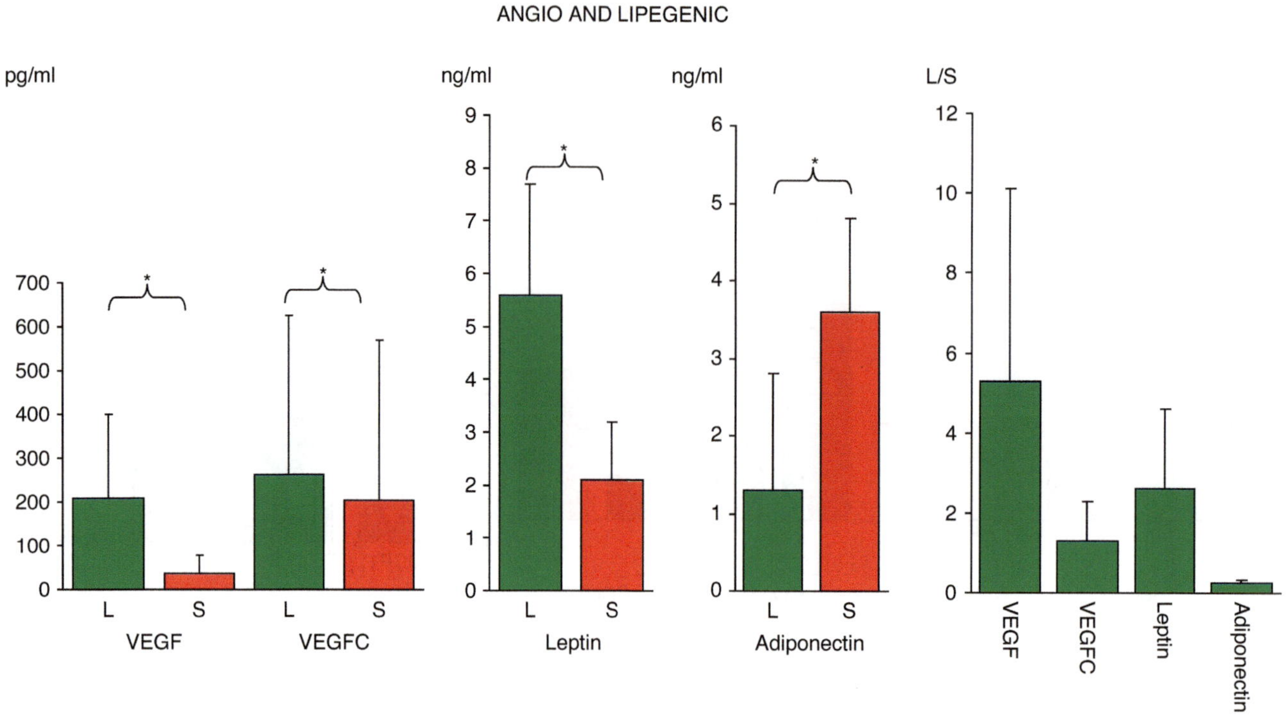

Fig. 14.8 The normal (N) and lymphedema leg (L) lymph growth hormones and lipogenic hormones concentration (mean, $n = 20$). Note high lymphedema lymph levels of VEGF, VEGF C, and leptin

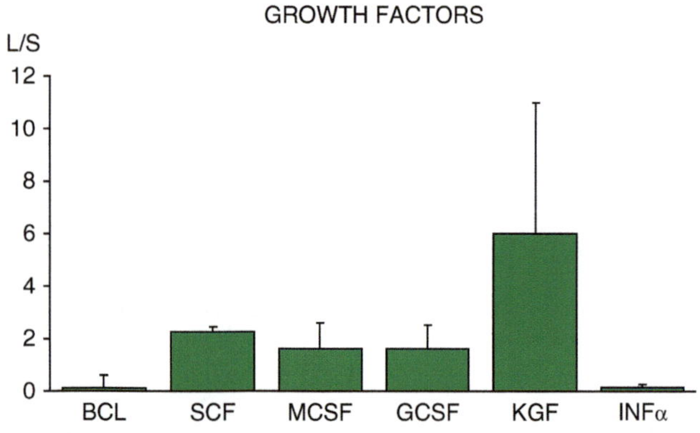

Fig. 14.9 The L/S ratio for the normal and leg lymphedema lymph (mean, $n = 20$). Note that there is increase in the lymphedema lymph values over normal lymph for ILRa, KGF, CCL2, VEGF, VEGF C, and leptin. There is the accumulation of these regulatory proteins in the tissue affecting cellular functions

inflammatory and anti-inflammatory cytokine. It is secreted by T cells and macrophages to stimulate the immune response. IL-6's role as an anti-inflammatory cytokine is mediated through its inhibitory effects on TNF-alpha and IL-1 and activation of IL-1ra and IL-10 [13]. IL-1Ra is secreted by immune cells, epithelial cells, and adipocytes. This protein inhibits the activities of interleukin 1 alpha and beta and modulates a variety of interleukin 1 related immune and inflammatory responses [14]. Tumor Necrosis Factor can cause cytolysis of certain tumor cell lines. It is involved in the induction of cachexia. It is a potent pyrogen, causing fever by direct action or by stimulation of interleukin-1 secretion. It can stimulate cell proliferation and induce cell differentiation under certain conditions [15]. Keratinocyte Growth Factor (KGF), also known as FGF7, is a growth factor present in the epithelialization -phase of wound healing. In this phase, keratinocytes are covering the wound, forming the epithelium. KGF binds to fibroblast growth factor receptor 2b (FGFR2b) [16]. TIMP metallopeptidase inhibitor 1, also known as TIMP1, a tissue inhibitor of metalloproteinases is a glycoprotein that is expressed from several tissues. In addition to its inhibitory role against most of the known MMPs, the encoded protein is able to promote cell proliferation in a wide range of cell types and may also have an anti-apoptotic function [17]. Monocyte chemotactic protein-1 (MCP-1) is a small inducible cytokine called CCL2 recruiting monocytes, T lymphocytes, dendritic cells to the sites of inflammation produced by either tissue injury or infection. It is produced by the lymphatic endothelial cells [18]. CCL21 is a small cytokine belonging to the CC chemokine family present in lymphatic endothelial cells of afferent vessels and lymph node sinuses. CCL21 elicits its effects by binding to a lymphocyte or dendritic cell surface chemokine receptor known as CCR7. It mediates Langerhans cell exit from the epidermis [19]. Vascular endothelial growth factor (VEGF) is a signal protein produced by cells that stimulate vasculogenesis and angiogenesis. It is important signaling proteins involved in both vasculogenesis (the de novo formation of the embryonic circulatory system) and angiogenesis (the growth of blood vessels from pre-existing vasculature). The members of VEGF family are VEGF-A, B, C, and D. VEGF C is regulating lymphangiogenesis [20]. Leptin is involved in the regulation of the inflammatory response, it has been further theorized that leptin's role as an inflammatory marker is to respond specifically to adipose-derived inflammatory cytokines. In terms of both structure and function, leptin resembles IL-6 [21]. Adiponectin is a protein exclusively secreted from adipose tissue, mainly subcutaneous, into the bloodstream and is very abundant in plasma relative to many hormones. Adiponectin is secreted into the bloodstream, where it accounts for approximately 0.01% of all plasma protein [22].

14.3 Lymphedema Serum Proteins in the Lymphedema Inflammatory Process in Skin and Subcutaneous Tissue

Obstruction of tissue fluid and lymph flow caused by obliteration of lymphatic outflow pathways brings about accumulation of filtered serum proteins, recirculating immune cells, cellular debris, metabolic waste products, and microbes colonizing deep tissues. Infection is the most common type of complication observed in lymphedema, and it is promoted by lymphatic system dysfunction, which causes locoregional and systemic immune disorders [23, 24]. DLA is a common and serious complication of obstructive lymphedema of limbs. Both processes as retention of waste products and chronic reaction to microbes bring about gradual destruction of skin and subcutaneous tissue recognized as hyperkeratosis of the epidermis, obliteration of lymphatic collectors and fibrosis of lymph nodes, immune cell infiltrates of epidermis, dermis, and subcutaneous tissue, fibrosis of the dermis and peri-lymphatic tissues and muscular fascia, increase in skin and fat tissue mass including fibroblasts secreting collagen and adipocytes [25].

The question arises whether these chronic processes affecting a large mass of limb tissues can be reflected in the serum by the appearance of specific proteins accumulating and released to circulation from the lymphedematous tissues. Direct analysis of tissue fluid/lymph proteins collected from swollen tissues would have given a better insight into the physiological as well pathological changes in tissues [26–32]. However, in the advanced stages of lymphedema with excess hypertrophied fibroblasts and adipocytes, there is scanty mobile fluid, and its volumes are not sufficient for clinical, biochemical evaluation. Serum concentration of proteins participating in cellular disintegration as caspase 1, HMGB1, Fas CD 95 L, and serpin, as well as, cell growth factors: cortisol, HGF, KGF, IGF were studied. Increased levels of these proteins would reflect the intensity of local processes in the lymphedematous tissues and prompted to control the inflammatory reaction.

14.3.1 Proteins Released from Tissues with Inflammatory Reaction

Serum caspase 1 level was increased approximately twice compared to normal, whereas soluble pro-apoptotic Fas/CD95 was ten times higher (Fig. 14.10). The level of serin protease inhibitor serpin was found twice above the normal values. In 22% of patients, it was higher over mean and 1 standard deviation. HMGB1 (high-mobility group box 1) playing role in autophagy, and the autophagic clearance of dysfunctional mitochondria reached levels twice as high as in normal serum (Fig. 14.10). In 22% of patients, it was higher over mean and 2 standard deviations.

Hormone regulating tissue reconstruction as serum cortisol was slightly elevated, whereas the insulin-like growth factor level was four times higher (Fig. 14.11). In 12% of patients, the values exceeded the mean by one standard deviation. The values of the human growth factor and keratinocyte growth factor remained within normal limits.

14.4 General Analysis

Proteins appearing in serum in high concentrations in patients with lymphedema without systemic clinical and biochemical signs of inflammation indicate that multiple processes of destruction and rebuilding proceed in the lymphedematous tissues. Measuring concentration of caspase 1, sFas, serpin, HMGB1 protein, adiponectin, and leptin give insight into these processes. Caspase-1/Interleukin-1 converting enzyme (ICE) is an evolutionarily conserved enzyme that proteolytically cleaves other proteins, such as the precursors of the inflammatory cytokines interleukin 1β and interleukin 18. It plays a central role in cell immunity as an inflammatory response initiator [33]. Fas ligand (FasL or CD95L) is a type-II transmembrane protein that belongs to the tumor necrosis factor (TNF) family. Its binding with its receptor induces apoptosis. Serpins are a superfamily of proteins with similar struc-

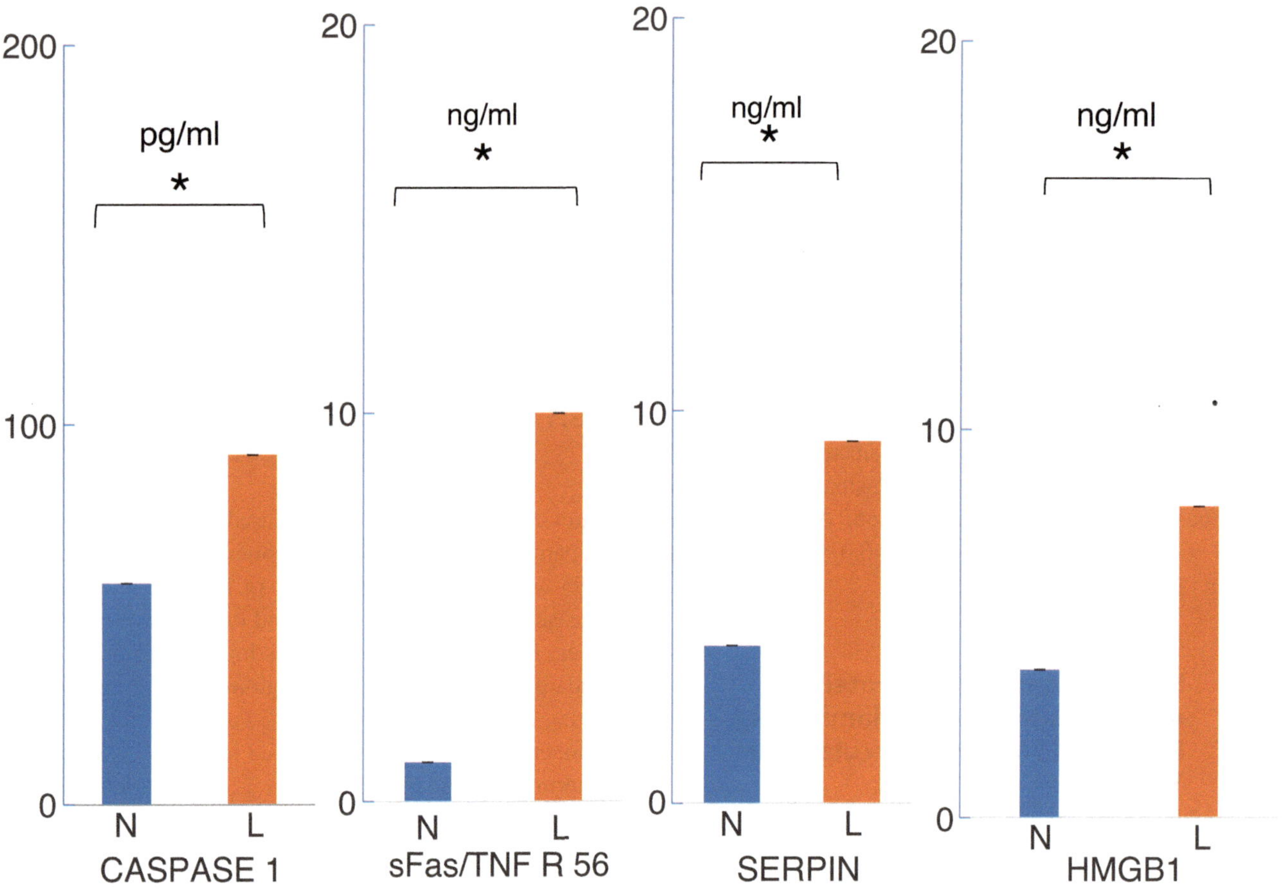

Fig. 14.10 Proteins participating in cellular disintegration in lymphedema and normal tissue fluid/lymph: caspase 1, serpin, fas CD 95 L, HMGB1 ($n = 25$, mean ± sd) *$p < 0.05$. The lymph level of all is higher than that in serum

tures that were identified for their protease inhibition activity. Protease inhibition by serpins controls coagulation and inflammation. Its high levels point to a chronic inflammatory processes in tissues [34]. HMGB1 (high-mobility group box 1) is among the most important chromatin proteins in the nucleus. HMGB1 interacts with nucleosomes, transcription factors, and histones. It is secreted by immune cells (like macrophages, monocytes, and dendritic cells) through leaderless secretory pathway. Activated macrophages and monocytes secrete HMGB1 as a cytokine mediator of Inflammation [35]. Cortisol functions to suppress the immune system, response. Cortisol prevents the release of substances in the body that cause inflammation. It inhibits the production of interleukin (IL)-12, interferon (IFN)-gamma, IFN-alpha, and tumor necrosis factor (TNF)-alpha by antigen-presenting cells (APCs) and T helper (Th1) cells but upregulates IL-4, IL-10, and IL-13 by Th2 cells [36]. Human Growth hormone (hGH), also known as somatotropin, is a peptide hormone that stimulates growth, cell reproduction, and cell regeneration in humans. It is thus important in human development. It is a type of mitogen which is specific only to certain kinds of cells [37]. Keratinocyte growth factor (KGF), also known as FGF7, is a growth factor present in the epithelialization phase of wound healing. In this phase, keratinocytes are covering the wound, forming the epithelium. KGF binds to fibroblast growth factor receptor 2b (FGFR2b). In lymphedema hyperkeratosis is the typical consequence of lymph stasis. In an indirect way KGF also stimulates fibroblasts proliferation [38]. IGF-1 is generated in the liver is the anabolic effector and linear growth-promoting hormone of the pituitary growth hormone (GH). IGF-1 acts on the proliferative cells. IGF-1 also induces organ and tissue growth [39].

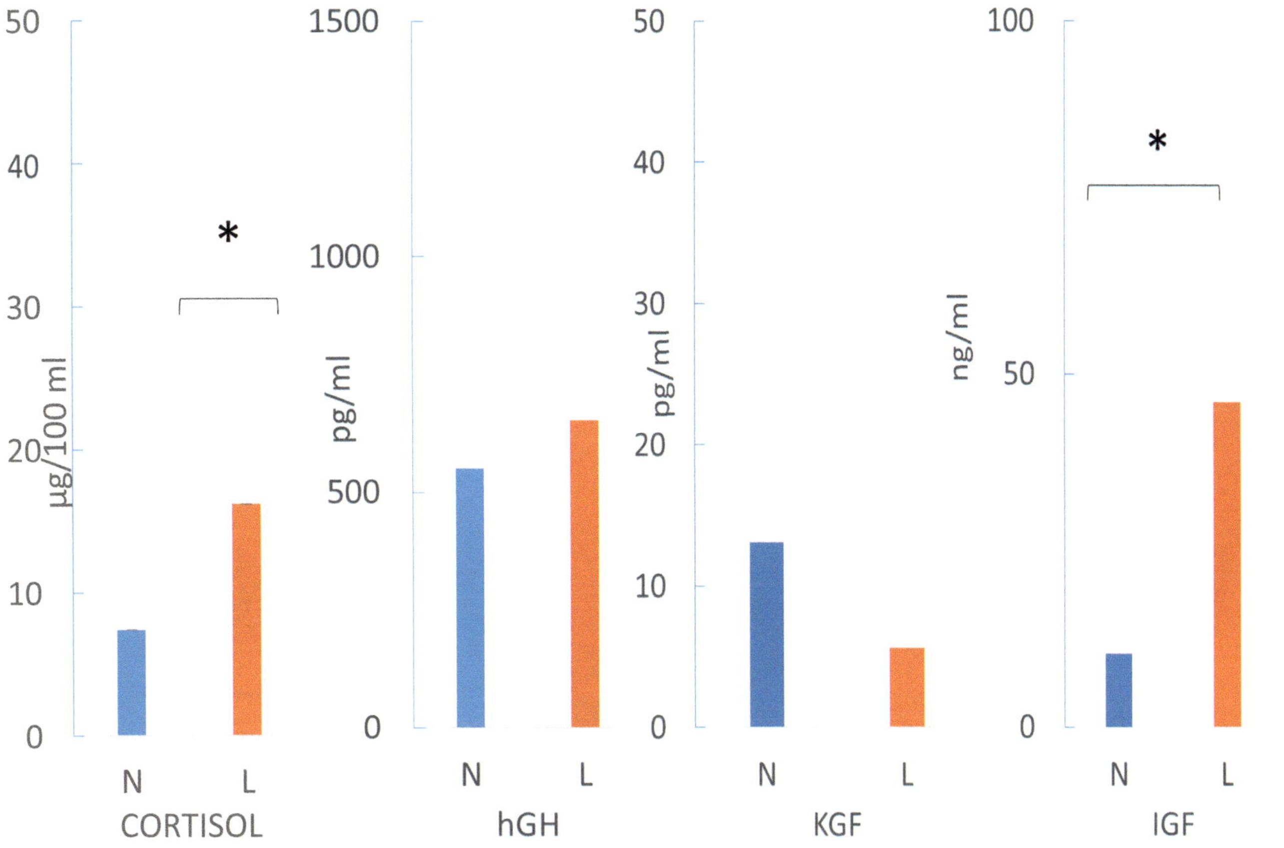

Fig. 14.11 Cell growth factors in lymphedema and normal tissue fluid/lymph: cortisol, hGF (human growth factor), KGF (keratinocyte growth factor), IGF1 (insulin growth factor) ($n = 25$, mean ± sd), $^*p < 0.05$. Cortisol and IGF1 level was higher than in serum

14.5 Lipids in Lymph of the Lymphedema Legs

The question arises whether excess lipids in tissue fluid/lymph in lymph drainage obstruction may lodge in adipocytes, increasing their volume and density. The tissue fluid contains lipoproteins, glycerol, choline, and enzymes as lipase, adipokines, and leptin. They all participate in subcutaneous adipogenesis. How are lipids filtered from blood at the exchange capillaries to the intercellular space and accumulate in the adipocyte liquid environment, as well as, how lipids contained in the stagnant tissue fluid/lymph in lymphedema are taken up by the resident adipocytes, needs more clarification.

Lipids are transported from the gut in a chemical form of lipoproteins as triglycerols and cholesterol, through the blood to tissues. This brings about a build-up of lipid concentration in the tissue cell environment. The in-tissue traffic of lipids is bidirectional. Blood-derived lipids are absorbed by adipocytes and other resident cells, and soon they leave cells in the reverse cholesterol transport mechanism back to tissue fluid/lymph and blood (Fig. 14.12) [40].

In this way, the body removes excess cholesterol from peripheral tissues and delivers it to the liver. From there it will be redistributed to other tissues or removed from the body by the gallbladder. The main lipoprotein involved in this process is the HDL-c. Thus, the type and volume of lipids in the tissue fluid surrounding cells and in lymph depend on influx to tissue as plasma filtrate and efflux from cells back to tissue fluid in the reverse cholesterol transport (Fig. 14.13).

The question arises: the lipid concentration and distribution of various lipid types in tissue fluid/lymph of limbs with obstructed lymphatics. It is well known that in the early stages of lymphedema, adipocyte hyperplasia is observed in regions where the tissue space is expanded by the interstitial fluid pressure and filled up by edema fluid.

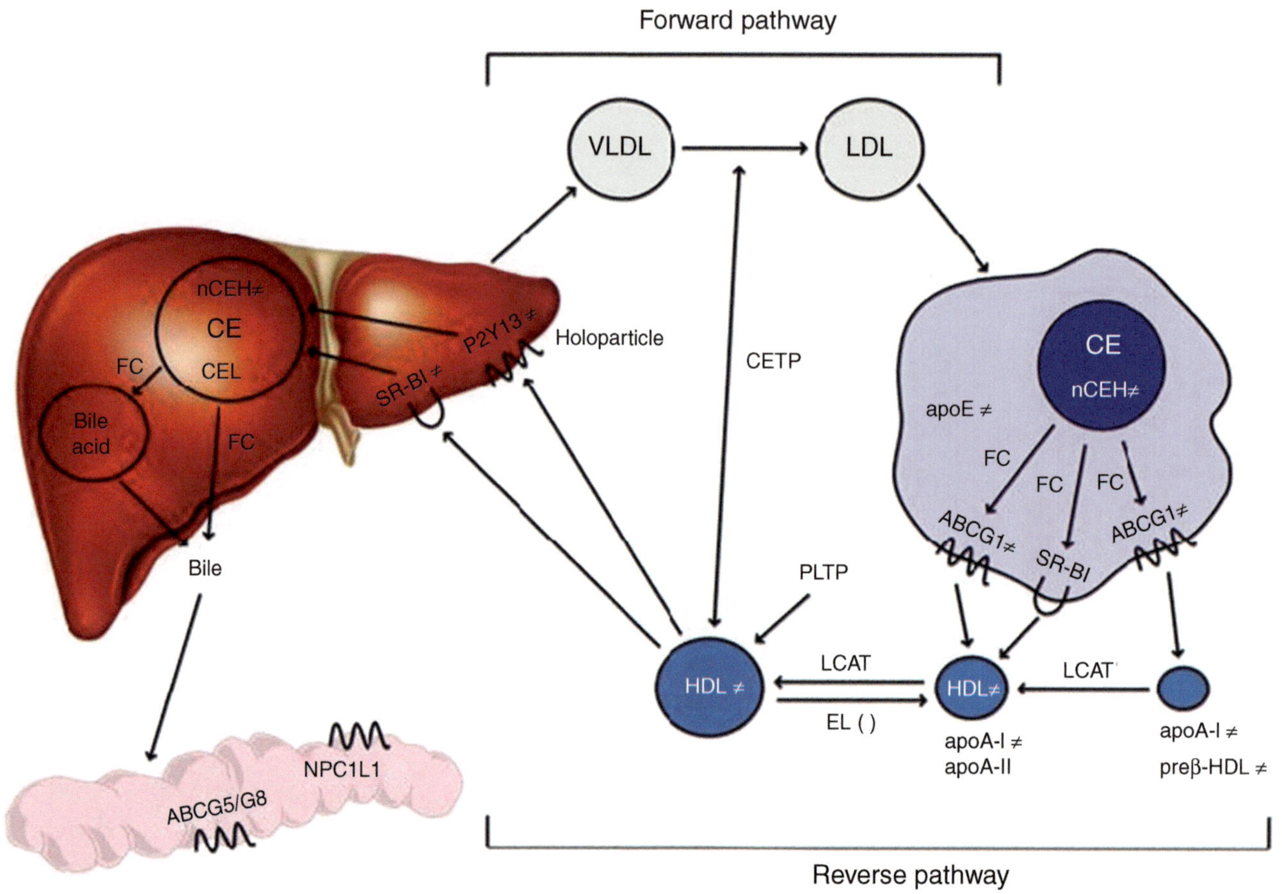

Fig. 14.12 Cholesterol transport pathways in humans. Cholesterol synthetized within the liver or intestine is secreted by hepatocytes in the form of apoB-containing lipoproteins in a forward pathway to supply cholesterol to tissue fluid and on this way to the peripheral cells. Free cholesterol can be effluxed binding transporter A1 (ABCA1) with apoA-I as acceptor or via ABCG1 with more mature spherical HDL particles serving as acceptor. Additional efflux capacity might be provided by scavenger receptor class B type 1 (SR-BI) or by so-called aqueous diffusion. Within HDL, cholesterol is esterified by lecithin cholesterol acyltransferase (LCAT). The reverse cholesterol transport of the effluxed cholesterol from cells is its transfer back to the liver. It is secreted first to the tissue fluid, further transported via lymphatics as lymph to the thorax venous angle and blood. The upper circle denotes the forward and the lower the reverse cholesterol transport in a pathway blood-tissue fluid/lymph-cells-tissue/fluid/lymph-blood (modified from 4). *apoA-I* apolipoprotein, *apoB* apolipoprotein, *CE* cholesterol esters, *CETP* cholesteryl ester transfer protein, *LDL* low-density lipoprotein, lecithin cholesterol acyltransferase, *LCAT* lecithin-cholesterol acyl transferase, *HDL* high-density lipoprotein, *SR-BI* scavenger receptor class B type 1, *VLDL* very low-density lipoprotein

14.5.1 Lymphedema Lymph Lipid Concentration

Concentration of tissue fluid/lymph cholesterol, HDL, LDL, triglycerides, and lipoproteins in lower limb plasma and tissue fluid/lymph is shown on Fig. 14.14.

Tissue fluid/lymph values were lower than in plasma. The difference was between 15 and 40% depending on the type of lipid. Concentration of Apo1A, ApoB, lipase, and total proteins in tissue fluid/lymph was at the ratio below 10% of plasma (Figs. 14.15 and 14.16)

14.5.2 Analysis of Lymph Lipid Concentration in the Aspect of Adipogenesis

We previously studied the tissue transport of lipids in the lymph of lower limbs of the healthy volunteers in the aspect of their role in atherogenesis. The normal mean tissue fluid/lymph level of cholesterol ester was 25 mg/dL, of triglyceride 26 mg/dL, and of lipoproteins 4.6 mg/dL. These data were used for comparison with those obtained from the lymphedema limbs. Interestingly, the proportions of various types of lipids were in tissue fluid/lymph different from those

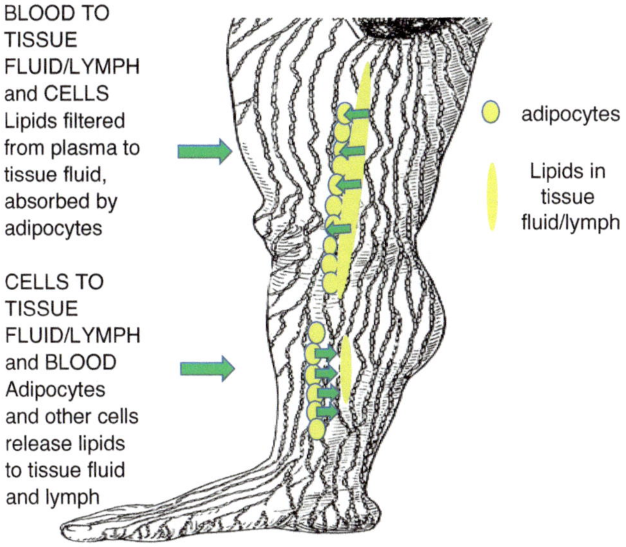

Fig. 14.13 A scheme of forward cholesterol transport in the human lower limb from blood to tissue fluid and cells and reverse from cells to tissue fluid/lymph and blood. Arrows show the pathways of lipid trafficking. In normal lymphatic drainage of tissues, lipids flow from blood to the tissue space and adipocytes (upper part of figure), and back from cells to tissue space and lymphatics and blood (lower part of figure)

in plasma. For example, the HDL cholesterol/nonHDL cholesterol ratio in lymph exceeded that in plasma. This suggested supplementing the blood-derived lipids with those released from adipocytes and other cells in reverse cholesterol transport. The obtained data illustrated a complex process of tissue adipogenesis [41].

The bidirectional movement of lipids in tissues cannot be accurately measured in terms of mass to-and-fro trafficking. However, a theoretical model can be constructed. Lipids are filtered to the extravascular space at the exchange capillary level. In their liquid form, they are taken up by resident cells, among them adipocytes. The reverse cholesterol transport drives them back from cells to the tissue space. Under normal conditions, with the functioning lymphatic system, they have transported away to the blood. Obstruction of the lymphatic drainage brings about accumulation of lipids in the tissue fluid from two sources. One is the unimpaired blood capillary supply system, and the other is the resident cells reverse transport. The influx from these sources to tissue fluid/lymph outweighs the efflux. As long as the interstitial space can expand, the tissue fluid concentration remains unchanged. Once the tissue space becomes filled up, the lipid

Fig. 14.14 Concentration of cholesterol, HDL, LDL, triglycerides, and lipoproteins in lower limb plasma and tissue fluid/lymph ($n = 20$, values are mean ± sd). The concentration of all lipids is higher in plasma than lymph, however, note a high level of tissue fluid/lymph cholesterol and triglyceride levels. *P* plasma, *L* tissue fluid/lymph, *CH* cholesterol, *HDL* high-density lipoproteins, *LDL* low-density lipoproteins, *TG* triglycerides, *Lp* lipoproteins

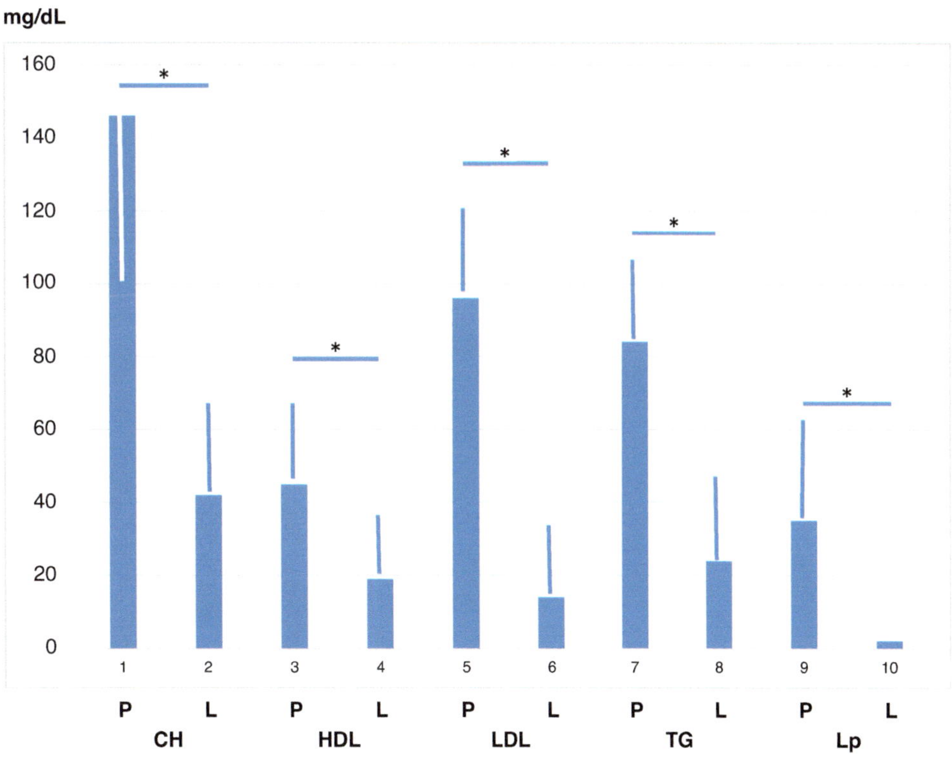

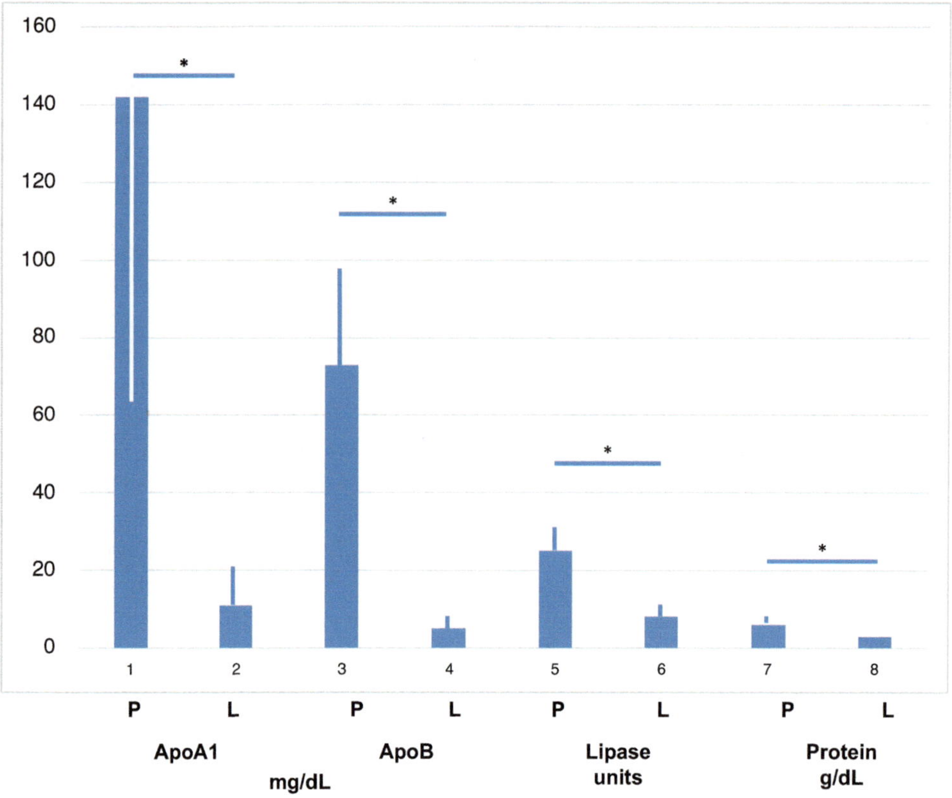

Fig. 14.15 Concentration of Apo1A, ApoB, lipase, and total proteins in patients with lymphedema/lipedema of lower limb ($n = 20$, values are means ± sd), *P* plasma, *L* tissue fluid/lymph. Low levels of tissue fluid/lymph of apolipoproteins and lipase is the result of their low transport through the blood capillaries

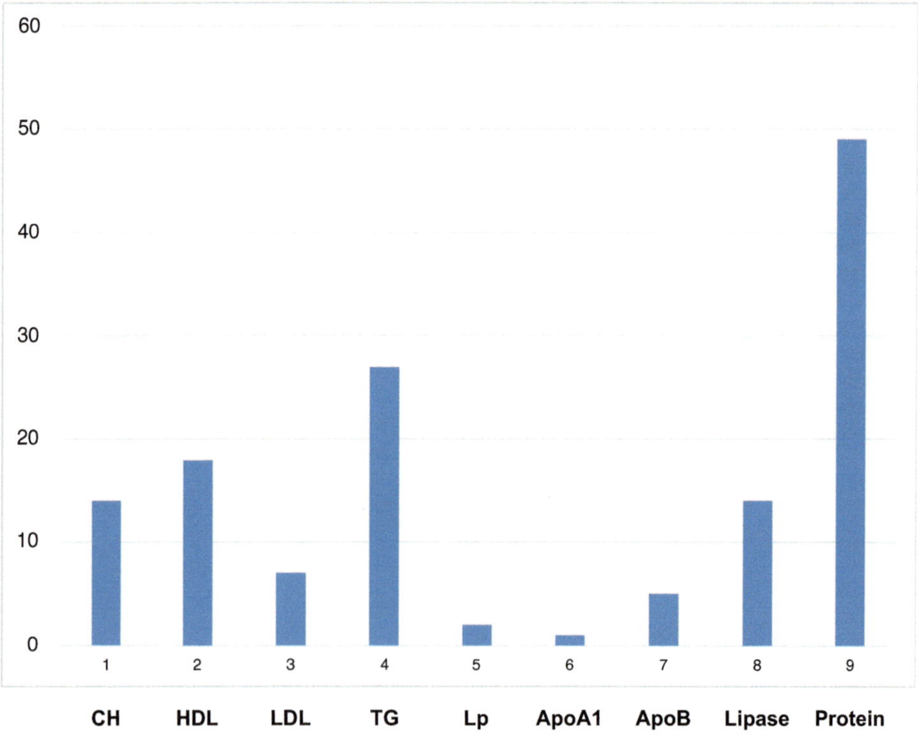

Fig. 14.16 Tissue fluid/lymph lipids to plasma ratio in patients with lower limb lymphedema/lipedema ($n = 20$, values are means ± sd). Note the relatively high ratio for CH, HDL, LDL, TG, and Lp

concentration rises, and most likely the reverse cholesterol transport is stopped. The effect is an increase in the adipocyte size.

Lipids are present in tissue fluid/lymph at lower than in serum but still relatively high concentrations, and the reverse cholesterol transport can be stopped in regions deprived of lymphatic drainage, resulting in gradual lipid accumulation in adipocytes and probably other resident cells. This may explain formation of excess adipose tissue in obstructive lymphedema.

References

General Analysis

1. Olszewski WL, Engeset A, Łukasiewicz H. Immunoglobulins, complement and lysozyme in leg lymph of normal men. Scand J Clin Lab Invest. 1977;37:669–74.
2. Olszewski WL, Engeset A. Immune proteins, enzymes and electrolytes in human peripheral lymph. Lymphology. 1978;11:156–64.
3. Olszewski WL. Immune proteins, cell interactions and immunoregulatory hormones: lymph versus blood. Lymphology. 1987;20:239–43.
4. Olszewski WL, Loe K, Engeset A. Immune proteins and other biochemical constituents of peripheral lymph in patients with malignancy and postirradiation lymphedema. Lymphology. 1992;25:166–71.
5. Olszewski WL, Jamal S, Łukomska B, Manokaran G, Grzelak I. Immune proteins in peripheral tissue fluid-lymph in patients with filarial lymphedema of the lower limbs. Lymphology. 1992;25:166–71.
6. Olszewski WL. Collection and physiological measurements of peripheral lymph and interstitial fluid in man. Lymphology. 1977;10:137–45.
7. Olszewski WL, Grzelak I, Ziółkowska A, Engeset A. Epidermal cell thymocyte activity factor/interleukin 1 (ETAF/IL)-like activity in lymph drained from normal human skin. Lymphology. 1988;21:118–23.
8. Olszewski WL, Grzelak I, Ziolkowska A, Engeset A. Effect of local hyperthermia on lymph immune cells and lymphokines of normal human skin. J Surg Oncol. 1989;11:109–16.
9. Olszewski WL, Pazdur J, Kubasiewicz E, Zaleska M, Cooke CJ, Miller NE. Lymph draining from foot joints in rheumatoid arthritis provides insight into local cytokine and chemokine production and transport to lymph nodes. Arthritis Rheum. 2001;44:541–9.
10. Olszewski WL, Engeset A, Sokołowski J. Lymph flow and protein in the normal male leg during lying, getting up, and walking. Lymphology. 1977;10:178–83.
11. Zaleska MT, Olszewski WL, Durlik M, Miller NE. Signaling proteins are represented in tissue fluid/lymph from soft tissues of normal human legs at concentrations different from serum. Lymphat Res Biol. 2013;11(4):203–10.
12. Blanton RA, Kupper TS, McDougall JK, Dower S. Regulation of interleukin 1 and its receptor in human keratinocytes. Proc Natl Acad Sci. 1989;86:1273–7.
13. Heinrich PC, Behrmann I, Haan S, Hermanns HM, Müller-Newen G, Schaper F. Principles of interleukin-6-type cytokine signalling and its regulation. Biochem J. 2003;374:1–20.
14. Dinarello CA. The interleukin-1 family: 10 years of discovery. FASEB J. 1994;8(15):1314–25.
15. Bashir MM, Sharma MR, Werth VP. TNF-alpha production in the skin. Arch Dermatol Res. 2009;30:87–91.
16. Rubin JS, Bottaro DP, Chedid M, Miki T, Ron D, Cheon G, Taylor WG, Fortney E, Sakata H, Finch PW, et al. Keratinocyte growth factor. Cell Biol Int. 1995;19(5):399–411.
17. Reichenstein M, Reich R, LeHoux JG, Hanukoglu I. ACTH induces TIMP-1 expression and inhibits collagenase in adrenal cortex cells. Mol Cell Endocrinol. 2004;215:109–14.
18. Mancardi S, Vecile E, Dusetti N, Calvo E, Stanta G, Burrone OR, Dobrina A. Evidence of CXC, CC and C chemokine production by lymphatic endothelial cells. Immunology. 2003;108:523–30.
19. Randolph GJ. Dendritic cell migration to lymph nodes: cytokines, chemokines, and lipid mediators. Semin Immunol. 2001;13:267–74.
20. Shin HY, Smith ML, Toy KJ, et al. VEGF-C mediates cyclic pressure-induced endothelial cell proliferation. Physiol Genomics. 2002;11:245–51.
21. Brennan AM, Mantzoros CS. Drug Insight: the role of leptin in human physiology and pathophysiology – emerging clinical applications. Nat Clin Pract Endocrinol Metab. 2006;2(6):318–27.
22. Díez JJ, Iglesias P. The role of the novel adipocyte-derived hormone adiponectin in human disease. Eur J Endocrinol. 2003;148:293–300.
23. Olszewski WL. Episodic dermatolymphangioadenitis (DLA) in patients with lymphedema of the lower extremities before and after administration of benzathine penicillin: a preliminary study. Lymphology. 1996;29(3):126–31.
24. Olszewski WL, Jamal S, Manokaran G, Pani S, Kumaraswami V, Kubicka U, Lukomska B, Dworczynski A, Swoboda E, Meisel-Mikolajczyk F. Bacteriologic studies of skin, tissue fluid, lymph, and lymph nodes in patients with filarial lymphedema. Am J Trop Med Hyg. 1997;57(1):7–15.
25. Olszewski W. Pathology and histochemistry. In: Lee BB, Bergan J, Rockson SG, editors. Lymphedema-A concise compendium of theory and practice. Cham: Springer; 2011. p. 75.
26. Olszewski WL, Jamal S, Lukomska B, Manokaran G, Grzelak I. Immune proteins in peripheral tissue fluid-lymph in patients with filarial lymphedema of the lower limbs. Lymphology. 1992;25(4):166–71.
27. Olszewski WL, Jamal S, Manokaran G, Gałkowska H, Grzelak I, Zaleska M. Lymph cytokines in obstructive lymphedema – a sign of chronic inflammatory reaction. Lymphology. 1998;31:126–31.
28. Olszewski WL, Pazdur J, Kubasiewicz E, Zaleska M, Cooke CJ, Miller NE. Lymph draining from foot joints in rheumatoid arthritis provides insight into local cytokine and chemokine production and transport to lymph nodes. Arthritis Rheum. 2001;44(3):541–9.
29. Olszewski WL. Pathophysiological aspects of lymphedema of human limbs: I. Lymph protein composition. Lymphat Res Biol. 2003;1(3):235–43.
30. Interewicz B, Olszewski WL, Leak LV, Petricoin EF, Liotta LA. Profiling of normal human leg lymph proteins using the 2-D electrophoresis and SELDI-TOF mass spectrophotometry approach. Lymphology. 2004;37(2):65–72.
31. Zaleska MT, Olszewski WL, Durlik M, Miller NE. Signaling proteins are represented in tissue fluid/lymph from soft tissues of normal human legs at concentrations different from serum. Lymphat Res Biol. 2013;11(4):203–10.
32. Zaleska MT, Olszewski WL. Serum immune proteins in limb lymphedema reflecting tissue processes caused by lymph stasis and chronic dermato-lymphangio-adenitis (Cellulitis). Lymphat Res Biol. 2017;15(3):246–51.
33. Denes A, Lopez-Castejon G, Brough D. Caspase-1: is IL-1 just the tip of the ICEberg? Cell Death Dis. 2012;3:e338.
34. Wajant H. The Fas signaling pathway: more than a paradigm. Science. 2002;296(5573):1635–6.
35. Silverman GA, Whisstock JC, Bottomley SP, Huntington JA, Kaiserman D, Luke CJ, Pak SC, Reichhart JM, Bird PI. Serpins

flex their muscle: I. Putting the clamps on proteolysis in diverse biological systems. JBiol Chem. 2010;285(32):24299–305.
36. Bianchi ME, Agresti A. HMG proteins: dynamic players in gene regulation and differentiation. Curr Opin Genet Dev. 2005;15(5):496–506.
37. Ranabir S, Reetu K. Stress and hormones. Indian J Endocrinol Metab. 2011;15(1):18–22.
38. Finch PW, Rubin JS. Keratinocyte growth factor/fibroblast growth factor 7, a homeostatic factor with therapeutic potential for epithelial protection and repair. Adv Cancer Res. 2004;91:69–136.
39. Laron Z. IGF-1 and insulin as growth hormones. Novartis Found Symp. 2004;262:56–77.

Lipids in Lymph of the Lymphedema Legs

40. Wijtske A, Tietge UW. Regulation of reverse cholesterol transport – a comprehensive appraisal of available animal studies. Nutr Metab. 2012;9:25.
41. Nanjee MN, Cooke CJ, Olszewski WL, Miller NE. Lipid and apolipoprotein concentrations in prenodal leg lymph of fasted humans: associations with plasma concentrations in normal subjects, lipoprotein lipase deficiency, and LCAT deficiency. J Lipid Res. 2000;41:1317–27.

Inflammation

15

Waldemar L. Olszewski and Marzanna T. Zaleska

Keywords

Lymphedema · Lymph · Bacteria · Antibiotics
Benzathine penicillin

15.1 Dermato-Lymphangio-Adenitis in Lymphedema

Summary (Figs. 15.1)
(Fig. 15.1): The functions of the lymphatic system include the detection, transport away, and neutralizing of microorganisms penetrating integuments. In lymphedema, most lymphatic collectors are obliterated, which cause stagnation of the tissue fluid containing microorganisms that permanently permeate sole and hand skin. These microbes grow up in tissue and evoke the immune reaction of the host. This inflammatory condition is called dermato-lymphangio-adenitis (DLA). Symptoms of acute DLA disappear after 3–7 days of wide-spectrum antibiotic therapy. However, some bacteria survived and, according to the literature, transform into the persister dormant form with very low metabolism. In this form, they do not respond to antibiotics. The most effective way to prevent the revival of dormant bacteria and decreasing the rate of acute DLA is the administration of low-dose for a long time benzathine penicillin [1].

W. L. Olszewski (✉)
Department of Vascular Surgery, Central Clinical Hospital, Ministry of Internal Affairs, Warsaw, Poland

M. T. Zaleska
Department of Vascular Surgery, Central Clinical Hospital, Ministry of Internal Affairs, Warsaw, Poland

Department of Applied Physiology, Mossakowski Medical Research Institute, Polish Academy of Sciences, Warsaw, Poland

15.1.1 Rationale for Using Term Dermato-Lymphangio-Adenitis

Tissues with chronic edema are the area of permanent inflammation called dermato-lymphangio-adenitis (DLA). About 50% of patients with lymphedema develop acute DLA, and 95% have chronic inflammation (Figs. 15.2 and 15.3). Acute inflammation of the skin and subcutaneous tissue (DLA) is known as erysipelas or cellulitis. Both terms are misnomer. Erysipelas is contagious disease caused by Streptococci. The term cellulitis often refers to the painful fat tissue in the lower limbs. DLA develops in tissues with tissue fluid/lymph stasis and is caused by bacteria that penetrate the skin (most often Staphylococci). Symptoms such as high fever, redness, and soreness of the skin subside after 3–5 days of antibiotic treatment. But they usually relapse. Long-term treatment with low-doses of benzathine penicillin reduces acute DLA recurrence to 3–5%. This protocol is effective, safe, and can be used for years in patients with chronic edema. No resistance to penicillin has been noted.

15.1.2 General Overview of Lymphedema Limbs Infections

Infections and inflammation of the skin and subcutaneous tissue are observe much more often on the legs and arms than in other part of the body. This is the result of the close the-contact of hands and feet with the environment in which microorganisms and chemical substances are present [1]. (Fig. 15.4).

The most frequently isolated bacteria strains from the skin surface are *S. epidermidis*, *S. aureus*, and Corynebacteria. These are the commensal bacteria that are always present on the skin surface and sweat glands and hair follicles. Pathogenic bacteria like Enterococcus, Enterobacter, Acinetobacter, Proteus, *E. coli*, and Pseudomonas are also found on the skin of calf and feet. They originate from the perineum region and fall with desquamated epidermal scales.

N. Liu (ed.), *Peripheral Lymphedema*, https://doi.org/10.1007/978-981-16-3484-0_15

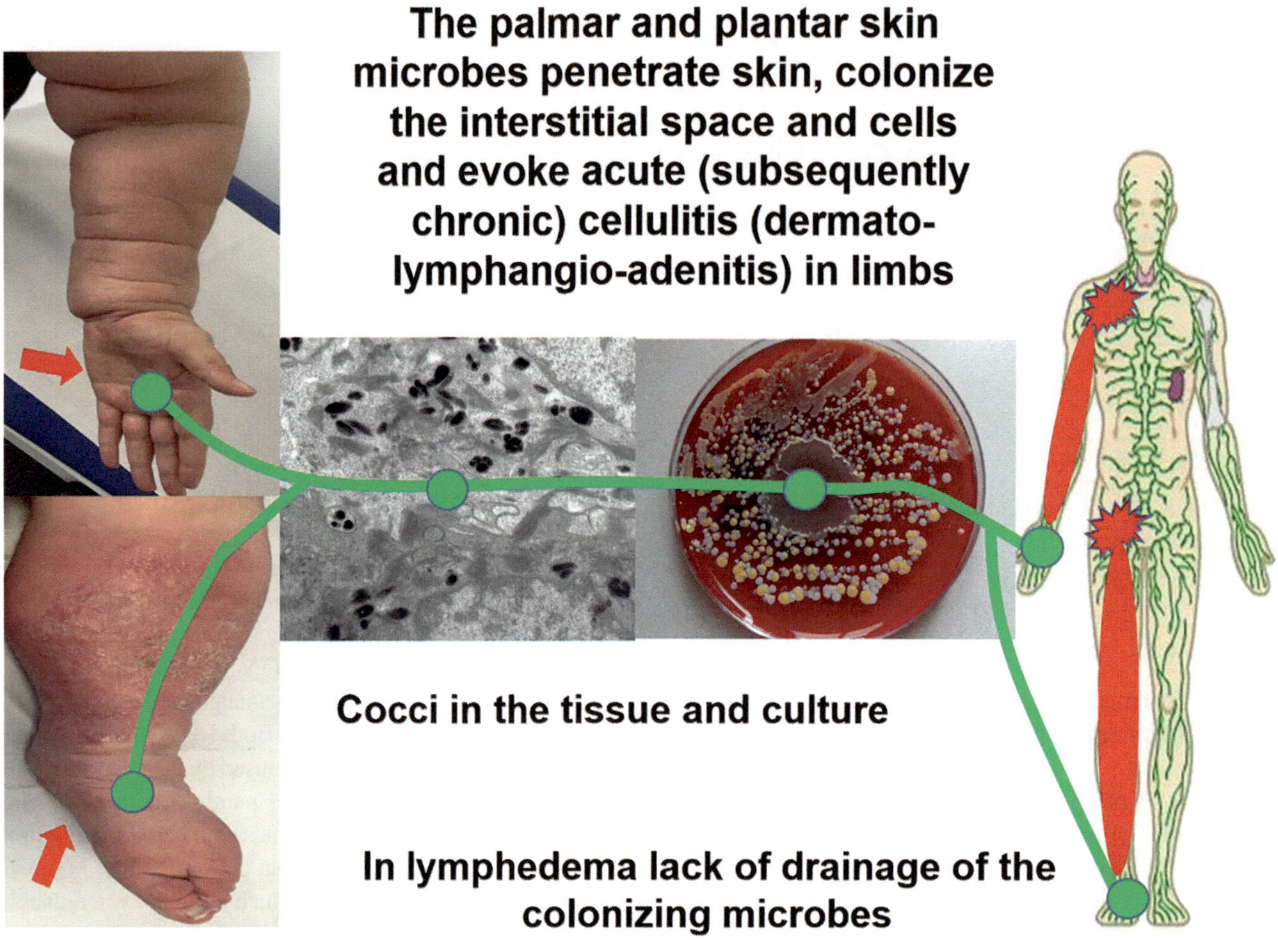

Fig. 15.1 Most lymphatic collectors are obliterated in lymphedema, which causes stagnation of the tissue fluid containing microorganisms that permanently permeate sole and hand skin. Therefore we can detect these microbes both in the tissues and in the tissue fluid

As long as the commensal bacteria remain on the skin surface, they are not pathogenic. However, even minor damage to the epidermis causes them to penetrate into the deeper layers of the skin and subcutaneous tissue and induce a local host response [2, 3]. The threshold which triggers a host response is the 105 mass of bacteria per gram of the tissue.

15.1.3 Clinical Aspects of Dermato-Lymphangio-Adenitis (DLA)

15.1.3.1 Lymphangitis

The initial symptoms of DLA are usually diagnosed as lymphangitis. In this condition, we observe red, warm, and painful strip along the course of the superficial lymphatics. There is also usually a fever. Initially, there is no inflammatory spreading of the lesion [4]. Lymphoscintigrams show the sites and extent of inflammatory changes (Fig. 15.5).

15.1.3.2 Chronic DLA

The non-treated lymphangitis often changed into a chronic form. This is DLA. Patients with lymphedema have a high risk of infection and chronic DLA due to impairment elimination of bacteria by the lymphatic vessels [5]. According to the literature, about 40% of patients with edema, regardless of etiology, suffer from infection of the skin and deep tissues. The recurrence rate of DLA is higher in patients with lower limb edema and among them with post-inflammatory etiology. Approximately 50% of these patients develop recurrent DLA attacks. In upper limb edema after mastectomy, infection in the form of acute and later chronic DLA are observed in 20–40% [6]. Presumably, it is due to the close contact of the lower limb with bacteria from the environment. Skin infections of various etiology (bacterial, fungal, or viral) develop more often there than in other regions of the body. The factor that increases the frequency of DLA attacks is the long duration of edema. Each episode of infection is associated with an increase in limb volume [1].

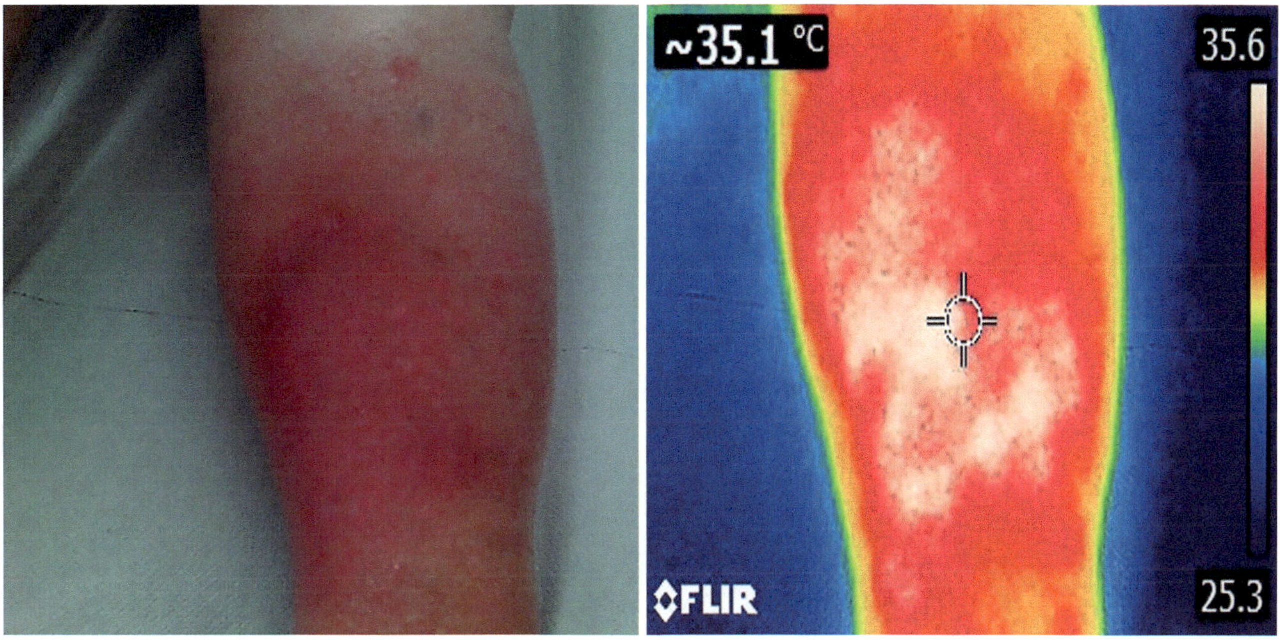

Fig. 15.2 Clinical picture of DLA of the lower limb with the erythema. Thermography shows increase of leg skin temperature. Specific for lymphedema is widespread inflammatory involvement of soft tissues of foot and calf, sometimes also thigh. This is different from erythema nodosum or venous dermatosclerosis with circumscribed foci

15.1.3.3 Acute DLA

Severe systemic symptoms during attacks of DLA resemble those of septicemia. The clinical signs include erythema and soreness of the skin, sometimes red streaks along the superficial lymphatic vessels, and enlargement and pain of LNs. In acute episodes there are also systemic symptoms like males, fever, and shivers. However, in subacute or latent course, only skin symptoms are observed. After each episode of DLA, swollen increases. Bacteremia also occurs in patients with acute DLA [7]. According to the literature, bacteria are isolated from the blood in 21% of cases with acute DLA and in 26% of cases with subacute DLA. Diversity of bacteria isolated from blood and tissues in these patients reveals their origin from the skin surface. After breaking the skin barrier, tissue colonization occurs and spreads into the blood. There are also fatal cases [1].

15.1.3.4 Differential Diagnosis of Lymphangitis, Erysipelas and Dermato-Lymphangio-Adenitis

These three terms are often used interchangeably, although they refer to various conditions. This may influence the choice of therapy. (a) Lymphangitis is a local change in the skin and subcutaneous tissue caused by the own bacterial flora. It has a mild clinical course, but at the site of inflammation, the lymphatic vessels may be damaged, and lymphedema may develop as a consequence. (b) Erysipelas is a primary acute local spreading condition in the skin with systemic reaction. It is caused by streptococci. It may be contagious. It either develops in lymphedematous tissues or is the primary factor for its development, (c) Dermato-lymphangio-adenitis is a secondary condition caused by own bacteria, mainly Staphylococci but not Streptococci. Developed as a complication of lymphedema. It is non-contagious [8]. The frequency of recurrences of DLA is high and increases with the duration of the edema. DLA is sometimes called cellulitis. This is a misnomer as cellulitis is a term referring to the accumulation of painful adipose tissue in the thigh and calf [1].

15.1.3.5 Pathomechanism of Tissue Infection and Inflammation in Lymphedema

Under physiological conditions, bacteria constantly inhabiting the surface of the skin and those from the environment after penetrating into the tissues are carried by lymphatic vessels to regional lymph nodes where they are eliminated (Fig. 15.4). The mass of bacteria is low and docs not elicit a clinically detectable reaction of the host. When lymphatic transport is impaired or totally halted, as in the lymphedema, bacteria colonize the tissues and proliferate. The increased mass of bacteria caused an inflammatory reaction. The histological pictures reveal lymphocytes and granulocytes, monocytes, and Langerhans´ cells infiltrating dermis and epidermis. If there is a rapid multiplication of bacteria, an inflammatory reaction of the skin and subcutaneous tissue of the limb develops with systemic septic symptoms and bacteremia [1]. (Fig. 15.6).

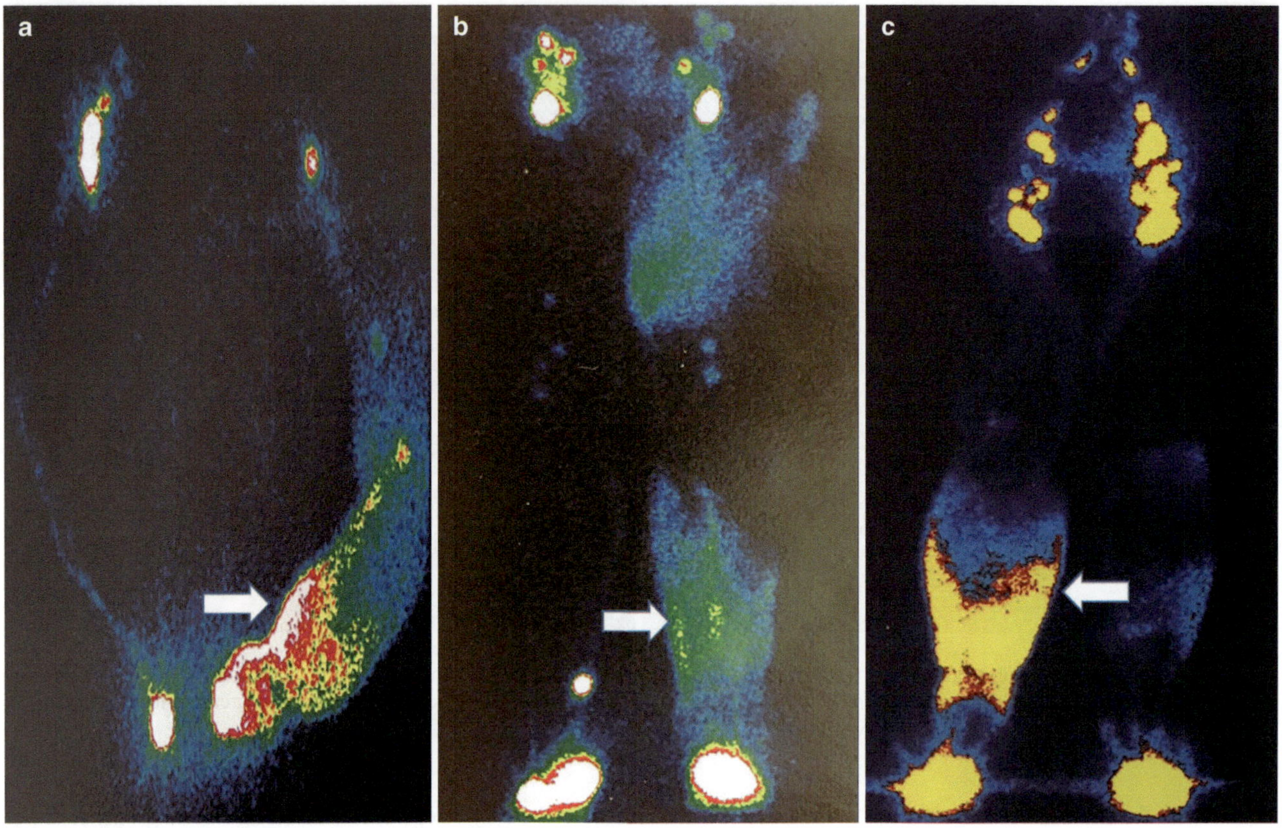

Fig. 15.3 Lymphoscintigraphic pictures of limbs affected by lymphedema and chronic DLA. (**a**) left upper limb, arrow shows a large focus of accumulation of edema fluid, (**b**) left lower limb with lymphedema after prostatectomy with pelvic lymphadenectomy and radiotherapy. The calf, thigh, and hypogastrium collect edema fluid (arrow). Skin is hot. (**c**) most common post-dermatitis right lower limb lymphedema, edema of the calf (arrow), recurrent DLA

15.1.4 Bacteriology of Lower Limb Skin

15.1.4.1 Bacterial Flora of Normal Foot and Calf Skin

The microbes are detected from all swabs taken from the skin surface of the feet and calves [1, 8]. The most frequently isolated species are Cocci (60%). 90% of them are *S. epidermidis* and other coagulase-negative strains. Among other, less frequent strains are *E. coli*, Citrobacter, Corynebacterium, Acinetobacter, Proteus, and *Bacillus cereus*. All strains are derived from patients skin, perineum, and anal area.

15.1.4.2 Bacterial Flora of Normal Leg Lymph

As our previous investigations on lymphatic lipid transport revealed in 12% of samples taken from healthy individuals, *S. epidermidis* was detected [1].

15.1.4.3 Bacterial Flora of Lymphedematous Leg Lymph

In European patients, Cocci are the most frequent (60% of simples) with the prevalence of *S. epidermidis* and *S. aureus* [1]. (Fig. 15.7).

15.1.5 Bacteria Persisters

Antibiotic therapy kills most bacteria. However, some of them survive and undergo modification into a persister form or small colony variants (SCV) with very low metabolism [1]. Figure 15.8).

In this form, without the division and incorporation of antibiotic, they remain in the tissues for months and years, and upon signals from the host, they return to their normal functions and start reproducing [9, 10]. The electron microscopy pictures reveal single widely dispersed Cocci (Fig. 15.9).

15.1.6 Sensitivity of Isolates to Antibiotics

Bacteria isolated from skin, subcutaneous tissue, lymph/tissue fluid, and lymph nodes both from patients with lymphedema and healthy subjects show susceptibility to most of the antibiotics. The surprise was the low susceptibility of bacteria to penicillin, although this antibiotic proved to be very efficient in the prevention of DLA recurrences in a

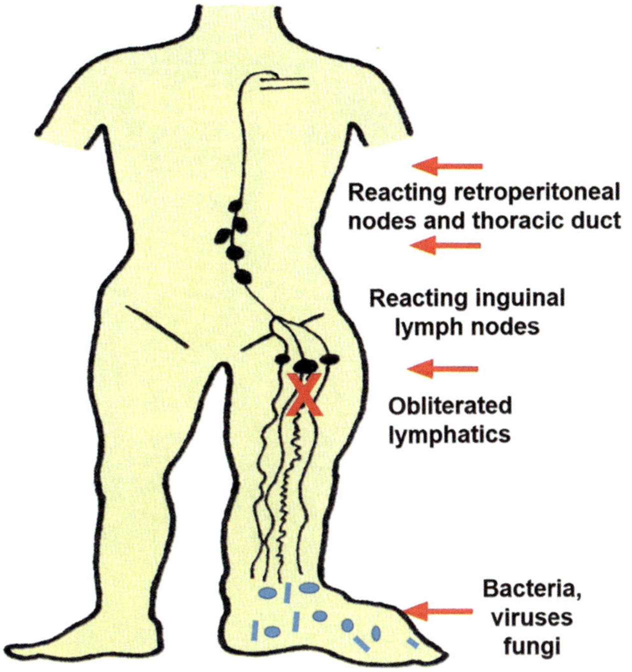

Fig. 15.4 Schematic presentation of events developing after penetration of microbes into the foot skin and subcutaneous tissue in a lymphedematous limb. The collecting lymphatics are obstructed. Collateral vessels open up and drain lymph to the inguinal lymph nodes. Immune reaction develops in inguinal and iliac lymph nodes. Thoracic duct may also be affected, as in some patients, the subclavian nodes at the venous angle become enlarged. DLA in the foot and calf is seen with the naked eye, but changes develop in inguinal, iliac, and retroperitoneal nodes. This is not a local but widespread inflammation reaction

long-term administration protocol. The susceptibility of bacteria to most antibiotics indicates their origins in the environment and not in hospitals [1].

15.1.7 Prophylaxis of Recurrent DLA

15.1.7.1 Chronic DLA

A chronic bacterial prophylaxis is necessary (Figs. 15.10 and 15.11).

Because the results of acute antibiotic therapy are short-time, prophylactic long-term administration of penicillin is necessary. The best efficacy is obtained with the intramuscular injunction of 1.2–2.4 million units of benzathine penicillin every 2–3 weeks. The alternative, although less effective, is oral therapy with penicillin V 2–four million units in 2–3 doses a day or 2 g amoxicillin with clavulanic acid for 3 days every 2–3 weeks [1, 11, 12]. Prolongation of the interval between doses of antibiotic lead to recurrences of DLA. In cases with ß-lactam allergy, the use of macrolide as, e.g., roxithromycin, is recommended.

Recent research data on benzathine penicillin prophylaxis. We studied the recurrence rate of DLA in lymphedema patients who receive prophylactic benzathine penicillin for a log time (Figs. 15.12 and 15.13).

In the entire investigated group with benzathine penicillin administration for 39.2 ± 38.7 (median 32) months, 23 out of 231 (10%) patients revealed DLA recurrence. There were 42 DLA incidents compared with 805 before the initiation of therapy (5.2%) (HR 0.05, CI 95% 0.034-0.079, $p < 0.01$) (Fig. 15.14).

Analysis of DLA Recurrence in Benzathine-Treated Patients The recurrence was observed in 6 patients out of 189 (4%) ($p < 0.01$) in the post-mastectomy, 4 out of 102 (2%) ($p < 0.01$) in the post-hysterectomy and 32 out of 514 (6%) (HR 0.031, CI 95% 0.01-0.089), (HR 0.039. CI 95% 0.013-0.122), and (HR 0.06, CI 95% 0.037-0.104), *all $p < 0.01$, respectively. Interestingly, among the patients with recurrence there was a decrease in the individual DLA episodes from 6.2 ± 3.6 to 1.7 ± 1.0%/patient (Figs. 15.15 and 15.16) There were no statistically significant differences in the recurrence rates between groups and depending on the stage of lymphedema (NS).

In summary, we showed that in patients with lymphedema experiencing multiple DLA episodes, administration of benzathine penicillin in a long follow-up of a median 38 months (with time range 5 to 156 months), decreases the recurrence of attacks by 95%. This study confirms the result reported in the literature, however, our follow-up has been much longer reaching in some cases a non-stop 30 years long penicillin administration. Recurrence of DLA episodes in the whole group, irrespective of the etiology of lymphedema, was 5.2%. It was caused in most patients by interruption of treatment for 4–6 weeks, leg trauma, or long-distance running. Interestingly, among the patients experiencing recurrence, despite penicillin administration, there was a decrease in the frequency of DLA episodes from 6.2 ± 3.6% to 1.7 ± 1.0%/patient.

15.1.8 Treatment of Acute DLA Attacks

All wide-spectrum antibiotics are efficient in the treatment acute DLA. We use 2 g of amoxicillin with clavulanic acid orally for 3–5 days and as a continuation of treatment, intramuscular administration of benzathine penicillin in the same protocol as with chronic DLA [1].

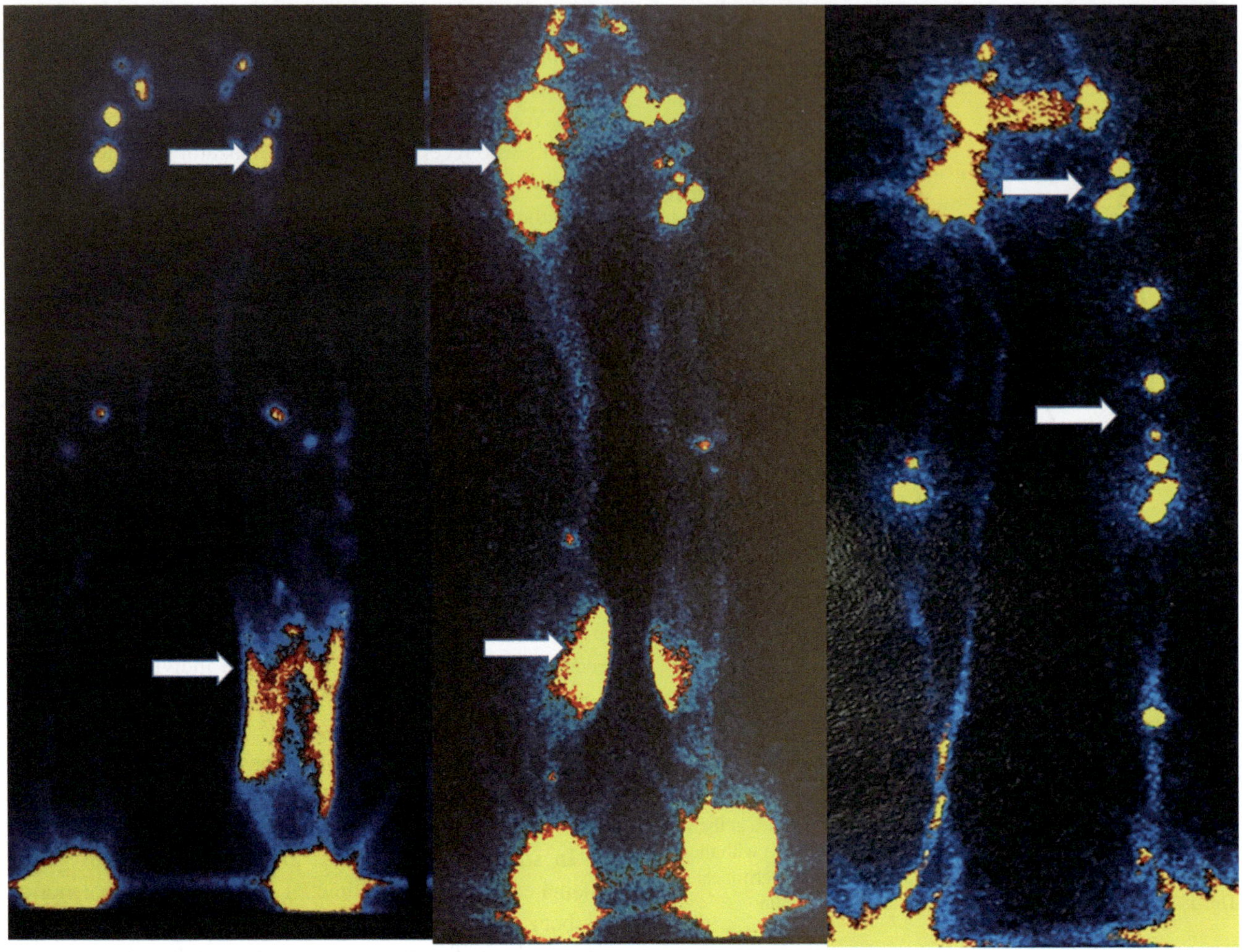

Fig. 15.5 Lymphoscintigraphic pictures are illustrating the inflammatory events in lower limbs. Left side—edema and inflammation in the calf (arrow), atrophy of inguinal lymph nodes (arrow), middle picture—edema and inflammatory focus in the calf (arrow), enlarged inguinal nodes (arrow), right side—multiple enlarged calves and thigh lymph nodes along the deep lymphatics in the popliteal and femoral vascular bundle (arrows)

15.1.9 Comments on the Mechanism of Persistence of Bacteria in Lymphedematous Tissues

Antibiotic therapy kills most the bacteria. However, some of them survive and undergo transition into "persister" or dormant form or small colony variants (SCV). In this form, they do not divide and do not incorporate antibiotics. They remain in tissues and begin to proliferate again in response to the hosts signal [9, 13]. Understanding this phenomenon prompts our search for methods preventing the reactivation of persisters by accidental signals as remote infection, trauma, viral invasion, pharmacological immuno- suppression in transplantation and oncology.

There are two possible explanations of this behavior of bacteria. According to the traditional "re-infection" hypothesis, the repeated episodes of inflammation at the same skin area are caused by modification in the tissues that occur during the first episode of cellulitis. The new explanation is based on the assumption that bacteria can survive as persister at the site of previous inflammation. It is well known that bacteria causing cellulitis (*Streptococcus pyogenes*, *Staphylococcus aureus*, *Escherichia coli*, *Pseudomonas aeruginosa*, *Acinetobacter baumannii*, etc.) may survive in the tissue intracellular or in biofilm. This mechanism of "relapsing" cellulitis should be taken into consideration when planning an effective antibiotic therapy [14].

How should we prevent the reactivation of the dormant bacteria? According to our previous experience, it should be

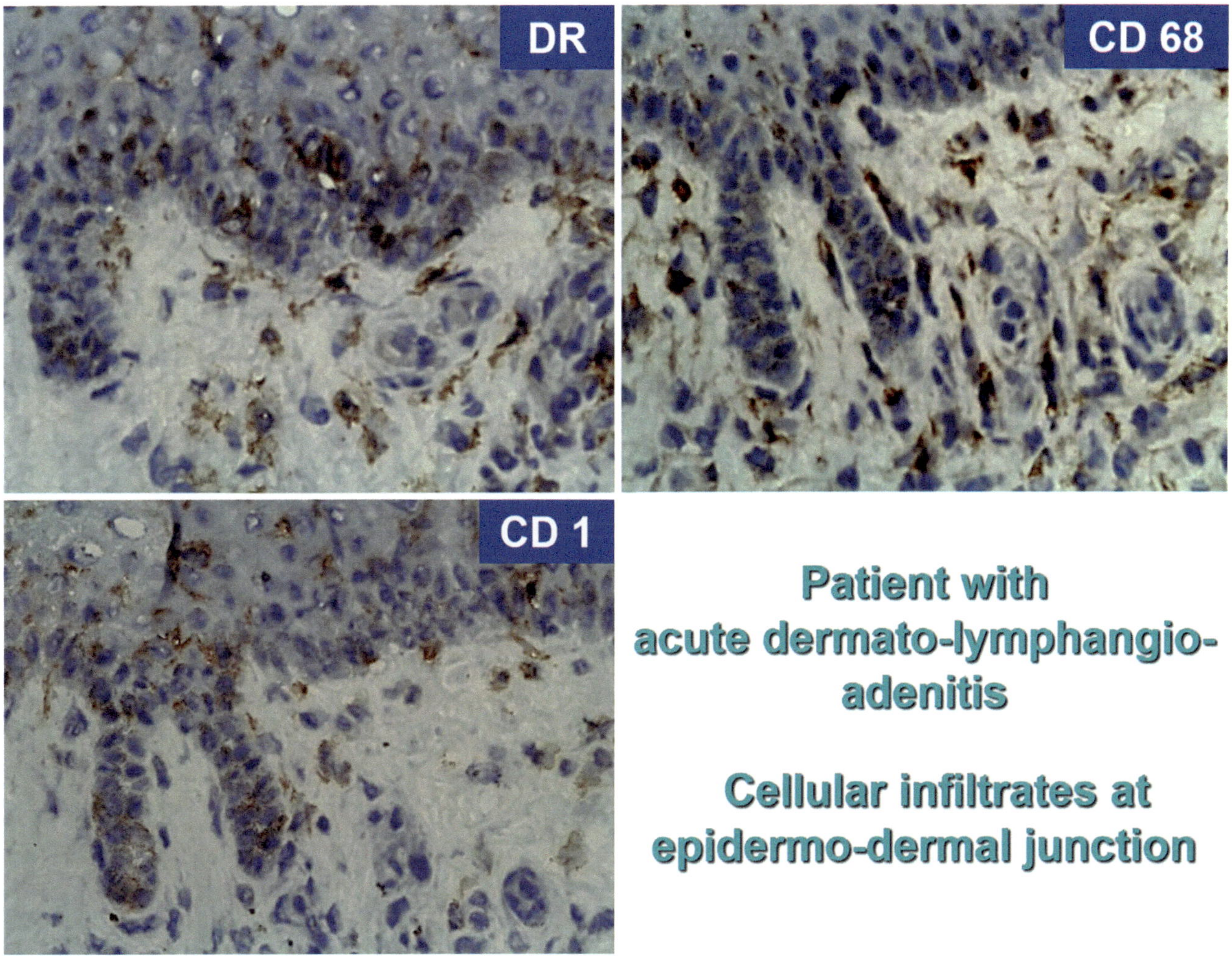

Fig. 15.6 Histological pictures of immune infiltrate in skin chronic DLA. The HLA DR-stained activated lymphocytes and Langerhans dendritic cells. The CD68 positive macrophages. The CD1 positive Langerhans cells. Note different location and density of the macrophage, dendritic cells, and lymphocytes, although they form a clinically common infiltrate

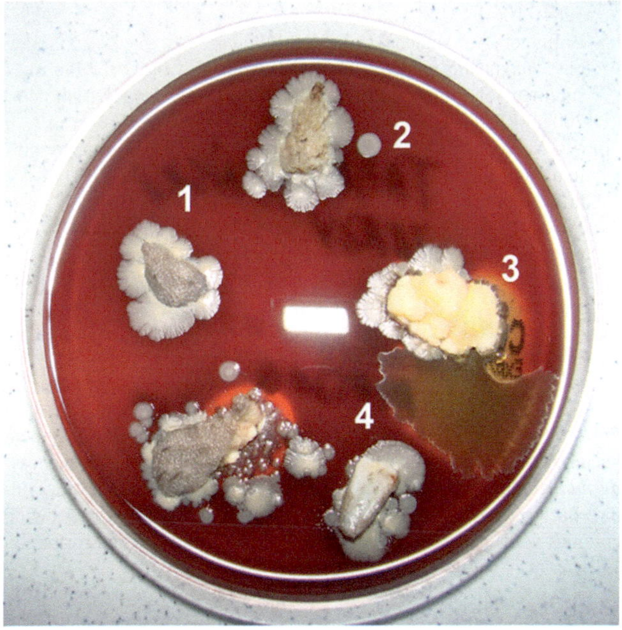

Fig. 15.7 The on-plate tissue fragments bacterial culture. 1—lymphedema disinfected leg skin with bacterial colonies around the specimen, 2—lymph node, 3—subcutaneous fat, 4—small vein fragment. Bacteria crawl out from specimens and create colonies around them

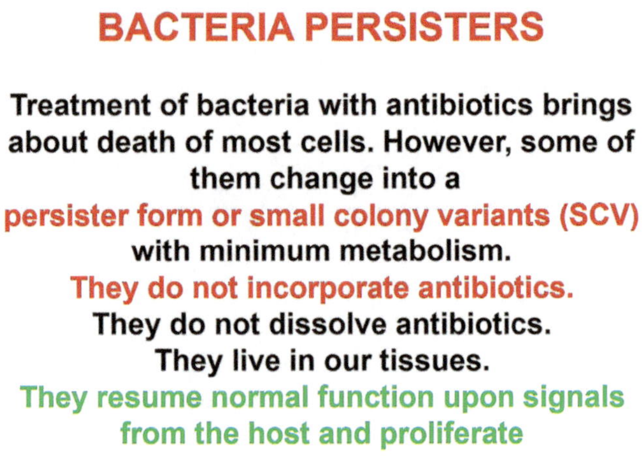

Fig. 15.8 Description of the persister bacteria present in the lymphedema tissues. This functional type of bacteria seems to be responsible for recurrence of acute DLA

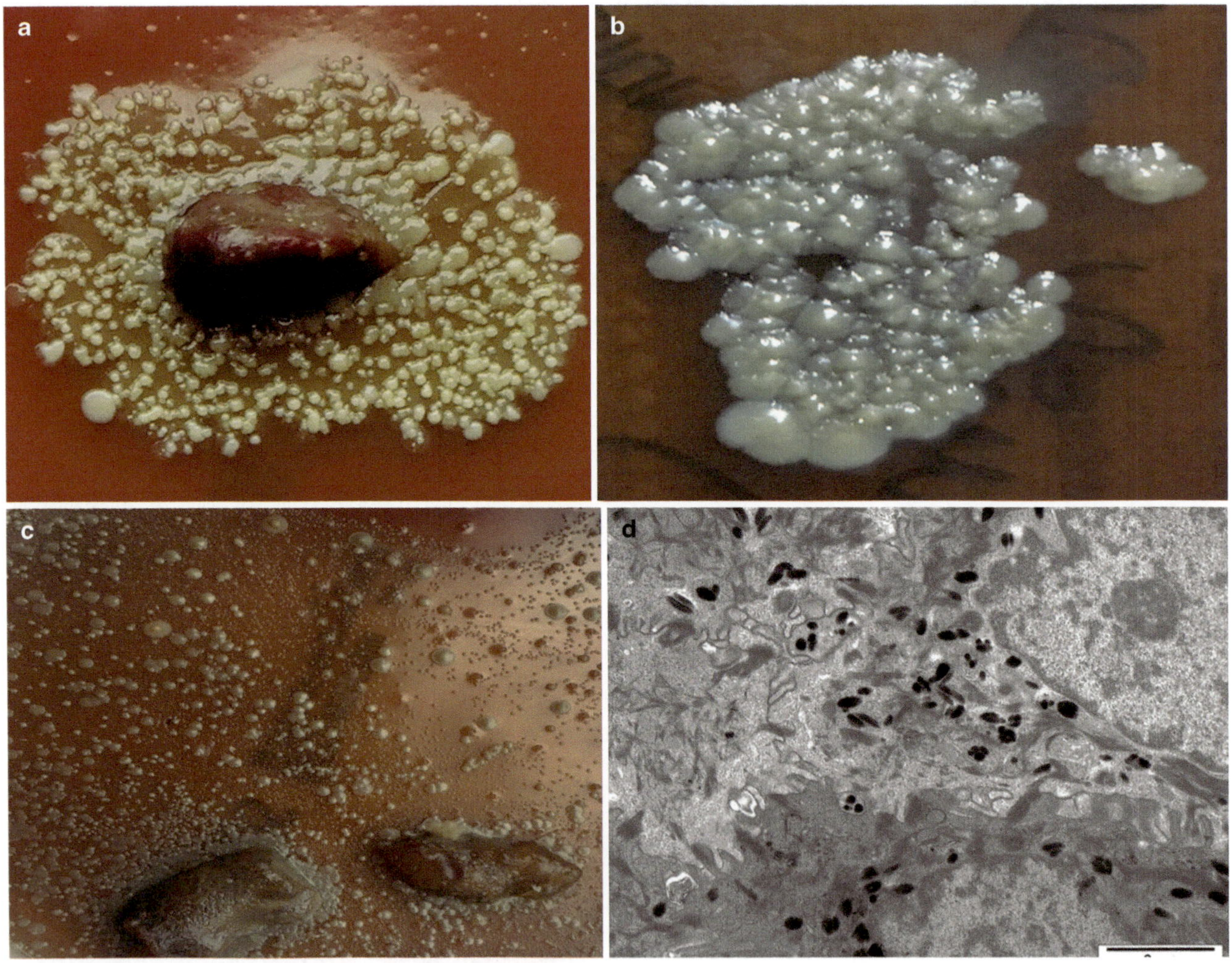

Fig. 15.9 The on-plate lymphedema inguinal lymph node fragment bacterial culture. (**a**) one week culture and dense *Staphylococcus epidermidis* colonies around the specimen. (**b**) in 2–3 weeks-lasting culture bacteria form confluent colonies. (**c**) supplementing the growing colonies with saline brings about to spread on the plate and formation of small persister colonies, these colonies are characterized by low level metabolism, they do not react to antibiotics, they stay separate and do not merge with other colonies. (**d**) electron-microscopic picture of bacteria in the fibroblast cytoplasm (black dot-like structures)

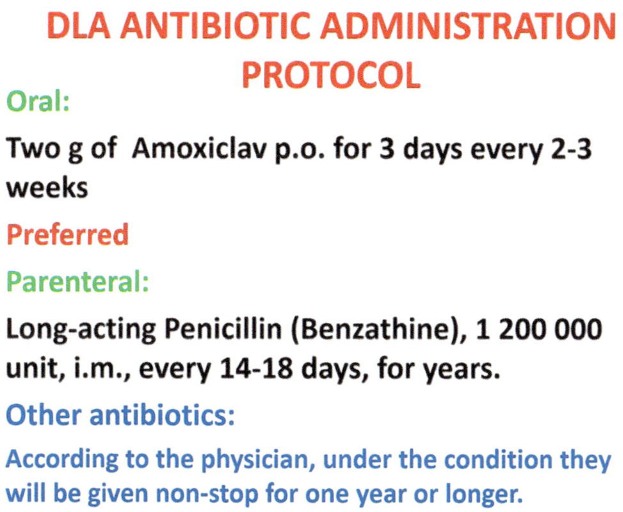

Fig. 15.10 Standard protocol for the treatment of acute and chronic DLA

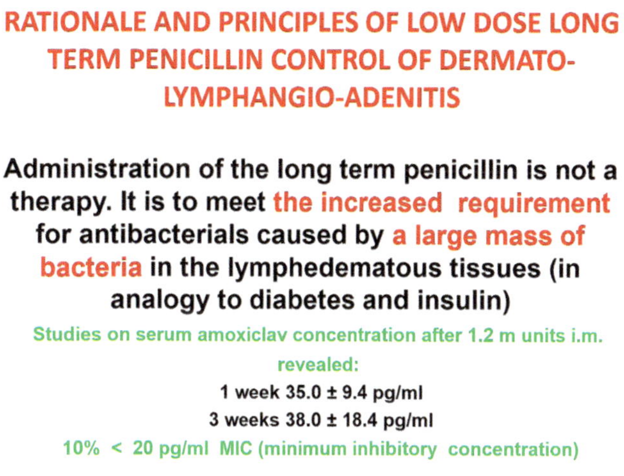

Fig. 15.11 The rationale and principles of low-dose long-term penicillin control of DLA

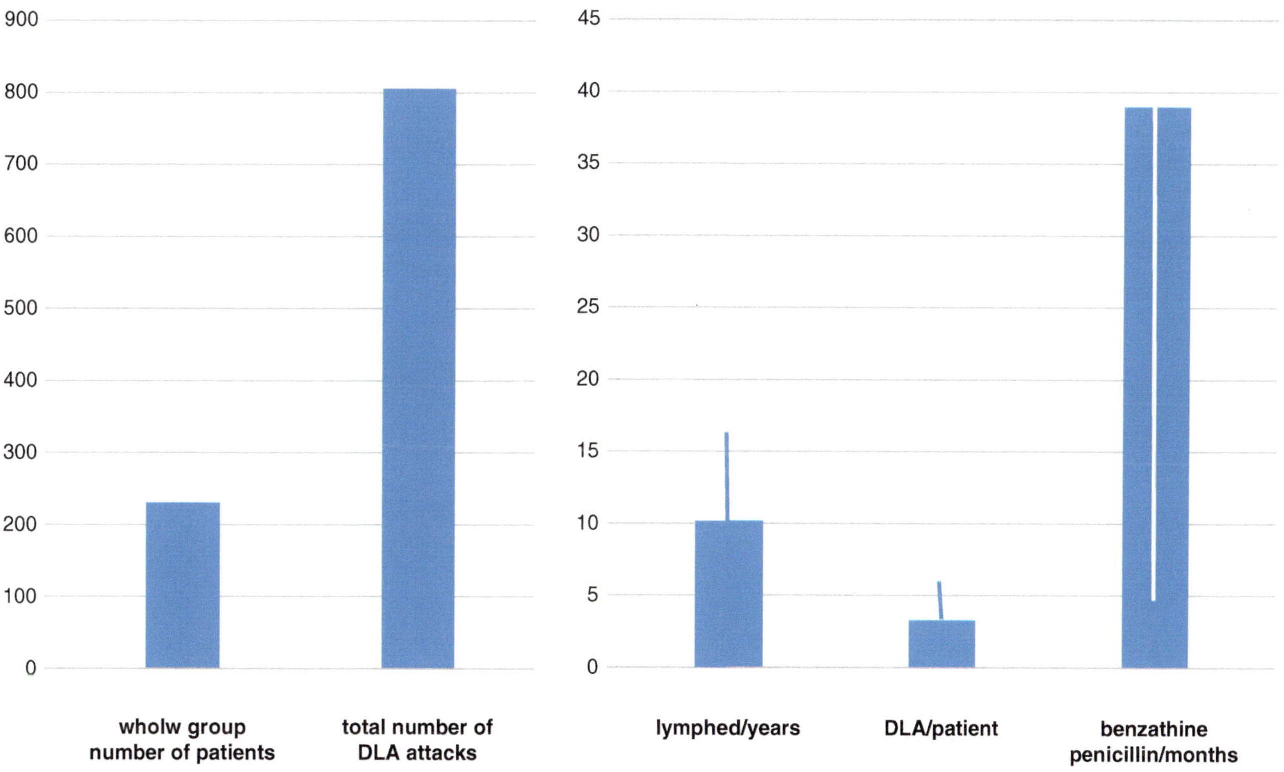

Fig. 15.12 The number of patients with limb lymphedema reporting acute DLA attacks and the total number of DLA attacks over the last 10 years. A mean of lymphedema duration, frequency of DLA per patient, and duration of benzathine penicillin therapy

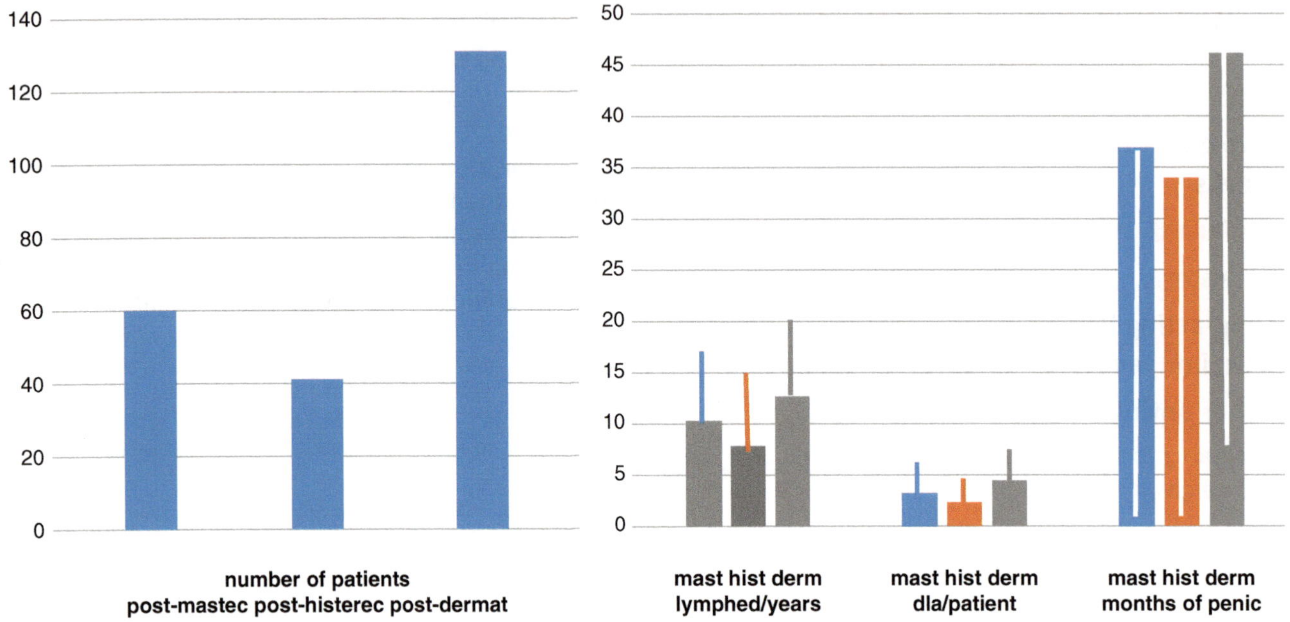

Fig. 15.13 The number of patients with the post-mastectomy, post-hysterectomy, and post-dermatitis DLA attacks. Mean time of lymphedema duration, number of DLA attacks per patient, and duration of benzathine penicillin therapy

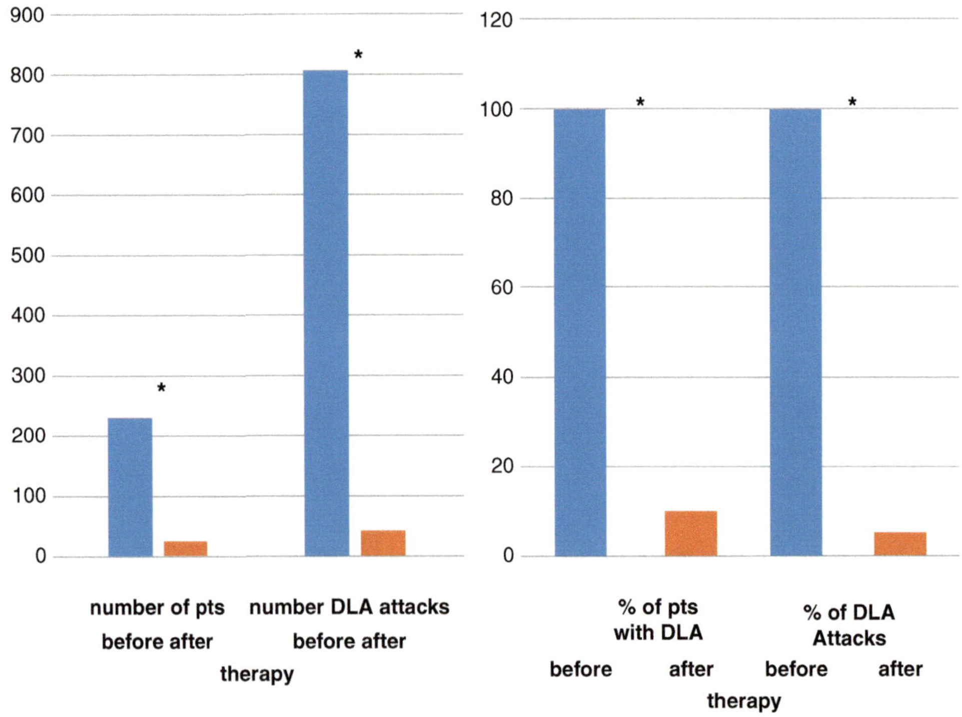

Fig. 15.14 The effects of benzathine penicillin therapy. The number of patients reporting the DLA attacks and the total number of DLA attacks significantly decreased (HR 0.05, CI 95% 0.034-0.079)

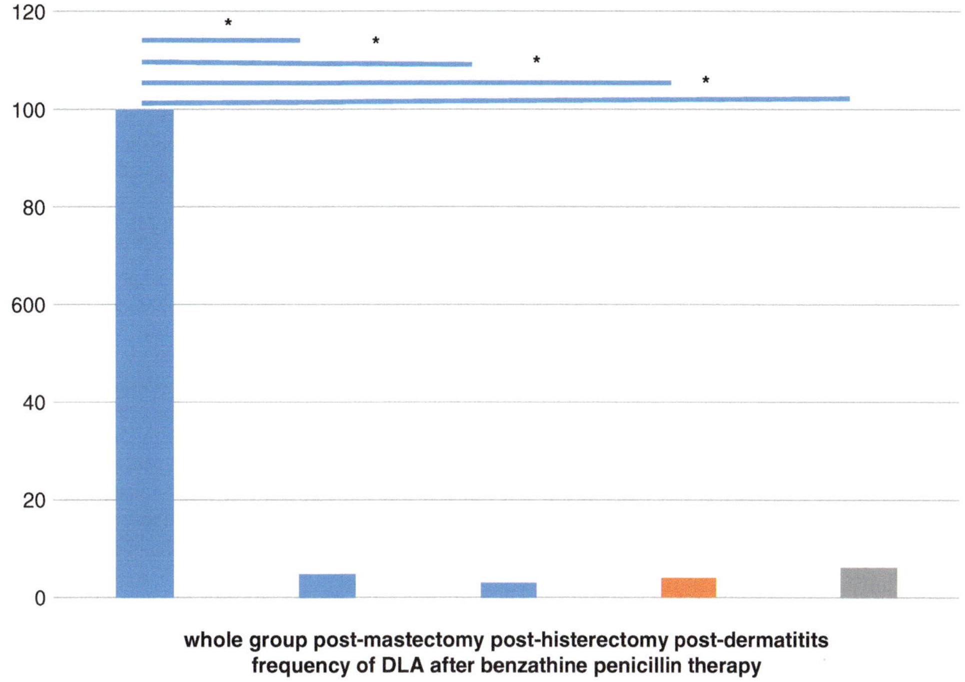

Fig. 15.15 The percent of DLA attacks after benzathine penicillin therapy in the whole group, post-mastectomy, post-hysterectomy, and post-dermatitis, (HR 0.031, CI 95% 0.01-0.089), (HR 0.039. CI 95% 0.013-0.122), and (HR 0.06, CI 95% 0.037-0.104), respectively

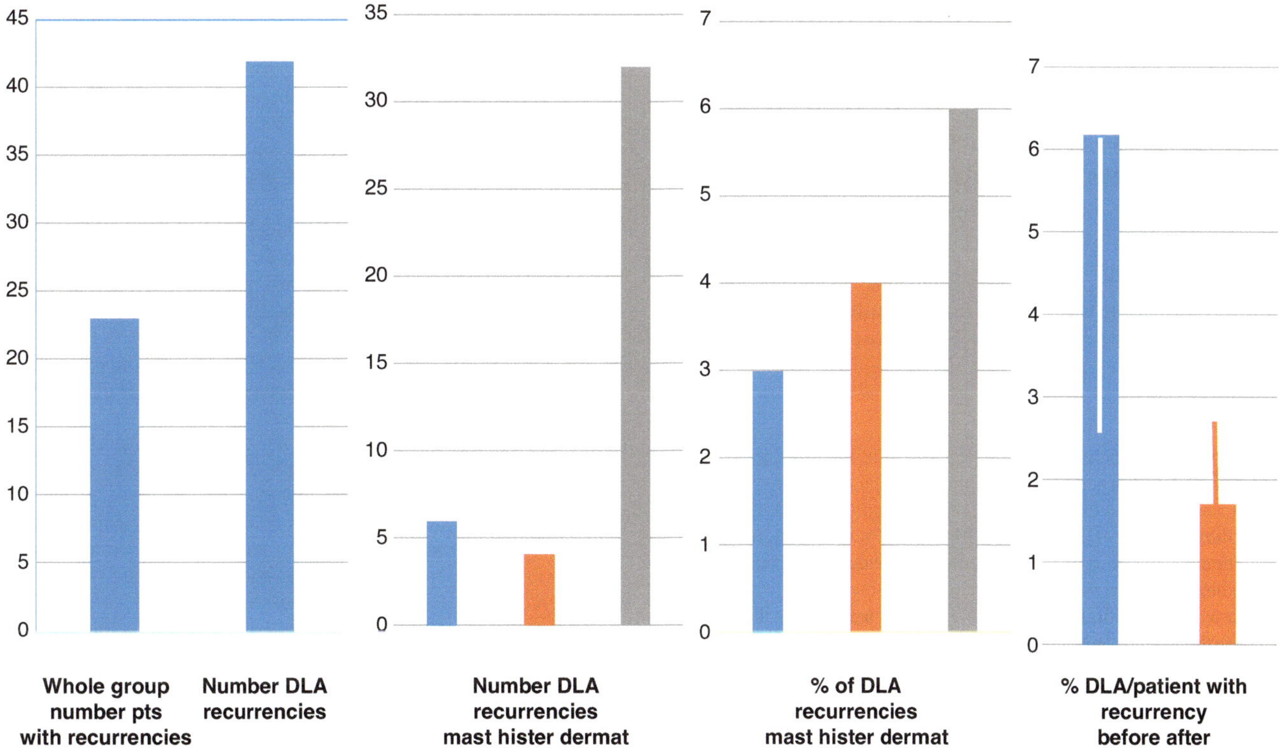

Fig. 15.16 Frequency of DLA recurrency during benzathine penicillin therapy. In the whole group, 10% of patients reported recurrence with 4.8% of attacks per affected patient. The number of DLA, % of DLA, and % DLA/patient with in the post-mastectomy, post-hysterectomy, and post-dermatitis groups. In the whole group of recurrent cases, the % of DLA/patient was lower after penicillin therapy compared with the pre-therapy data

a long duration or even permanent prophylaxis by administration of long-term antibiotics. Therefore, intramuscular administration of benzathine penicillin at a dose of 1.2–2.4 million units every 2–3 weeks with local anesthetic is the best solution and has proven better efficacy than any oral protocols. In concert with the views on bacterial dormancy in limb tissues, we investigated the clinical course of lymphedema in terms of the prevalence of DLA in patients receiving injections of long-acting penicillin for long periods of time. Already in 1996, we found that recurrent episodes of DLA in a one-year treated penicillin-treated group decreased from 100% to 9% ($p < 0.002$) (15.11).

What concerns the reaction of different bacterial strains during penicillin prophylaxis? We observed more Cocci and gram-positive bacilli and fewer gram-negative bacilli from the surface of the food and calf skin. At the same time, among the strains isolated from the lymph and deep tissues of the lower limbs, a redaction of the spread of gram-positive cocci and gram-negative bacilli was noted. No emergence of resistance to both the penicillin and other tested antibiotic was noted. All bacteria isolated from the skin, deep tissues, lymph, and lymph nodes, both lymphedema patients and healthy individuals, were susceptible to most antibiotics. Unexpectedly, the least susceptible was observed to penicillin, although this antibiotic was very effective. The susceptibility of bacteria to most antibiotics indicates their origins in the environment and not in hospitals [15].

Positive results of prophylactic effectiveness of benzathine penicillin on lymphedema DLA episodes are also accumulating from multiple sources. In the pertinent literature, the decrease in the DLA recurrency ranges between 46% and 100% when long-term penicillin is administered over 1 year [14–23]. None of the studies reported severe adverse effects to antibiotics [11, 12, 17, 24].

References

1. Olszewski WL. Diagnosis and Management of Infection in lymphedema. In: Lee BB, et al., editors. Lymphedema. Springer; 2018. p. 465–81.
2. Dreyer G, Addiss D, Gadelha P, et al. Interdigital skin lesions of the lower limbs among patients with lymphoedema in an area endemic for bancroftian filariasis. Tropical Med Int Health. 2006;11:1475–81.
3. McPherson T, Persaud S, Singh S, et al. Interdigital lesions and frequency of acute dermatolymphangioadenitis in lymphoedema in a filariasis-endemic area. Br J Dermatol. 2006;154:933–41.
4. Karonidis A, Chen HC. Preservation of toes in advanced lymphedema: an important step in the control of infection. Ann Plast Surg. 2010 Apr;64(4):446–50.
5. Gabillot-Carré M, Roujeau JC. Acute bacterial skin infections and cellulitis. Curr Opin Infect Dis. 2007 Apr;20(2):118–23.
6. Dreyer G, Medeiros Z, Netto MJ, et al. Acute attacks in the extremities of persons living in an area endemic for bancroftian filariasis: differentiation of two syndromes. Trans R Soc Trop Med Hyg. 199(93):413–7.
7. Olszewski WL, Jamal S, Manokaran G, et al. Bacteriological studies of blood, tissue fluid, lymph and lymph nodes in patients with acute dermatolymphangioadenitis (DLA) in course of 'filarial' lymphedema. Acta Trop. 1999;73:217–24.
8. Olszewski WL, Jamal S, Manokaran G, et al. Bacteriologic studies of skin, tissue fluid, lymph, and lymph nodes in patients with filarial lymphedema. A J Trop Med Hyg. 1997;57:7–15.
9. Lewis K. Persister cells. Ann Rev Microbiol. 2010;64:357–72.
10. Singh R, Ray P, Das A, Sharma M. Role of persisters and small-colony variants in antibiotic-resistance of planktonic and biofilm-associated Staphylococcus aureus: an in vitro study. J Med Microbiol. 2002;58:1067–73.
11. Olszewski WL. Episodic dermatolymphangioadenitis (DLA) in patients with lymphedema of the lower extremities before and after administration of benzathine penicillin: a preliminary study. Lymphology. 1996;29:126–31.
12. Olszewski WL, Jamal S, Manokaran G, et al. The effectiveness of long-acting penicillin (penidur) in preventing recurrences of dermatolymphangioadenitis (DLA) and controlling skin, deep tissues, and lymph bacterial flora in patients with "filarial" lymphedema. Lymphology. 2005;38:66–80.
13. Olszewski WL, Zaleska M, Stelmach E, Swoboda-Kopec E, Jain P, Agrawal K, Gogia S, Gogia A, Andziak P, Durlik M. Cryptic bacteria of lower limb deep tissues as a possible cause of inflammatory and necrotic changes in ischemia, venous stasis and varices, and lymphedema. Surg Infect. 2015 Jun;16(3):313–22.
14. Chaniotakis I, Bassukas ID. The first disease episode: a strategic treatment target to prevent cellulitis relapses. Published online: January 22, 2020 Dermatology. https://doi.org/10.1159/000505538.
15. Haque N, Hossain MA, Bilkis L, Musa AK, Mahamud C, Bari MS, et al. Antibiotic susceptibility pattern of Staphylococcus Epidermidis. Mymensingh Med J. 2009 Jul;18(2):142–7.
16. Oh CC, Ko HCH, Lee HY, et al. Antibiotic prophylaxis for preventing recurrent cellulitis: a systematic review and metaanalysis. J Infect. 2014;69:26–34.
17. Dalal A, Eskin-Schwartz M, Mimouni D, Ray S, Days W, Hodak E, Leibovici L, Paul M. Interventions for the prevention of recurrent erysipelas and cellulitis. Cochrane Database Syst Rev. 2017 Jun 20;6:CD009758. https://doi.org/10.1002/14651858.CD009758.pub2.
18. Wang JH, Liu YC, Cheng DL, et al. Role of benzathine penicillin G in prophylaxis for recurrent streptococcal cellulitis of the lower legs. Clin Infect Dis. 1997;25:685–9.
19. Rob A, Herzegova J. Benzathine penicillin G once-every-3-week prophylaxis for recurrent erysipelas a retrospective study of 132 patients. J Dermatol Treat. 2018;29:39–43.
20. Vignes S, Dupuy A. Recurrence of lymphoedema-associated cellulitis (erysipelas) under prophylactic antibiotherapy: a retrospective cohort study. J Eur Acad Dermatol Venereol. 2006;20:818–22.
21. Lau JCY, Kiss C, Roberts E, Horne K, Korman TM, Woolley I. Surveillance of life-long antibiotics: a review of antibiotic prescribing practices in an Australian healthcare network. Ann Clin Microbiol Antimicrob. 2017;16:3.
22. Lau JCY, Kiss C, Roberts E, Horne K, Korman TM, Woolley I. Cellulitis in adult patients: a large, multicenter, observational, prospective study of 606 episodes and analysis of the factors related to the response to treatment. PLoS One. 2018;13(9):e0204036.
23. Thomas KS, Crook AM, Nunn JA, Foster KA, Mason JM, Chalmers JR, Nasr JM, Brindle JR, English J, Meredith SK, Reynolds NJ, Berker D, Mortimer PS, Williams CH. Penicillin to prevent recurrent leg cellulitis. N Engl J Med. 2013;368:18.
24. Chen HM, Li YL, Liu YM, et al. The experience of intramuscular benzathine penicillin for prophylaxis of recurrent cellulitis: a cohort study. J Microbiol Immunol Infect. 2017 Oct;50(5):613–8.

Tissue Overgrowth in Lymphedema

16

Waldemar L. Olszewski and Marzanna T. Zaleska

Keywords

Lymphedema · Lymph · Fibrosis · Hyperkeratosis
Immune cells

Summary (Fig.16.1)
(Fig.16.1): Lymphedema develops because of pathological occlusion of the main lymphatic pathways draining limbs and organs. Lymphedema is a symptom and not a separate entity. It is not only pathological cumulation of tissue fluid in the intracellular space, but also overgrowth of fibroblasts and adipocytes and retention of microorganisms that permanently penetrate the skin surface and can provoke chronic inflammation. The most common reasons for lymphatic damage are bacterial infections of limb skin and subcutaneous tissue, tissue injuries, lymphadenectomy, and radiation therapy for cancer treatment. Less common are chronic venous insufficiency with dermatosclerosis and filariasis. The histopathological images show a lymphatic collector completely or partially filled up with collagen deposits and other non-cellular masses, and absence of endothelial and muscular cells, dilated subepidermis lymphatics, extended tissues spaces with fluid, hyperkeratosis, fibrosis of dermis, subcutaneous tissue, and facia. Electromicroscopic pictures confirm the inherence of bacteria in intracellular fluid and opened interendothelial junctions in subepidermal lymphatics [1].

Note on the figure a. lymphedematous skin and subcutaneous tissue with excess adipose tissue, b. hyperkeratosis of epidermis and fibrosis of dermis, c, fibrosis of muscular fascia, and d. obliterated lymphatic collector. Understanding the type and kinetics of changes is necessary for establishing a rational preventive therapy.

16.1 Classification of Lymphedema of Lower Limbs

Lymphedema develops because of pathological occlusion of the main lymphatic pathways draining limbs and organs. The damaged lymphatic vessels do not regenerate. Lymphangiogenesis occurs only at the level of lymphatic capillaries (initial lymphatics), which is visible during the wound healing process. The pathological changes in the tissue in the course of lymphedema depend on the primary etiological factor. They can be seen in lymphoscintigraphy, MRI, and in histological specimens. Since lymphedema is only a symptom, the term “lymphedema” should be supplemented with the etiological factor (Fig. 16.2). Patients with lymphedema are all over the world. However, the most advanced cases remain in Asia, Africa, and South America. These cases demonstrate all the clinical and histological changes that occur in the obstruction of the lymph flow [1].

16.2 Morphological Changes in Lymphedema

During lymphedema, there are the accumulation of the tissue fluid, overgrowth of keratinocytes, fibroblast, and adipocytes. Thus, the entire mass of a limb in lymphedema consists of both increase in fluid and tissue volume. Some of the fluid can be removed using compression therapy, but the tissue that has grown up will remain. This is why, despite removal of mobile edema fluid, the limb size remains large (Figs.16.3, 16.4, and 16.5).

W. L. Olszewski (✉)
Department of Vascular Surgery, Central Clinical Hospital, Ministry of Internal Affairs, Warsaw, Poland

M. T. Zaleska
Department of Vascular Surgery, Central Clinical Hospital, Ministry of Internal Affairs, Warsaw, Poland

Department of Applied Physiology, Mossakowski Medical Research Institute, Polish Academy of Sciences, Warsaw, Poland

N. Liu (ed.), *Peripheral Lymphedema*, https://doi.org/10.1007/978-981-16-3484-0_16

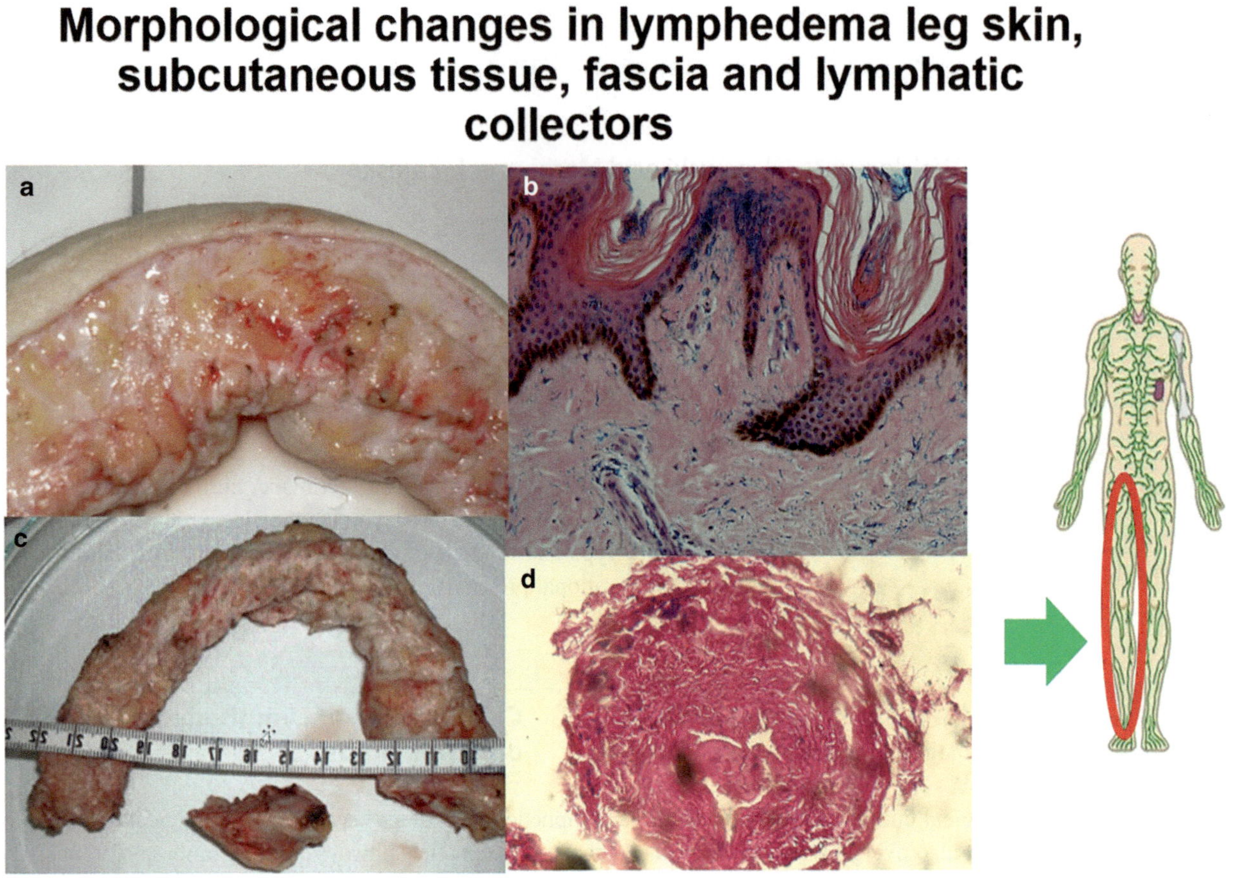

Fig. 16.1 Morphological changes in lymphedema leg skin, subcutaneous tissue, fascia, and lymphatic collectors, (**a**) Skin and subcutaneous tissue with excess adipose tissue, (**b**) hyperkeratosis of epidermis and fibrosis of dermis, (**c**) fibrosis of muscular fascia, (**d**) obliterated lymphatic collector

CLASSIFICATION OF LYMPHEDEMA

1. POSTINFLAMMATORY (DERMATITIS, LYMPHANGITIS, LYMPHADENITIS OF VARIOUS ETIOLOGIES)
2. POSTSURGICAL (AFTER GROIN AND AXILLARY DISSECTION ALSO INCLUDING RADIOTHERAPY, ARTERIAL RECONSTRUCTIONS AND SAPHENOUS VEIN HARVESTING FOR CORONARY BYPASSES)
3. POSTTRAUMATIC (CLOSED AND OPEN LIMB INJURIES WITH IMMOBILIZATION)
4. MIXED LYMPHATICO-VENOUS TYPE IN CHRONIC VENOUS INSUFFICIENCY
5. IDIOPATHIC (PRIMARY)
6. PARASITIC (FILARIAL)

Fig. 16.2 Classification of types of limb lymphedema according to the etiological factors. The order of types responds to the frequency rate in the world. The most common is the post-dermatitis, then post-surgical in oncology, and post-traumatic lymphedema. The idiopathic or primary lymphedema should be listed as the malformations with lack of developed initial lymphatics. There should be genetic confirmation. Filarial lymphedema is common in the geographical areas where filarial is common in the environment, however, the dominating factor is a bacterial infection of the foot with subsequent lymphatic damage in the barefoot walking population

16.3 Microscopic Changes of Soft Tissues in Lymphedema

Macroscopic changes in limbs include fibrosis of the skin, overgrowth of fibrous and adipose tissue (Figs. 16.6, 16.7, and 16.8).

16.3.1 Lymphatics

The histological pictures of lymphatics and tissues differ depending on what was the primary cause of damage. They depend upon where the primary causative factor damaged lymphatics. In the post-dermatitis lymphedema, changes develop in the distal parts of the limb. In post-surgical lymphedema, obstructive changes arise at the surgical procedure sites. In post-traumatic lymphedema, damage to lymphatic is located at the site of injury. Destructive changes develop in a die-back process in the periphery, most likely due to lack of microorganism transport away. At the advanced stage of lymphedema tissue, histological changes are similar in all etiological lymphedema forms.

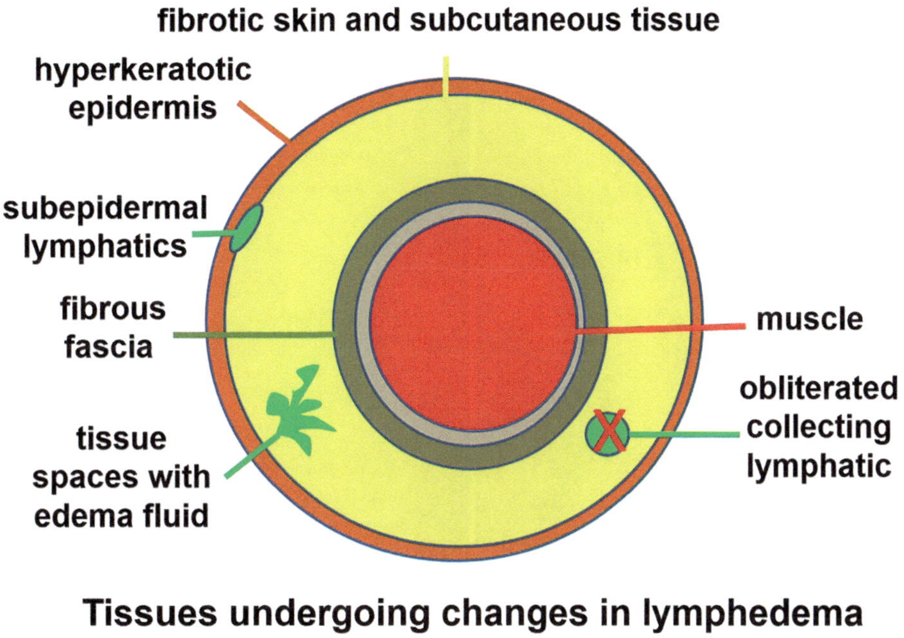

Fig. 16.3 Schematic presentation of topography and type of tissue changes in lymphedema. This scheme is useful for the interpretation of pictures of computer tomography, ultrasonography, MRI and isotope, and fluorescent lymphography. It may also be helpful in the determination of advancement and staging of lymphedema, as well as, in evaluating the therapy effects

DIFFERENT PROPORTIONS OF FIBROUS TISSUE
AND MOBILE TISSUE FLUID VOLUME
AT VARIOUS LEVELS
OF LYMPHEDEMATOUS LIMB

SKIN	SUBCUTIS	FASCIA
SOFT	SOFT FAT +++ FIBROSIS Ø TF Ø	SOFT FIBROSIS Ø
THICK +	FIBROSIS + FAT ++ TF +++	FIBROSIS ++
THICK ++	FIBROSIS ++ FAT + TF ++	FIBROSIS ++
THICK +++	FIBROSIS +++ FAT + TF +	FIBROSIS +++

Fig. 16.4 Scheme presenting the progression of tissue changes in lymphedema of lower limbs in distal and proximal limb levels. Skin, subcutis, and muscular fascia are most affected in the distal parts of limbs. The mechanism of it is not entirely clear. Factors as tissue (edema) fluid pressure (TF), volume of the accumulated fluid, and skin-derived infection should be accounted. The therapeutic hint is efforts to prevent foot and lower calf fibrosis, papillomatosis, fluid leakage, and ulcerations. Antibacterial and antifungal medicaments are strongly recommended

16.3.2 Skin, Subcutaneous Tissue, and Nodes

All pathological transformation that occurs under the influence of inflammation or trauma in the lymphatic vessels leads to their obliteration by fibroblasts. This is the cost of the lymphatic system performing the function of removing microorganisms and own impaired cells in the body. The inflammatory process is also destructive for the body's own cells and tissues. (Figs. 16.9, 16.10, 16.11, 16.12, 16.13, 16.14, and 16.15).

16.4 General Analysis

A summary list of histological changes: (1) obliteration of lymphatic collectors and fibrosis of lymph nodes, (2) hyperkeratosis of epidermis, (3) immune cell infiltrates of epidermis, dermis, and subcutaneous tissue, (4) fibrosis of the dermis, perilymphatic tissues, and muscular fascia, (5) proliferation of skin and fat tissue (fibroblasts secreting collagen, adipocytes accumulating lipids) [1–8]. Changes in peripheral lymphatic vessels following lymphadenectomy take place in three stages: ectasis, contraction, and sclerosis. During the first stage, the increased intralymphatic pressure (pressure inside the lymphatics) leads to the flattering of the endothelial cells lining the lymphatic vessels. In the second stage, smooth muscle cells are converted into synthetic cells to promote the for-

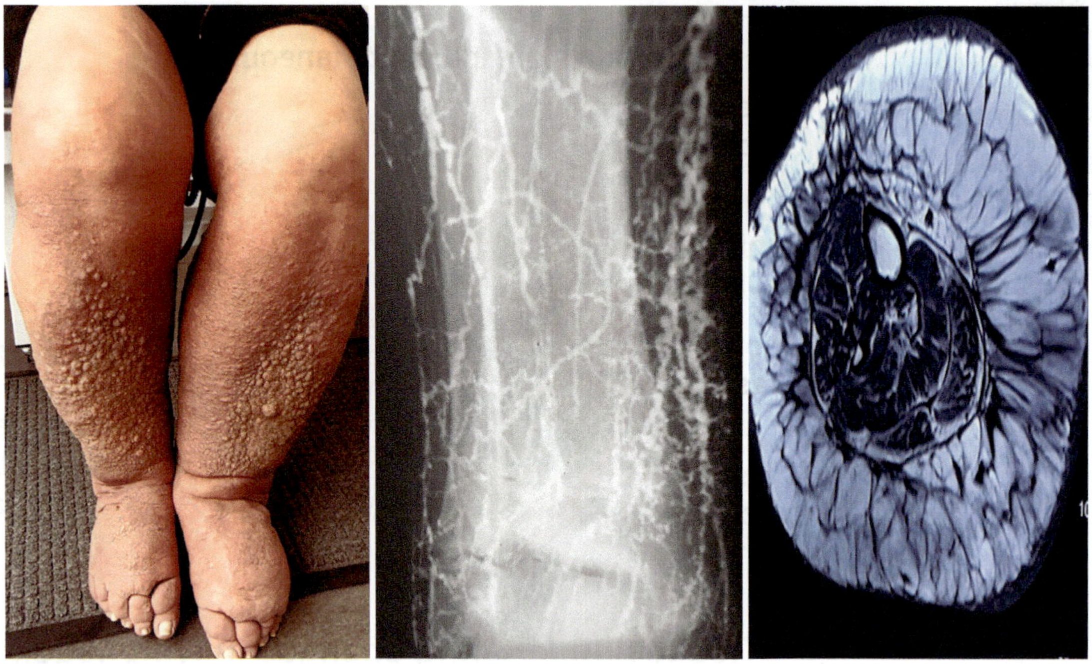

Fig. 16.5 The basic clinical and visualization changes in lymphedema are caused by obstruction of the main lymphatics draining lower limbs. Left side- swollen legs with fibrosis and papillomatosis of skin, middle part- dilated subepidermal lymphatics bypassing the obstructed main collectors (previously called "dermal backflow"), right side-overgrown adipose tissue

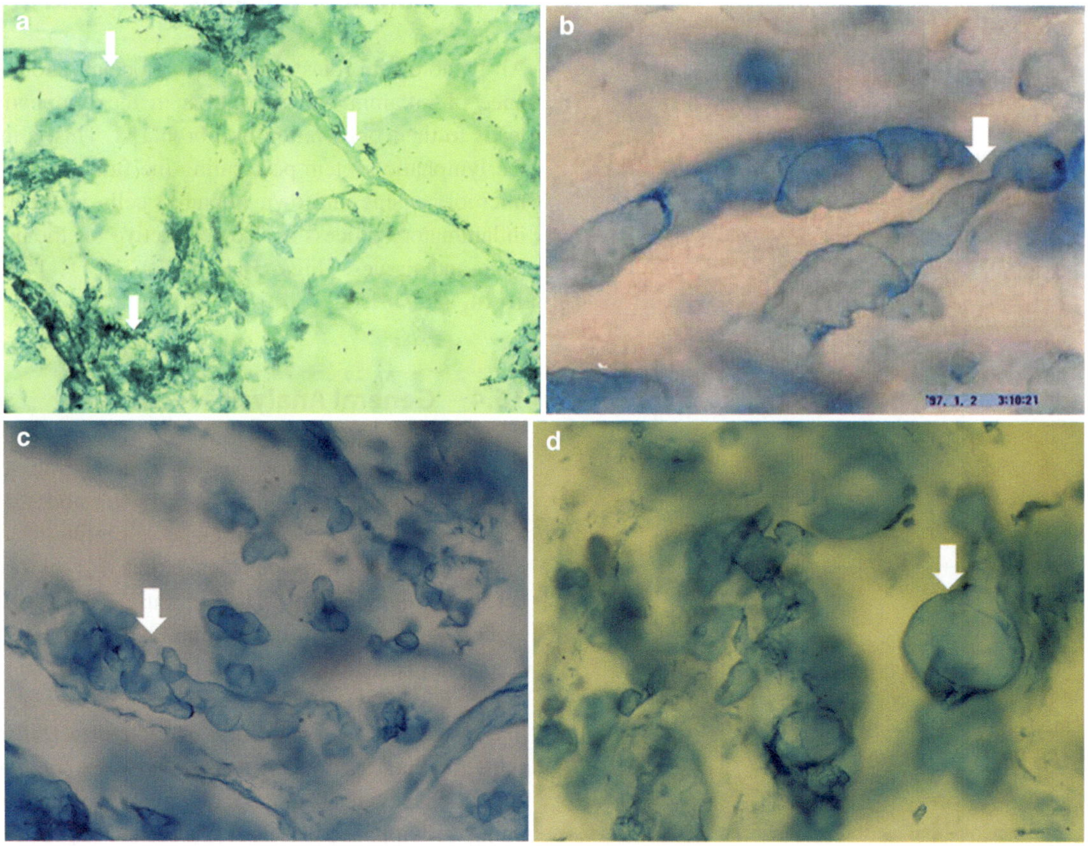

Fig. 16.6 Pictures demonstrating changes in the subepidermal lymphatics are bypassing the obstructed collectors. (**a**) dense, irregular pattern of dilated large (arrow), minor 100 micron-wide (arrow), and a network of minute lymphatics (arrow) is shown. Under higher magnification depicted (**b**) dilated lymphatics with valves (arrow points to the stricture), likely to be followed soon by total obstruction, (**c**) more advanced stage with "varices" budding off from minor lymphatics, and d. dilated isolated bullous fragments of lymphatics

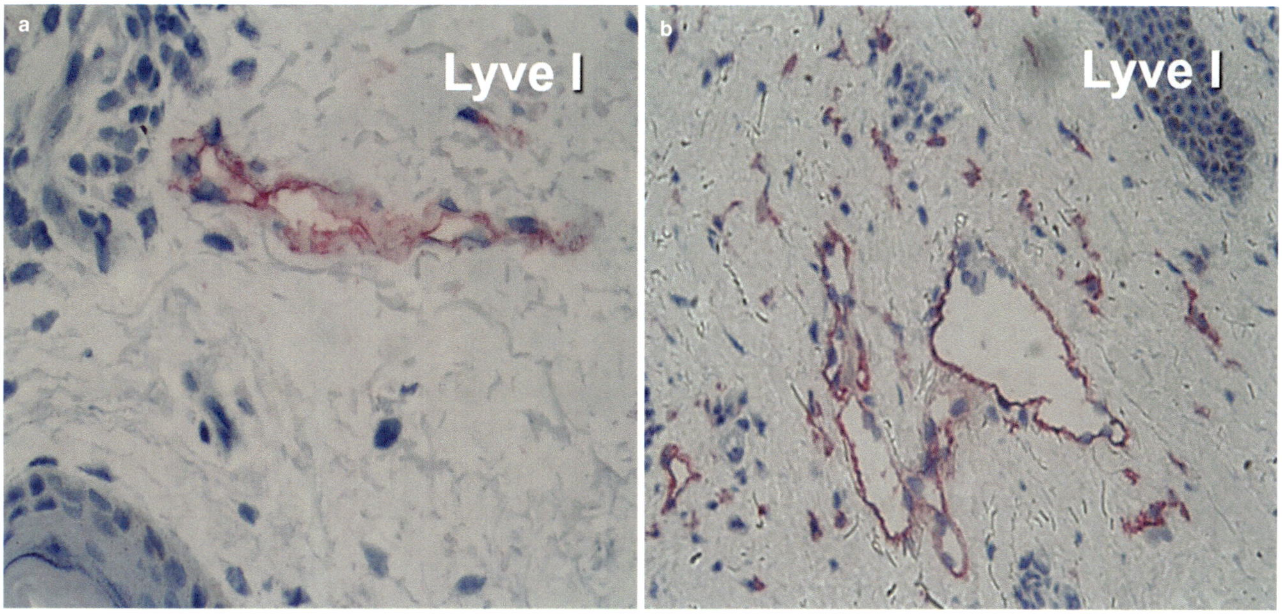

Fig. 16.7 Biopsy pictures of LYVE 1-stained (hyaluronate receptor) dermal lymphatics, (**a**) normal, (**b**) dilated due to lymph flow obstruction (magn. × 40)

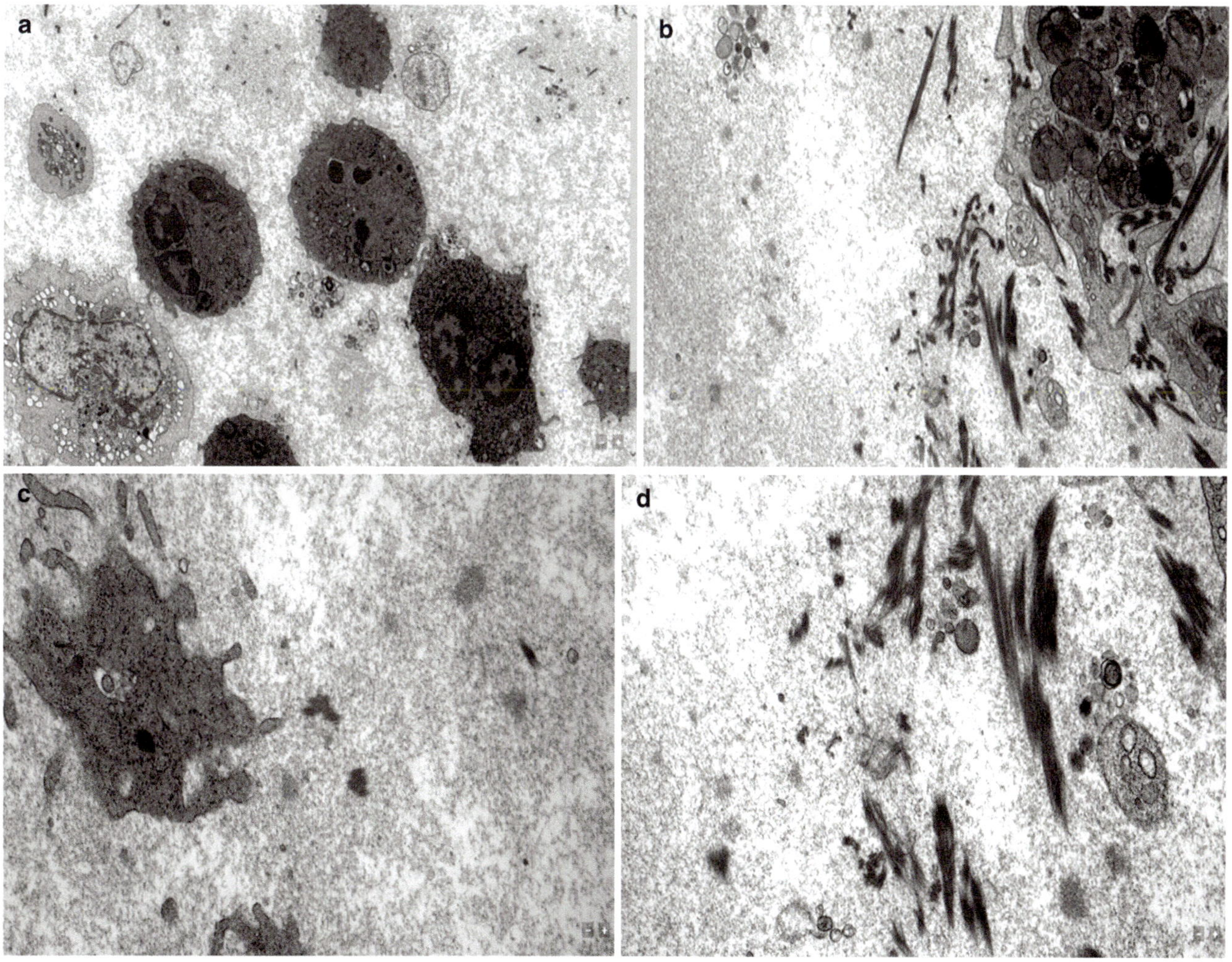

Fig. 16.8 Dilated dermal lymphatics contain in their lumen not only stagnant lymph fluid but also ground matrix and cellular debris. This material accumulates in lymphatics and plays its role in the process of tissue changes. (**a**) live and apoptotic lymphocytes, (**b**) fragments of collagen fibers and mitochondria, (**c**) destructed Langerhans cell (EM magn. × 1000). Background with minute dispersed protein particles

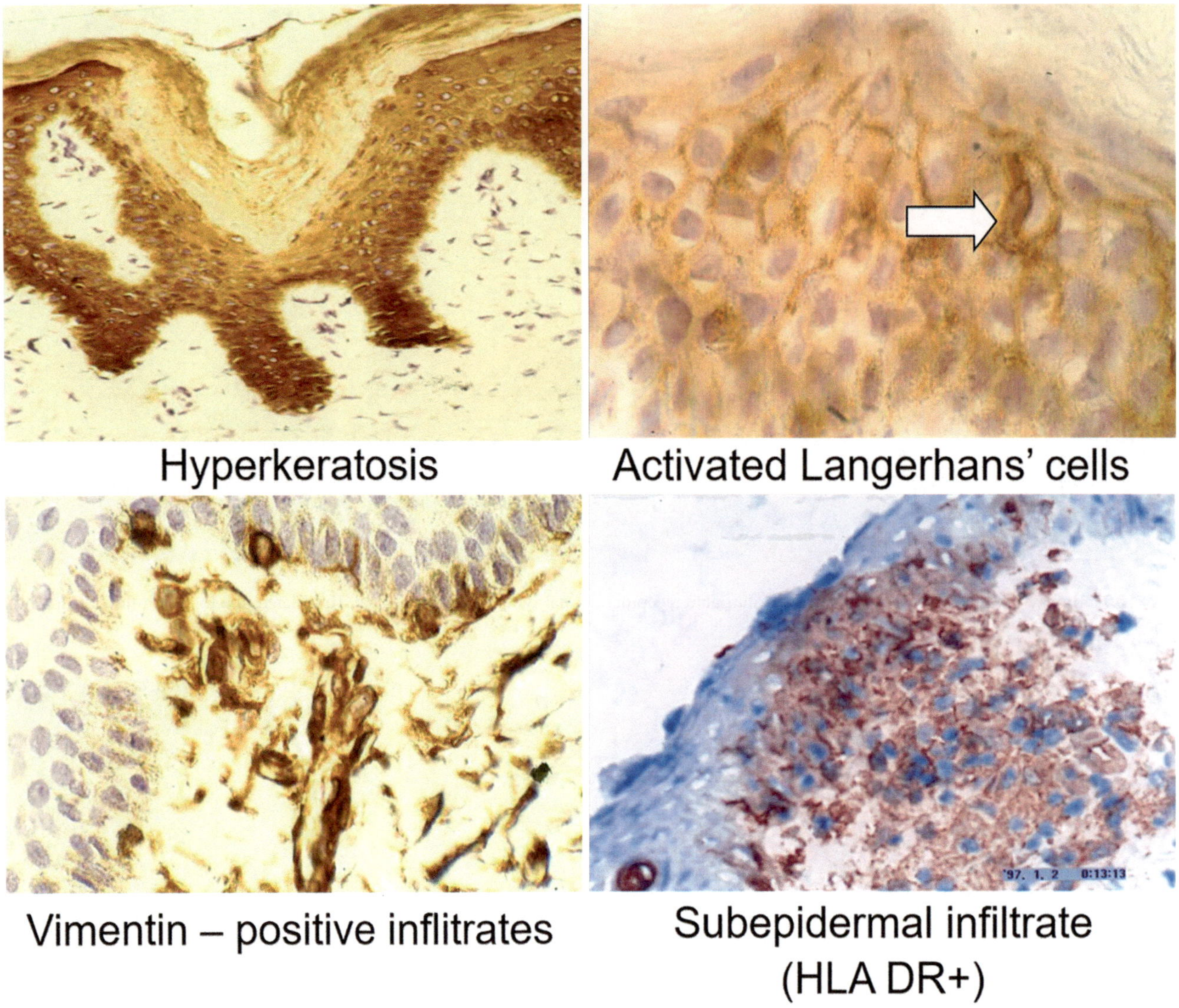

Fig. 16.9 Tissue histological pictures of changes developing in the skin of the lymphedematous limbs (anti-keratin, anti CD1, vimentin, and HLA DR monoclonal antibodies, magn. × 40)

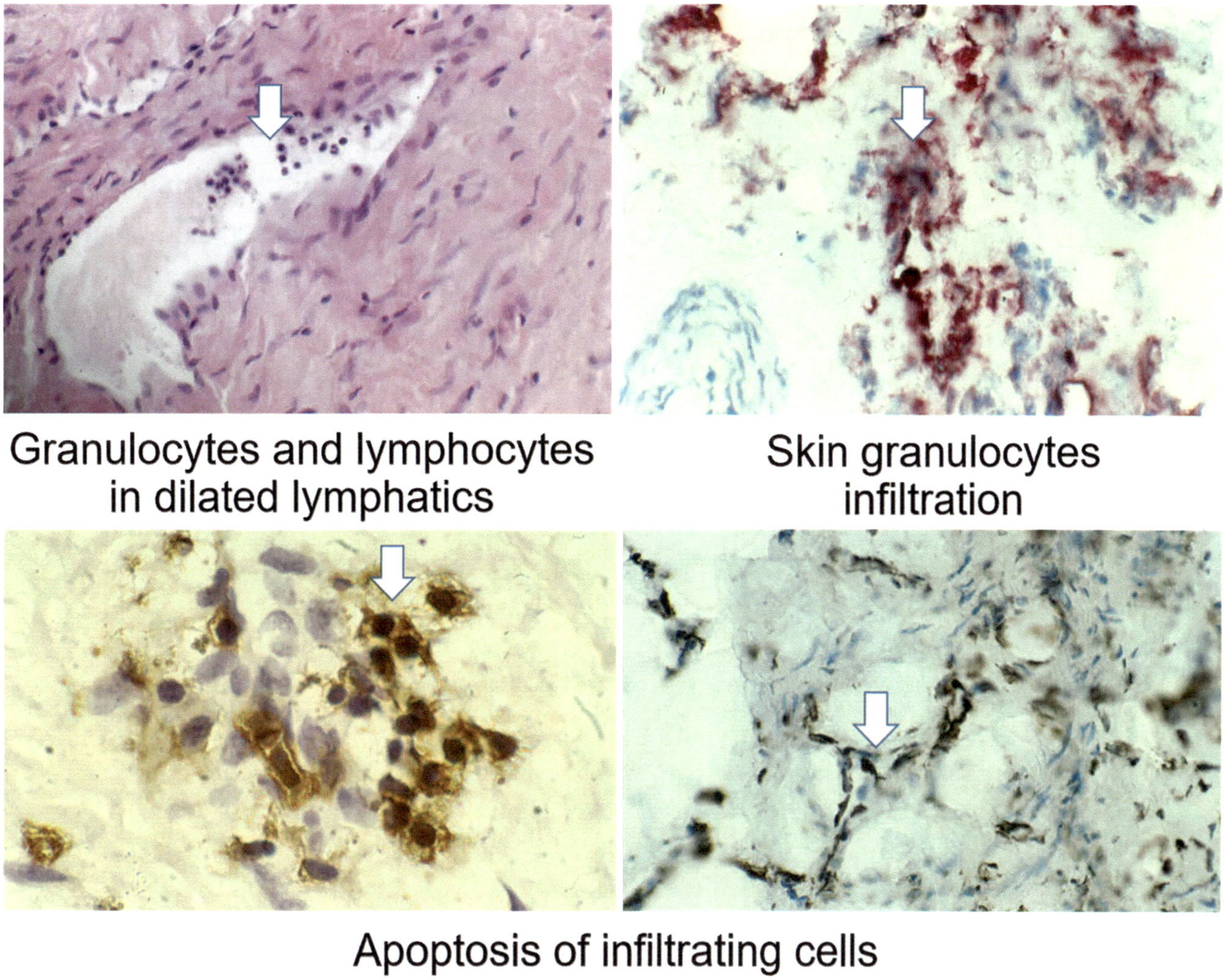

Fig. 16.10 Cellular changes are developing in the skin of the lymphedematous limbs. Granulocytes and recirculating lymphocytes are stuck in the non-conductive, dilated dermal lymphatics and fibrous and adipose tissue. Some of these cells undergo apoptosis. Their debris is not removed (hematoxylin-eosin, HIS 48 anti-granulocyte, anti-DNA fragmentation monoclonal antibodies, magn. × 40)

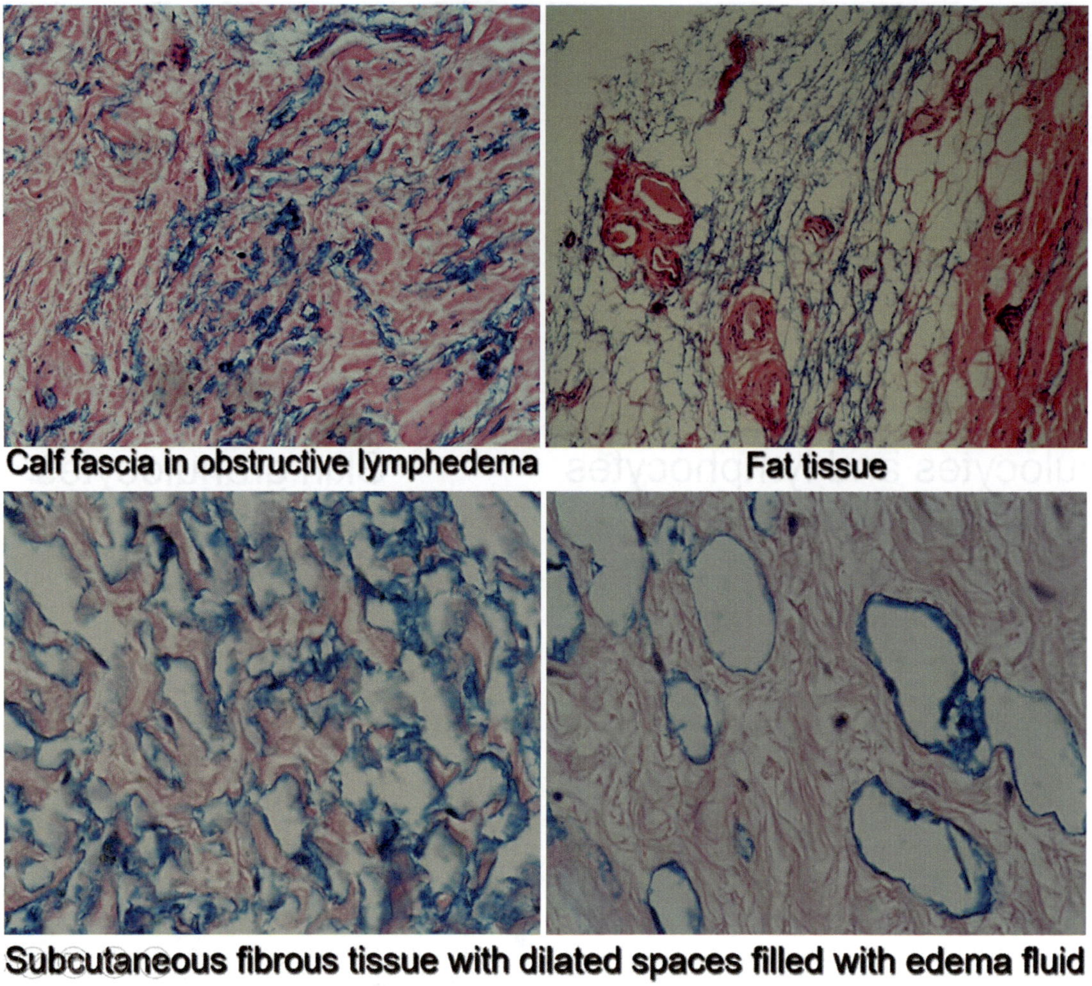

Fig. 16.11 Muscular fascia and subcutaneous tissue changes in the lymphedematous limbs. Deformed tissue with spontaneously formed tissue spaces (Paris Blue stained) filled up with edema fluid. Hyperplastic adipocytes are seen. (hematoxylin-eosin, × 20 and 40)

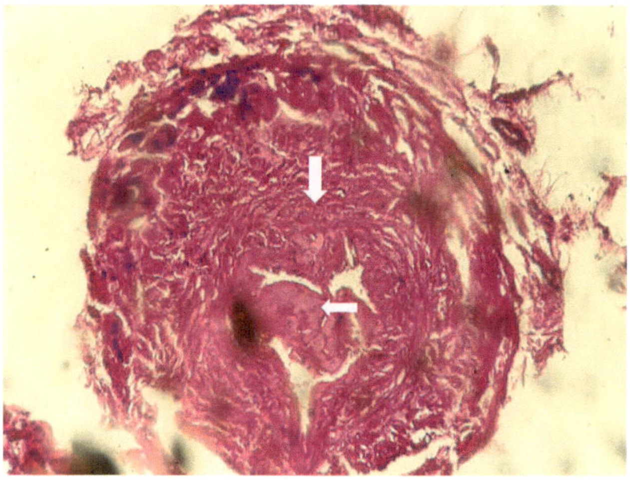

Fig. 16.12 Lymphatic collector with the occluded lumen. The upper arrow shows the irregular thick layer of collagen fibers, lower arrow points to an organized clot or acellular hyaline-like mass filling up the lumen. (hematoxylin-eosin, magn. × 40)

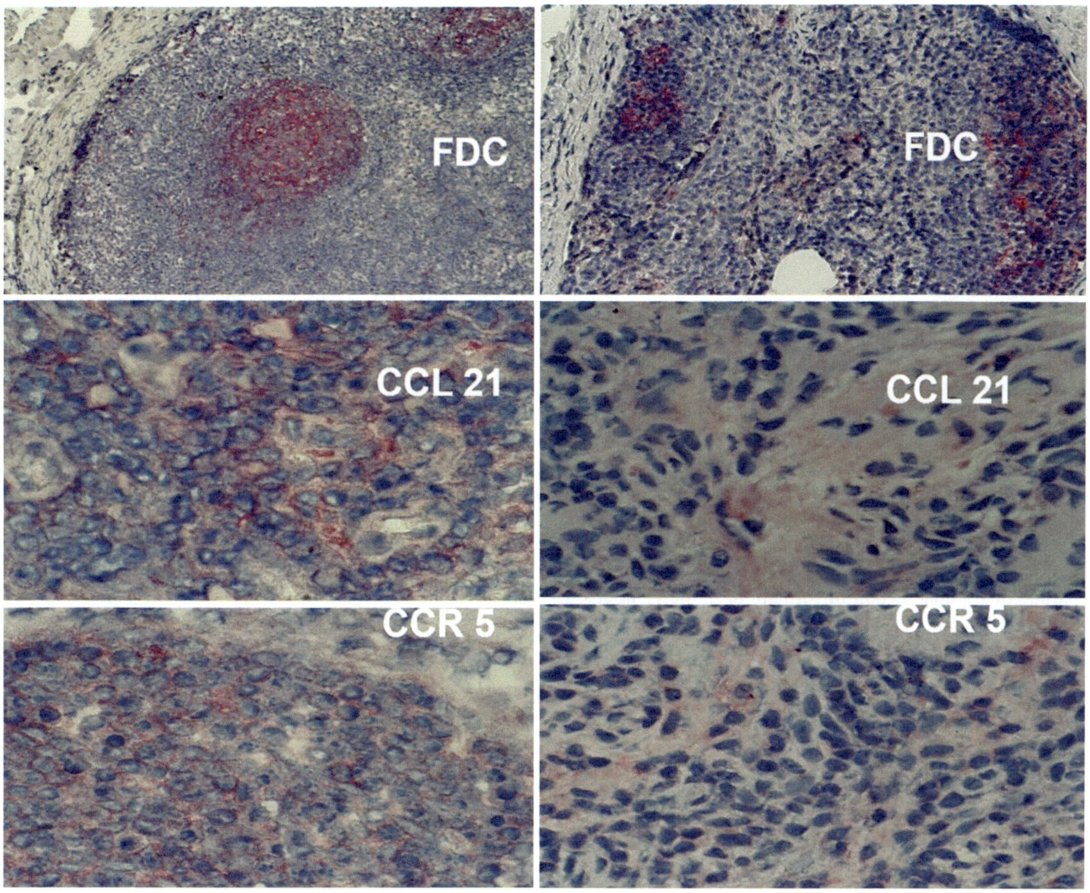

Fig. 16.13 Histological pictures of normal and lymphedema inguinal lymph nodes. Upper panel. Follicle with follicular dendritic cells (FDC) in the mid part of a normal node. In lymphedema, FDC is absent. Lack of follicle structure. Mid panel. The CLL21-positive para-cortical T cells in a normal node and lack of them in a lymphedema node. Lower panel. The CCL5-positive B cells in the follicle in a normal node. Lack of these cells in the lymphedema node. Obstruction of lymphocyte recirculation blood-interstitial space-lymphatics-lymphoid tissue-blood results in lack of influx of lymphocytes and dendritic cells into tissues. This may affect local immunity (monoclonal antibody to FDC-M1, CCL 21, and CCL5 cell antigens, magn × 40)

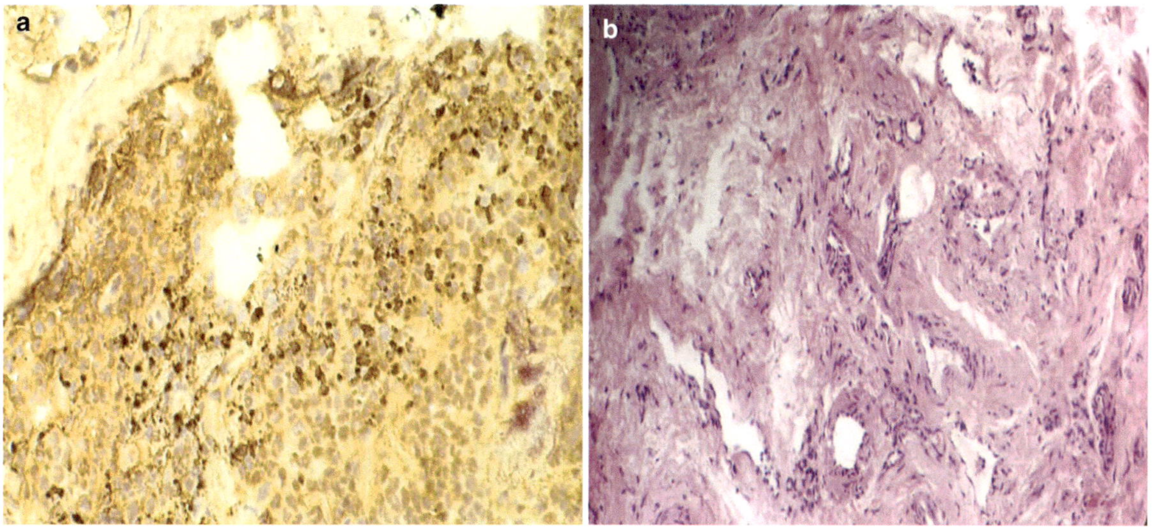

Fig. 16.14 Histological pictures of an inguinal lymph node in lymphedema. (**a**) apoptotic lymphocytes stained dark, (**b**) fibrosis of lymph node with lack of lymphoid tissue. In advanced stages of lymphedema lymph nodes undergo atrophy. There is no lymphocyte traffic through the node and no influx of antigens from the peripheral tissues (monoclonal antibodies to DNA fragments, hematoxylin-eosin stain, magn. × 40)

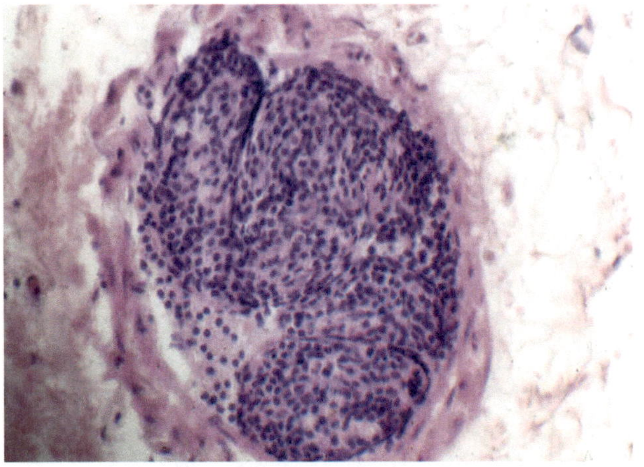

Fig. 16.15 Histological picture of a newly formed lymph node from the popliteal region in a lymphedematous limb. New lymphoid follicles arise in the periphery along the remaining patent deep lymphatics, usually along the popliteal and femoral artery and vein. An apparently paradoxical phenomenon of formation of "new" nodes in the lymphedematous tissues caused by bacterial antigenic stimulation of the pre-existing lymphoid follicles (hematoxylin-eosin, magn, × 40) (WLO de novo)

mation of collagen. In the third stage, the cells of the vessel wall are replaced with fiber elements. They become stiff, and their interior is limited or completely closed [1].

During lymphedema, the mass of keratinocytes, fibroblasts, and adipocyte cells increases. The intracellular matrix mass also increases due to production by resident cells of proteins and lipids and lack of transport away. The chronic inflammatory process proceeding with immune cell infiltrates and focal lymphocyte agglomerations.

References

1. Olszewski WL. Pathology and biochemistry. In: Lee BB, et al., editors. Lymphedema. London Limt: Springer-Verlag; 2011. p. 75–80.
2. Olszewski WL. Cells in lymph. In: Lymph stasis: pathophysiology, diagnosis and treatment. Boca Raton, FL: CRC Press; 1991. p. 259–83.
3. Olszewski WL, Engeset A, Romaniuk A, Grzelak I, Ziolkowska A. Immune cells in peripheral lymph and skin of patients with obstructive lymphedema. Lymphology. 1990;23:23–33.
4. Olszewski WL, Jamal S, Manokaran G, Lukomska B, Kubicka U. Skin changes in filarial and non-filarial lymphoedema of the lower extremities. Trop Med Parasitol. 1993;44(1):40–4.
5. Olszewski W, Machowski Z, Sokolowski J, Sawicki Z, Zerbino D, Nielubowicz J. Primary lymphedema of lower extremities. I. Lymphangiographic and histological studies of lymphatic vessels and lymph nodes in primary lymphedema. Pol Med J. 1972;11:1564–72.
6. Fumiere E, Leduc O, Fourcade S, Becker C, Garbar C, Demeure R, Wilputte F, Leduc A, Delcour C. MR imaging, proton MR spectroscopy, ultrasonographic, histologic findings in patients with chronic lymphedema. Lymphology. 2007;40:157–62.
7. Mihara M, Hara H, Hayashi Y, Narushima M, Yamamoto T, Todokoro T, Iida T, Sawamoto N, Araki J, Kikuchi K, Murai N, Okitsu T, Kisu I. Isao Koshima pathological steps of cancer-related lymphedema: histological changes in the collecting lymphatic vessels after lymphadenectomy. PLoS One. 2013;8(5):10.137.
8. Olszewski WL. De novo lymph node formation in chronic inflammation of the human leg. Ann N Y Acad Sci. 2002 Dec;979:166–77.

Part V

Diagnosis of Lymphedema: Assistant in Diagnosis

Clinical Diagnosis and Differential Diagnosis

17

Ningfei Liu

Abstract

The diagnosis of lymphedema is generally easy, especially when the patient has a family genetic history, history of surgery or radiotherapy, trauma, or infection. Congenital or early-onset primary lymphedema needs to be distinguished from the limb hypertrophy and vascular and bone deformities that are associated with some syndromes. In individuals with late-onset swelling, especially symmetrical swelling of both extremities, involvement of the heart or kidney and liver dysfunction must be excluded. Rapid developments in modern medical technology, especially imaging modalities for the lymphatic system, have made the diagnosis and differential diagnosis of lymphedema much easier.

Keywords

Peripheral lymphedema · Diagnosis
Differential diagnosis · Lymphatic system imaging
Genetic diagnosis

The diagnosis of lymphedema is based on the history and signs. When the patient has a family history of lymphedema or had experienced cancer treatment as surgery or radiation therapy, the diagnosis may not be difficult. The onset and progress of lymphedema are slowly and generally occurs in one of the arms or legs. The swelling caused by lymphedema ranges from early pitting and mild in a short period of time to late elephantiasis for years to decades. Primary lymphedema and anomalies of the lymphatic system can be accurately diagnosed with various individual or combined imaging modalities, including MR lymphangiography, lymphoscintigraphy, and or indocyanine green lymphography [1, 2, 3, 4, 5]. Developments in modern medicine and progress in the genetic study of lymphedema have made molecular diagnosis for both primary and secondary lymphedema possible. More than 20 genes that are pathogenic for primary lymphedema have been found thus far [6], as have some genes that increase susceptibility to secondary lymphedema, such as breast cancer-related lymphedema [7, 8]. An accurate diagnosis can lead to precise selection of treatment.

The following diseases can be confused with chronic lymphedema and should be included in the differential diagnosis:

1. Chronic varicose vein and valve dysfunction. This often involves the legs and results in skin pigmentation and sclerosis.
2. Acute deep venous thrombosis. Characteristics include acute onset, commonly unilateral, painful, Homan's sign positive. Associated pulmonary embolism can be fatal. The thrombosis can be diagnosed using Doppler ultrasound.
3. Cardiac edema. Pitting edema is confined to the distal regions of both lower extremities. Swelling may reduce after the elevation of the lower limbs.
4. Lipedema. This is more common in women and manifests as symmetrical or asymmetrical involvement of the lower limb(s) and trunk with no swelling in the feet. There is no cellulitis, and the skin is sensitive without keratosis (Fig. 17.1).
5. Myxedema. This is generally considered to be related to hypothyroidism. The patient has a history of treatment for hyperthyroidism. It involves both lower limbs with nodular hyperplasia of the skin (Fig. 17.2).
6. Benign tumor, such as neurofibroma. Although neurofibromas may appear somewhat similar to lymphedema, these benign tumors grow slowly, there is no history of infection, and the tumors are soft in marked contrast to the hardness of lymphedematous tissue. There is no skin keratosis with neurofibromas (Fig. 17.3), and there are characteristically associated brown spots or striations.

N. Liu (✉)
Department Plastic and Reconstructive Surgery,
Shanghai Ninth People's Hospital, Shanghai Jiao Tong University
School of Medicine, Shanghai, China

N. Liu (ed.), *Peripheral Lymphedema*, https://doi.org/10.1007/978-981-16-3484-0_17

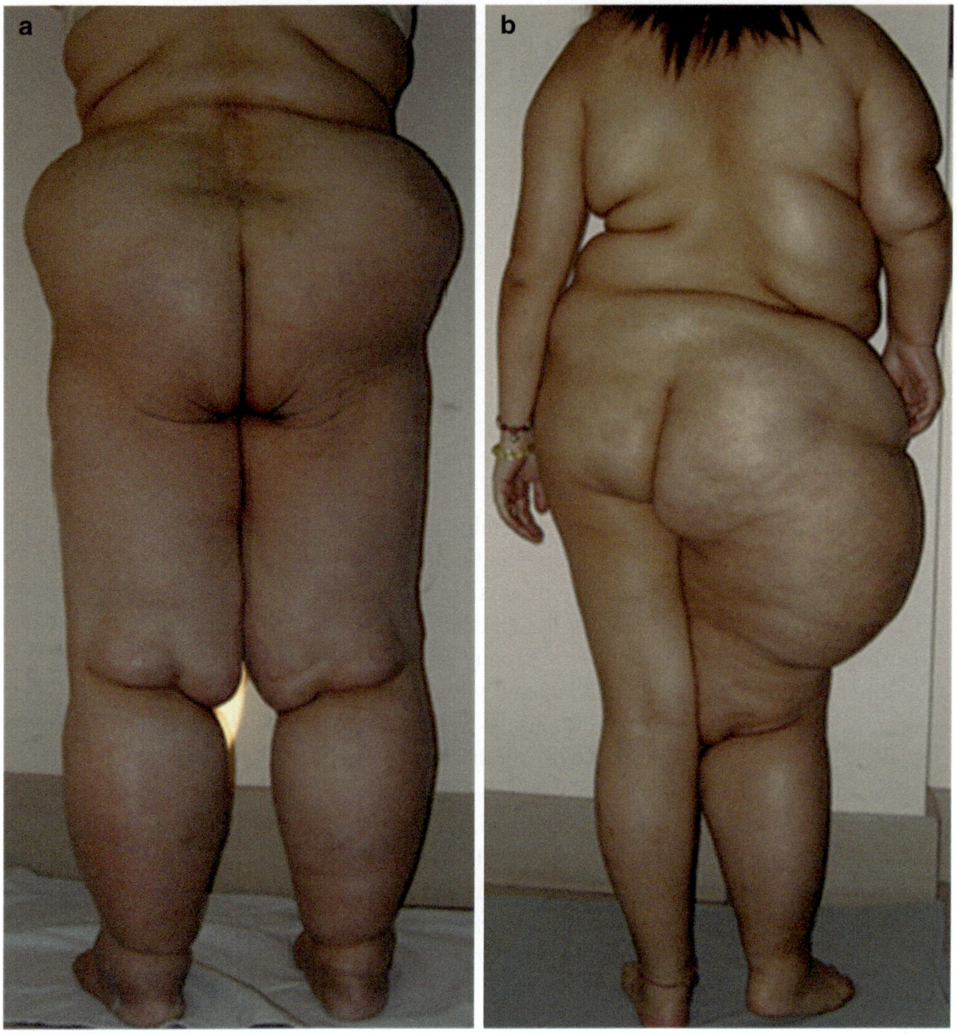

Fig. 17.1 (**a**) A woman with symmetrical lipedema of the trunk and lower limbs. (**b**) A woman with asymmetrical lipedema

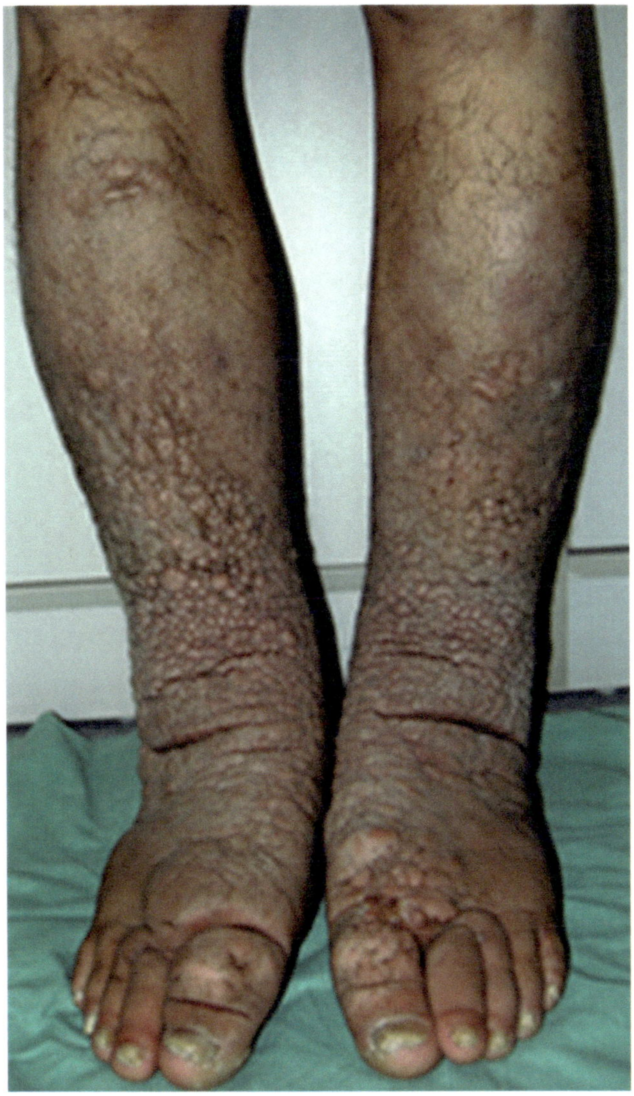

Fig. 17.2 Myxedema in the bilateral calf

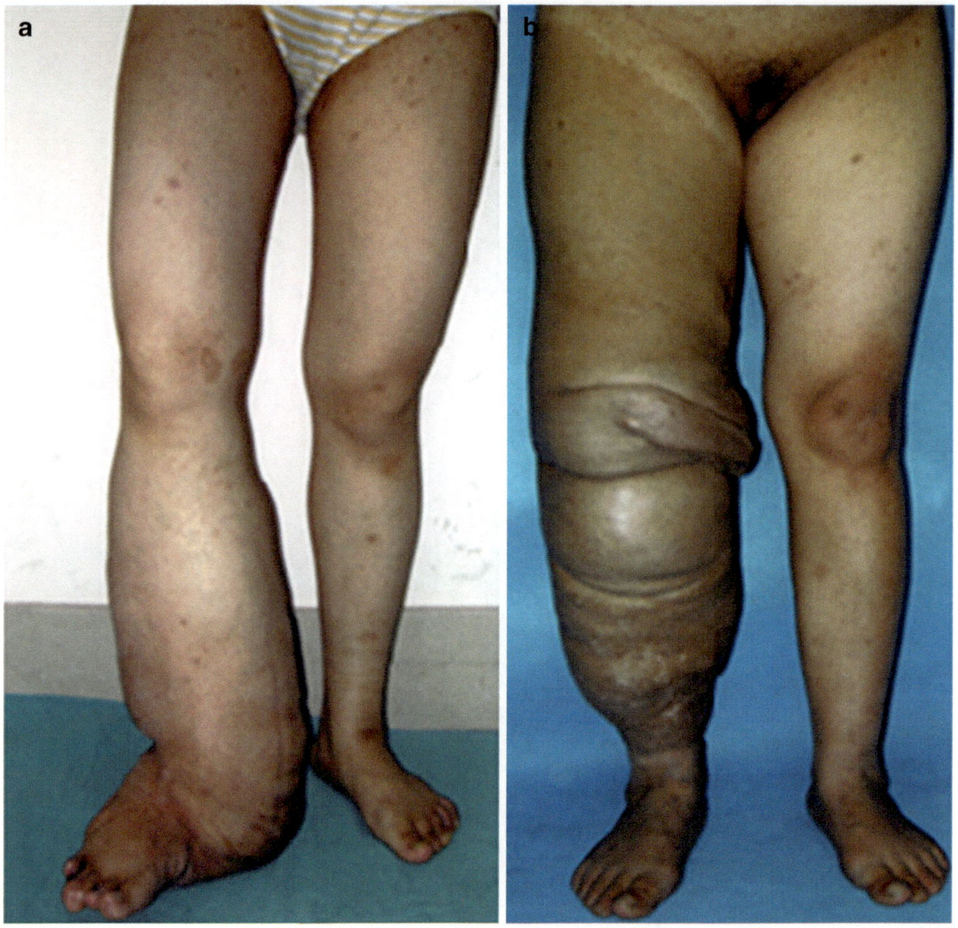

Fig. 17.3 (**a**) A woman with neurofibroma of right lower leg and foot. (**b**) A woman with neurofibroma of right thigh and calf

References

1. Liu NF, Lu Q, Jiang ZH, Wang CG, Zhou JG. Anatomic and functional evaluation of the lymphatics and lymph nodes in diagnosis of lymphatic circulation disorders with contrast magnetic resonance lymphangiography. J Vasc Surg. 2009;49(4):980–7.
2. Szuba A, Shin W, Strauss HW, Rockson S. The third circulation: radionuclide lymphoscintigraphy in the evaluation of lymphoedema. J Nucl Med. 2003;44(1):43–57.
3. Barrett T, Choyke PL, Kobayashi H. Imaging of the lymphatic system: new horizons. Contrast Media Mol Imaging. 2006;1(6):230–45.
4. Yu ZY, Sun D, Wang L, Chen J, Han LH, Liu NF. Diagnosis of primary lymphedema with indocyanine green lymphography. Chin J Plast Surg. 2018;34(4):256–9.
5. Yamamoto T, Yamamoto N, Doi K, Oshima A, Yoshimatsu H, Todokoro T, Ogata F, Mihara M, Narushima M, Iida T, Koshima I. Indocyanine green-enhanced lymphography for upper extremity lymphedema: a novel severity staging system using dermal backflow patterns. Plast Reconstr Surg. 2011;128(4):941–7. https://doi.org/10.1097/PRS.0b013e3182268cd9.
6. Michelini S, Paolacci S, Manara E, Eretta C, Mattassi R, Lee BB, Bertelli M. Genetic tests in lymphatic vascular malformations and lymphedema. J Med Genet. 2018;55(4):222–32. https://doi.org/10.1136/jmedgenet-2017-105064.
7. Brouillard P, Boon L, Vikkula M. Genetics of lymphatic anomalies. J Clin Invest. 2014;124(3):898–904. https://doi.org/10.1172/JCI71614.
8. Finegold DN, Schacht V, Kimak MA, Lawrence EC, Foeldi E, Karlsson JM, Baty CJ, Ferrell RE. HGF and MET mutations in primary and secondary lymphedema. Lymphat Res Biol. 2008;6(2):65–8. https://doi.org/10.1089/lrb.2008.1524.

MR Lymphangiography (MRL)

18

Ningfei Liu

Abstract

Magnetic resonance lymphangiography (MRL) is a relatively new imaging modality in the diagnosis of lymphatic disorders. Our experience with 4000 cases shows that MRL can provide high-quality imaging of structural anomalies of both lymphatic vessels and lymph nodes because of its high resolution. It is also possible to demonstrate functional changes in the lymphatic vessels and lymph nodes by tracing paramagnetic contrast injected intradermally into the distal part of the affected limb. We here provide details of the methodology of the MRL examination.

Keywords

MR lymphangiography · Dynamic imaging · Lymphatic vessel · Lymph node · Lymphedema · Lymphatic disorders · Morphology · Functional test · Paramagnetic contrast

Contrast magnetic resonance lymphangiography (MRL), a new means of imaging the lymphatic system, quickly and adequately demonstrates the lymphatic pathways and draining lymph nodes and can provide both a morphological and functional assessment [1, 2, 3, 4]. Paramagnetic contrast mediums like gadobenate dimeglumine that are used for MRL are commercially available and widely used. The contrast is injected intracutaneously into the interdigital webs of the dorsum of the foot or hand.

Following is a description of how we perform dynamic 3D-MRL. We use a 3.0 T MR unit with a maximum gradient strength of 80mT/m and a slew rate of 200mT/m/ms. The patient is placed in a supine position. A six-element phased array sensitivity encoding (SENSE) cardiac reception coil is used. The scanning starts from the patient's foot or hand and proceeds proximally in three or four separate and successive stages according to the length of the affected limb.

Before injection of contrast agent, a 3D heavily T2-weighted MRI is performed. The serial turbo sequences include fat saturation and half-scan acquisition single-shot fast spin-echo sequences using the following parameters: TR 2820 ms, TE740 ms, field of view 360 mm × 285 mm, matrix 240 × 190, slice thickness 2 mm, 55–85 slices. A series of maximum intensity projection (MIP) images are then constructed. For dynamic MRL, 3D fast spoiled gradient-recalled echo T1-weighted images with a fat saturation technique (T1 High-Resolution Isotropic Volume Excitation) are acquired at 5, 10, 15, 20, 25, and 30 min after injection of contrast. The MR imaging parameters are as follows: TR/TE 3.5/1.7 ms, flip angle 25°, the field of view 360 mm × 320 mm, matrix 300 × 256, slices 55–95, voxel size 1.5 mm × 1.2 mm × 1.2 mm, average number of signals 2, acquisition time 0 min 40s. We then use a maximum intensity projection (MIP) technique to construct 3D MR images from the post-contrast coronal images at each time point. The examination takes about one and half hours per patient. The appearance and pattern of distribution of lymphatic pathways in the affected extremities and the morphological characteristics of the inguinal or axillary nodes on pre- and post-contrast MR images are then analyzed.

Quantitative analysis includes:

- Assessment of the time course of enhancement of lymph flow in vessels directly draining from the injection site(s). The length of the enhanced vessel on the final image is recorded, and the speed of contrast movement calculated using the following formula:

N. Liu (✉)
Department Plastic and Reconstructive Surgery,
Shanghai Ninth People's Hospital, Shanghai Jiao Tong University School of Medicine, Shanghai, China

N. Liu (ed.), *Peripheral Lymphedema*, https://doi.org/10.1007/978-981-16-3484-0_18

$$\text{Speed (cm/min)} = \frac{\text{Total length of visualized lymph vessel (cm)}}{\text{Examination time (min)}}$$

Assessment of enhancement of the inguinal or axillary lymph nodes to which the injection site(s) directly drain. The ratio of the signal intensity (SI) of the lymph node to the signal intensity of adjacent muscle is calculated to evaluate the enhancement of these lymph nodes. Operator-defined regions of interest (ROIs) are drawn on coronal post-contrast images. In the case of the lower limb, the ROI for muscle is in the upper portion of the thigh near the inguinal region and of approximately the same size as the lymph node. The ratio of node/muscle SI on post-contrast MR images is compared between the lymphedematous and contralateral limb. The dynamic enhancement of contrast in the nodes bilaterally is estimated and wash-in and wash-out curves are derived from the designated ROI. The peak enhancement time and lymph node/muscle SI ratio at peak time are then directly compared.

18.1 Lymphatic Images

18.1.1 Lymphatic Drainage Patterns

Enhancement of lymphatic vessels with contrast is seen soon after injection.

The contrast agent enables the generation of clear images with low background of lymphatic vessels and lymph nodes. Generally, there are no contrast-enhanced or discontinuous lymphatic vessels in non-edematous healthy limbs. In lymphedematous limbs, contrast-enhanced lymphatics with the various pattern are demonstrated. Enhancement of these lymphatic pathways persists throughout the examination time of around 40 min. The signal intensity increases, and the channels gradually become totally opacified with time. Dermal back flow is another pathological feature of lymphatics in individuals with lymphedema. The number of contrast-enhanced lymphatics in primary lymphedematous limbs varies from single to numerous. Their irregular shapes, non-uniform diameters, and twistedness (Fig. 18.1a) make it easy to distinguish them from veins. In limbs with secondary lymphedema after tumor surgery, the lymphatics are dilated but not increased in number. In acute lymphedema, the diameters of the obstructed lymphatic channels are greatly increased (Fig. 18.2). The co-existence of accumulation of edema fluid in the subcutaneous tissues and visualization of contrast-enhanced lymphatic vessels is important in diagnosing lymphatic disorders.

18.1.2 Transportation of Contrast Within Lymphatic Channels

On post-contrast MR images of the lower limb, enhanced lymphatic vessels around the ankle are clearly visualized soon after injection. The flow of contrast within the vessels is detected on a series of dynamic images. The length of a relatively straight representative opacified lymphatic vessel with prominently enhanced lymph flow is then measured (Fig. 18.3a). The speed of contrast transportation can then be calculated and is expressed as cm/min. The speed of enhanced lymph flow in this study ranged from 0.301 to 1.48 cm/min in 23 patients (Fig. 18.3b). The real-time observation of the lymph flow in the lymph collectors of obstructed lymphedema lower limb demonstrated dynamic lymph leakage (Fig. 18.4).

18.2 Lymph Node Imaging

18.2.1 Morphologic Characteristics of Inguinal Lymph Nodes

Morphological changes, including nodal size, internal lymph node architecture, and lymph node borders, are evaluated. Inguinal lymph nodes on the contralateral side and in healthy volunteers characteristically number from two or three to seven or eight, are spherical or oval, and around 1.0 cm in diameter (Fig. 18.5). However, the shape, number, and volume of regional nodes in primary lymphedematous extremities vary greatly. Compared with the contralateral limb, the abnormalities of inguinal nodes in edematous limbs failure to visualize any nodes; small nodes; nodes with irregular borders and homogeneous architecture; irregular shape with homogeneous architecture; and increased numbers of enlarged nodes (Fig. 18.5).

18.2.2 Transportation of Contrast in Lymph Nodes

The filling function of inguinal nodes can be assessed 30–40 min after intracutaneous injection of the contrast agent. The lymph node to muscle signal intensity ratio is compared between nodes of the edematous limb and the contralateral nodes. Post-contrast MR images showed remarkably asymmetrical accumulation of contrast between the nodes of the edematous and contralateral limbs of patients with unilateral lymphedema (Fig. 18.6). The post-contrast enhancement of node/muscle SI ratio is significantly lower in lymphedematous limbs than in the contralateral limbs.

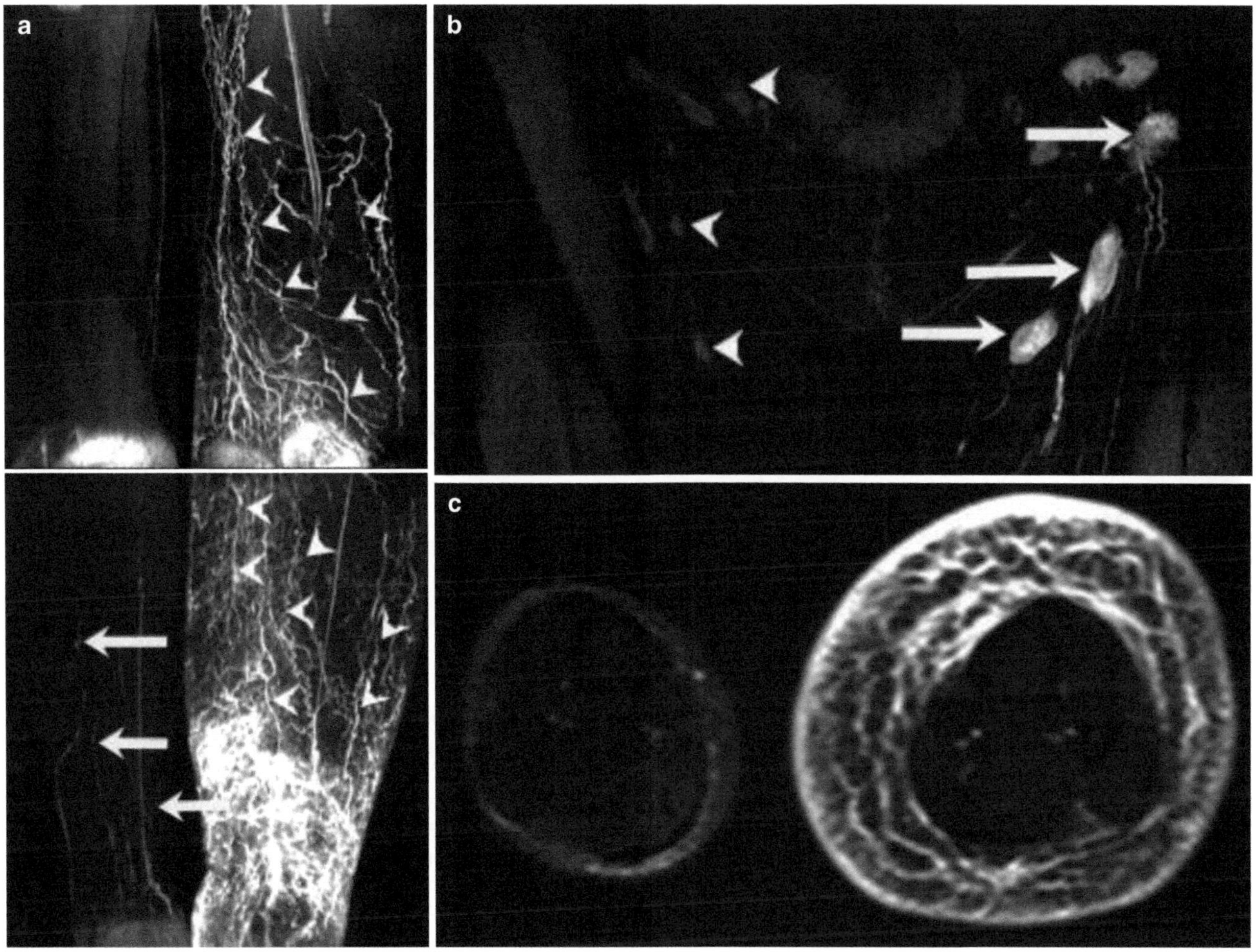

Fig. 18.1 (**a**) A 36-year-old woman with primary lymphedema of left lower limb, numerous tortuous and dilated lymph vessels (arrowheads) were demonstrated in contrast with contralateral no edema right limb with a few light lymphatic vessels (arrows) on postcontrast MRL imaging. (**b**) Enlarged inguinal lymph node with heterogeneous appearance and inhomogeneous enhancement in edema limb (arrows) in contrast with the contralateral nodes that were evenly enhanced (arrowheads). (**c**) Axial section of T2-weighted MR image shows the thickness and edema of the subcutis (high signal intensity) of the left lower limb

The specificity of absorption and transportation of the contrast agent by the lymphatic system makes it possible to visualize fine details of morphological changes in lymphatics and regional lymph nodes by high-resolution MR imaging. The rapid transportation of contrast agent by draining lymphatic and regional lymph node ensures the opportunity to consecutively and in real-time examine the transportation function of the lymphatics and lymph nodes within a reasonable length of time. Tracing the movement of enhanced flow within lymphatic vessels allows quantitative assessment of abnormal lymph flow kinetics. Comparison of dynamic nodal enhancement between the edematous and contralateral limbs and analysis of the time-signal intensity curves can clarify whether transport of lymph is delayed or absent in individual nodes, allowing quantitative assessment of abnormal nodal lymph flow kinetics. The combination of the lymphatic and lymph node images can then provide an integrated picture of the affected lymphatic system [5, 6, 7].

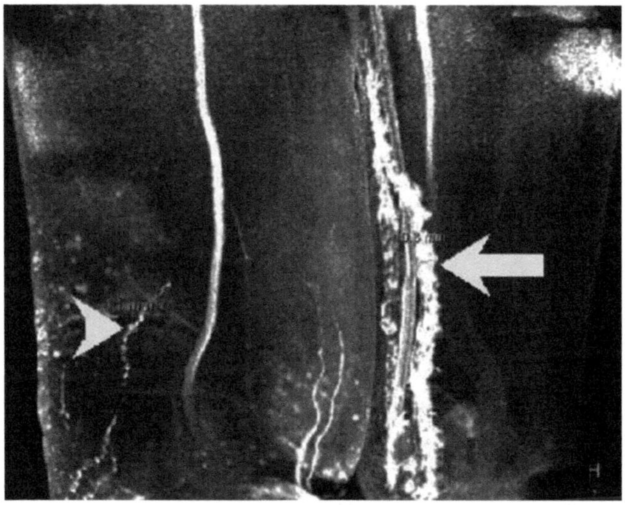

Fig. 18.2 MRL imaging in a woman with malignant lymphedema due to inguinal lymph node metastases. The arrow head in the right limb points to a lymphatic with 1.1 diameter, and the arrow in the left limb points to an extremely dilated lymphatic 10 mm in diameter

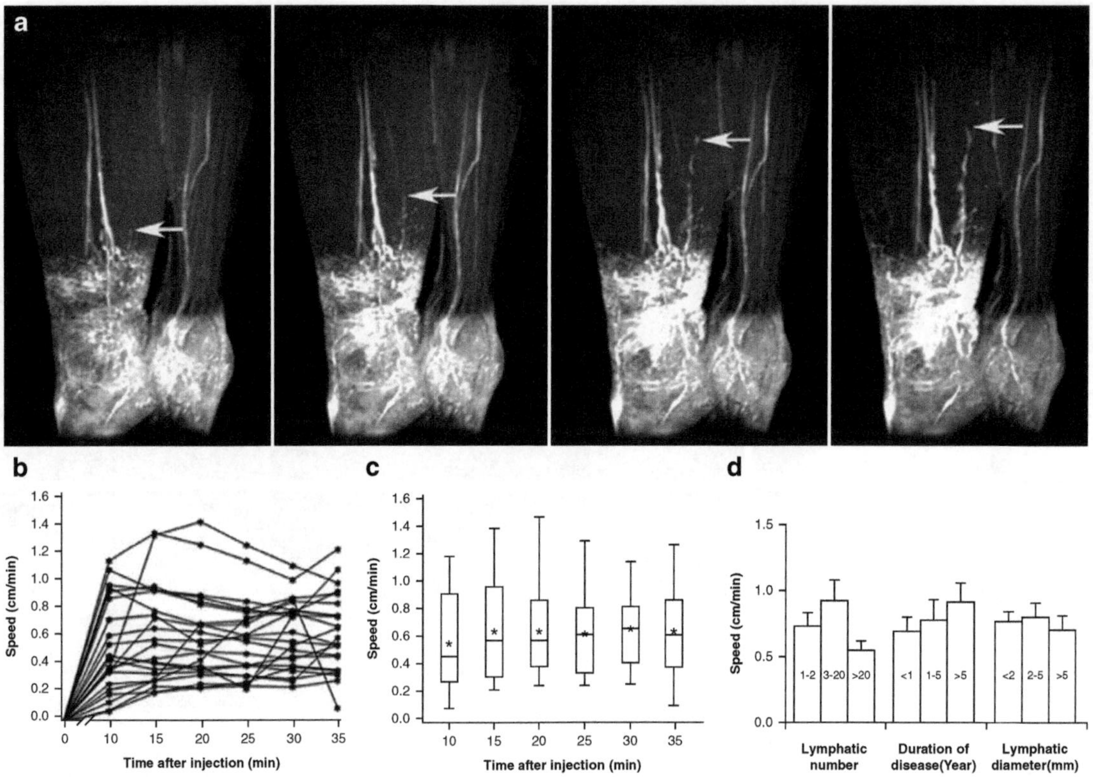

Fig. 18.3 Dynamic images of enhanced lymph flow. (**a**) Observation of movement of contrast-enhanced flow in a lymphedematous limb. (**b**) Enhanced flow speed (cm/min) at a series time points is shown for of 23 lymph vessels of lymphedematous limbs. (**c**) Mean flow speed is charted at each time point of 23 tested vessels.* The horizontal line in the middle of each box indicates the median; the top and bottom borders of the box mark the 75th and 25th percentiles, respectively. The whiskers mark the 90th and percentiles. (**d**) Comparison of lymph speed in three groups with various vascular diameters, vascular numbers, and disease durations. Data are presented with the standard deviation

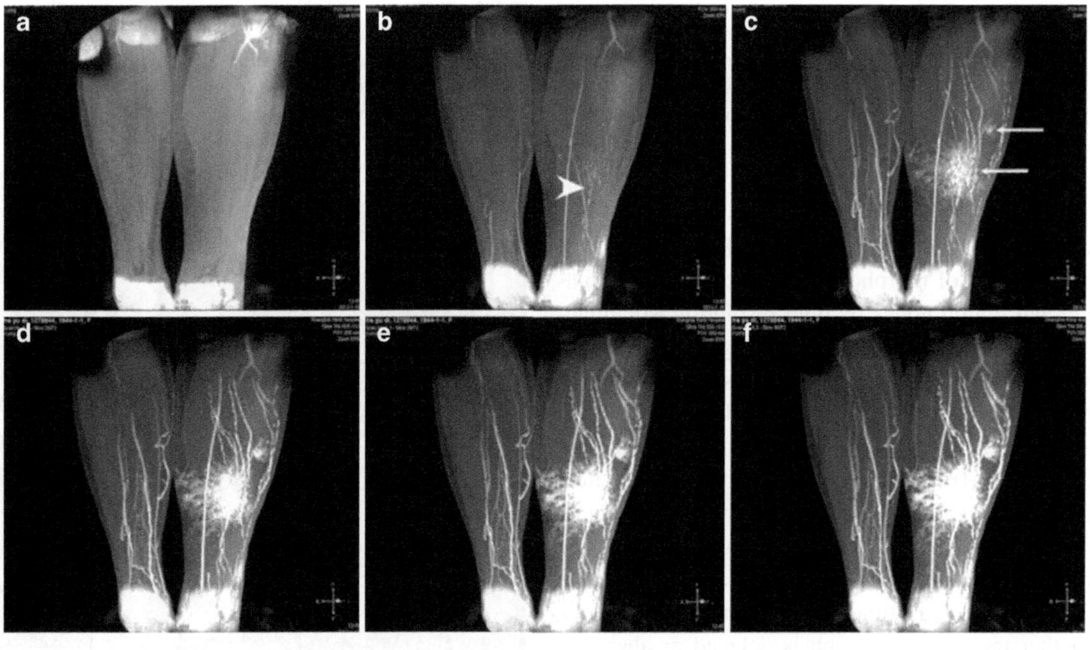

Fig. 18.4 Dynamic imaging MR lymphangiogram shows lymphatic disruption and lymph leakage in the left lower leg. (**a**) No lymph vessels were visualized on initial inspection. (**b**) Lightly enhanced collecting vessels (arrow head) were observed in the distal part of the lower leg at 8 min. (**c-f**) Anterior tibial lymphatic disruptions and lymph leakage (arrows) were displayed and extravasation of contrast and the enhancement of lymph vessels became evident over time (last image was at 18 min.)

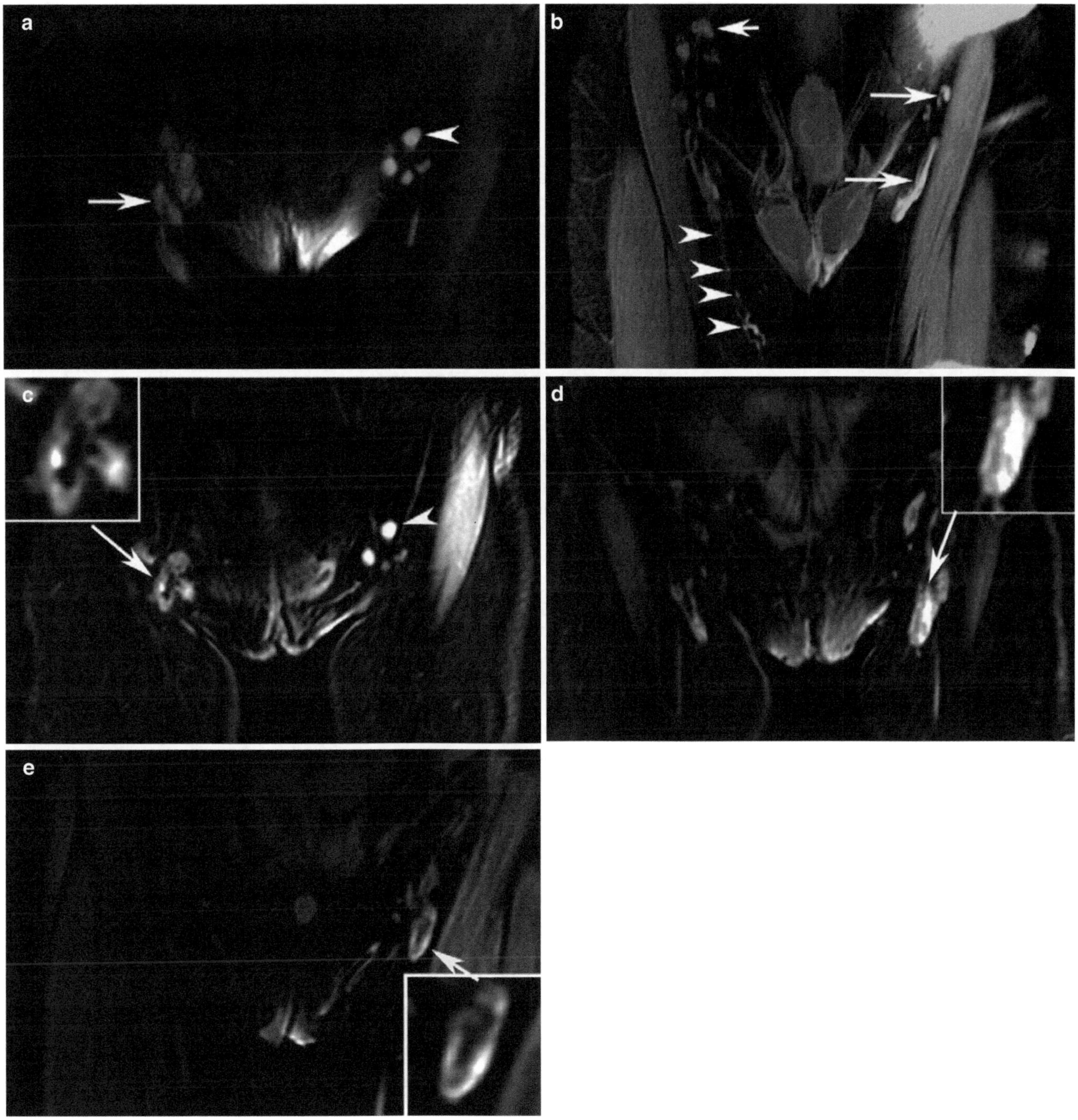

Fig. 18.5 Contrast magnetic resonance lymphangiographic imaging of inguinal lymph nodes. (**a**) asymmetrical accumulation of contrast between the nodes with heterogeneous appearance and poor enhancement in the edematous limb (arrow) and contralateral nodes that were evenly enhanced (arrowhead). (**b**) Contrast-enhanced flow is detained in afferent collectors (arrowheads) of a limb with lymphangiectasia without enhancement in the drainage nodes (short arrow) in contrast to highlighted nodes (arrow) in a limb without edema. (**c**) Contrast-enhanced central part of nodes (arrow) that are irregularly shaped are compared with evenly enhanced contralateral healthy nodes (arrowhead). (**d**) Central region of the enhanced node. Ee, (**e**) Contrast enhancement of contrast in the marginal region of the nodes and left central region unenhanced

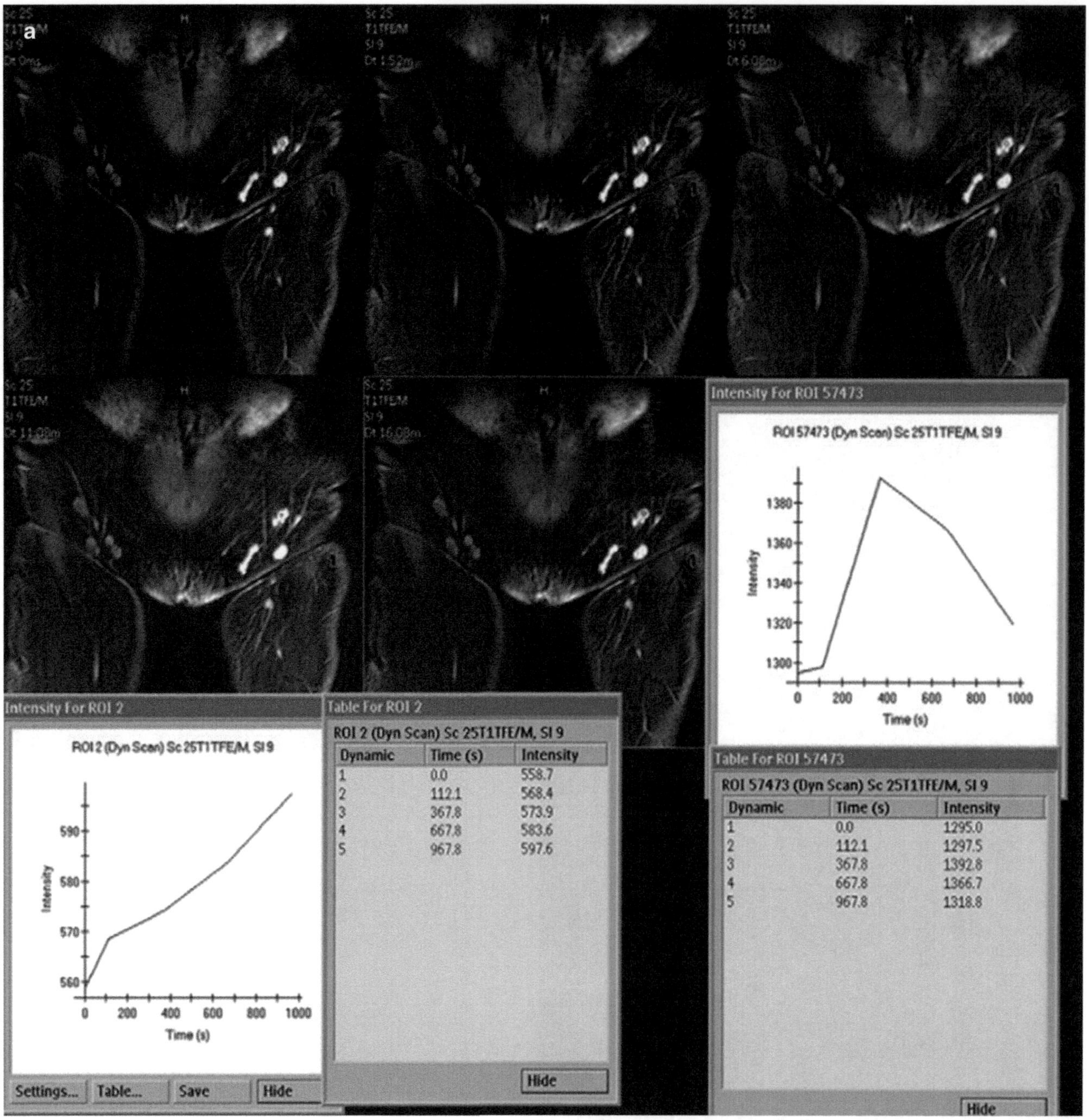

Fig. 18.6 Coronal images of dynamic enhancement of lymph nodes after contrast injection. (**a**) Real-time record of comparison of nodal enhancement in edematous (arrow) and non-edematous (arrowhead) limbs in a series of images. The wash-in curve was prolonged in (left) the affected limb in contrast with a quick wash-in and wash-out curve in (right) the unaffected limb. (**b**) Peak time node vs. muscle signal intensity ratios in affected limbs were significantly lower than that of unaffected limbs. (**c**) Nodes of edematous limbs displayed significantly longer time to peak enhancement

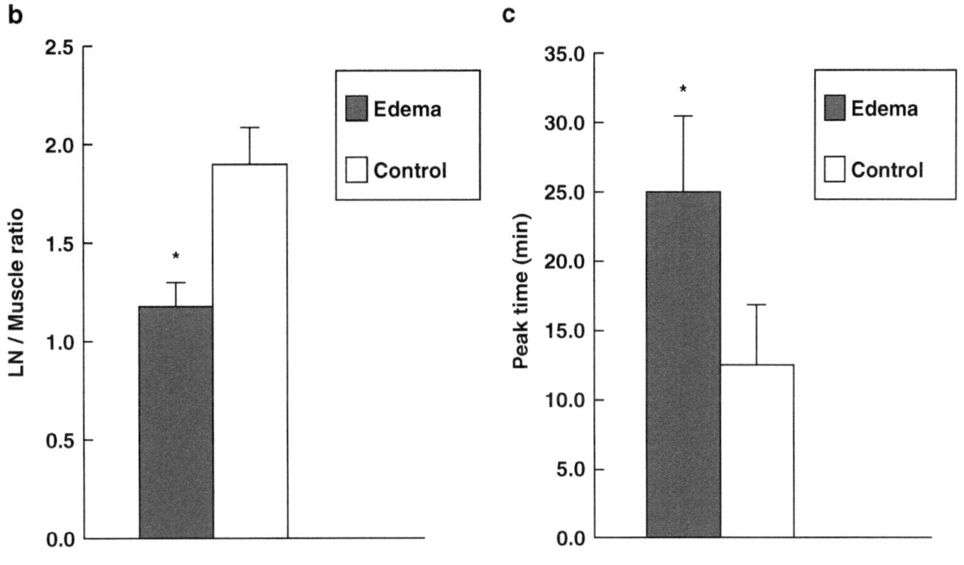

Fig. 18.6 (continued)

Furthermore, contrast-enhanced 3D MR not only demonstrates the lymphatics and lymph nodes, but also identifies extra-lymphatic abnormalities such as the location of edema in tissues and deposition of fat tissue, enabling differentiation of different types of edema. Because of the limitation of scanning by the MR unit, the feet are not included in routine tests, which is a limitation of MRL. In patients with lymphatic dysfunction, the slow enhancement of lymphatics in the dorsum of the foot may not be visualized. We, therefore, recommend additional ICG lymphography to help differentiate lymphatic aplasia/hypoplasia from lymphatic dysfunction in patients in whom these disorders are suspected.

References

1. Liu NF, Lu Q, Jiang ZH, Wang CG, Zhou JG. Anatomic and functional evaluation of the lymphatics and lymph nodes in diagnosis of lymphatic circulation disorders with contrast magnetic resonance lymphangiography. J Vasc Surg. 2009;49(4):980–7.
2. Barrett T, Choyke PL, Kobayashi H. Imaging of the lymphatic system: new horizons. Contrast Media Mol Imaging. 2006;1(6):230–45.
3. Lohrmann C, Felmerer G, Speck O, Keck T, Foeldi E, Langer M. Postoperative lymphoceles: detection with high-resolution MR lymphangiography. J Vasc Interv Radiol. 2006;17(6):1057e62.
4. Lu Q, Xu J, Liu N. Chronic lower extremity lymphedema: a comparative study of high-resolution interstitial MR lymphangiography and heavily T2-weighted MRI. Eur J Radiol. 2010;73(2):365e73. https://doi.org/10.1016/j.rad.2008.10.041.
5. Liu NF, Lu Q, Wang CG, Zhou JG. Magnetic resonance imaging as a new method to diagnose protein losing enteropathy. Lymphology. 2008;41(3):111–5.
6. Lu Q, Bui D, Liu NF, Xu JR, Zhao XH, Zhang XF. Magnetic resonance Lymphography at 3T: a promising noninvasive approach to characterise inguinal lymphatic vessel leakage. Eur J Vasc Endovasc Surg. 2012 Jan;43(1):106–11. https://doi.org/10.1016/j.ejvs.2011.09.007.
7. Liu N, Zhang Y. Magnetic resonance lymphangiography for the study of lymphatic system in lymphedema. J Reconstr Microsurg. 2016;32(1):66–71. https://doi.org/10.1055/s-0034-1384213.

19 Nuclear Medicine Imaging in the Diagnosis of Peripheral Lymphedema: Lymphoscintigraphy

Feng Xu

Abstract

Lymphoscintigraphy has been used to study the lymphatic system by injecting radiolabeled tracers for decades. It was an easy and safe method to evaluate the lymphatic system. Furthermore, it can be performed on patients of any age with extremely low radiation exposure and making dynamic observation of tracer distribution possible. Lymphoscintigraphy was usually performed by a γ-camera with low-energy high-resolution collimators, which is available at most centers worldwide. Lymphoscintigraphy was carried out in our section (Nuclear Medicine, Shanghai Ninth People's hospital) since the year 2007 when dual-head SPECT/CT was introduced in our hospital. In this part, we introduce the common tracers, methods, and typical images of lymphoscintigraphy.

Keywords

Lymphoscintigraphy · Diagnosis · Peripheral Lymphedema

Lymphoscintigraphy has been used to study the lymphatic system by injecting of radiolabeled tracers since the 1950s [1]. It offers an objective and reliable approach to diagnose and characterize the severity of lymphedema [2]. Lymphoscintigraphy can be performed by a γ-camera with low-energy high-resolution collimators, which is available at most centers. General application of lymphoscintigraphy was to distinguish lymphatic from venous edema [3], evaluate the efficacy of treatment [4, 5], identify sentinel nodes in patients with melanoma [6] or breast [7], identify the inguinal lymph nodes in patients with pelvic tumor, or quantify lymphatic flow [8].

The kind of radiotracers for lymphoscintigraphy was various. They were mainly divided into two types: colloidal and noncolloidal radiotracers [9]. These tracers differ based on particle size. The best particle size for lymphoscintigraphy is considered to be between 50 and 70 nm [10]. The most commonly used tracers are summarized in Table 19.1. They are all ^{99m}Tc-labeled tracers which are suitable for nuclear imaging with a suitable energy peak (140 kev) and a half-life of 6.02 h. The liver and kidneys take up the tracers physiologically and excreted to the bladder. Nowadays, in China, ^{99m}Tc-sulfur colloids and ^{99m}Tc-dextan were the most frequently used tracers for lymphoscintigraphy [7, 11, 12].

The protocol for lymphoscintigraphy is not standardized till now due to the choice of the radiotracer, the type and site of injection, the use of dynamic and static acquisitions, and the acquisition time, which made it difficult to compare the findings across the studies [9].

Both subcutaneous and intradermal injections are used in routine lymphoscintigraphy. Which way is better is still in controversial. Suga K et al. indicated that intradermal administration of noncolloidal agents (^{99m}Tc-human serum albumin) is associated with rapid lymphatic transport, facilitating rapid evaluation and better quantification of lymphatic flow [5].

In our section, the tracer was administrated intradermally into the first three web spaces of both feet (0.3 mL, 37 MBq in total) for the patient with lower extremity lymphedema or first three web space of each hand for the patient with upper limb swelling, three injections for each limb in total. Each injection site was covered with a cotton ball to prevent leakage of tracer through the needle puncture site. Feet or hands were gently massaged for at least 5 min at the injection sites to promote uptake of the tracer into lymphatic channels and lymphatic flow. The procedure is safe as tracers rarely cause an allergic reaction [13].

Rezende et al. suggested that most axillary lymph nodes were seen in 1 h after ^{99m}Tc-dextan was subcutaneously

F. Xu (✉)
Department of Nuclear Medicine, Shanghai Ninth People's Hospital, Shanghai JiaoTong University School of Medicine, Shanghai, China

N. Liu (ed.), *Peripheral Lymphedema*, https://doi.org/10.1007/978-981-16-3484-0_19

injected on the dorsum of the hand in preoperative patients with breast cancer [14]. In our section, lymphoscintigraphy with ^{99m}Tc-dextan was usually performed 1 hour after injection of ^{99m}Tc-dextan. As shown in Table 19.1, the particle size of ^{99m}Tc-dextan was much smaller than ^{99m}Tc-sulfur colloids, the large particle size of ^{99m}Tc-sulfur colloid contributes to the minimal absorption and slow transit [15]. Therefore, lymphoscintigraphy with ^{99m}Tc- sulfur colloids was performed usually 3 h after injection. All lymphoscintigraphy was completed by a SPECT/CT scanner with low-energy high-resolution collimators from the feet to liver (or head when necessary) for lower extremity lymphedema and from the lower abdomen to head for the patient with upper limb swelling, the parameters of the scan included an energy peak of 140 keV, window width of 20%, acquisition speed of 5 cm/min, acquisition matrix of 512 × 512, and magnification of 1. Lymphoscintigraphy with ^{99m}Tc-dextan or ^{99m}Tc-sulfur colloids was repeated several times with the same method in 24 hours after injection when dynamic observation of tracer distribution was needed.

Table 19.1 Frequently used radiotracers in China and their particle size

Type	Agent	Particle size
Colloidal	^{99m}Tc-sulfur colloids	100–1000 nm
	^{99m}Tc-phytate	200–1000 nm
Noncolloidal	^{99m}Tc-dextan	6–7 nm
	^{99m}Tc-human serum albumin	2–3 nm

In our section, lymphoscintigraphy with ^{99m}Tc-sulfur colloids was performed 3 h after injection because of its large particle size. Bilateral inguinal lymph nodes were demonstrated clearly in patients with no lymphedema on the lower extremity (Fig. 19.1a). Asymmetry of inguinal lymph nodes, dermal backflow, and abnormal deep collateral flow partial such as popliteal lymph nodes can be seen on patients with partial obstruction(Fig. 19.1b–d). Lymphoscintigraphy also demonstrated the area where the lymph chain was disrupted by operation (Fig. 19.1e). In our experience, the images achieved by ^{99m}Tc-dextan were almost the same as ^{99m}Tc-sulfur colloids (Fig. 19.2). The main difference was the acquisition time, in most cases with no limb lymphedema, inguinal, or axillary lymph nodes appeared clearly about one hour after an injection of ^{99m}Tc-dextan. Three hours later, the inguinal or axillary lymph nodes became heavier. Suehiro et al. indicated that earlier visualization of inguinal or axillary lymph nodes was suggestive of a high output status of the lymphatic system of one's legs or arms by using lymphoscintigraphy with ^{99m}Tc-human serum albumin [3], which was consist with our findings with ^{99m}Tc-sulfur colloids

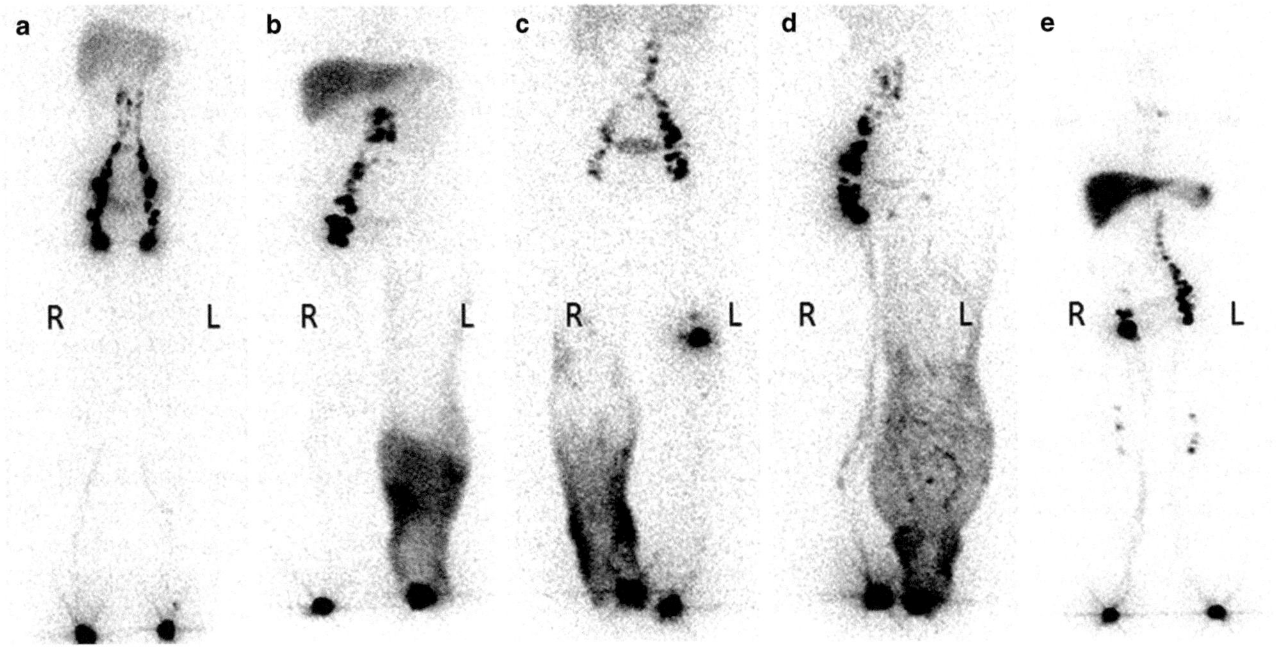

Fig. 19.1 Lymphoscintigraphy with 99mTc-sulfur colloids. Three hours after injection of ^{99m}Tc-sulfur colloids. (**a**) Patient with no lymphedema on both legs; Bilateral inguinal lymph nodes, iliacs lymph nodes, and lumbar trunk were demonstrated clearly. (**b**) Patient with lymphedema in left leg; Dermal backflow was seen in the left shank with no lymph node displayed in the left leg. (**c**) Patient with lymphedema on both legs; Dermal backflow was seen in the right shank, meanwhile, the right inguinal lymph nodes imaged poorly. No dermal backflow was seen in the left leg; however, the inguinal lymph nodes and iliacs lymph nodes were not demonstrated clearly as normal, and the popliteal lymph node was seen. (**d**) Patient with lymphedema on left leg; Dermal backflow was seen in the whole left leg with no lymph nodes displayed. (**e**) Woman developed swelling in her right upper thigh after right inguinal lymph nodes dissection due to endometrial carcinoma. The right lymph chain was disrupted in the inguinal area

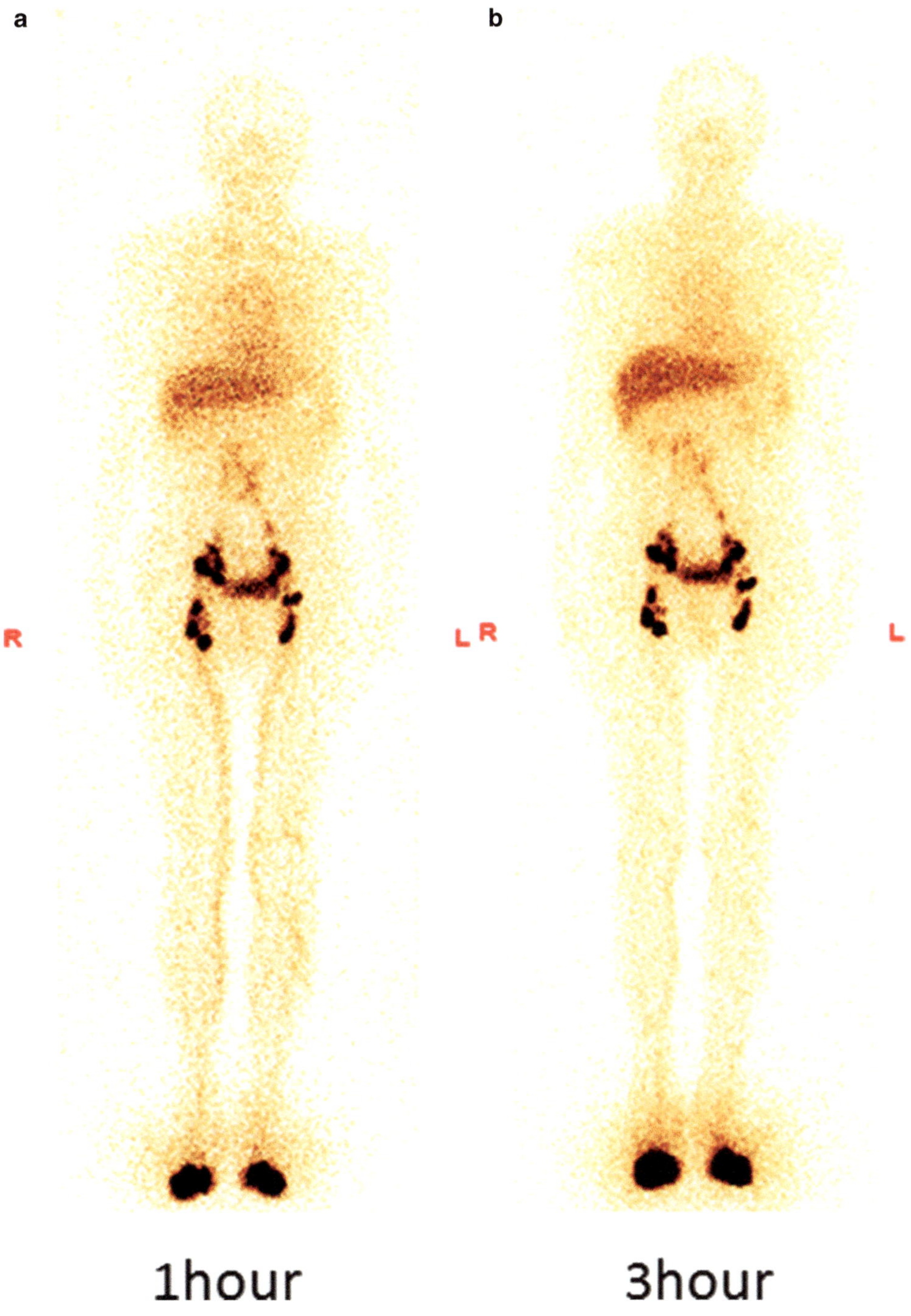

Fig. 19.2 Normal distribution of ^{99m}Tc-dextan in the lower extremity in a 76-year man. One hour after injection (**a**), bilateral inguinal and iliac lymph nodes were seen as well as lymph vessels. Liver and bladder were appeared; Three hours later (**b**), bilateral lymph vessels cleared away, the lymph nodes were almost the same as the previous exam

(Fig. 19.1b–d) and ^{99m}Tc-dextan (Figs. 19.3, 19.4, 19.5, and 19.6). Meanwhile, the absence of inguinal lymph nodes does not indicate the obstruction of the whole limb (Fig. 19.7), in order to make it clear, the proximal area should be injected with tracer additionally (Figs. 19.7 and 19.8). Lymphoscintigraphy can also be performed in the area of the head and neck as well as the limbs. The findings were the same as the limbs (Fig. 19.9).

Compare to the lymph nodes imaged in the lymphoscintigraphy, the lymph vessels were not imaged as clear as lymph nodes (Fig. 19.6). For one thing, the best acquisition time for lymph vessels were correlated to one's output status of the lymphatic system. The higher the output status, the earlier acquisition time is needed. For another, the spatial resolution of lymphoscintigraphy was low. Compared to lymphoscintigraphy, MRI lymphangiography is more suitable to demonstrate the lymph vessels [16].

Some authors [9, 17, 18] attempted to propose a staging/scoring system for patients with lymphedema by the images of lymphoscintigraphy, unfortunately, they are not widely

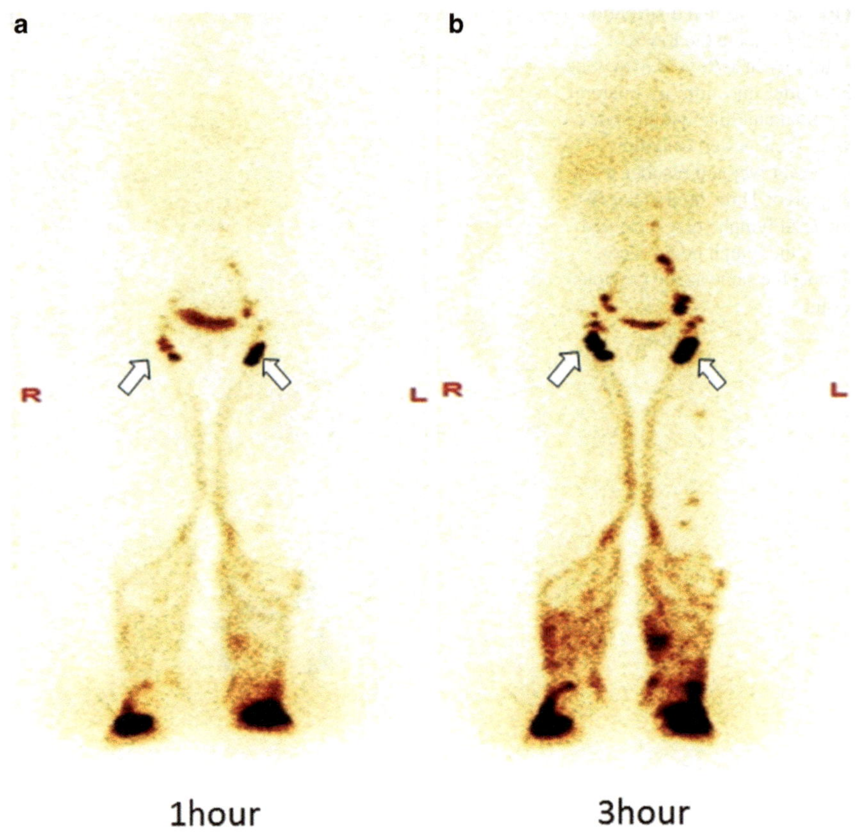

Fig. 19.3 Bilateral edema of shanks and ankles (mainly on the right side) occurred in a 24-year young woman more than 20 years. One hour after injection (**a**), dermal backflow was seen in both shanks; meanwhile, bilateral lymph vessels and inguinal lymph nodes were appeared; however, the right inguinal lymph node was not as clear as the left side (white arrows); Three hours later (**b**), dermal backflow and bilateral lymph vessels became heavier. Inguinal lymph nodes were clear as normal

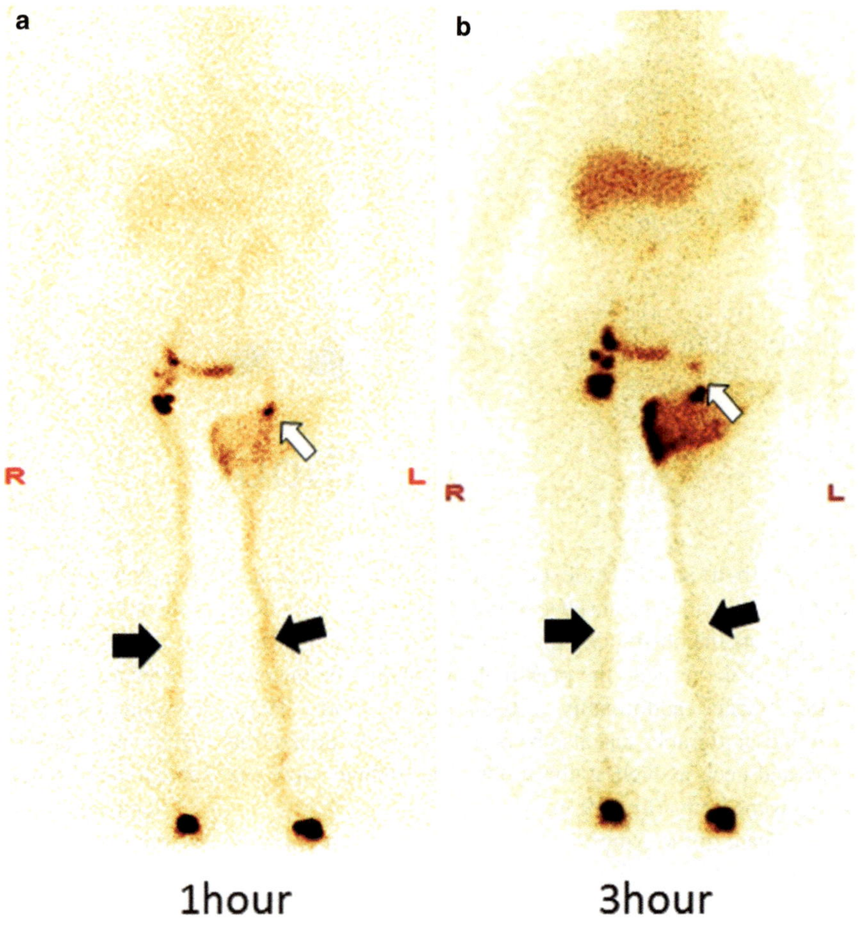

Fig. 19.4 Left thigh edema occurred in a 46-year female 3 months after left inguinal lymph nodes dissection due to cervical cancer. One hour after injection (**a**), bilateral lymph vessels were appeared (black arrow), and dermal backflow was seen in the left thigh; meanwhile, the left inguinal lymph nodes imaged poorly (white arrow) compared to the opposite side. Three hours later (**b**), bilateral lymph vessels cleared away slowly (black arrow). Dermal backflow became heavier. More inguinal lymph nodes imaged in the left side, but still not clear as normal (opposite side)

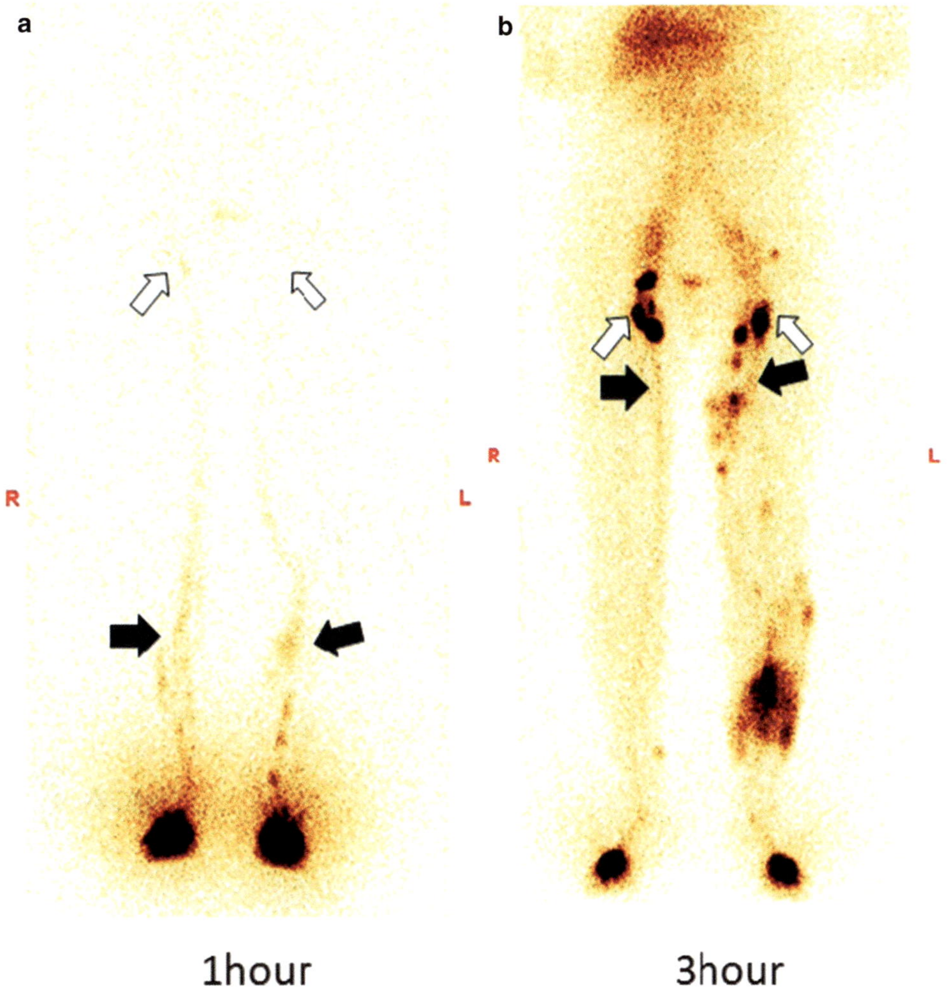

Fig. 19.5 Eight years after the operation of the left knee joint in a 74-year-old woman, the infection occurred twice a year during the period. Bilateral edema occurred in her lower limbs (Mainly on the left side). One hour after injection (**a**), bilateral lymph vessels were seen (black arrows) in the shanks; meanwhile, the bilateral inguinal lymph nodes were not seen (white arrows). Three hours later (**b**), bilateral lymph vessels cleared away in the shanks and appear in the thigh (black arrows). Dermal backflow was seen in the left shank. Bilateral inguinal lymph nodes were seen (white arrows)

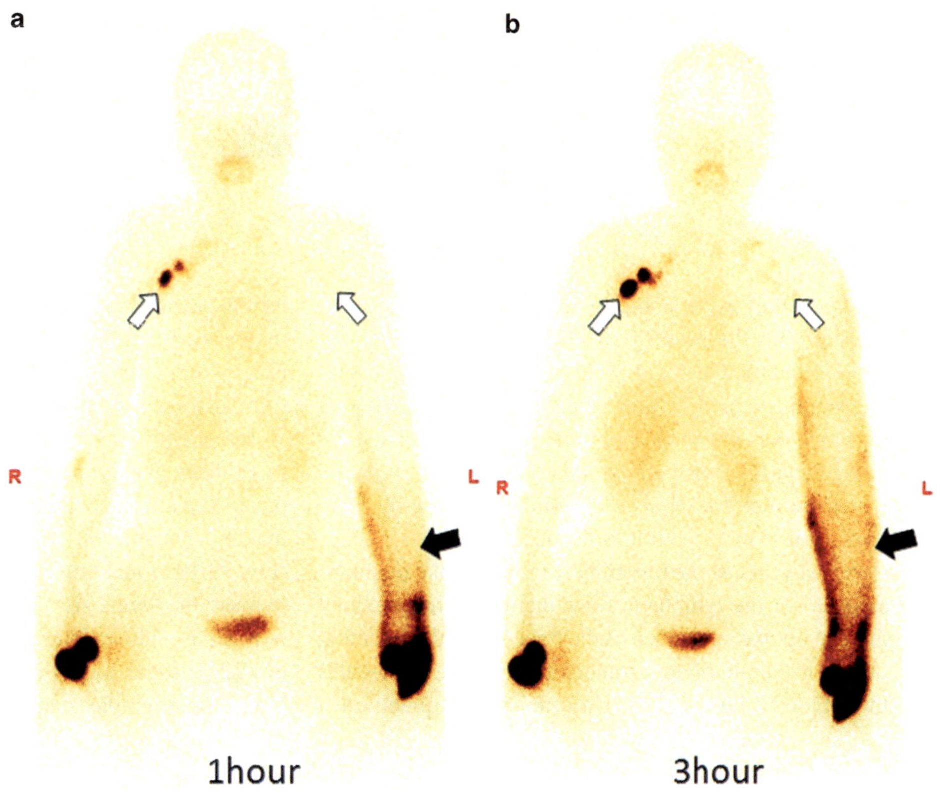

Fig. 19.6 Edema with red skin of left upper limb occurred in a 74-year-old woman for 4 months. One hour after injection (**a**), the right axillary lymph nodes were seen, while the left axillary lymph nodes were not seen (white arrows), meanwhile, dermal backflow was seen in her left upper limb (black arrow). Three hours later (**b**), dermal backflow became heavier in the whole upper limb (black arrow), and the left axillary lymph nodes were still not appeared

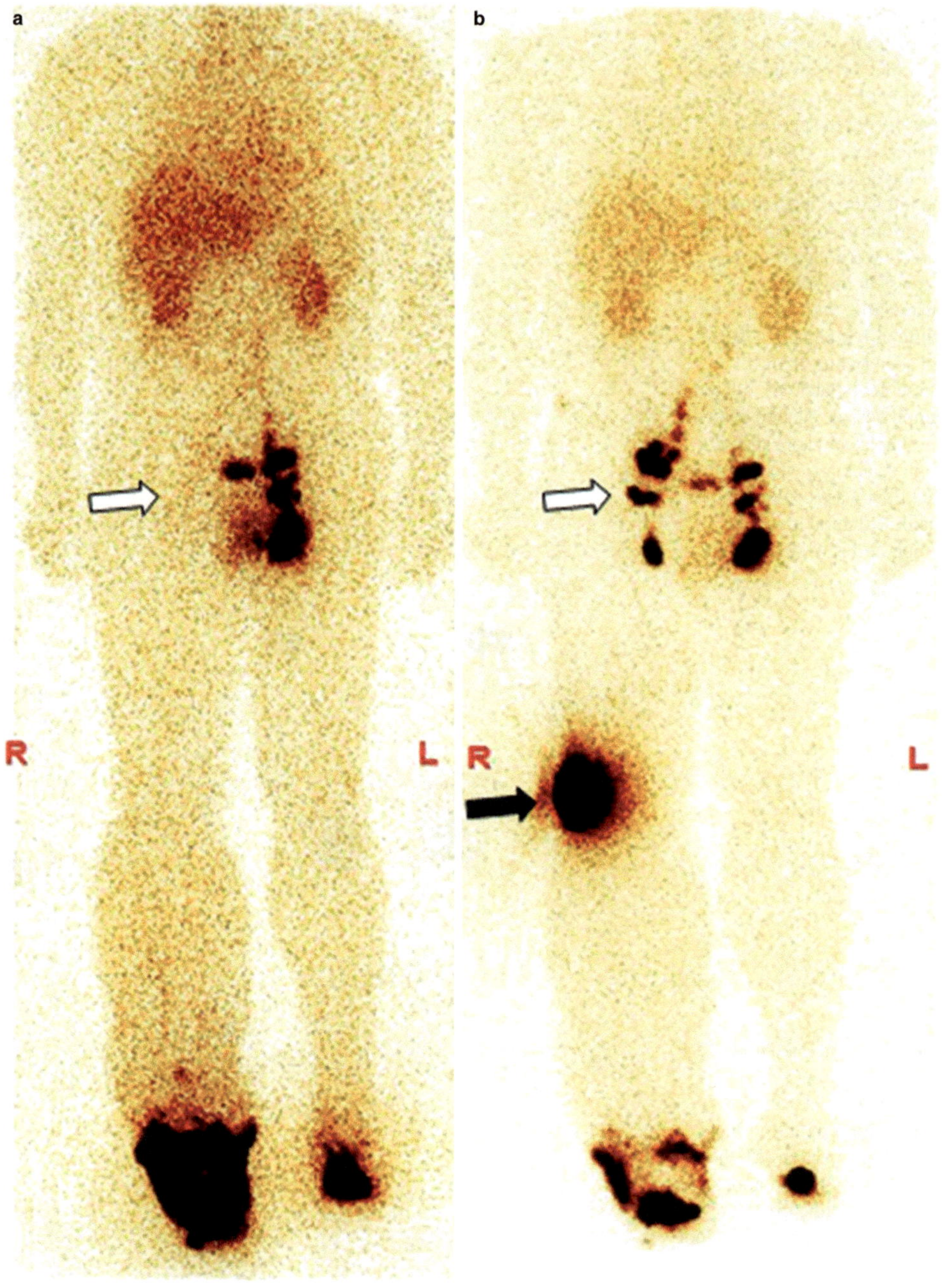

Fig. 19.7 A 44-year-old man was involved in an accident 17 years ago. Edema of his right shank occurred and became heavier afterwards. Three hours after injection (**a**), the left inguinal lymph nodes were appeared; however, no lymph node was seen on the right side (white arrow); ^{99m}Tc-dextan was injected intradermally on the right popliteal space immediately (black arrow), one hour later (**b**), the right inguinal lymph appeared (white arrow)

used because they were complex, and there were no clear relationship with the severity of the disease and treatment response. Recently, Cheng et al. invited a new lymphoscintigraphy staging named Taiwan Lymphoscintigraphy Staging (TLS), which was based on three major findings (visualization of proximal/intermediate lymph nodes, linear lymphatic ducts, and dermal backflow) on lymphoscintigraphy [19]. However, further investigation is needed.

In the past years, some researchers tried to make quantitative analyses of the lymphatic flow, including the proximal lymph node uptake, clearance of the tracer from the injection site, and an even rate of appearance of the soluble molecules in the blood [20, 21]. Unfortunately, quantitative lymphoscintigraphy analyses sometimes demonstrated inconsistent results, additionally, they are time-consuming [22]. Therefore, quantitative lymphoscintigraphy was not routinely used in clinical practice.

In conclusion, lymphedema was an easy and safe method to evaluate the lymphatic system, it can be performed on patients of any age with extremely low radiation exposure and making dynamic observation of tracer distribution possible (Fig. 19.10). Qualitative visualization of the images is enough to make the diagnosis of lymphedema [23]. The main limitation for lymphoscintigraphy was the spatial resolution was low [24], some foci (Fig. 19.11), and lymph vessels in the lymphoscintigraphy cannot be identified correctly. In addi-

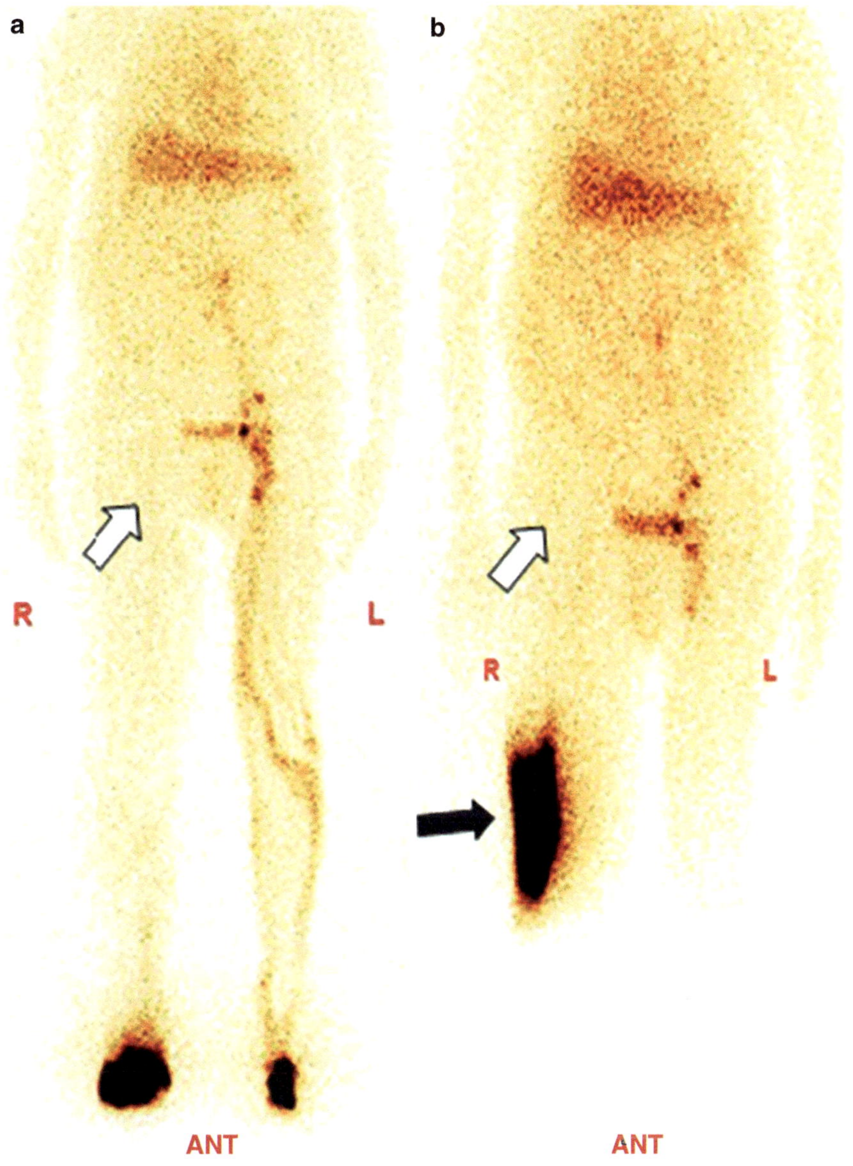

Fig. 19.8 Edema of the right lower extremity continued to worsen in a 74-year-old man for 6 years. Three hours after injection (**a**), the left inguinal lymph nodes were appeared; however, no lymph node was seen on the right side (white arrow); ^{99m}Tc-dextan was injected intradermally on the right popliteal space immediately (black arrow), one hour later (**b**), the right inguinal lymph still not appeared (white arrow)

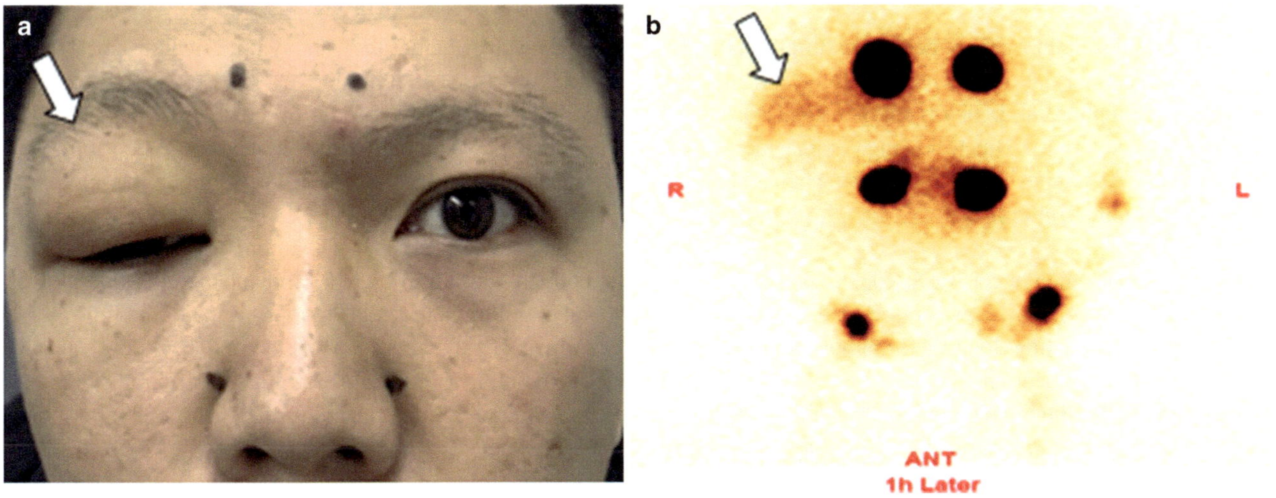

Fig. 19.9 Right maxillofacial swelling occurred in a 31-year male after the operation due to parotid gland carcinoma. ^{99m}Tc- dextan was injected intradermally in four black spots (**a**). One hour after injection (**b**), lymphoscintigraphy showed lymphatic insufficiency of the right side, dermal backflow in the right eyelid was seen (white arrows)

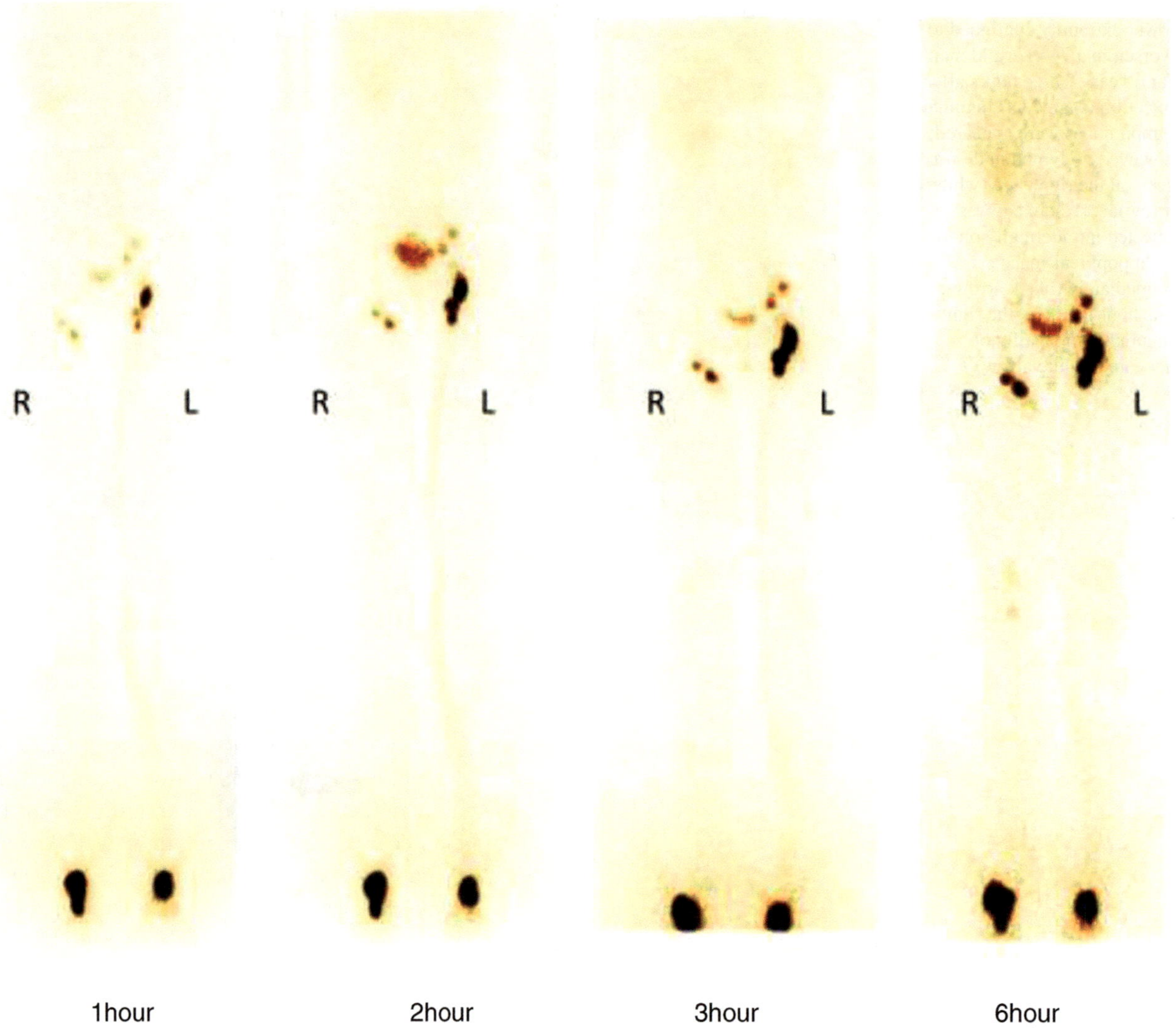

Fig. 19.10 Dynamic observation of tracer distribution in a patient with lymphedema in the right leg. Compared to the right leg, earlier visualization of inguinal lymph nodes was seen in the left leg with the iliac lymph nodes demonstrated clearly. The iliac lymph nodes on the right side were not seen throughout the process

tion, lymphoscintigraphy cannot be used to differentiated primary and secondary lymphedema [20], and the imaging protocol for lymphoscintigraphy is still not standardized.

Finally, we summarize the following points which help to make the correct diagnosis of lymphedema when reading the images of lymphoscintigraphy:

1. Make it clear which tracer was used.
2. Make it clear which place was injected.
3. Make it clear for how long the lymphoscintigraphy was performed after injection.
4. Pay attention to the bilateral inguinal lymph nodes for the lower limb (axillary lymph nodes for the upper limb). Make sure whether they are symmetrical or not, whether they were appeared in time.
5. Are there any lymph nodes of the deep lymphatic system (i.e., popliteal lymph node) appeared? When they were seen, it indicated the slow drainage of the lymphatic system.
6. Is there any presence of "dermal backflow?" The presence of "dermal backflow" indicated abnormal displacement of lymphatic ducts to the surface of the limb.
7. Above all, the presence of "dermal backflow" and the asymmetry of inguinal (or axillary) lymph nodes are the most important parameters for the diagnosis of peripheral lymphedema.

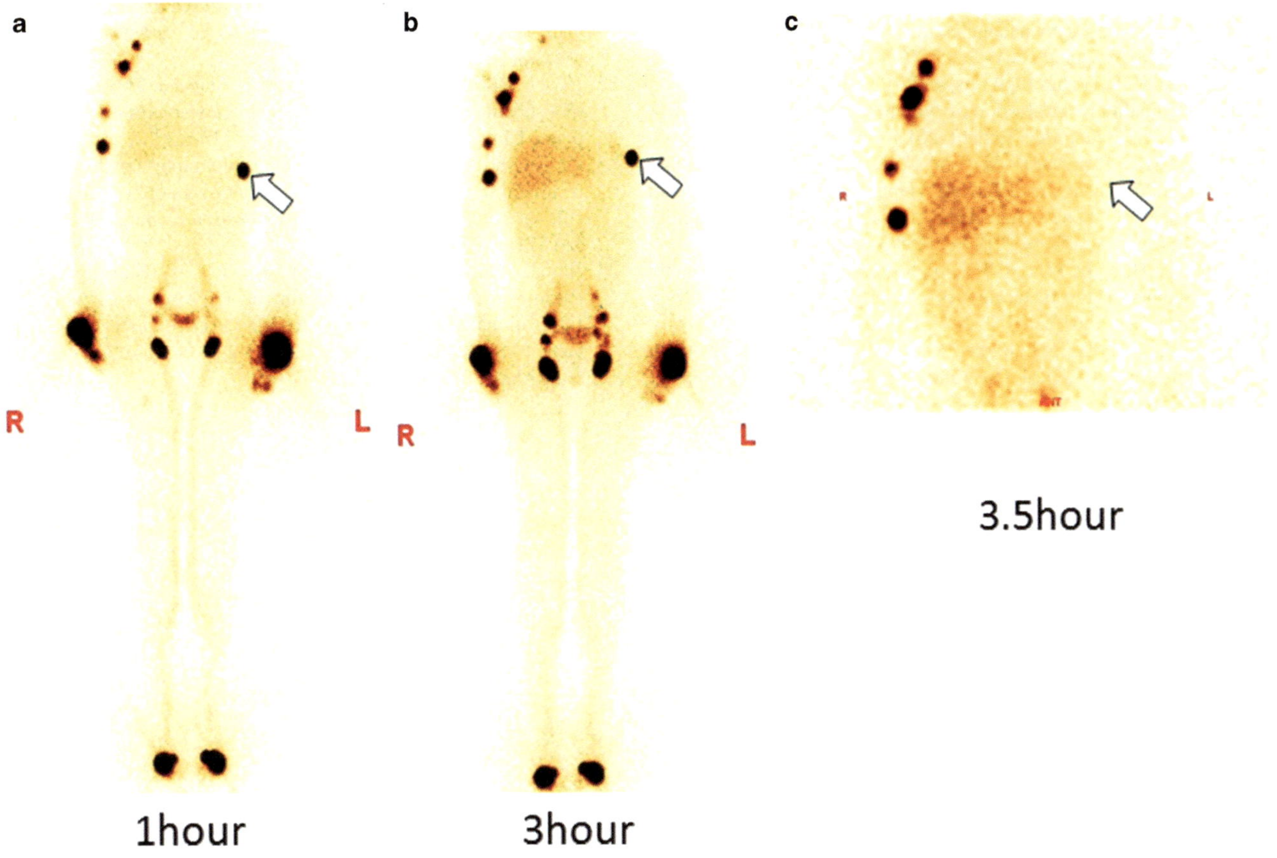

Fig. 19.11 False positive foci were seen on the images of lymphoscintigraphy (**a** and **b**). Physician suspected the foci to be a contaminated point made by tracer on the clothe. The patient removed the clothing, and regional lymphoscintigraphy was performed for the third time (**c**). The foci disappeared, which confirmed the doctor's suspicions (white arrows)

References

1. Walker LA. Localization of radioactive colloids in lymph nodes. J Lab Clin Med. 1950 Sep;36(3):440–9.
2. Weissleder H, Weissleder R. Lymphedema: evaluation of qualitative and quantitative lymphoscintigraphy in 238 patients. Radiology. 1988 Jun;167(3):729–35.
3. Suehiro K, Morikage N, Murakami M, Yamashita O, Harada T, Ueda K, et al. Differentiation of high and low output lymphatic failure using qualitative Lymphangioscintigraphy. Ann Vasc Dis. 2015;8(2):93–9.
4. Greene AK, Voss SD, Maclellan RA. Liposuction for swelling in patients with lymphedema. N Engl J Med. 2017 Nov 2;377(18):1788–9.
5. Suga K, Uchisako H, Nakanishi T, Utsumi H, Yamada N, Oohara M, et al. Lymphoscintigraphic assessment of leg oedema following arterial reconstruction using a load produced by standing. Nucl Med Commun. 1991 Oct;12(10):907–17.
6. Schuitevoerder D, Grinlington L, Stevens J, Nance R, Fortino J, Vetto JT. Nonvisualized sentinel lymph nodes on lymphoscintigraphy in melanoma: predictive factors and surgical outcomes. Nucl Med Commun. 2017 May;38(5):383–7.
7. Wei L, Chen F, Zhang X, Li D, Yao Z, Deng L, et al. (99m) Tc-dextran lymphoscintigraphy can detect sentinel lymph node in breast cancer patients. Exp Ther Med. 2015 Jan;9(1):112–6.
8. Yoo JN, Cheong YS, Min YS, Lee SW, Park HY, Jung TD. Validity of quantitative lymphoscintigraphy as a lymphedema assessment tool for patients with breast cancer. Ann Rehabil Med. 2015 Dec;39(6):931–40.
9. Szuba A, Shin WS, Strauss HW, Rockson S. The third circulation: radionuclide lymphoscintigraphy in the evaluation of lymphedema. J Nucl Med. 2003 Jan;44(1):43–57.
10. Strand SE, Bergqvist L. Radiolabeled colloids and macromolecules in the lymphatic system. Crit Rev Ther Drug Carrier Syst. 1989;6(3):211–38.
11. Wen Z, Tong G, Liu Y, Meeks JK, Ma D, Yang J. The lymphoscintigraphic manifestation of (99m)Tc-dextran lymphatic imaging in primary intestinal lymphangiectasia. Nucl Med Commun. 2014 May;35(5):493–500.
12. Zhang W, Wu P, Li F, Tong G, Chen X, Zhu Z. Potential applications of using 68Ga-Evans blue PET/CT in the evaluation of lymphatic disorder: preliminary observations. Clin Nucl Med. 2016 Apr;41(4):302–8.
13. Yoshida RY, Kariya S, Ha-Kawa S, Tanigawa N. Lymphoscintigraphy for imaging of the lymphatic flow disorders. Tech Vasc Interv Radiol. 2016 Dec;19(4):273–6.
14. Rezende LF, Pedras FV, Ramos CD, Gurgel MS. Preoperative upper limb lymphatic function in breast cancer surgery. Rev Assoc Med Bras (1992). 2011 Sep-Oct;57(5):540–4.
15. Hung JC, Wiseman GA, Wahner HW, Mullan BP, Taggart TR, Dunn WL. Filtered technetium-99m-sulfur colloid evaluated for lymphoscintigraphy. J Nucl Med. 1995 Oct;36(10):1895–901.
16. Notohamiprodjo M, Weiss M, Baumeister RG, Sommer WH, Helck A, Crispin A, et al. MR lymphangiography at 3.0 T: correlation with lymphoscintigraphy. Radiology. 2012 Jul;264(1):78–87.

17. Maegawa J, Mikami T, Yamamoto Y, Satake T, Kobayashi S. Types of lymphoscintigraphy and indications for lymphaticovenous anastomosis. Microsurgery. 2010 Sep;30(6):437–42.
18. Ebrahim M, Savitcheva I, Axelsson R. Reliability of a scoring system for qualitative evaluation of lymphoscintigraphy of the lower extremities. J Nucl Med Technol. 2017 Sep;45(3):219–24.
19. Cheng MH, Pappalardo M, Lin C, Kuo CF, Lin CY, Chung KC. Validity of the novel Taiwan lymphoscintigraphy staging and correlation of Cheng lymphedema grading for unilateral extremity lymphedema. Ann Surg. 2018 Sep;268(3):513–25.
20. Tomczak H, Nyka W, Lass P. Lymphoedema: lymphoscintigraphy versus other diagnostic techniques--a clinician's point of view. Nucl Med Rev Cent East Eur. 2005;8(1):37–43.
21. Pain SJ, Nicholas RS, Barber RW, Ballinger JR, Purushotham AD, Mortimer PS, et al. Quantification of lymphatic function for investigation of lymphedema: depot clearance and rate of appearance of soluble macromolecules in blood. J Nucl Med. 2002 Mar;43(3):318–24.
22. Jensen MR, Simonsen L, Karlsmark T, Bulow J. The washout rate of a subcutaneous 99mTc-HSA depot in lower extremity lymphoedema. Clin Physiol Funct Imaging. 2012 Mar;32(2):126–32.
23. Pappalardo M, Cheng MH. Lymphoscintigraphy for the diagnosis of extremity lymphedema: current controversies regarding protocol, interpretation, and clinical application. J Surg Oncol. 2020 Jan;121(1):37–47.
24. Jimenez-Heffernan A, Ellmann A, Sado H, Huic D, Bal C, Parameswaran R, et al. Results of a prospective multicenter International Atomic Energy Agency sentinel node trial on the value of SPECT/CT over planar imaging in various malignancies. J Nucl Med. 2015 Sep;56(9):1338–44.

20 Indocyanine Green Lymphography

Ziyou Yu

Abstract

Indocyanine green (ICG) lymphography is becoming increasingly popular in the diagnosis and evaluation of lymphedema. Studies have found ICG lymphography as a reliable and sensitive approach for detecting lymphedema and real-time observation of lymph flow. Since ICG lymphography is minimally invasive, lack of radiation exposure, safe, and easy to perform, it is increasingly being used in the diagnosis and surveillance of lymphedema in the past decade. In this chapter, we will focus on ICG lymphography in the diagnosis of chronic lymphedema of extremities.

Keywords

Indocyanine green lymphography · Chronic lymphedema Diagnosis

20.1 Introduction

Indocyanine green (ICG) is a tricarbocyanine, and near-infrared dye which can be excited between 750–800 nm and fluorescence imaged at a longer emission wavelength (over 800 nm) [1]. ICG has been used for over 50 years in monitoring cardiac output, hepatic function, liver blood flow, and retinal angiography. ICG can be fast removed from circulation and can be injected several times if needed. In addition, there has been a growing interest in the use of ICG angiography for intraoperative monitoring of blood flow, for example, in neurosurgery, bypass coronary surgery, flap operations in reconstructive surgery, etc. In recent years, with the advancement of imaging techniques, near-infrared fluorescence imaging using ICG has the opportunity to imaging the lymphatic system.

ICG has a molecular weight of 751.4 Da. It is taken up by the lymphatics after intradermal injection and can therefore be used to observe lymphatic flow using an infrared camera system. Since the penetration depth of near-infrared is around 2 cm under the skin, this technique is suitable for visualizing superficial lymphatic channels and lymph nodes. The use of ICG for lymphatic mapping was first reported by Kitai in 2005 for intraoperative identification of sentinel lymph nodes in breast cancer patients [2]. In 2007, Unno et al. first introduced ICG lymphography for the diagnosis of lymphedema and reported characteristic dermal backflow images in secondary lymphedema patients compatible with lymphoscintigraphic findings [3]. Recently, a growing body of research has shown that ICG lymphography is a reliable and sensitive approach for detecting lymphedema and real-time observation of lymphatic flow. Since ICG lymphography is minimally invasive, lack of radiation exposure, safe, and easy to perform, it is increasingly being used in diagnosis and surveillance of lymphedema, preoperative determination of functional lymphatic vessels before lymphaticovenular anastomosis, and real-time observation of lymphatic vessels during surgery. In this chapter, we will focus on the diagnostic value of ICG lymphography and imaging findings in chronic lymphedema of extremities.

20.2 ICG Lymphographic Findings in Healthy Subjects

ICG is usually injected intradermally into the interdigital space on the dorsum of the hands or foot (0.1–0.2 ml/injection site, a total of 2–5 injection sites). Immediately or within a few minutes after ICG injection, enhanced lymphatic collectors can be clearly delineated from the injection site and drained upward in healthy limbs toward the lymph nodes in the axilla or groin. The vessels could still be observed 30 min after injection [4]. Typical fluorescence images representing

Z. Yu (✉)
Department of Plastic and Reconstructive Surgery, Shanghai Ninth People's Hospital, Shanghai Jiao Tong University School of Medicine, Shanghai, China

N. Liu (ed.), *Peripheral Lymphedema*, https://doi.org/10.1007/978-981-16-3484-0_20

the lymphatics of normal subjects are shown Fig. 20.1. Lymphatic vessels in the thigh are usually blurry and may not detectable in the obese subject. Lymphatic vessel contraction and propulsion can be observed in most subjects (usually more clear below the midcalf level). We found in 97% of healthy subjects, the lymphatic vessel can be visualized dur-

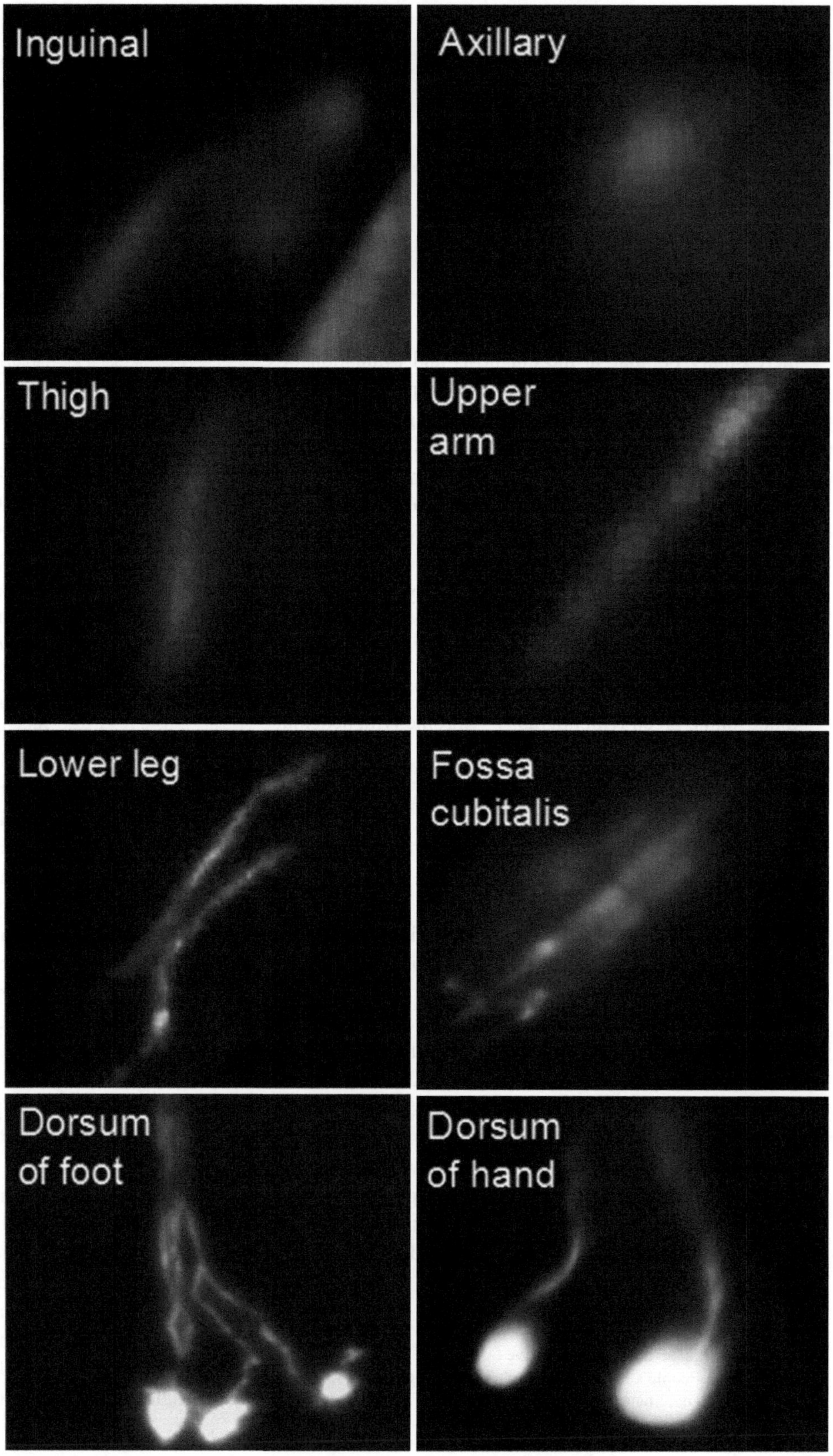

Fig. 20.1 ICG lymphographic findings in healthy limbs. Lymphatic collectors developed from the injection site and drained upward into the lymph nodes in the axilla or groin can be observed within a few minute after injection

ing the administration of ICG dye (unpublished data), indicating the contrast agent can be rapidly taken up by the capillary lymphatics. As the movement of ICG dye from the injection site toward the proximal region can be traced by the fluorescent signal, researchers have using ICG lymphography to assess lymph function by measuring the transit time and calculating the ICG velocity [5, 6] Mean transit time from foot to groin in healthy subjects was reported to be 357 ± 289 and 653 ± 564 seconds for the right and left legs respectively in standing position. The transit time from hand to axilla was reported to be 2.25 ± 1.00 minutes.

20.3 ICG Lymphographic Findings in Chronic Lymphedema

In the lymphedematous limb, both the lymphatic drainage pattern and speed have changed dramatically. The characteristic imaging feature is dermal backflow, which is retrograde lymph filling in the skin as a result of lymphatic blockage or dysfunction. As lymphographic image continues to change after ICG dye injection due to impaired lymphatic drainage, it is necessary to observe the lymphatic flow dynamically. In our experience, observing immediately or within a few minutes after injection (T0) would allow identifying the functional or aberrant lymphatic vessels and their contractile function. After T0 observation, patients were asked to walk on a treadmill. Images were obtained again at 30 min after ICG dye injection (T1). T1 images reflect more generalized distribution of ICG dye, usually dermal backflow or subcutaneous contrast diffusion shown in the skin and may mask the enhanced lymphatic vessel. Although dermal backflow is the typical feature of both primary and secondary lymphedema, there are varying imaging characteristics based on different etiology.

20.4 Primary Lymphedema

Primary lymphedemas have no clearly identifiable cause. ICG lymphography can therefore be used as a screening examination. Images in primary lymphedematous limb exhibit various morphological and functional abnormalities, including delayed or absent enhancement of lymphatic vessels and lymph nodes, dermal backflow and subcutaneous contrast diffusion, and abnormal lymphatic architecture.

Due to the dysfunction of the lymphatics, uptake and transportation of the ICG dye is severely delayed. We recently investigate 77 extremities with primary lymphedema and found delayed lymphatic drainage exhibit in 94.8% of limbs (unpublished data). In most cases, the fluorescent signal can only be detected below the level of ankle at T0 and no ICG fluorescence visible above the level of knee as well as the inguinal region T1. Lymph nodes can hardly be observed in the majority of primary lymphedema cases. We found, in several subjects, no fluorescent signal could be detected even 12 or 24 h post ICG dye injection, and we assume this may indicate lymphatic hypoplasia. Except for these fluorescence negative patients, all lymphedematous limbs showed dermal backflow and subcutaneous contrast diffusion at T1. Figure 20.2 shows imaging findings of a 35-year-old male patient with primary lymphedema of the left lower limb (stage I). Lymphatic vessels can be observed at the anterior surface of the limb below the level of knee at

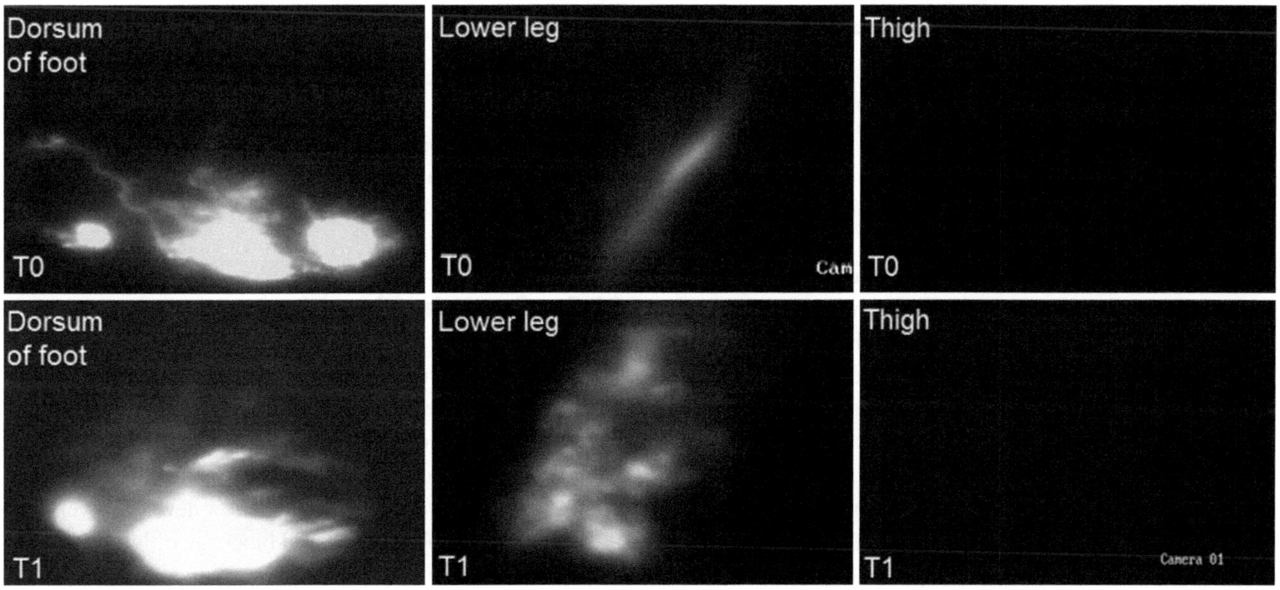

Fig. 20.2 Imaging findings of a 35-year-old male patient with primary lymphedema of left lower limb (stage I). Lymphatic vessels can be observed at the anterior surface of the limb below the level of knee at T0. Massive dermal backflow masks the lymphatic vessel image at T1, and no fluorescent signal could be detected above the level of knee. T0, immediately after injection; T1, 30 min after injection

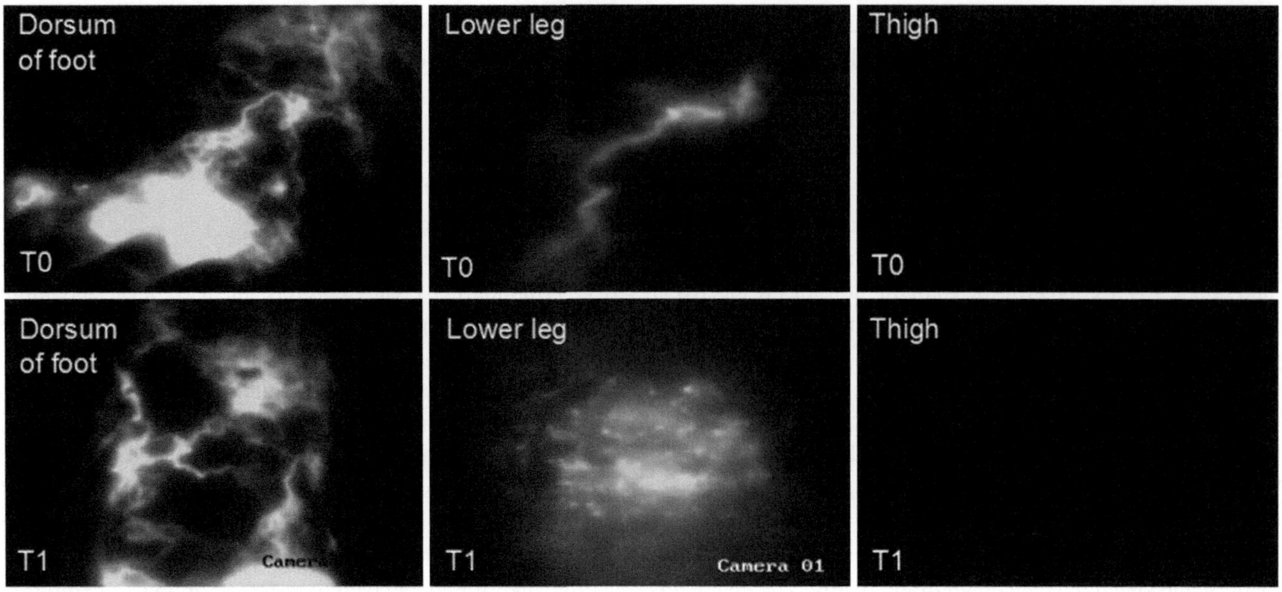

Fig. 20.3 Imaging findings of a 42-year-old male patient with 12 years' onset of primary lymphedema of the right lower limb (stage II). Torturous lymphatic vessel network could be observed at dorsum of foot at T0, and massive dermal backflow occurred in the lower leg at T1. T0, immediately after injection; T1, 30 min after injection

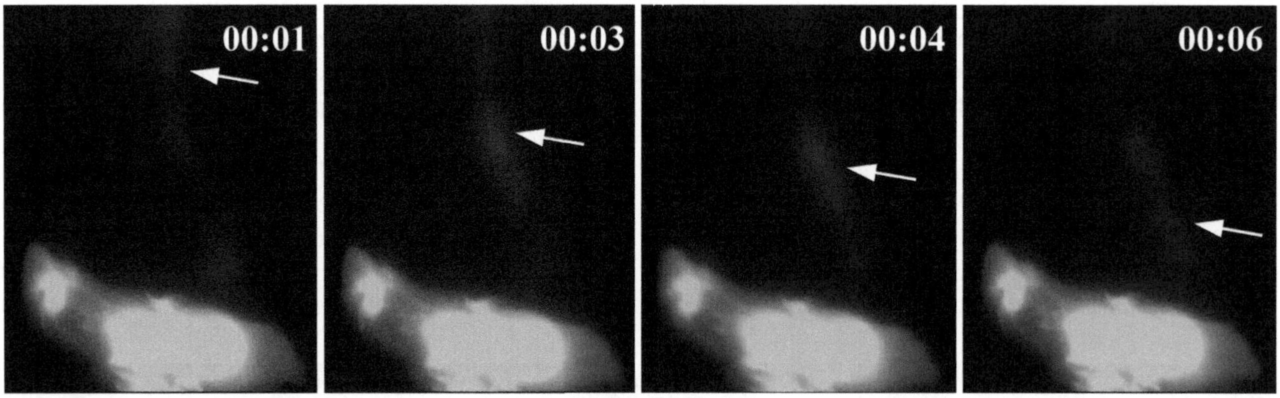

Fig. 20.4 Lymph reflux was detected in a 13-year-old female patient with primary lymphedema of unilateral lower limb (stage I). Lymph reflux toward the distal part can be observed at dorsum of the feet. Arrows, lymph reflux

T0. However, massive dermal backflow masks the lymphatic vessel image at T1, and no fluorescent signal could be detected above the level of the knee.

Aberrant lymphatic architecture could often be observed in patients with primary lymphedema, which may indicate structural abnormalities in primary lymphedema. Figure 20.3 shows the ICG images of a 42-year-old male patient with 12 years' onset of primary lymphedema of the right lower limb (stage II). Torturous lymphatic vessel network could be observed at dorsum of foot at T0, and massive dermal backflow occurred in the lower leg at T1. Lymph reflux could also be detected by real-time observation of lymphatic vessels. Figure 20.4 shows imaging findings at dorsum of the feet in patient with stage I unilateral lower limb lymphedema. Contraction of lymphatic vessels pushing lymph upward accompanied with lymph reflux towards the feet can be observed.

20.5 Secondary Lymphedema

Patients with secondary lymphedema have a previously adequate and functional lymphatic system. Normal or dilated lymphatic vessels could usually be observed at T0. Fluorescent signal could also be detected at the proximal of the extremity in most cases. However, dermal backflow developed very rapidly as a result of obstruction and blockage of lymphatic vessels. Dermal backflow and massive contrast diffusion often present throughout the entire extremity at T1. Figure 20.5 is an example of ICG lymphographic imaging of a 56-year-old

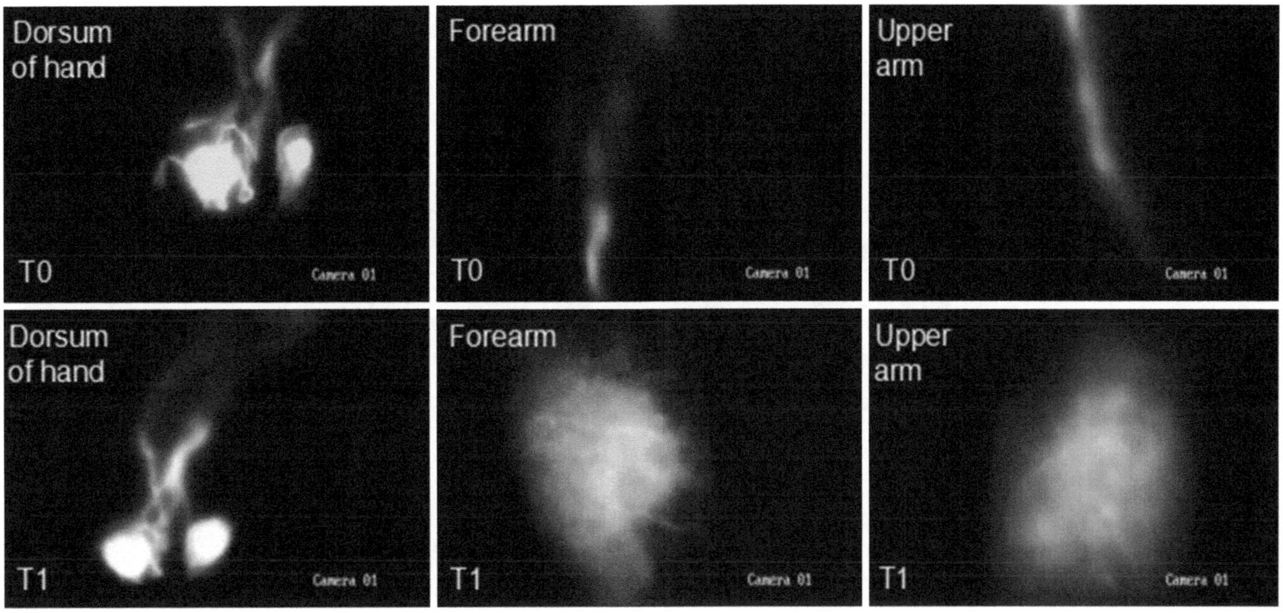

Fig. 20.5 ICG lymphographic imaging of a 56-year-old women with secondary lymphedema (stage II). Enhanced lymphatic vessel drained toward the axilla could be observed at T0. Massive dermal backflow, as well as enhanced dermal lymphatic capillaries, were shown at T1. T0, immediately after injection; T1, 30 min after injection

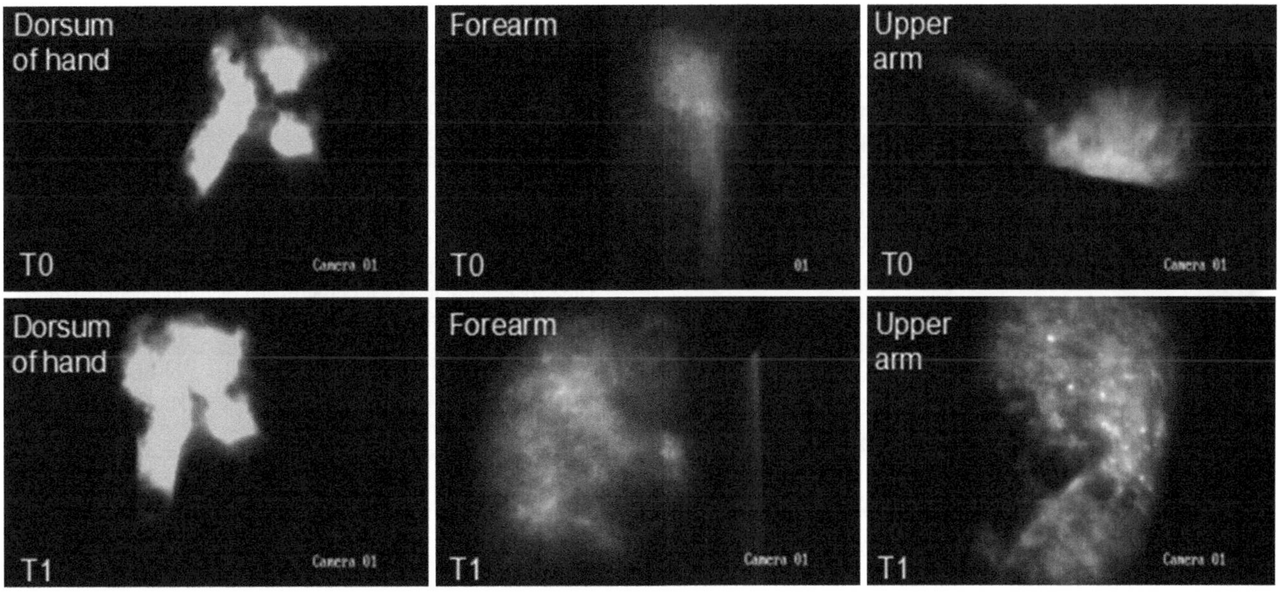

Fig. 20.6 Imaging findings of a patient with stage III secondary lymphedema of the upper limb. Dermal backflow and extravascular deposition of ICG could be observed at T0. Massive high signal intensity of ICG deposition could be observed in the upper arm at T1. T0, immediately after injection; T1, 30 min after injection

women who developed unilateral secondary lymphedema 3-years post-mastectomy (stage II). Enhanced lymphatic vessel drained toward the axilla could be observed at T0. Typical dermal backflow, as well as enhanced dermal lymphatic capillaries, were shown at T1, indicating lymph reflux and compromised lymphatic function. Figure 20.6 shows imaging of a patient with stage III secondary lymphedema of the upper limb. Dermal backflow and extravascular deposition of ICG could be observed at T0 with the extent increasing with time. Massive high signal intensity of ICG deposition (some researchers described as "Milky Way" or "stardust") could be observed in the upper arm at T1. Figure 20.7 shows the generalized distribution of ICG in another patient with stage III secondary lymphedema of the upper limb.

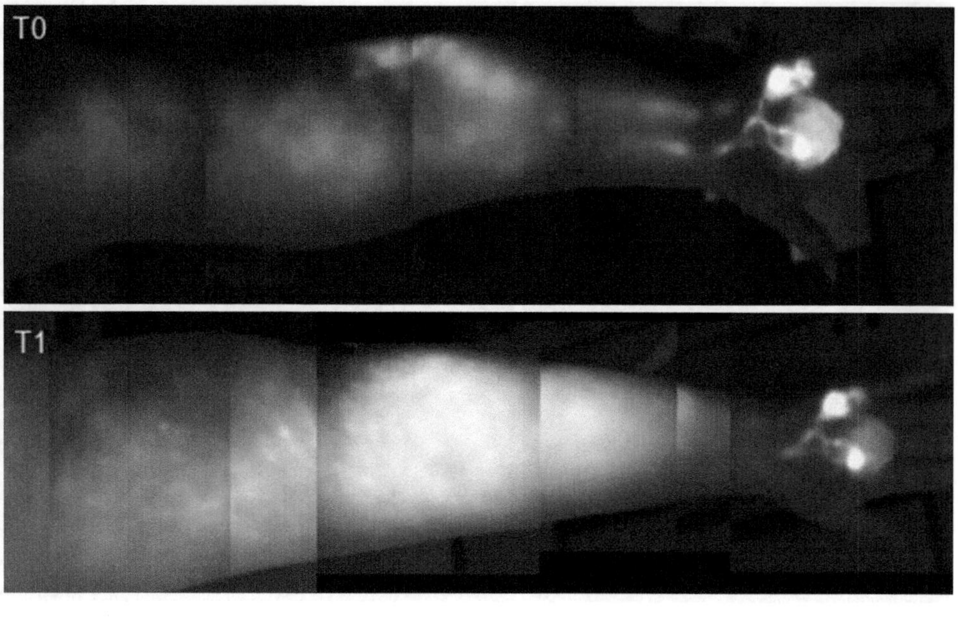

Fig. 20.7 Generalized distribution of ICG in patient with stage III secondary lymphedema of upper limb. T0, immediately after injection; T1, 30 min after injection

Dermal backflow may appear in various patterns in the affected limb. Yamamoto et al. [7–9] classified different dermal backflow patterns as "splash, stardust and diffuse" which are correlated with the severity of lymphedema. However, different patterns may be observed in the same extremity and continue to change with time. Both the extent and site of dermal backflow are also variable among patients. Quantitative methods for the analysis of ICG dynamics need to be developed for more accurately assessing the severity of the disease. Recently, researchers have found that ICG velocity decreases as the lymphedema severity stage progresses [4]. Measurement of ICG velocity may be used for the evaluation of lymphatic drainage function. Computational development work is still needed to facilitate ICG imaging analysis.

20.6 Advantages and Disadvantages

Compare with other examination methods, ICG lymphography is less invasive, lack of radioactivity, and cost-effective. ICG lymphography is sensitive for detecting lymphedema even at the latent stage and could therefore be used for early detection and surveillance of lymphedema. ICG lymphography can be easily performed in an outpatient setting and can be used as a screening examination. This technique also allows real-time observation of lymphatic flow and lymphatic pumping, thus furthers our understanding of pathophysiological alterations of lymphatic disorders. Limited penetration of near-infrared is the main disadvantage of this approach. ICG lymphography cannot visualize lymphatic vessels deeper than 2 cm from the skin surface and cannot well evaluated in obese patients.

References

1. Alander JT, Kaartinen I, Laakso A, Patila T, Spillmann T, Tuchin VV, et al. A review of indocyanine green fluorescent imaging in surgery. Int J Biomed Imaging. 2012;2012:940585.
2. Kitai T, Inomoto T, Miwa M, Shikayama T. Fluorescence navigation with indocyanine green for detecting sentinel lymph nodes in breast cancer. Breast Cancer. 2005;12(3):211–5.
3. Unno N, Inuzuka K, Suzuki M, Yamamoto N, Sagara D, Nishiyama M, et al. Preliminary experience with a novel fluorescence lymphography using indocyanine green in patients with secondary lymphedema. J Vasc Surg. 2007;45(5):1016–21.
4. Yamamoto T, Narushima M, Yoshimatsu H, Yamamoto N, Oka A, Seki Y, et al. Indocyanine green velocity: lymph transportation capacity deterioration with progression of lymphedema. Ann Plast Surg. 2013;71(5):591–4.
5. Unno N, Nishiyama M, Suzuki M, Yamamoto N, Inuzuka K, Sagara D, et al. Quantitative lymph imaging for assessment of lymph function using indocyanine green fluorescence lymphography. Eur J Vasc Endovasc Surg. 2008;36(2):230–6.
6. Yamamoto T, Narushima M, Yoshimatsu H, Yamamoto N, Kikuchi K, Todokoro T, et al. Dynamic Indocyanine green (ICG) lymphography for breast cancer-related arm lymphedema. Ann Plast Surg. 2014;73(6):706–9.
7. Yamamoto T, Matsuda N, Doi K, Oshima A, Yoshimatsu H, Todokoro T, et al. The earliest finding of indocyanine green lymphography in asymptomatic limbs of lower extremity lymphedema patients secondary to cancer treatment: the modified dermal backflow stage and concept of subclinical lymphedema. Plast Reconstr Surg. 2011;128(4):314e–21e.
8. Yamamoto T, Narushima M, Doi K, Oshima A, Ogata F, Mihara M, et al. Characteristic indocyanine green lymphography findings in lower extremity lymphedema: the generation of a novel lymphedema severity staging system using dermal backflow patterns. Plast Reconstr Surg. 2011;127(5):1979–86.
9. Yamamoto T, Yamamoto N, Doi K, Oshima A, Yoshimatsu H, Todokoro T, et al. Indocyanine green-enhanced lymphography for upper extremity lymphedema: a novel severity staging system using dermal backflow patterns. Plast Reconstr Surg. 2011;128(4):941–7.

21 Nuclear Medicine Imaging in the Diagnosis of Peripheral Lymphedema: Single-Photon Emission Computed Tomography/Computed Tomography (SPECT/CT)

Feng Xu

Abstract

The superiority of Single-Photon Emission Computed Tomography/Computed Tomography (SPECT/CT) over scintigraphy alone has been proven in various diseases, including the lymphatic system. SPECT/CT provides much more information than lymphoscintigraphy alone, not only the function but also the morphology of the lymphatic system. As shown in the part of "Lymphoscintigraphy," the images of lymphoscintigraphy were lack of precise location of foci. SPECT/CT solved the problem perfectly. Whether SPECT/CT was necessary for patients with lymphedema usually depend on nuclear medicine physician, considering the added value of the SPECT/CT. In this part, we introduce the tracers, methods, and typical images for lymphoscintigraphy combined SPECT/CT.

Keywords

SPECT/CT · Diagnosis · Peripheral Lymphedema

The superiority of SPECT/CT over scintigraphy alone has been proven in various diseases, including the lymphatic system [1–3]. SPECT/CT provides much more information than lymphoscintigraphy alone, not only the function but also the morphology of the lymphatic system. As shown in the part of "Lymphoscintigraphy," the images of lymphoscintigraphy were lack of precise location of foci. SPECT/CT solved the problem perfectly. In many centers, SPECT/CT is performed for sentinel lymph nodes biopsy in some anatomic regions to provide visual information to the surgeon, even if it causes mild additional radiation exposure [4, 5]. Recently, Thomas et al. introduced that characterization of lymphatic drainage in oropharyngeal squamous cell carcinoma is feasible using a nonoperative injection technique and SPECT-CT [6]. Whether SPECT/CT was necessary for patients with lymphedema usually depends on nuclear medicine physician, considering the added value of the SPECT/CT.

All ^{99m}Tc-labeled tracers for lymphoscintigraphy were suitable for SPECT/CT imaging. Here, we introduce the use of SPECT/CT with ^{99m}Tc-dextan.

SPECT/CT was usually performed shortly after lymphoscintigraphy in the first 24 h after injection (depends on different situations). In our section, SPECT/CT (Discovery NM/CT 670, GE Medical system, Hayozma, Israel) was performed during the same session as lymphoscintigraphy with the patient in the same position. A SPECT study with a matrix of 128 × 128 was acquired; zoom factor of 1.2–1.5, according to the individual patient; and a rotation of 360° (180° per head) 30-s images (one image every 6°). Next, spiral CT was performed using the following parameters: tube voltage of 120 kVp, tube current of 180 mA, beam collimation of 20 mm, table speed of 37 mm/s, tube rotation time of 0.5 s, and pitch of 0.938:1.

There were few reports about the use of SPECT/CT in the lymphatic system. Compared to lymphoscintigraphy, SPECT/CT was higher in emission and anatomic resolution. Limura et al. reported that ^{99m}Tc-phytate SPECT/CT was valuable to evaluate the therapeutic effect of lower limb edema [1]; Saad et al. indicated that ^{99m}Tc-nanocolloid SPECT/CT may improve the accuracy of diagnosis of the lymph node metastasis of penile cancer [2]; Yang et al. found that ^{99m}Tc-sulfur colloids lymphoscintigraphy combined with SPECT/CT help to made a correct diagnosis of chylous leakage in a 7-month-old girl [3]. Recently, Gentileschi et al. reported that ^{99m}Tc-albumin nanocolloids SPECT/CT combined with ultrasound fusion imaging is feasible for the preoperative identification of groin efferent lymph node for vessel-to-venous anastomosis [7]. Furthermore, Dionyssiou et al. suggested a new technique named "Selected Lymph Node" which is a safe and effective technique in selecting the most suitable lymph nodes, minimizing the donor-site

F. Xu (✉)
Department of Nuclear Medicine, Shanghai Ninth People's Hospital, Shanghai JiaoTong University School of Medicine, Shanghai, China

N. Liu (ed.), *Peripheral Lymphedema*, https://doi.org/10.1007/978-981-16-3484-0_21

morbidity, and decreasing the overall operating time by using SPECT/CT [8].

In our experience, we found that lymphoscintigraphy and SPECT/CT were complements. The advantage of lymphoscintigraphy is that it can be completed in a relatively short time (within 10 min) with a wide range and low radiation dose to patients, which was especially useful for those infants and young children. In addition, it can be performed many times without increasing the radiation dose to patients, and the dynamic distribution of tracers in the lymphatic system can be observed. However, lymphoscintigraphy still had has its own drawbacks. On the images of lymphoscintigraphy, we can see tracer in the liver, kidney, bladder, urine, some non-lymphoid tissues, in addition, "dermal backflow" is common in patients with lymphedema, therefore some important lymph nodes and lymphatic vessels may difficult to be identified. Fortunately, these problems can be solved by SPECT/CT (Figs. 21.1 and 21.2). However, SPECT/CT had limitations too: Firstly, patients may expose to extra radiation from the CT component, which might be harmful to those radiosensitive infants and young children [5]. Secondly, SPECT/CT is not suitable for dynamic imaging also because of the radiation from CT. Finally, the scanning range of SPECT/CT is relatively limited (about 20 cm field of view), and the imaging time is relatively long (10 min one bed).

How to make the patients with lymphedema benefit most from lymphoscintigraphy and SPECT/CT remains a clinical project to be solved. In our experience, lymphoscintigraphy is the main investigation to establish the lymphedema diagnosis. Dynamic observation of tracer distribution in the lymphatic system by using lymphoscintigraphy several times is a useful method for further understanding of the lymphatic

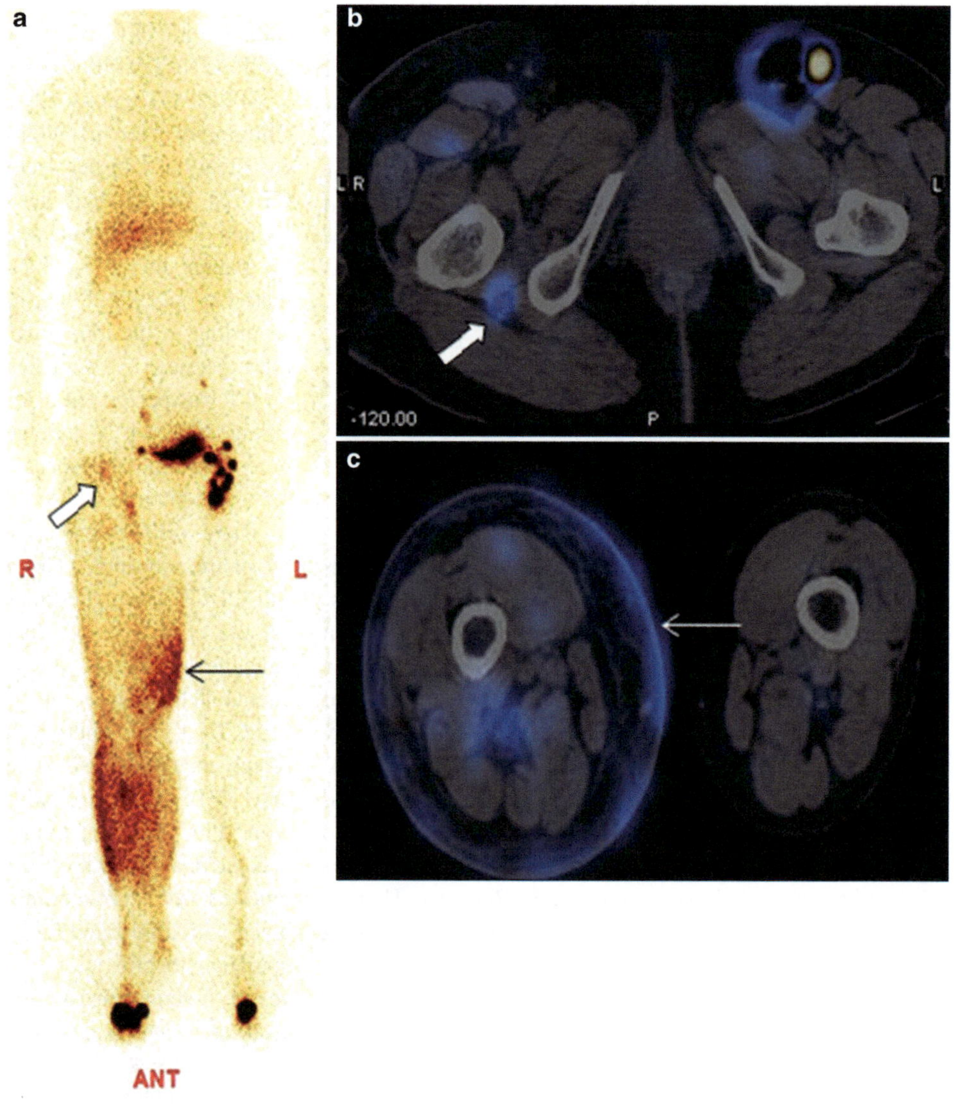

Fig. 21.1 Edema of the right lower extremity occurred in a 54-year-old woman for 1 month due to cervical cancer. Three hours after injection (**a**), dermal backflow was seen in the whole right leg, meanwhile, we were not sure whether the foci on the lymphoscintigraphy (open arrow) were the right inguinal lymph nodes or not and whether there was lymph-vessel inside the dermal backflow or not (arrow). SPECT/CT made the two problems clear that the foci were not the inguinal lymph nodes (**b**) and there were no lymph-vessel inside the dermal backflow (**c**)

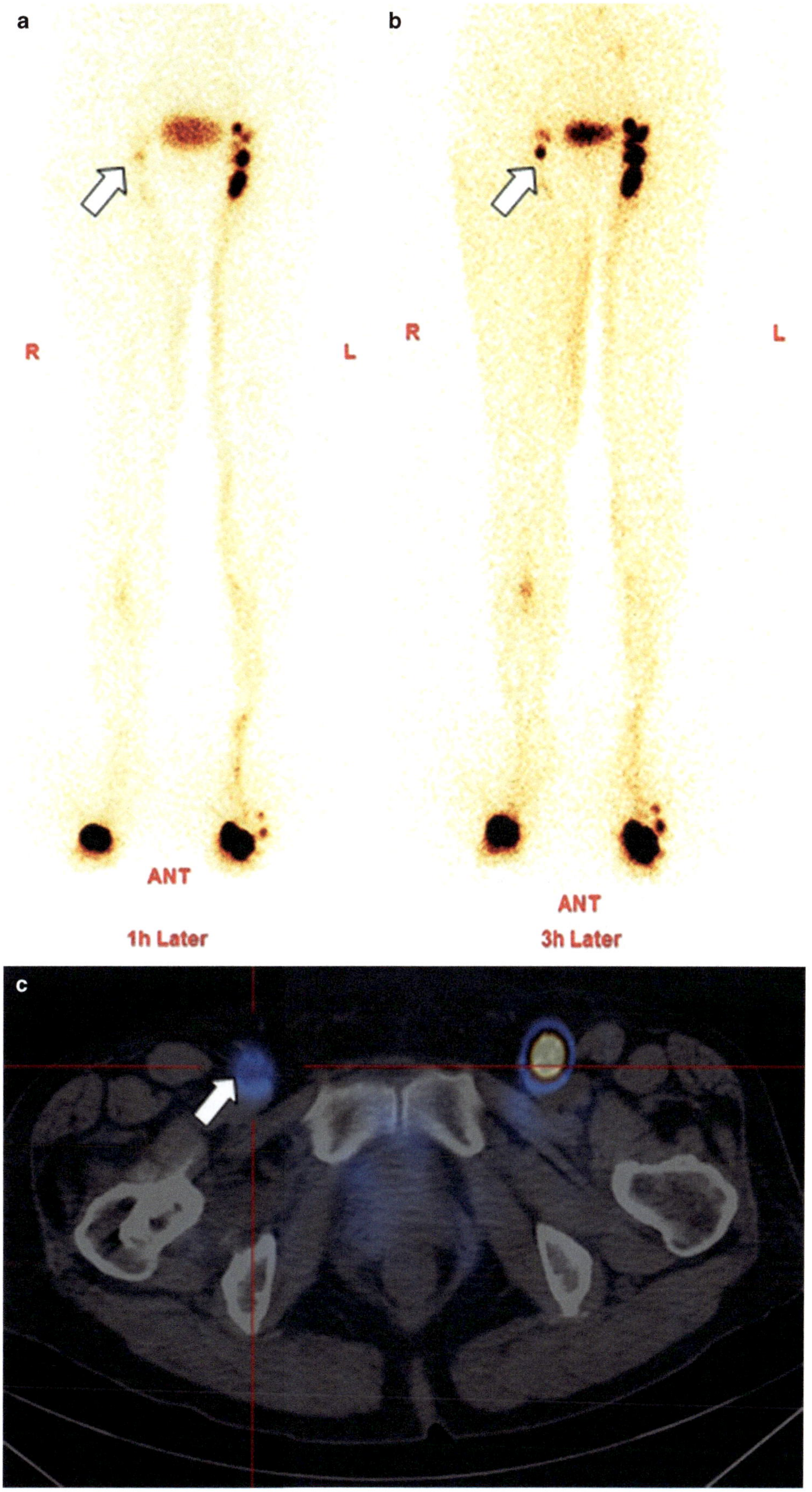

Fig. 21.2 Edema of right lower extremity occurred in 71-year-old woman due to operation of uterine cancer 10 years ago. In order to make it clear whether the foci in the right inguinal region (**a**, **b**) was lymph node or not (white arrows), SPECT/CT was performed. It showed the inguinal lymph nodes took up the tracer (**c**)

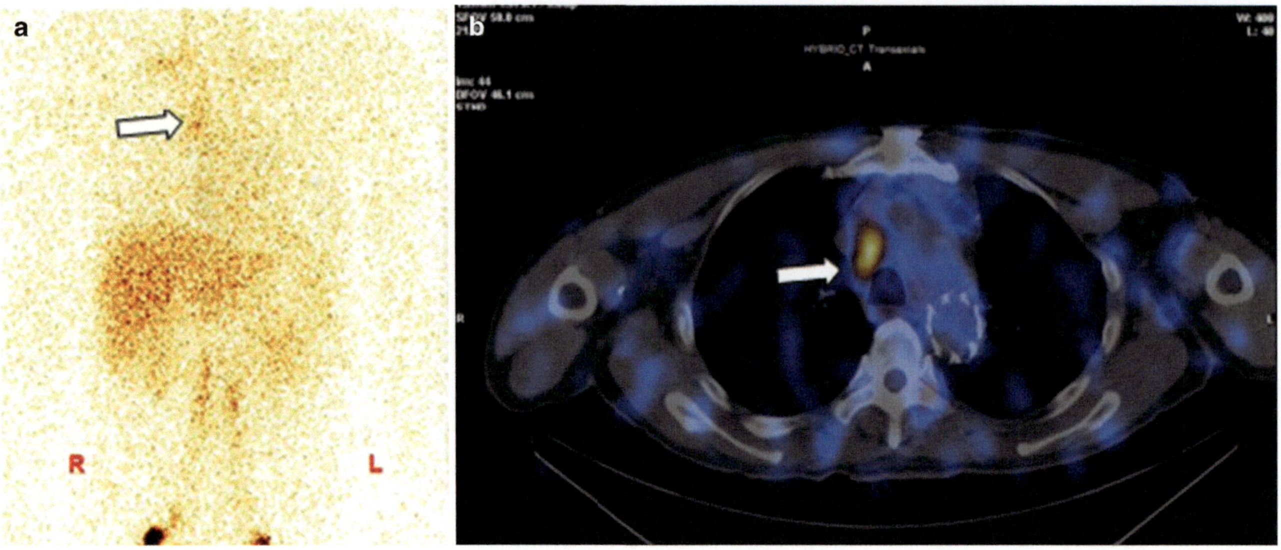

Fig. 21.3 Intrathoracic chylous leakage occurred after aortic replacement in a 47-year male. Three hours after injection on feet, we found there was foci in the chest area (open arrow) on the image of lymphoscintigraphy with ^{99m}Tc-dextan (**a**), SPECT/CT made its more clear (**b**)

system, especially for those young children. Usually, SPECT/CT was performed when lymphoscintigraphy was completed, and it is suitable for evaluating undetermined but very important lymph nodes (usually in the inguinal or axillary region), identifying the lymphatic vessels, or localizing the lymphatic leakage in lymphoscintigraphy (Fig. 21.3).

References

1. Iimura T, Fukushima Y, Kumita S, Ogawa R, Hyakusoku H. Estimating Lymphodynamic conditions and Lymphovenous anastomosis efficacy using (99m)Tc-phytate lymphoscintigraphy with SPECT-CT in patients with lower-limb lymphedema. Plast Reconstr Surg Glob Open. 2015 May;3(5):e404.
2. Saad ZZ, Omorphos S, Michopoulou S, Gacinovic S, Malone P, Nigam R, et al. Investigating the role of SPECT/CT in dynamic sentinel lymph node biopsy for penile cancers. Eur J Nucl Med Mol Imaging. 2017 Jul;44(7):1176–84.
3. Yang J, Codreanu I, Zhuang H. Minimal lymphatic leakage in an infant with chylothorax detected by lymphoscintigraphy SPECT/CT. Pediatrics. 2014 Aug;134(2):e606–10.
4. Jimenez-Heffernan A, Ellmann A, Sado H, Huic D, Bal C, Parameswaran R, et al. Results of a prospective multicenter International Atomic Energy Agency sentinel node trial on the value of SPECT/CT over planar imaging in various malignancies. J Nucl Med. 2015 Sep;56(9):1338–44.
5. Fairbairn N, Munson C, Khan ZA, Butterworth M. The role of hybrid SPECT/CT for lymphatic mapping in patients with melanoma. J Plast Reconstr Aesthet Surg. 2013 Sep;66(9):1248–55.
6. Thomas CM, Khan MN, Mohan R, Hendler A, Hosni A, Chepeha DB, et al. Lymphatic mapping with SPECT-CT for evaluation of contralateral drainage in lateralized oropharyngeal cancers using an awake injection technique. Head Neck. 2019 Nov 28.
7. Gentileschi S, Albanese R, Pino V, Stefanizzi G, Fragomeni S, Zagaria L, et al. SPECT/CT and fusion ultrasound to target the efferent groin lymph node for lymphatic surgery. Microsurgery. 2019 Oct;39(7):605–12.
8. Dionyssiou D, Demiri E, Sarafis A, Goula CO, Tsimponis A, Arsos G. Functional lymphatic reconstruction with the "selected lymph node" technique guided by a SPECT-CT lymphoscintigraphy. J Surg Oncol. 2019 Nov;120(6):911–8.

Comparison of Current Imaging Methods in Diagnosis of Peripheral Lymphedema

22

Ningfei Liu

Abstract

Lymphoscintigraphy (LSG), MR lymphangiography (MRL), and indocyanine green lymphography (ICG) are the three most commonly used forms of imaging for diagnosing lymphedema. Because different contrast agents are used, and these different modalities have different working principles, the imaging findings may not be consistent. Knowing the advantages and disadvantages of those diagnostic modalities is helpful in promoting objective understanding of this condition.

Keywords

Lymphoscintigraphy (LSG) · MR lymphangiography (MRL) · ICG lymphography (LCG) · Lymphedema Lymphatic system · Lymph vessel · Lymph node Dysfunction · Dermal backflow · Lymphatic imaging

The clinical diagnosis of lymphedema in an extremity is not usually difficult, particularly in the late stages of the disease. However, the history and clinical examination do not always indicate the nature or extent of the underlying abnormality. Radionuclide lymphoscintigraphy was introduced by Sherman and TerPogossian in the 1950s [1]. This method, which uses various 99 m Tc-labeled molecules, was the standard means of evaluating lymphatic disease for many decades. It is relatively safe, repeatable, and easy to do [2]. Nevertheless, radionuclide-based imaging has the disadvantage of poor resolution. Since 2007, dynamic magnetic resonance lymphangiography (MRL) using the paramagnetic contrast agent gadobenate dimeglumine was adopted routinely in the clinic to assess lymphatic system architecture and lymph drainage in extremities affected by lymphedema and to guide treatment of this disorder [3–6]. Since then, indocyanine green lymphography has been gradually implemented, mainly to diagnose secondary lymphedemas such as breast cancer-related lymphedema and primary lymphedema [7–9], an advantage being that it is sensitive and easy to perform. These three forms of imaging are currently the most commonly used to investigate lymphatic disorders. Because the contrast agents, equipment, and working principles differ between these tests, the imaging results may be inconsistent. Each examination has its own unique advantages and disadvantages. A comparison of the utility of the three tests for the diagnosis of lymphatic disorders based on 500–20,000 patients for each test is provided below.

1. Contrast absorption and transportation.
   LSG: the isotopic tracer may remain at the injection point and not be absorbed.
   MRL: fast and consistent.
   ICG: fast and consistent.
2. Real-time observation of enhanced lymph flow/functional testing.
   LSG: not possible.
   MRL: can be included in the whole testing set and the enhanced lymph flow/lymph node filling can be recorded for later analysis.
   ICG: sensitive for testing lymphatic function; real-time lymph flow and lymphatic contraction can both be visualized during the procedure and recorded.
3. Imaging of lymphatic vessels.
   LSG: can demonstrate the thoracic duct and lymph vessels of the extremities, but not of the foot.
   MRL: can demonstrate the lumbar trunks, thoracic duct, and lymph vessels of the extremities, but not of the foot.
   ICG: can demonstrate the superficial lymph vessels in all regions of the body.

N. Liu (✉)
Department Plastic and Reconstructive Surgery, Shanghai Ninth People's Hospital, Shanghai Jiao Tong University School of Medicine, Shanghai, China

N. Liu (ed.), *Peripheral Lymphedema*, https://doi.org/10.1007/978-981-16-3484-0_22

4. Inguinal/iliac lymph nodes imaging.
   LSG: possible provided the tracer is absorbed from the injection point.
   MRL: always possible.
   ICG: possible to visualize the inguinal lymph nodes.
5. Resolution of enhanced lymphatic imaging.
   LSG: poor resolution imaging of lymphatic trunks because of the radioactive shadow.
   MRL: high resolution imaging of lymphatic trunks.
   ICG: clarity of imaging of lymphatic vessels depends on the thickness of the subcutaneous tissue and severity of the edema.
6. Resolution of enhanced lymph node imaging.
   LSG: possible to visualize lymph nodes provided the tracer is absorbed; poor resolution of nodal structure because of radioactive shadow.
   MRL: high resolution of lymph nodes with clear demonstration of morphological and pathological changes in them.
   ICG: poor resolution of lymph nodes; unable to visualize nodal structure.
7. Localization of pathological changes (swelling, fibrosis, fat) in surrounding tissues.
   LSG: not possible.
   MRL: can clearly demonstrate the extent of edema, fibrotic tissue, and fat deposition.
   ICG: not possible.
8. Demonstration of both superficial and deep lymphatic system.
   LSG: possible to visualize popliteal, iliac, and lumbar lymph nodes and the thoracic duct.
   MRL: possible to visualize both superficial and deep lymphatic systems.
   ICG: visualizes only the superficial lymphatic system.
9. Scope of scan.
   LSG: possible for lymphatic system throughout the body.
   MRL: mostly segmental examinations but separate tests to examine more regions are possible.
   ICG: localized examination only.
10. Ease of performance.
    LSG: specialized preparation of the apparatus by a radiologist needed.
    MRL: specialized preparation of the apparatus by a radiologist needed.
    ICG: can be performed by a clinician or nurse (therapist).
11. Adverse effects.
    LSG: no adverse effects except radiation exposure.
    MRL: none.
    LCG: allergy is very rare.

LSG, MRL, and ICG can all be regarded as interstitial lymphangiography techniques because the contrast agent is injected intra- or subcutaneously and absorbed through the primary lymphatic vessels [10]. There are, however, differences between each modality in the imaging of lymphatic system abnormalities in limbs affected by lymphedema. These differences are likely to be attributable to technical and physiological differences [11]. For example, the higher resolution of MRL compared with LSG and ICG may result in differences in the imaging results of the three modalities. Radionuclide and fluorescent-based imaging are unable to display distinct anatomical and structural changes within the lymphatic system. MRL clearly depicts lymph vessels with various morphological abnormalities, in both small solitary vessels (1 mm in diameter), and in networks of tortuous and dilated lymphatic trunks (10 mm in diameter) [10] (Fig. 22.1). The quality of MRL imaging in the mapping of lymphatic patterns is comparable to that of direct lymphangiography with the use of an iodine oil contrast agent and thus enables classification of anatomic abnormalities in lymphatics. The rate of detection of lymphatic vessels and lymph nodes is much higher with MRL than with LSG [11, 12] (Fig. 22.2). LCG lymphography is better than LSG imaging for the same reason. Minimal or complete lack of absorption from the injection site and slow transportation of radiotracer may both contribute to the lower rate of detection of LSG imaging. Another disadvantage of LSG is the heavy density of "dermal backflow" in the images, which is due to the overlapping of the shadows of dilated vessels filled with radionuclide tracer (Fig. 22.3). Lymphatic imaging by ICG inspection can vary according to the duration of the change test. Enhanced lymph vessels may be visualized immediately after contrast injection; however, the image can be obscured by the contrast diffusing into the edema fluid in the subcutaneous layer within 5 or 10 min (Fig. 22.4). The disadvantage of ICG lymphography is that its use is limited to lymphatic vessels less than 2 cm deep in the sub-cutaneous tissue [9]. However, ICG is able to detect functional lymphatics in any location in the body. It is noteworthy that failure to detect any lymphatic vessels by MRL imaging may denote lymphatic aplasia or hypoplasia and that failure to detect any lymphatic vessels by LSG imaging may denote the failure of tracer uptake. Lymphatic dysfunction or a transporting anomaly in which only the lymphatics in the dorsum of the foot (the region that is not covered in MRL nor LSG inspections) are affected can be detected by ICG lymphography [9]. Therefore, in patients with a diagnosis of lymphatic aplasia/hypoplasia, a combination of MRL and ICG examinations are suggested to differentiate between lymphatic dysfunction and lymphatic aplasia/hypoplasia.

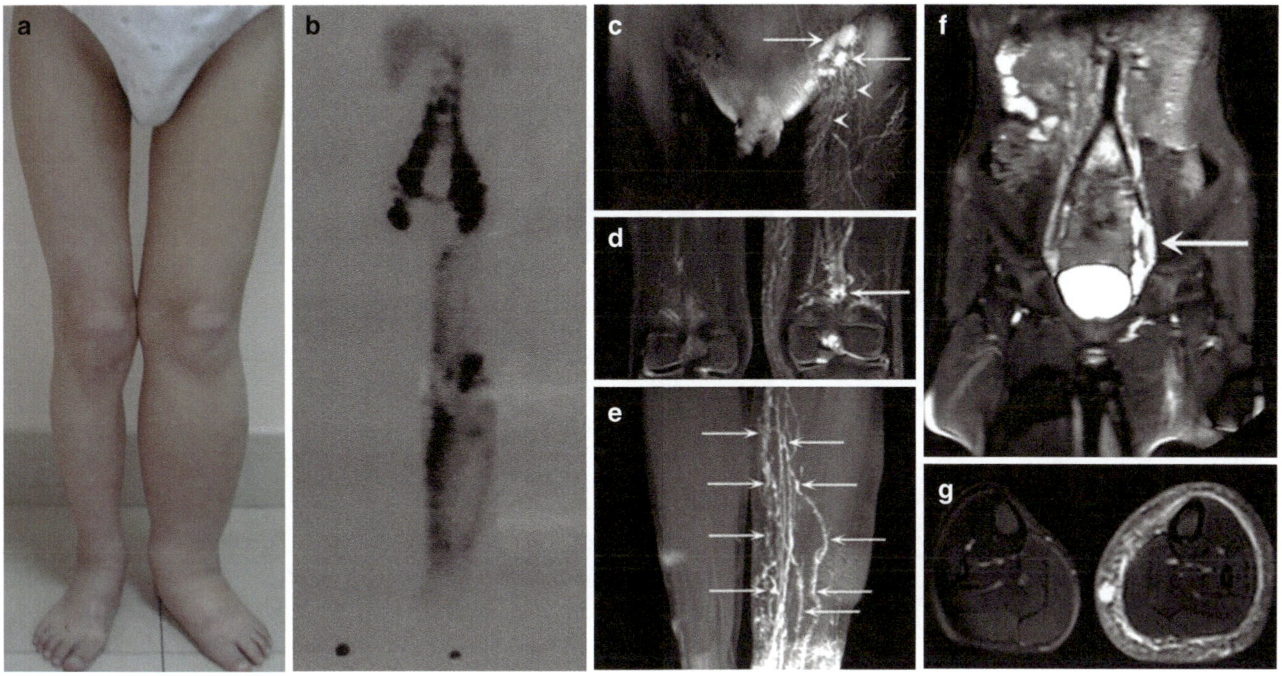

Fig. 22.1 (**a**) Patient age 12, three-month history of swelling of the whole of left leg. (**b**) Lymphoscintigram showing dermal backflow in the lateral and medial part of lower leg and inner aspect of thigh. (**c**) MRL showing contrast-enhanced inguinal and iliac lymph node (arrow) and prominent afferent lymphatics (arrowhead). (**d**) Enhanced deep lymphatic vessels (arrow) in the popliteal fossa. (**e**) Tortuous and dilated lymphatic vessels (arrow) were clearly displayed on post-injection MRL imaging. (**f**) Contrast-enhanced pelvic lymph vessels and nodes (arrow). (**g**) MR imaging showing edema fluid encircling the limb and disperse within subcutaneous tissue

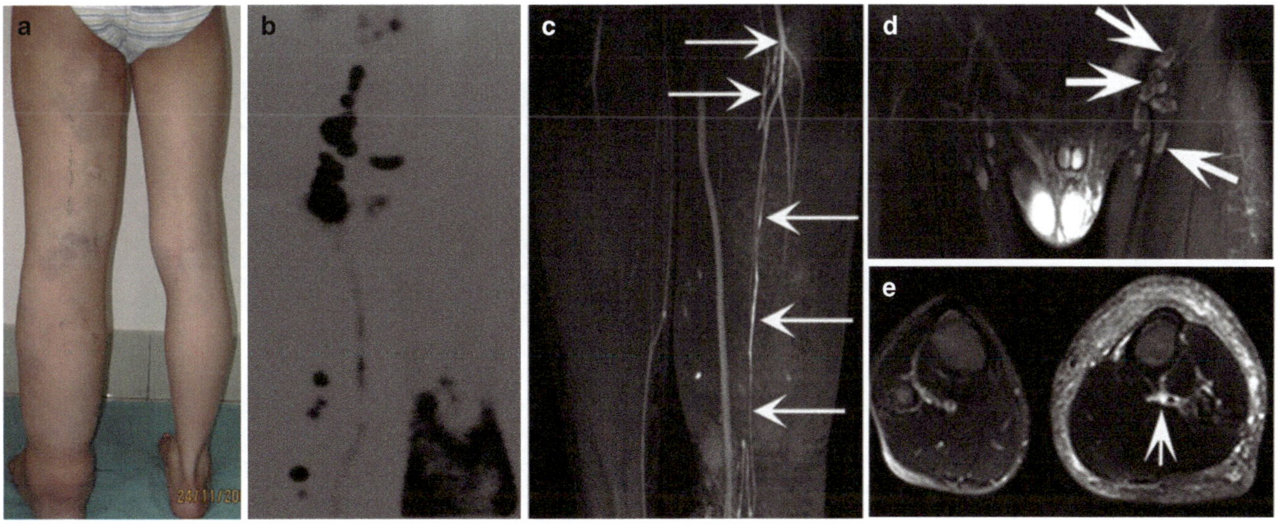

Fig. 22.2 (**a**) Patient age 12 with chief clinical features of KTS of left lower limb. (**b**) LSG showing dermal backflow up to the knee level. No inguinal lymph node and identifiable lymph vessel are visualized in the affected leg. (**c**) A solitary deep lymphatic vessel (arrow) was seen parallel with the vein on MR lymphangiogram. (**d**) MRL imaging showing the heterogeneous texture of inguinal lymph nodes with higher signal intensity in the cortex region (arrow). Edema fluid was dispersed in the subcutaneous layer and intramuscular space (small arrow) on the axial section of MRI

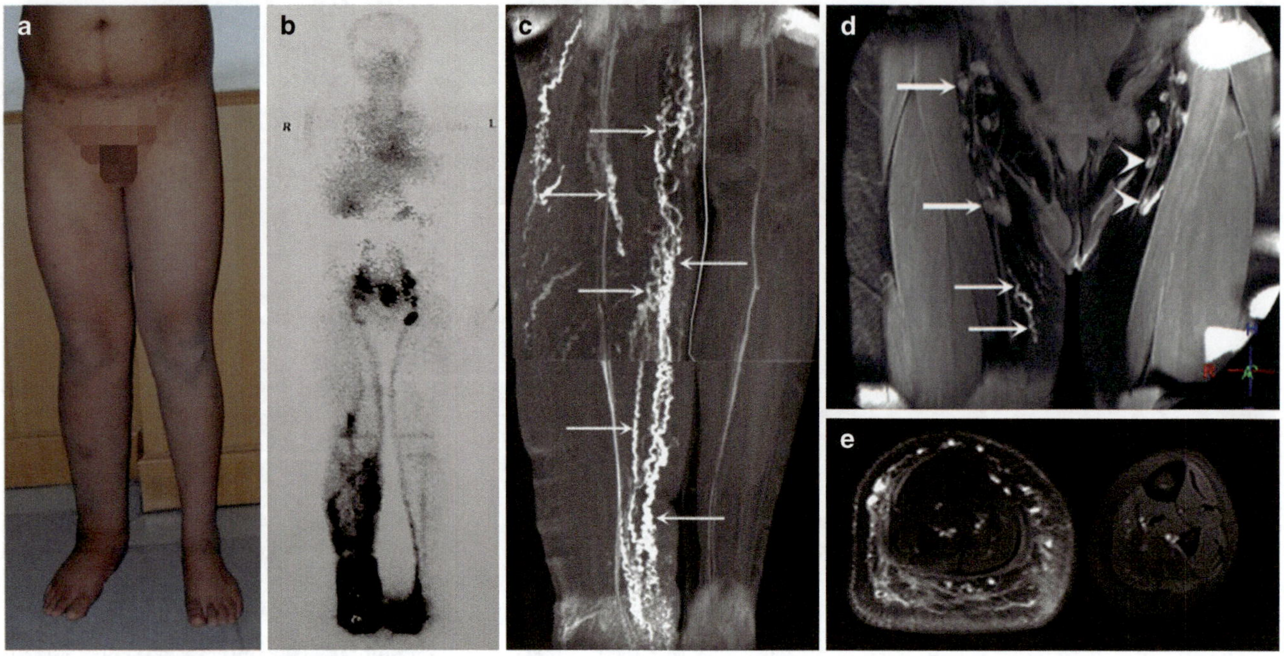

Fig. 22.3 (**a**) Patient age 17, six-year history of swelling of the right lower leg. (**b**) LSG showing dermal backflow in the lower leg and asymmetry of inguinal lymph nodes with the faintness of the node images. (**c**) MRL imaging delineates bundles of lymphatic vessels of the whole limb. (**d**) Contrast-enhanced the afferent lymph vessels (small arrow) but not the inguinal nodes (large arrow) in lymphedematous limb in contrast with intense enhancement of nodes on the controlateral side (arrowhead). (**e**) Cross-section of MRI showing dilated lymphatic vessels and edema fluid dispersing in the subcutaneous layer

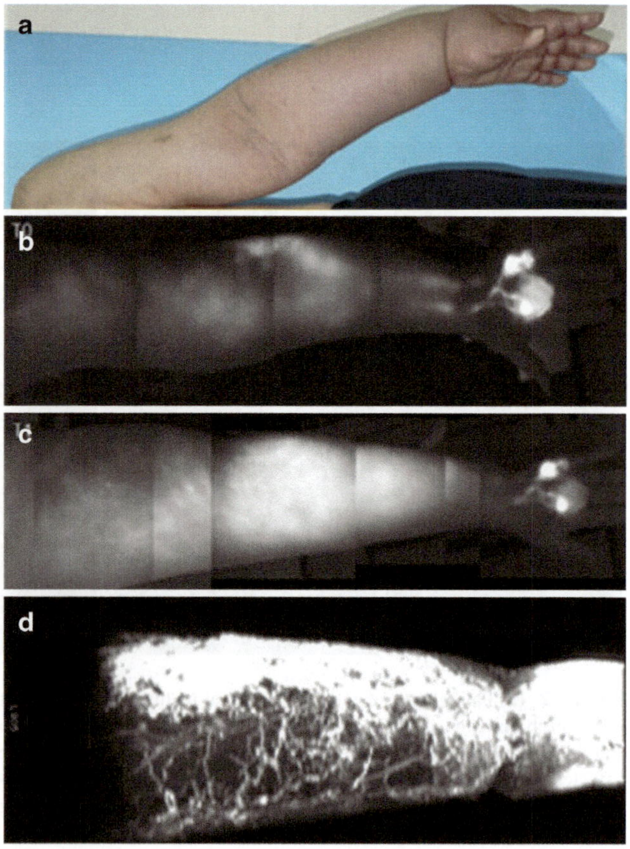

Fig. 22.4 Comparison of ICG lymphogram and MRL imaging of lymphatics in BCRL limbs. (**a**) A 56 years-old woman with BCRL of the left arm of 5 years. (**b**) The imaging of ICG lymphography immediately after the contrast injection showed 2 lymphatic collectors in the dorsum of the hand and forearm. (**c**) The imaging of ICG lymphography 5 min after the contrast injection on which massive dermal backflow in the forearm and upper arm and no clear lymphatics could be visualized. (**d**) MRL clearly demonstrated massively dilated lymph collectors in the affected upper extremity

References

1. Sherman DC, Ter-Pogossian M. Lymph node concentration of radioactive colloidal gold following interstial injection. Cancer. 1953;6(6):1238–45.
2. Szuba A, Shin W, Strauss HW, Rockson S. The third circulation: radionuclide lymphoscintigraphy in the evaluation of lymphoedema. J Nucl Med. 2003;44(1):43–57.
3. Liu NF, Lu Q, Wang CG, Zhou JG. Magnetic resonance imaging as a new method to diagnose protein losing enteropathy. Lymphology. 2008;41(3):111–5.
4. Liu NF, Lu Q, Jiang ZH, Wang CG, Zhou JG. Anatomic and functional evaluation of the lymphatics and lymph nodes in diagnosis of lymphatic circulation disorders with contrast magnetic resonance lymphangiography. J Vasc Surg. 2009;49(4):980–7. https://doi.org/10.1016/j.jvs.2008.11.029.
5. Lu Q, Xu J, Liu N. Chronic lower extremity lymphedema: a comparative study of high-resolution interstitial MR lymphangiography and heavily T2-weighted MRI. Eur J Radiol. 2010;73(2):365–73. https://doi.org/10.1016/j.ejrad.2008.10.041.
6. Lu Q, Bui D, Liu NF, Xu JR, Zhao XH, Zhang XF. Magnetic resonance Lymphography at 3T: a promising noninvasive approach tocharacterise inguinal lymphatic vessel leakage. Eur J Vasc Endovasc Surg. 2012 Jan;43(1):106–11. https://doi.org/10.1016/j.ejvs.2011.09.007.
7. Yamamoto T, Yamamoto N, Doi K, Oshima A, Yoshimatsu H, Todokoro T, Ogata F, Mihara M, Narushima M, Iida T, Koshima I. Indocyanine green-enhanced lymphography for upper extremity lymphedema: a novel severity staging system using dermal backflow patterns. Plast Reconstr Surg. 2011;128(4):941–7. https://doi.org/10.1097/PRS.0b013e3182268cd9.
8. Mihara M, Hara H, Araki J, Kikuchi K, Narushima M, Yamamoto T, Iida T, Yoshimatsu H, Murai N, Mitsui K, Okitsu T, Koshima I. Indocyaninegreen (ICG) lymphography is superior to lymphoscintigraphy for diagnostic imaging of early lymphedema of the upper limbs. PLoS One. 2012;7(6):e38182. https://doi.org/10.1371/journal.pone.0038182.
9. Yu ZY, Sun D, Wang L, Chen J, Han LH, Liu NF. Diagnosis of primary lymphedema with indocyanine green lymphography. Chin J Plast Surg. 2018;34(4):256–9.
10. Barrett T, Choyke PL, Kobayashi H. Imaging of the lymphatic system: new horizons. Contrast Media Mol Imaging. 2006;1(6):230–45.
11. Liu NF, Lu Q, Liu PA, Wu XF, Wang BS. Comparison of radionuclide lymphoscintigraphy and dynamic magnetic resonance lymphangiography for investigating extremity lymphedema. Br J Surg. 2010 Mar;97(3):359–65. https://doi.org/10.1002/bjs.6893.
12. Notohamiprodjo M, Weiss M, Baumeister RG, Sommer WH, Helck A, Crispin A, Reiser MF, Herrmann KAMR. Lymphangiography at 3.0 T: correlation with lymphoscintigraphy. Radiology. 2012;264(1):78–87.
13. Olszewski WL, Liu NF. Magnetic resonance lymphography (MRL): point and count-point. Lymphology. 2013;46(4):202–7.

Part VI

Treatment of Lymphedema: Conservative Treatment

23 Compression Therapy

Etelka Foeldi

Abstract

Compression therapy has been applied for the treatment of peripheral lymphedema for more than 100 years. Adequate compression therapy enables not only the mobilization of the increased tissue fluid but also the reduction or regression of the resulting tissue alterations as the thickening of the cutis, sclerotic alterations of the subcutis, and fatty tissue. This chapter introduces the principles and the implementation of compression therapy, as well as the structure of lymphological compression bandaging and stocking.

Keywords

Lymphedema · Physical decongestive therapy · Compression therapy · Compression stockings · Compression bandaging · Proinflammatory genes

Compression therapy is the application of mechanical pressure on the skin over various regions of the body, with the aim of alleviating symptoms of disease. The most familiar effects are decongestion, pain relief, and the reduction of swelling and inflammation. In Lymphology, compression therapy has been consistently applied for the treatment of peripheral lymphedema, i.e., lymphedema of the extremities, for more than 100 years.

Lymphedema is a disease associated with chronic inflammatory processes in the interstitium, and is caused by a disturbance to the balance between the lymphatic load, the volume of ultrafiltrated fluid, and the lymph drainage system's reabsorption capacity. The resultant swelling is not, however, simply caused by an increased volume of tissue fluid, but is also due to the disturbed homeostasis in the interstitium: disturbances to the cell population, the expression of proinflammatory factors, and extracellular components such as collagen fibers. The disease is characterized by tissue alterations as the disease progresses, independent of the original location and etiology. In the first stage of lymphedema, in addition to the increase of interstitial fluid (clinical observations would be soft, pitting edema), processes already take place in the interstitium which lead to the following clinical symptoms:

- Thickening of the cutis, broadening of the skin folds.
- Fibrotic, sclerotic alterations of the subcutis including the fascia.
- Occasionally there is also an increase in fatty tissue.

In many cases, lymphostatic hyperkeratoses develop, as well as papillomatoses and varicose protruberences (stages 2 and 3 of lymphedema).

Adequate compression therapy enables not only the mobilization of the increased tissue fluid but also the reduction or regression of the resulting tissue alterations, too.

23.1 How Are the Principles for the Effects of Compression Therapy?

The materials used in order to create compression pressure also influence skin temperature. Interstitial pressure is raised through the application of mechanical pressure on the skin. Fluid, as is well known, cannot be compressed, so that intravasal and extravasal flow (along tissue pathways) increase.

This effect enables the mobilization of the increased tissue fluid, as lymphatic flow in the lymph vessels is also accelerated as well as the uptake of free tissue fluid into the lymph capillaries. The indirect positive effects of compression therapy on venous diseases are also of great significance: The increased venous flow is not only a prophylaxis against

E. Foeldi (✉)
Földiklinik GmbH & Co.KG, Hinterzarten, Germany
e-mail: etelka.foeldi@foeldiklinik.de

N. Liu (ed.), *Peripheral Lymphedema*, https://doi.org/10.1007/978-981-16-3484-0_23

thromboses, but it also reduces ambulatory venous hypertension, which in turn reduces ultrafiltration. Furthermore, the increased interstitial pressure leads to the reabsorption of fluid via terminal blood capillaries.

23.2 How We Use Compression Therapy?

Compression therapy is the most important component of complex physical decongestive therapy (CDT). CDT is conducted in two phases, depending on the dosage of therapeutic measures: Phase 1 is the daily application of therapeutic measures and compression therapy is conducted with compression bandaging. Phase 2, also known as the maintenance phase, compression therapy is conducted with fitted medical compression garments.

23.3 How Is the Structure of Lymphological Compression Bandaging?

According to the appropriate curative and protective skincare procedure, a tubular dressing made from cotton wool is wrapped around the skin to protect it. Padding materials are applied over the cylindrical bandage: a padding bandage made of synthetic fibers or thin layers of foam for an even distribution of pressure (Fig. 23.1). Uneven foam padding materials can be used, too, in order to achieve a micro-massage effect during movement. Compression pressure is finally secured with short stretch elastic bandages. It should be taken into account that as well as the layer of protective padding material, skin wrinkles, and indentations must be filled with made-to-measure pieces of foam. Fingers and toes are wrapped with double layers of elastic bandages.

Table 23.1 shows the application of compression bandaging, depending on the age of the patient and the stage of the lymphedema.

The medical compression stockings are custom-made, flat-knitted garments, which are meant to prevent the re-accumulation of edema fluid. Their stretchability should match that of the elastic bandages. Patients with chronic lymphedema must wear medical compression stockings their whole life (Fig. 23.2), even if the lymphedema can be successfully reduced to its latent state with therapy. The type of compression stockings a patient requires shows Table 23.2. The form of compression garments what the patient required, can change over the course of his or her life, relative to the receding of the lymphedema or the occurrence of intercurrent diseases (orthopedic, neurological, etc.).

In a clinical study, we examined the therapeutic effects of compression therapy during phase 1, both with regard to the reduction of the expression of proinflammatory genes, as well as the positive effects on the thickness of skin. Ultrasound was used to measure skin thickness before and after phase 1 of therapy, and the expression of proinflammatory genes was measured in the blood. A follow-up examination was performed at the end of phase 1 of therapy. Diagrams 23.1 and 23.2 show the results.

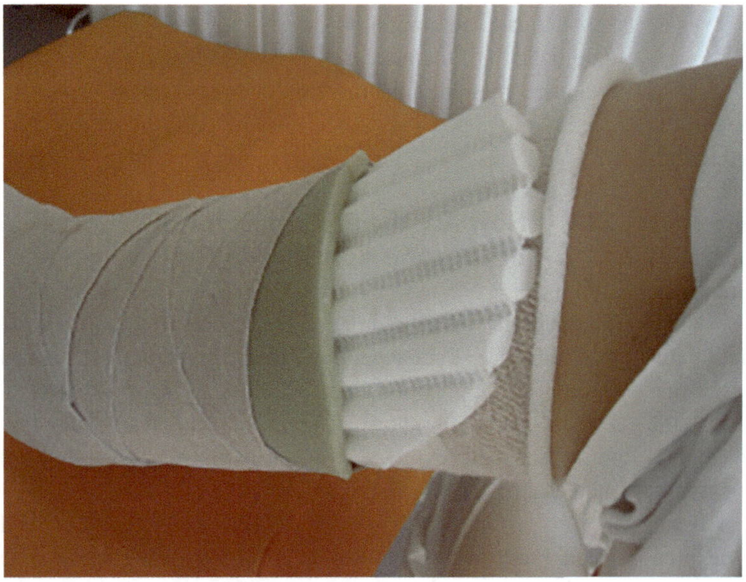

- Skin protection via tube cotton bandage
- Padding material – even or uneven –
- Textile elastic (short stretch) bandaging

Fig. 23.1 Apply compression padding material and short stretch bandaging to a lower extremity

Table 23.1 Application of compression bandaging, depending on the age of the patient and the stage of the disease

		Pressure	Padding		Max. application time
Children	6 months–2 years	10–20 mmHg	Smooth (padding bandages/foam)		12–16 h
	2–6 years	20–30 mmHg	Smooth	Padding bandage	16–20 h
			Uneven	Foam	
	6–12 years	20–30 mmHg	Smooth	Padding bandage	16–20 h
			Uneven	Foam	
Adults	Stage I	20–30 mmHg	Smooth	Padding bandage	12–16 h
			Smooth	Foam	
	Stage II	30–46 mmHg	Smooth	Padding bandage	18–22 h
			Uneven	Foam	
	Stage III	46 mmHg and stronger	Smooth	Padding bandage	18–22 h
			Uneven	Foam	
	Lymphedema combination forms	Individual	Individual		Individual
Geriatric	60–70 years	30–46 mmHg	Smooth	Padding bandage	18–22 h
			Uneven	Foam	
	Over 70 years	20–30 mmHg	Smooth	Padding bandage	12–16 h

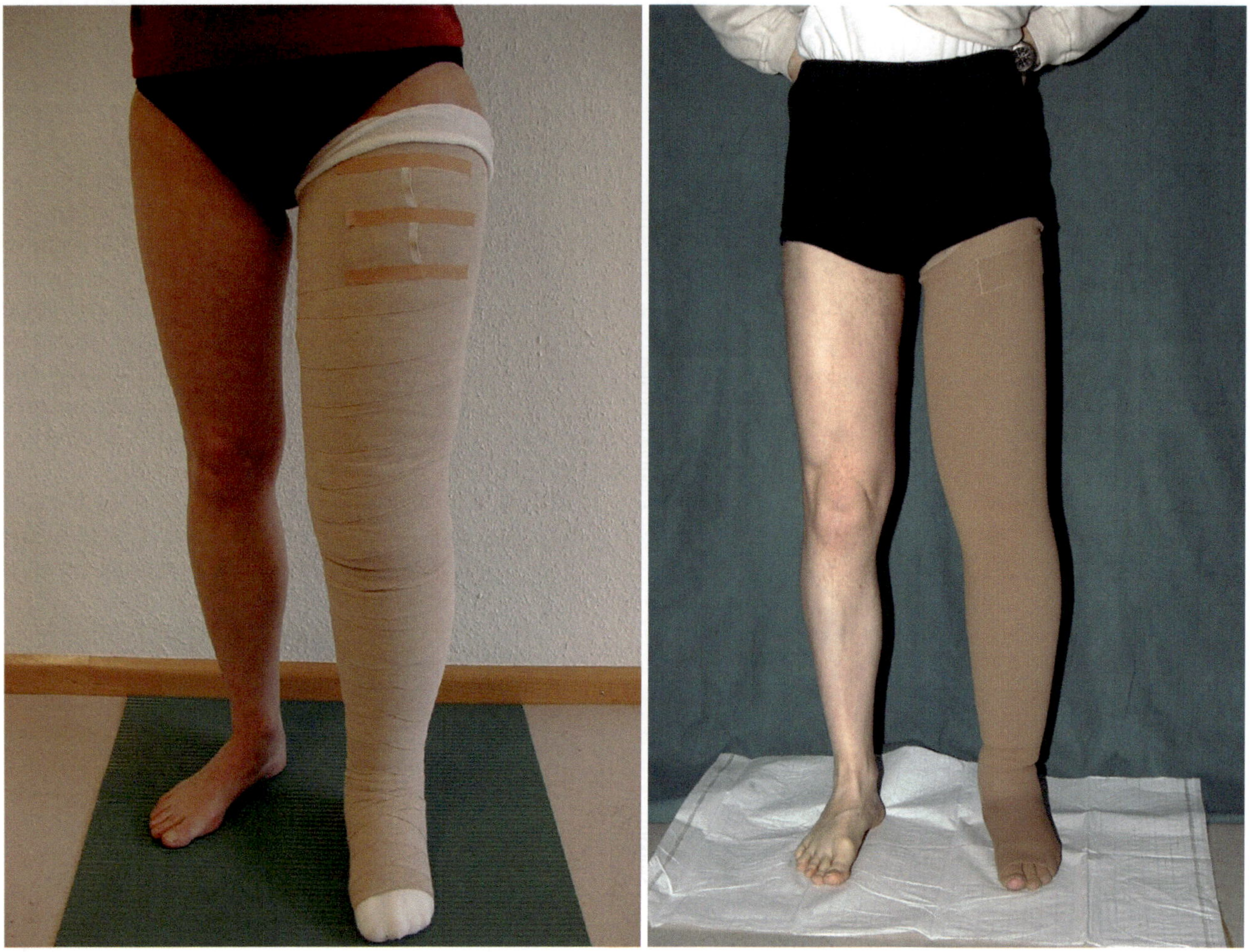

Fig. 23.2 Compression bandaging is completed of the lower limb (left); wear medical compression stockings (right)

Table 23.2 Compression stockings depend on the stage and location of the lymphedema

Location	Stage I	Stage II	Stage III
Toes/foot	Toe caps CCl. I	Toe caps CCl. I	Toe caps CCl. I
	Socks CCl. I	Socks CCl. II	Socks CCl. III
Lower leg + toes/foot	Toe caps CCl. I	Toe caps CCl. I	Toe caps CCl. I
	Knee stockings CCl. II	Knee stockings CCl. II	Knee stockings CCl. IV
Whole leg + toes/foot	Toe caps CCl. I	Toe caps CCl. I	Toe caps CCl. I
	Groinal stocking CCl. II	Groinal stocking CCl. III	Groinal stocking CCl. IV
Truncal quadrant + both legs + toes/foot	Toe caps CCl. 1	Toe caps CCl. I	Toe caps CCl. I
	Tights with one leg CCl. II	Tights with one leg CCl. III	Tights with one leg of CCl. IV
		Truncal garment CCl. II	Truncal garment CCl. II
Truncal quadrant + both legs + toes/foot	Toe caps CCl. I	Toe caps CCl. I	Toe caps CCl. I
	Tights CCl. II	(a) Knee stockings CCL. III	(a) Knee stockings CCl. IV
		(b) Half-hose CCl. II	(b) Half-hose CCl. II/III
Lower arm + hand	Long glove CCl. I	Long glove CCl. II	Long glove CCl. II or III
Whole arm + hand	Sleeve CCl. I	Sleeve CCl. II	Sleeve CCl. II or III
	Glove CCl. I	Glove CCl. II	Glove CCl. II

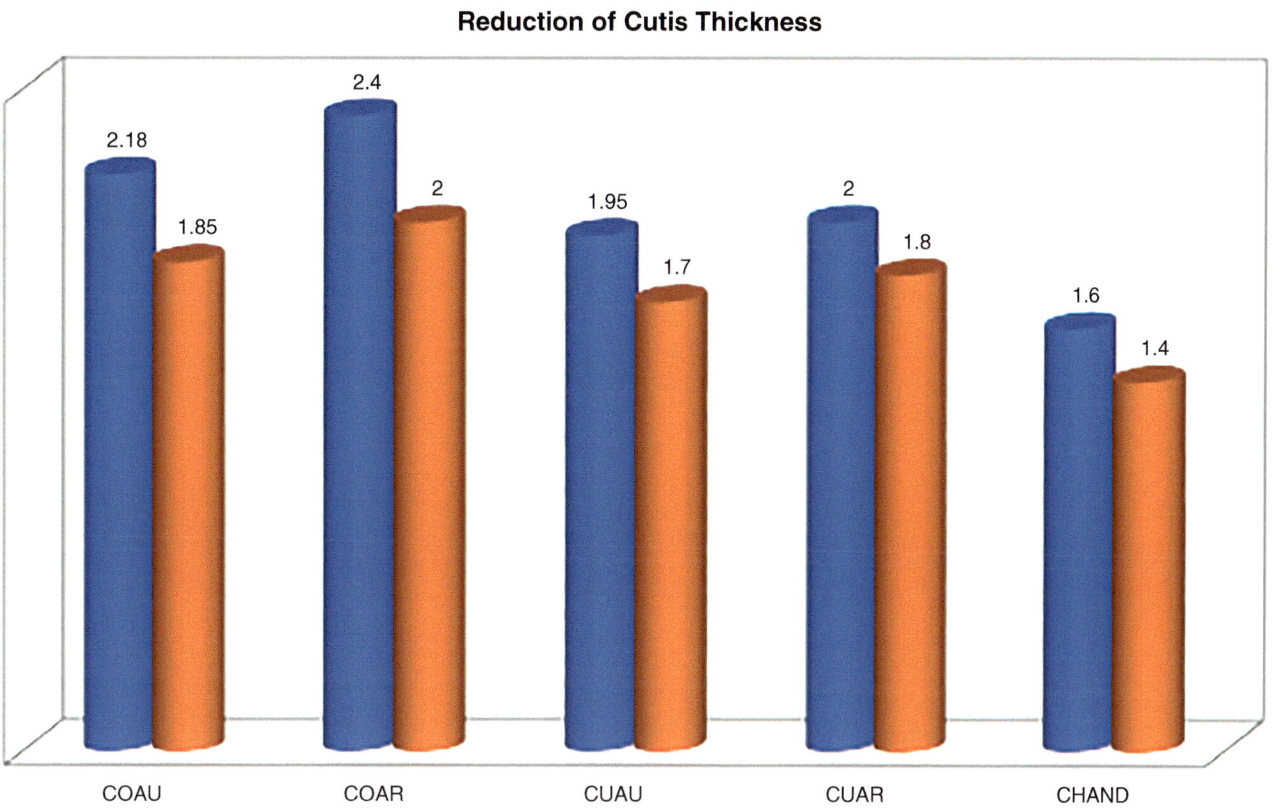

Diagram 23.1 Skin thickness measurements

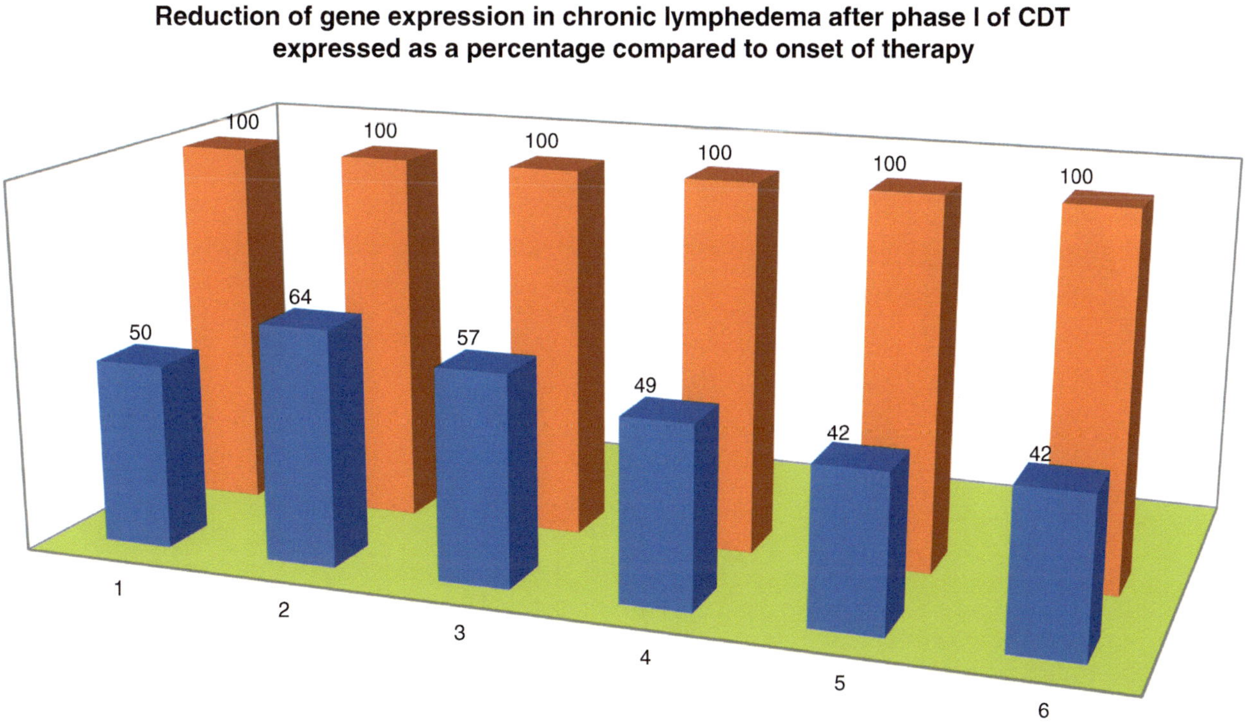

Diagram 23.2 Reduction of proinflammatory genes

24 Complex Physical Decongestive Therapy for Lymphedema (CDT)

Etelka Foeldi

Abstract

Complex Physical Decongestive Therapy (CDT) is the standard therapy for lymphedema. The aim of treatment is to cause the lymphedema to regress to a clinically edema-free stage or at least to decrease the stages of lymphedema. CDT as the basic therapy for lymphedema encompasses five elements as skin care, manual lymph drainage, compression therapy, decongestive exercise, and self-treatment education. The dosage, indications, and contraindications of individual components depend on the stage of lymphedema, the age of patient, and comorbidities. The long-term success of therapy depends on cooperation along the therapeutic chain of doctors, physiotherapists, and ensuring adequate medical compression garments.

Keywords

Complex physical decongestive therapy (CDT) · Primary lymphedema · Secondary lymphedema · Multicausal lymphedema · Skin care · Manual lymph drainage · Exercise therapy

Lymphedema can manifest in numerous parts of the body. It can affect the extremities, trunk, head, and genitals, with the internal organs only rarely affected.

Pathophysiologically, lymphedema is defined as a disturbance in the balance between the flow of fluid into the interstitium from the blood vessels (lymphatic load), and the disturbed or insufficient lymphatic transport (transport capacity of the lymphatic vessels). Lymphedema is characterized by subsequent alterations to the connective tissue in areas affected by lymphatic congestion [1]; in the extracellular spaces, and in the cells themselves (Fig. 24.1). Without adequate therapy, the alterations will progress with swelling of the affected region, transformation of the connective tissue, with resultant fibroses, scleroses, and/or fatty tissue deposition as the clinical consequences.

Lymphedema may occur in any age group, and is a chronic disease. Primary forms of lymphedema dominate in children and younger patients, with secondary lymphedema dominating with increasing age. From a clinical point of view, particularly in geriatric patients with lymphedema that is slow to manifest, we also define a third form of lymphedema: multicausal lymphedema. It is well known that numerous chronic diseases which increase with age (metabolic, orthopedic, neurological diseases, etc.) lead to disturbances in the permeability of blood capillaries, which leads to a long-term increase in lymphatic load. The lymph vascular system can compensate for this for a time, but the constant overloading eventually leads to decompensation and the tissue alterations typical for lymphedema eventually occur [2–12].

Complex physical decongestive therapy (CDT) is the standard therapy for lymphedema. CDT is also medically indicated for surgical treatment in suitable cases. The aim of treatment is to cause the lymphedema to regress to a clinically edema-free stage (which is not to be understood as healing of the disease) or at least to decrease the stages of lymphedema. A general medical, lymphological, and psychological evaluation at the outset of treatment is essential for the successful application of CDT.

CDT as the basic therapy for lymphedema encompasses the following coordinated components:

- Guidelines for skin care and sanitation.
- Manual lymph drainage, with additive physiotherapy techniques as required.
- Compression therapy with specialist multilayer, compression bandaging, and/or lymphological compression stockings.
- Decongestive sport and exercise therapy.

E. Foeldi (✉)
Földiklinik GmbH & Co.KG, Hinterzarten, Germany
e-mail: etelka.foeldi@foeldiklinik.de

N. Liu (ed.), *Peripheral Lymphedema*, https://doi.org/10.1007/978-981-16-3484-0_24

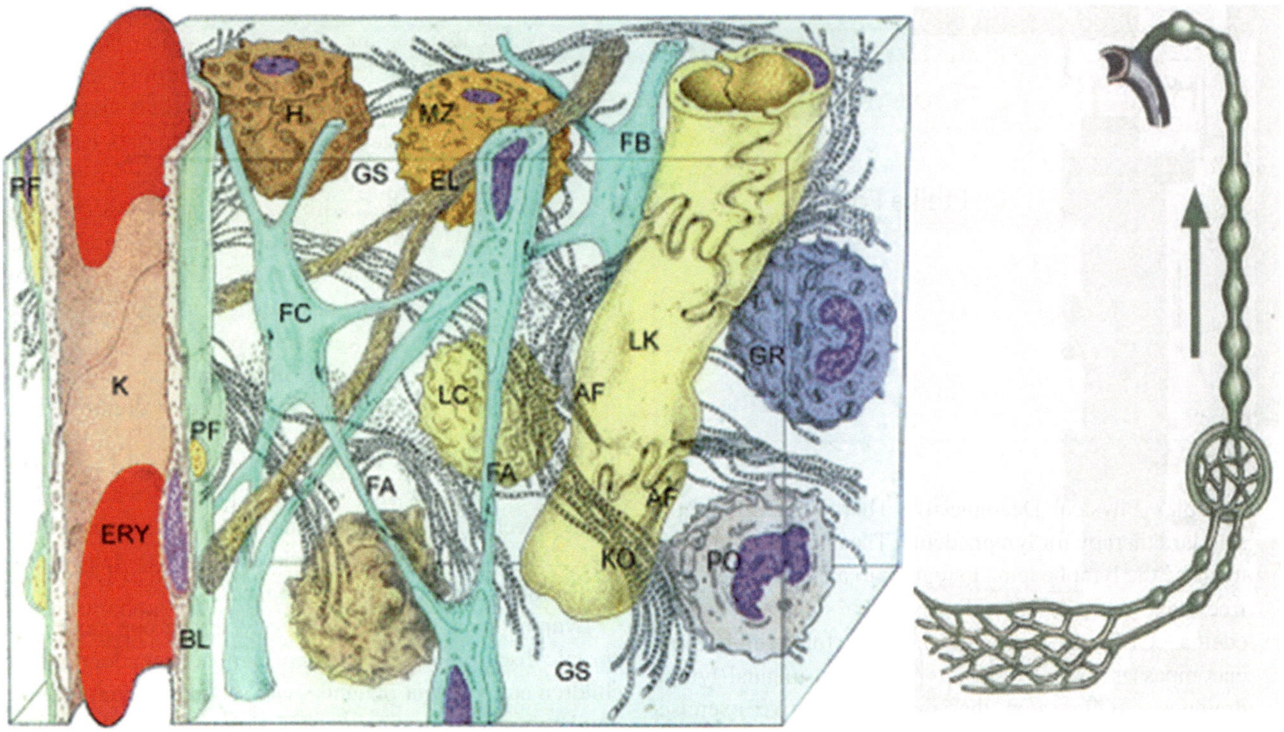

Fig. 24.1 Disturbances to lymph formation and lymphatic flow alter ECM and different cells like fibroblasts, macrophages with the following consequences: fluid accumulation and fibrosis; therefore CDT has to be more than just the mobilization of fluid; it has to normalize the homeostasis in the interstitium

- Education and schooling in individual self-treatment measures.

The dosage, indications, and contraindications of individual components depend on numerous factors:

- The stage of lymphedema in which therapy is initiated.
- Comorbidities.
- Age of the patient and individual living circumstances.

24.1 CDT Is Applied in Two Phases

In Phase I treatment measures are highly dosed in order to mobilize the increased tissue fluid—1–3× per day. The treatment can take place on an in-patient basis in highly specialized medical facilities with the necessary infrastructure (lymphologically trained doctors, nursing staff, qualified physiotherapists). In milder cases, Phase I of therapy can take place on an out-patient basis, if the conditions for successful treatment are met.

Phase II of CDT encompasses adapted components based on the individual patient's needs with the aim of preventing renewed swelling, and to optimize the therapeutic results of Phase I. Components may be applied continuously (compression therapy, exercise, etc.), on a weekly basis, or in series. A repeat Phase I of therapy may be required depending on the progression of the disease, particularly when intercurrent diseases occur (Table 24.1).

CDT should be applied in its entirety during Phase I and Phase II, as far as living circumstances and/or contraindications permit.

At the outset of CDT, the clinical picture should be precisely documented, and the therapeutic goals defined on the basis of these findings. Lymphedema aggravating comorbidities should be treated as far as is possible and taken into consideration when applying CDT. The long term success of therapy depends on cooperation along the therapeutic chain, from:

- Doctors
- Physiotherapists
- Ensuring adequate medical compression garments (bandaging material and prescribed and fitted compression garments)

Therapeutic goals in childhood:

The patient's parents are instructed and integrated into the application of CDT, with the aim of ensuring the patient's ability to complete schooling and professional training, and in order to reduce the psychiatric impact of living with the disease.

Table 24.1 Prevention and phases treatment of lymphedema within CDT

	Symptoms	Phase I decongestion	Phase II optimization	Phase III preservation
Stage 0	No swelling, pathological lymphoscintigram	Prevention when lymphedema risk factors present		
Stage I	Edema of soft consistency, raising of the limb reduces swelling	MLD: 1× per day, compression bandaging, exercise, duration 14–21 days		MLD: in series, compression garments as required or consistent in the long-term
Stage II	Edema with secondary tissue alterations, raising of the limb without effect	MLD: 2× per day, compression bandaging, exercise, duration 24–28 days	MLD: 1–2× per week for the duration of 2–5 years, compression garments and bandaging, exercise, repetition of phase I	MLD: in series or 1× per week, compression garments are worn consistently in the long-term, exercise
Stage III	Elephantiastic hard swelling, often of lobular form with typical skin alterations	MLD: 2–3× per day, compression bandaging, exercise, duration 28–35 days	MLD: 2–3× per week for the duration of 5–10 years, compression garments and bandaging, exercise, repetition of phase I	MDL: In series or 1–2× per week, compression stockings worn consistently in the long-term, exercise, repetition of phase I

Therapeutic goals in adult patients:

The aim of CDT in adults is to prevent lymphedema complications such as erysipelas, to preserve the patients' ability to work, and to improve their quality of life.

Geriatric therapeutic goals:

Adequate, holistic care, preservation of mobility, and the prevention of care dependency in these patients.

In daily practice, the following clinical symptoms are observed following CDT:

Considerable reduction in the swelling of the affected region, reduction of congestive complaints such as feelings of heaviness or tautness, an increase in mobility, normalization of lymphostatic skin alterations including the reduction of fibroscleroses.

The mechanisms of action and dosage of the individual components of CDT are described below.

24.2 Skin Care/Skin Protection

Compression materials can stress the skin, with a subsequent reduction in moisture and fat content. Skin protection and skin care are thus important components of therapy in the long term, and should take place daily. An important role is played by the choice of basic skin care products. Creams with a high lipid content should be chosen, i.e., moisturizing and fat replenishing products.

24.2.1 Skin Sanitation

In lymphedema, injuries to the skin can lead to superinfections and may cause progression in the edema. Wounds, ruptured cysts, and fistulae should thus be disinfected as soon as possible (e.g., Polyvidon, Octenidin). Causative treatment is required for interdigital, or deep skin fold macerations. Allergic skin reactions, e.g., after insect bites, can be temporarily treated with antihistamines after disinfection; cortisone may be required for severe cases. Additional skin diseases such as psoriasis and neurodermititis should be systematically treated as required, and care must be taken to choose suitable compression material.

24.3 Manual Lymph Drainage, with Additive Manual Techniques as Required

Manual lymph drainage is a specialist therapy, consisting of four basic techniques which exact a stretch stimulus on the cutis and subcutis including the fascia (Fig. 24.2). The walls of the lymph vessels are stretched, which leads to an increase in lymphangiopulsation with the following effects: The velocity of lymph flow in the collectors is increased, with a consecutive increase in lymph formation (the uptake of tissue fluid into the initial lymph vessels). The pathologically increased interstitial fluid is thus reduced. Additive manual techniques should be used in stages II and III with the aim of softening indurated tissue. Further additional manual techniques are indicated for the improvement of functional deficits in orthopedic/neurological diseases.

24.4 Compression Therapy with Specialist Multilayer, Compression Bandaging, and/or Lymphological Compression Stockings

See Chap. 6.

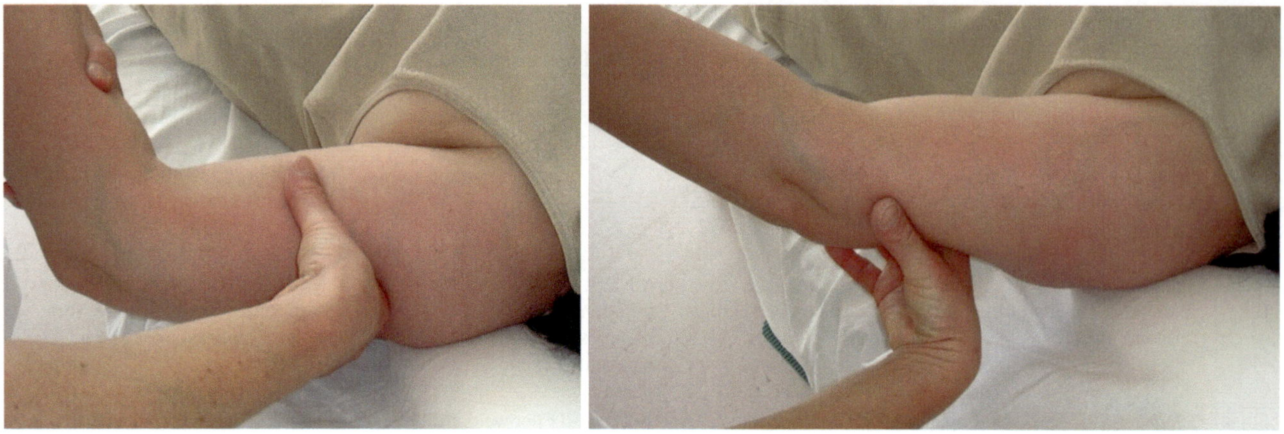

Fig. 24.2 Manual lymph drainage

24.5 Decongestive Sports and Remedial Exercise Therapy

Remedial exercise therapy and an active lifestyle are additional effective components of CDT. From the lymphological point of view, we differentiate between targeted movement in order to activate the muscle and joint pumps in the congested area, and an active sporty lifestyle for the preservation of general health. Targeted exercise leads to contraction and relaxation of the skeletal musculature, with subsequent changes in interstitial pressure. The changes in pressure in the interstitium are increased with contraction/relaxation against firm resistance (targeted external compression) with the effect of increasing lymphangiomotoricity. Intensive breathing exercises also increase venous blood flow and cause an increase in lymphatic flow. An individual remedial exercise program should be established in Phase I of CDT, which is then continued in Phase II of CDT. The program should be adapted to the age and general health of the patient. The following types of exercise have proven particularly effective: Walking and Nordic walking, cycling, exercise bike, swimming and water gymnastics, medical training therapy, moderate or strength training, under the guidance of physiotherapists in a fitness studio if required. These measures, in combination with a calorie-controlled diet, can also help to preserve normal body weight [13–19].

24.6 Individual Self-Treatment

CDT can be arduous and time consuming for the patient, particularly in the beginning. Psychological stress is also caused by the fact that lymphedema is an incurable disease, and CDT is required as a life-long treatment. Patients often feel profoundly helpless if the therapeutic results they hope for are not attainable, or if intercurrent diseases occur which lead to worsening of the lymphedema. This can lead to a reduction in compliance with the unfortunate consequence of a further worsening of the lymphedema. It is thus essential to provide patients with a detailed explanation about the functionality of the lymph vascular system and the causes of lymphedema, as well as the effectiveness of individual therapy components. Consultations with therapeutic professionals are an important factor in helping patients to organize their daily lives. Written information materials are helpful in the beginning. The contents should encompass skin care/sanitation, breathing techniques, decongestive physiotherapy, and self-bandaging. Some patients require psychological support in order to stay motivated and remain consistent with daily therapy [20–27].

24.7 Medical Reasons for the Modification of Individual Components of CDT, Including Indications and Contraindications

- Age: Compression therapy in children should only be applied after 6 months of age, with greatly reduced compression pressure, in order to avoid damage to the skin. The same principle applies to geriatric patients.
- Comorbidities: Comorbidities that are present in addition to the lymphedema may necessitate modifications to the application of CDT. Additive physiotherapy measures may also be indicated. The following comorbidities are known to be absolute contraindications for CDT:
  - Acute decompensated cardiac insufficiency
  - Acute phlebothrombosis
  - Acute erysipelas
  - Severe arterial blood flow disorders
  - Peripheral arterial occlusive disease

If the comorbidity improves, it may be possible to apply CDT in a modified form. Of note is lymphedema in cancer relapse patients, as this is a palliative situation. If metastases are successfully treated, CDT can be successfully applied and the therapeutic goals achieved [28–31].

The following measures can also be applied in addition to CDT:

- In obesity-associated lymphedema, bariatric interventions can improve the therapeutic results for lymphedema.
- Mechanical intermittent compression/pneumatic compression may be used in an adjuvant therapy form of CDT, particularly for lymphedema of the arms and legs with distal emphasis.

Nutrition:

A special lymphological diet is only medically indicated for rare combination forms (lymphedema with other lymph vessel malformations): the MCT diet is prescribed for chylous effusions and/or lymphostatic enteral protein loss.

Lymph tape:

Elastic tape can be applied as an additive measure in combination with compression therapy [32].

Medication:

There is currently no drug that can treat the cause of lymphedema. Lymphedema comorbidities may be treated with the relevant medication.

Thermotherapy, soft laser:

There has been insufficient proof of effectiveness for these methods so far.

References

1. Liu NF, Zhang LR. Changes of tissue fluid hyaluronan (hyaluronic acid) in peripheral lymphedema. Lymphology. 1998;31(4):173–9.
2. Zvonik M, Földi E, Felmerer G. The effects of reduction operation with genital lymphedema on the frequency of erysipelas and the quality of life. Lymphology. 2011;44(3):274–8.
3. Greene AK, Grant FD, Slavin SA, Maclellan RA. Obesity-induced lymphedema: clinical and lymphoscintigraphic features. Plast Reconstr Surg. 2015;135(6):1715–9.
4. Kaiserling E. Morphologische Befunden beim Lymphödem. In: Földi M, Földi E, editors. Lehrbuch Lymphologie. München: Urban und Fischer; 2010. p. 132–3.
5. Mouta C, Heroult M. Inflammatory triggers of lymphangiogenesis. Lymphat Res Biol. 2003;1(3):201–18. https://doi.org/10.1089/153968503768330247.
6. Casley-Smith JR, Clodius L, Piller NB. Tissue changes in chronic experimental lymphoedema in dogs. Lymphology. 1980;13(3):130–41.
7. Radhakrishnan K, Rocson SG. The clinical spectrum of lymphatic disease. Ann NY Acad Sci. 2008;1131:155–84.
8. Stemmer R. Das klinische Zeichen zur Früh- und Differentialdiagnose des Lymphödems. Vasan. 1979;5:261–2.
9. Schellong SM, Wollina U, Unger L, Machetanz J, Stelzner C. Das geschwollene Bein. Internist. 2013;54(11):1294–303.
10. Yamamoto T, Yamamoto N, Doi K, Oshima A, Ogata F, Mihara M, et al. Characteristic indocyanine green lymphography findings in lower extremity lymphedema: the generation of a novel lymphedema severity staging system using dermal backflow patterns. Plast Reconstr Surg. 2011;128(4):941–7.
11. Liu N, Wang C, Sun M. Noncontrast three-dimensional magnetic resonance imaging vs lymphoscintigraphy in the evaluation of lymph circulation disorders: a comparative study. J Vasc Surg. 2005;41:69–75.
12. Lohrmann C, Földi E, Barthomolä JP, Langer M. MR imaging of the lymphatic system: distribution and contrast enhancement of gadodiamide after intradermal injection. Lymphology. 2006;39(4):156–63.
13. Dayes IS, Whelan TJ, Julian J, Parpia S, Pritchard KL, D'Souza DP, et al. Randomized trial of decongestive lymphatic therapy for the treatment of lymphedema in women with breast cancer. J Clin Oncol. 2013;31(30):3758–63.
14. Lee BB, Andraden M, Bergan J, Boccardo NF, Campisi C, Damstra R, et al. Diagnose und Behandlung des primären Lymphödems. Vasomed. 2010;22(6):302–3.
15. Földi E, Sauerwald A, Henning B. Effect of complex decongestive physiotherapy on gene expression for the inflammatory response in peripheral lymphedema. Lymphology. 2000;33(1):19–23.
16. Brunner U, Frei-Fleischlin C. Gegenwärtiger Stand der KPE beim primären und sekundären Lymphödem der Beine. Vasa. 1993; 22(1).
17. Földi E. The current state of chronic lymphedema therapy. Top Geriatr Rehabil. 2012;28(4):240–2.
18. Yamamoton T, Todo Y, Kaneuchi M, Handa Y, Watanabe K, Yamamoto R. Study of edema reduction patterns during the treatment phase of complex decongestive physiotherapy for extremity lymphedema. Lymphology. 2008;41(2):80–6.
19. Brenke R, Freund R, Strössenreuther R.Adjuvante physikalische Therapie beim Lymphödem sowie bei ausgewählten Begleiterkrankungen am Bewegungsapparat. In: Földi M, Földi E, editors. Lehrbuch der Lymphologie. 7. Aufl. München: Elsevier, Urban & Fischer; 2010. p. 507–9.
20. Schöhl J, Rössler J, Földi E. Primary lymphedema—long term study and quality of life in patients undergoing complex physical decongestive therapy. LymphForsch. 2013;17(2):88–93.
21. Schöhl J. Das primäre Lymphödem des Kindes: Langzeittherapieverlauf und Lebensqualität. Inaugural-Dissertation. Freiburg; 2010.
22. Noori S, Petereit R, Rindermann J, Jungkunz HW. Reduktion der lymphostatischen Fibrosklerose verschiedener Hautschichten während der KPE: Aktuelle Ergebnisse einer randomisierten kontrollierten Studie mit 88 Patienten. Lymphologie in Forschung und Praxis. 2014;18(1):13.
23. Hwang JH, Kwonn JY, Lee KW, Choi JY, Kim BT, Lee BB, et al. Changes in lymphatic function after complex physical therapy for lymphedema. Lymphology. 1999;32(1):15–21.
24. Franzeck UK, Spiegel I, Fischer M, et al. Combined physical therapy for lymphedema evaluated by fluorescence microlymphography and lymph capillary pressure measurements. J Vasc Res. 1997;34(4):306–11.
25. Jullien P, Somé J, Brantus P, et al. Efficacy of home-based lymphoedema management in reducing acute attacks in subjects with lymphatic filariasis in Burkina Faso. Acta Trop. 2011; Suppl 1:55–61.
26. Földi M, Strössenreuther R. Grundlagen der manuellen Lymphdrainage. 2., überarb. Aufl. München: Urban und Fischer; 2000.

27. Huang TW, Tseng SH, Lin CC, Bai CH, Chen CS, Hung CS, et al. Effects of manual lymphatic drainage on breast cancer-related lymphedema: a systemic review and metaanalysis of randomized controlled trials. World J Surg Oncol. 2013;11:15.
28. Partsch H, Partsch B, Braun W. Interface pressure and stiffness of readymade compression stockings: comparison of an in vivo and in vitro measurements. J Vasc Surg. 2006;44(4):809–14.
29. Hanna R, Bohbot S, Connolly N. A comparison of interface pressure of three compression bandage systems. Br J Nurs. 2008;17(20):16–24.
30. Forster R, Sonderegger A. Übungsbeispiele zur entstauenden Gymnastik bei Beinlymphödemen. In: Földi M, Földi E, editors. Lehrbuch der Lymphologie: Für Mediziner, Masseuren und Physiotherapeuten. 7. Aufl. München: Elsevier, Urban & Fischer; 2010. p. 604–8.
31. Sörensen S. Kongressvortrag: KPE bei Herzinsuffizienz—immer eine absolute Kontraindikation? Kongress DGL Halle; 2014.
32. Liebl M, Preiß S, Pögel S, Pinnow J, Schwedtke C, Taufmann I, et al. Elastisches Tape als therapeutische Interventionn in der Erhaltungsphase der Komplexen Physikalischen Entstauungstherapie (KPE Phase II) von Lymphödemen. Phys Rehab Kur Med. 2014;24(01):34–41.

25 Far Infrared Radiation Thermotherapy

Ningfei Liu

Abstract

Far infrared radiation thermotherapy (FIRT) is one of the few effective conservative treatments for chronic extremity lymphedema. FIRT combined with bandaging is effective in reducing the amount of edema, skin thickness, and size of the affected limb. A distinctive effect of FIRT/bandaging is reduction in the frequency of dermatolymphangioadenitis. FIRT reduces tissue fibrosis and improves skin elasticity. The mechanisms by which FIRT reduces chronic lymphedema include increasing the biological effects of the microcirculation of lymph and blood in the skin and enhancing tissue immune function. FIRT has been shown over 5 years of follow-up to be a safe means of treating malignant tumors.

Keywords

Far infrared radiation thermotherapy (FIRT)
Lymphedema · Extremity · Dermatolymphangioadenitis (DLA) · Lymphedematous tissue · Skin fibrosis
Immune dysfunction · Cytokines

Far infrared radiation thermal therapy (FIRT) was first described by Chang in 1964 [1]. This treatment was originally devised by village doctors in southern China to alleviate or resolve the common complications of chronic lymphedema, namely recurrent erysipelas or cellulitis, and was found incidentally to also reduce the edema. Because FIRT has the unique effect of reducing infection, this treatment has been applied for half a century in the author's hospital and in some European and other Asian countries. The specially designed FIRT machine contains six far infrared ray tubes for producing heat and a regulator for controlling the temperature (Fig. 25.1). The patients are treated for 2 h daily at a temperature of 42 °C for 4 weeks for a total of 20 sessions. Better results can be achieved by repeating the treatment annually for 3–5 years.

Several studies on the efficacy and underlying mechanisms of this treatment have been published [2–5]. Infrared is invisible, being adjacent to the visible light region on the electromagnetic spectrum. Infrared radiation transfers energy, in the form of heat, to the target tissues and is perceived as heat by thermoreceptors in the surrounding skin [4, 5]. FIRT can penetrate the skin and gradually transfer energy into deep tissue through a resonance absorption mechanism of organic and water molecules [6, 7]. In an animal study, a significant increase in skin blood flow after, but not during, FIR exposure was found, which demonstrates that FIR therapy promotes and improves skin microcirculation via a biological, not a hyperthermic, mechanism [8].

Clinical studies have demonstrated that FIRT combined with bandaging is effective in alleviating edema and reducing skin thickness and the size of the affected limb (Figs. 25.2 and 25.3). Therapeutic results can be achieved with one course of this treatment. Recent studies have demonstrated that FIRT/bandaging reduces the frequency of dermatolymphangioadenitis (DLA). A retrospective study of 64 patients with chronic lower limb lymphedema after resection of gynecological tumors showed that the frequency of DLA decreased significantly following treatment [9], 78% of patients having no recurrences of DLA in the year subsequent to treatment. A controlled study has shown that FIRT/bandaging treatment reduces the incidence of DLA more effectively than bandaging alone [10] (Fig. 25.4). Improvement in immune function in local tissue may account for reduced inflammation. Samples from FIRT-treated patients have shown an increase in serum concentration of interleukin (IL)-1β after FIRT therapy and reduced local tissue fluid concentrations of the inflammatory cytokines IL-2, IL-10, and IL-18. Additionally, significant changes in anti-

N. Liu (✉)
Department Plastic and Reconstructive Surgery,
Shanghai Ninth People's Hospital, Shanghai Jiao Tong University School of Medicine, Shanghai, China

N. Liu (ed.), *Peripheral Lymphedema*, https://doi.org/10.1007/978-981-16-3484-0_25

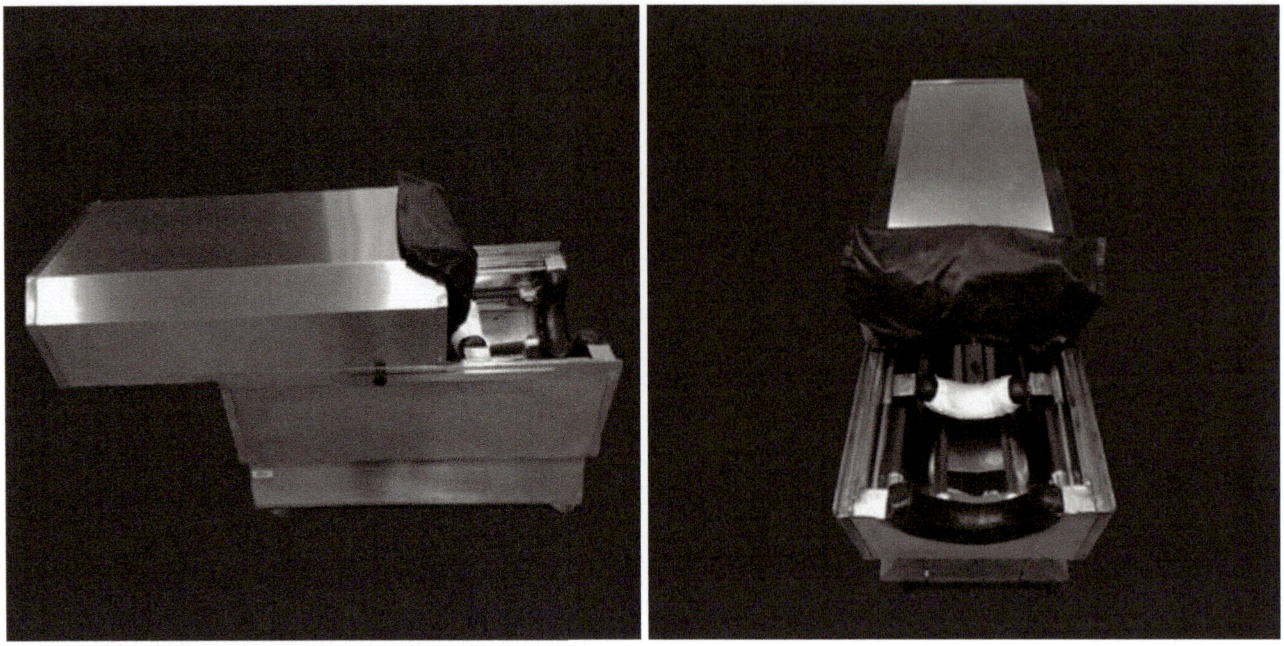

Fig. 25.1 The machine used can produce far-infrared ray (6–14 lm wavelengths) in its cabin. Patients place their extremities in the cabin for treatment

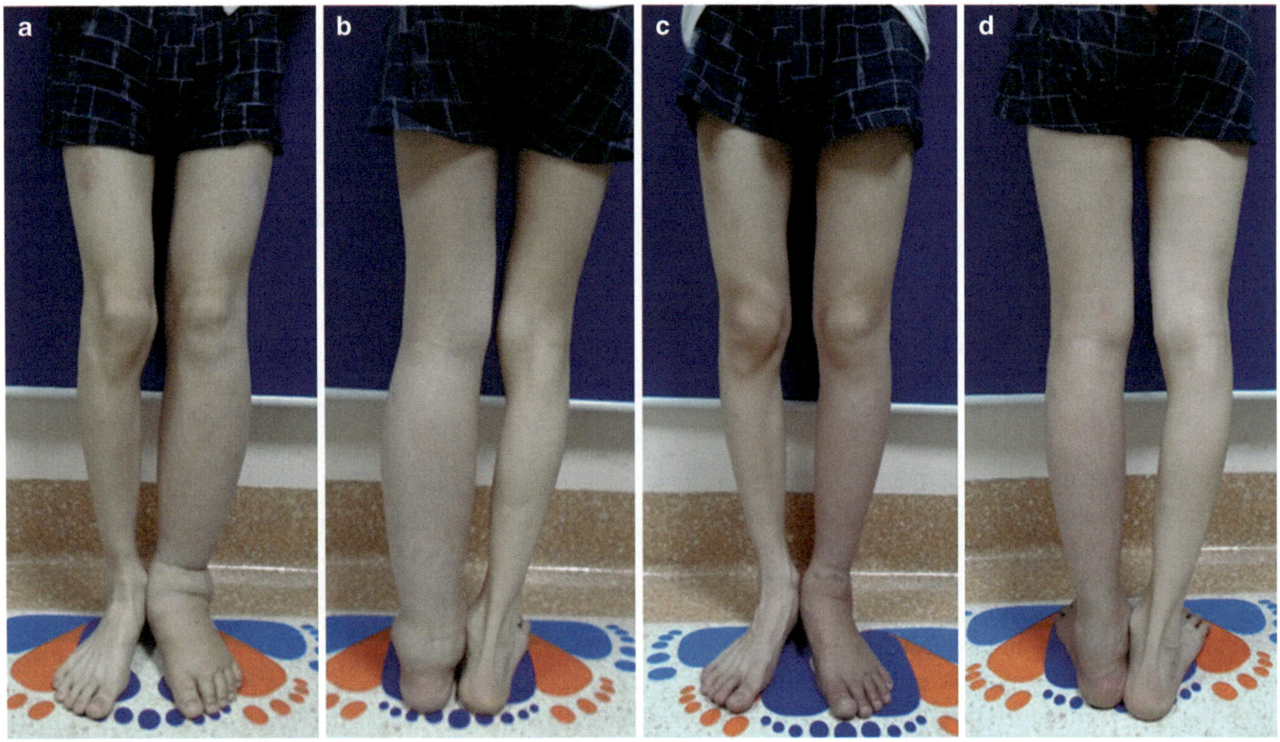

Fig. 25.2 A photographic image shows the improvement of a patient pre- (**a** and **b**) and post-treatment (**c** and **d**)

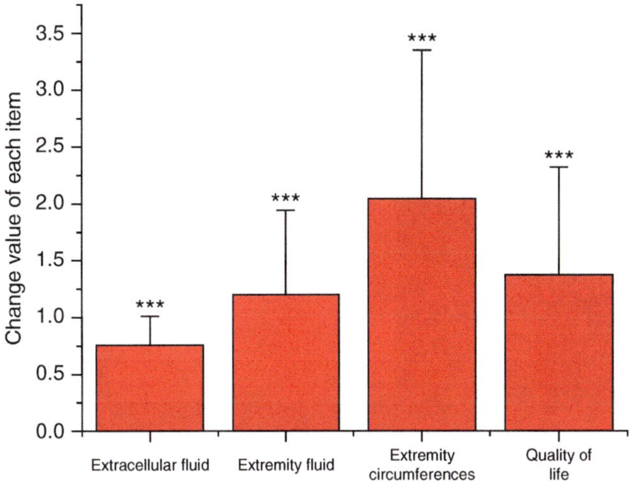

Fig. 25.3 Change value of extracellular fluid, extremity fluid, extremity circumferences, and quality of life after treated by far-infrared radiation. ***$p < 0.001$

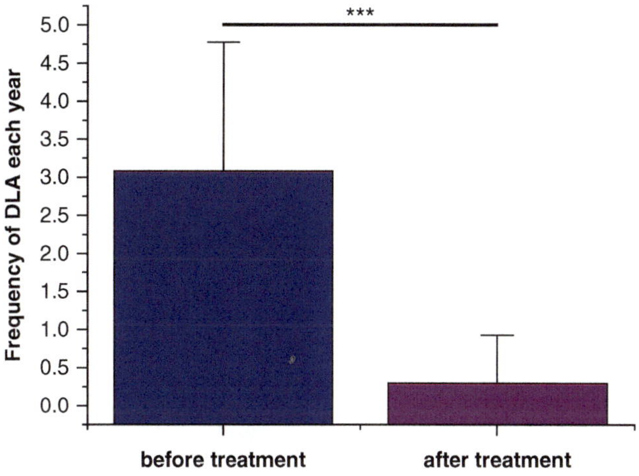

Fig. 25.4 The changes of frequency of DLA after treatment. In group 1 (HBT group) and group 2 (SBT group), the frequency of DLA reduced. The frequency of DLA in group 1 reduced significantly compared with the reduction in group 2.*$p < 0.05$; **$p < 0.01$; ***$p < 0.001$; HBT, heating and bandage treatment; SBT, single bandage treatment

gens in skin epidermal cells and fibroblasts have been reported after FIRT treatment [7]. Thus, FIRT reduces inflammation by improving and enhancing the immune function of local tissues through mechanisms that are not as yet fully understood.

A recent study investigating the biological effects of FIRT on promoting skin fibrosis has shown that FIRT treatment not only reduces extracellular water, but also reduces skin fibrosis, as evidenced by significant improvement in the elasticity of lymphedematous skin, obvious reduction in fiber and dense material [11] (Fig. 25.5), and a significant decrease in local tissue fluid concentrations of transforming growth factor-β1 and IL-18 (Table 25.1), both of which are cytokines that are responsible for tissue inflammation and fibrosis (Fig. 25.6).

A recent study on the oncological safety of FIRT in the treatment of cancer-related lymphedema demonstrated that there were no increase in tumor marker (CA153, CA125) concentrations after treatment with FIRT [12]. Furthermore, none of the treated patients were subsequently diagnosed with lymphadenectasis or newly enlarged lymph nodes. An in vitro experiment showed that FIRT does not affect the viability, proliferation, cell cycle, or apoptosis of fibroblasts, MCF-7, and MDA-MB-231 cells. Thus, FIRT should be considered feasible and safe for the treatment of breast cancer-related lymphedema more than 5 years after mastectomy and treatment of other malignant tumors. FIRT does not promote recurrence or metastasis of breast cancer (or other tumors) and is a well-tolerated therapy with no adverse reactions.

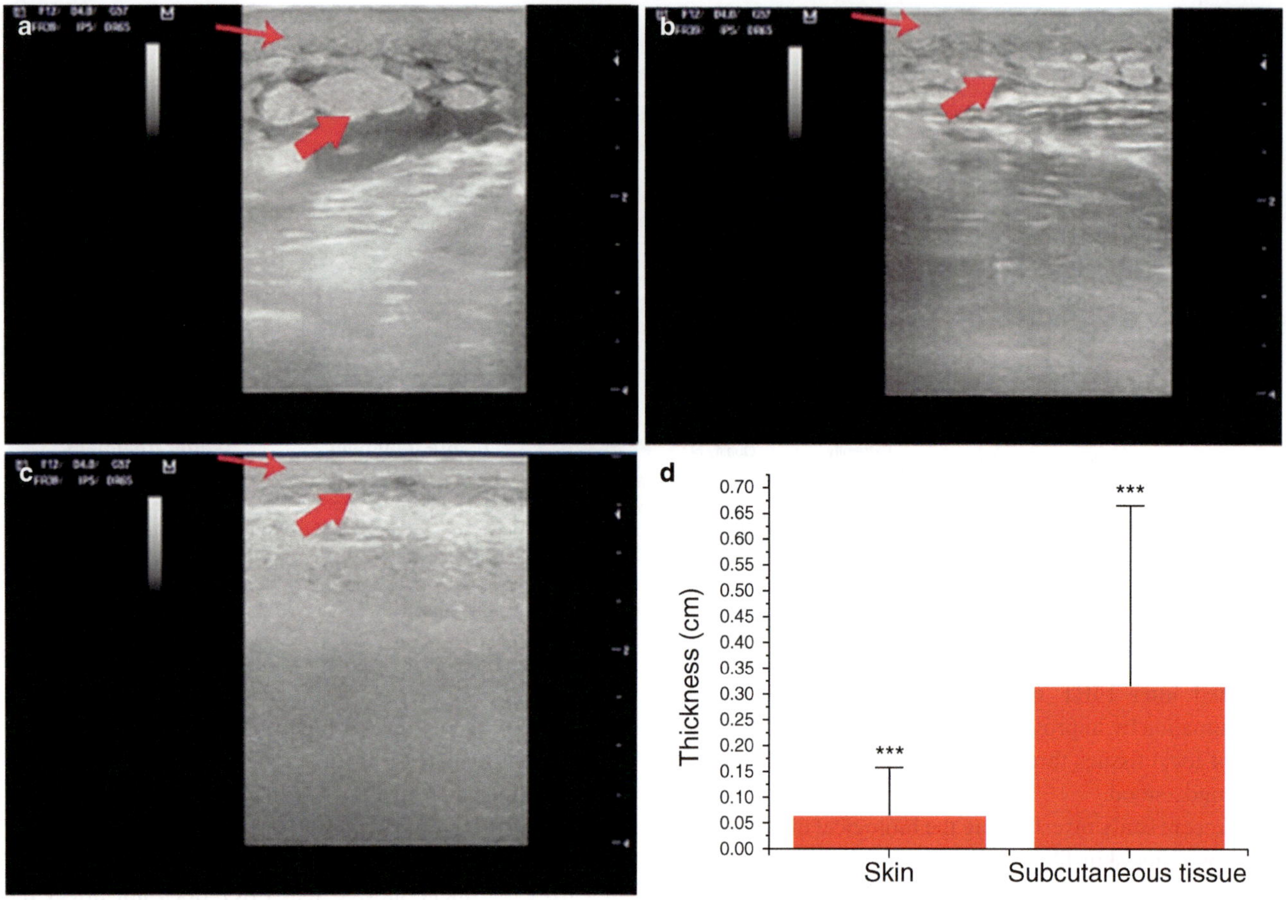

Fig. 25.5 The performance of ultrasound. The thickness of skin and subcutaneous tissue reduced after being treated by far-infrared radiation. At the same time, the scope of dark space reduced and the echogenic line became clearer. Small arrow, the layer of skin; large arrow, the layer of subcutaneous tissue. (**a**) The extremity with lymphedema before far-infrared radiation treatment. (**b**) The extremity with lymphedema after far-infrared radiation treatment. (**c**) The healthy extremity. (**d**) The change value of thickness of skin and subcutaneous tissue in extremity with lymphedema. ***$p < 0.001$

Table 25.1 The statistics on laboratory outcomes about fibrosis

Items	*p* (serum)	*p* (tissue fluid)
TGF-b1	Undetectable	0.041*
IL-1b	0.198	0.243
IL-4	0.256	0.498
IL-18	0.153	0.049*
Caspase-1	0.490	0.164

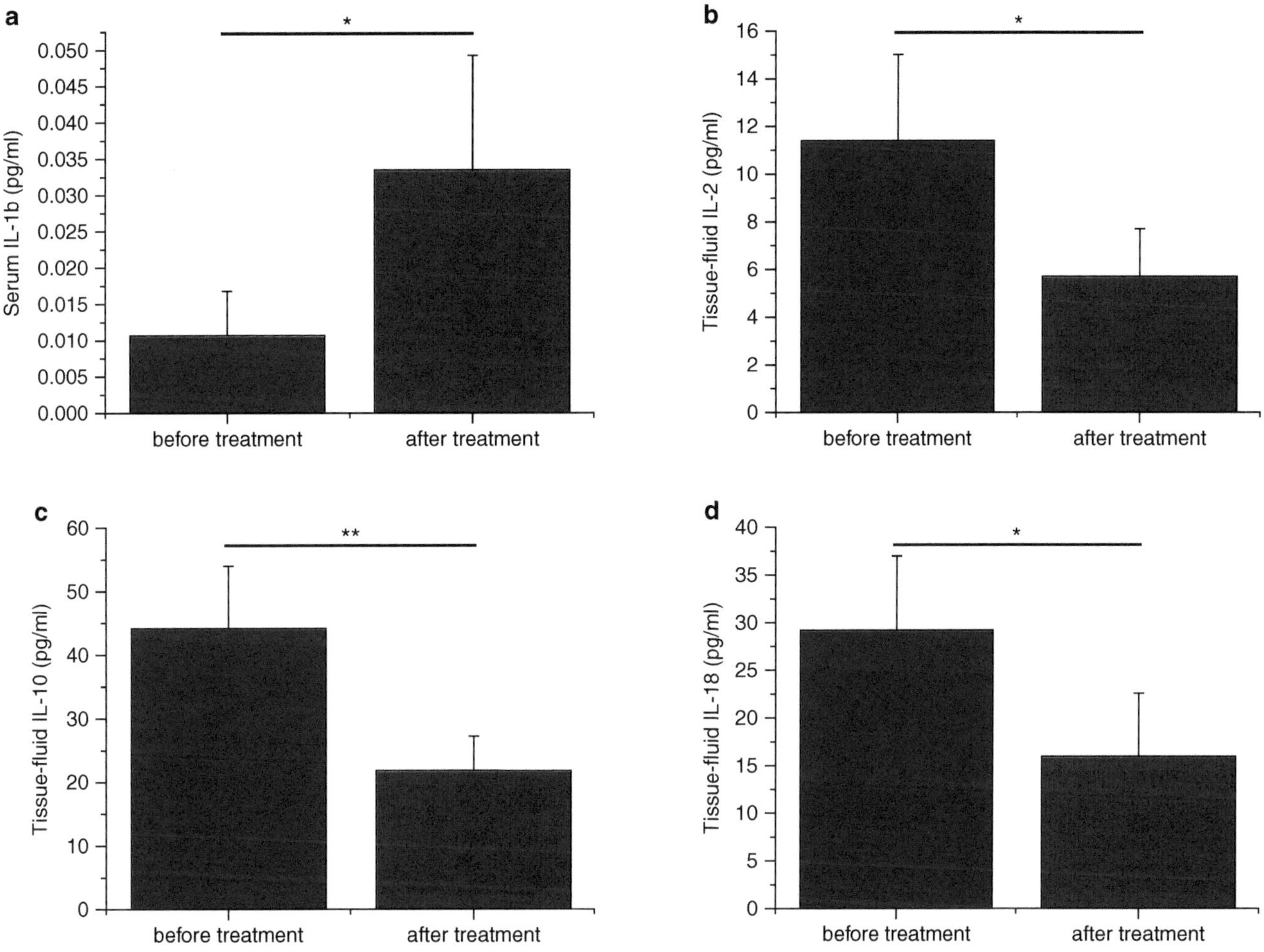

Fig. 25.6 Concentration of inflammatory factors in serum and tissue fluid. (**a**) The concentration of IL-1b in serum before and after treatment; (**b**) the concentration of IL-2 in tissue fluid before and after treatment; (**c**) the concentration of IL-10 in tissue fluid before and after treatment; (**d**) the concentration of IL-18 in tissue fluid before and after treatment. $*p < 0.05$; $**p < 0.01$

References

1. Zhang DS. Heating and bandaging treatment of chronic lymphedema: a 1045 cases report. Chin J Surg. 1985;23(1):13–6.
2. Chang CJ, Cormier JN. Lymphedema interventions: exercise, surgery and compression devices. Semin Oncol Nurs. 2013;29(1):28–40.
3. Zhou JG, Liu NF, Cao WG, Li SL. Effect of different compression materials on the heating and bandaging treatment of chronic lymphedema. Chin J Tissue Eng. 2009;5(4):229–30.
4. Chang TS, Han LY, Gan JL, Huang WY. Microwave: an alternative to electric heating in the treatment of peripheral lymphedema. Lymphology. 1989;22(1):20–4.
5. International Society of Lymphology. The diagnosis and treatment of peripheral lymphedema: 2013 consensus document of the international society of lymphology. Lymphology. 2013;46(1):1–11.
6. Leung TK. In vitro and in vivo studies of the biological effects of bioceramic (a material of emitting high performance far-infrared ray) irradiation. Chin J Physiol. 2015;58(3):147–55.
7. Liu NF, Olszewski W. The influence of local hyperthermia on lymphedema and lymphedematous skin of the human leg. Lymphology. 1993;26(1):28–37.
8. Yu SY, Chiu JH, Yang SD, Hsu YC, Lui WY, Wu CW. Biological effect of far-infrared therapy on increasing skin microcirculation in rats. Photodermatol Photoimmunol Photomed. 2006;22(2):78–86.
9. Li K, Xu H, Liu NF, Sadigh P, Evans V, Zhang YX. Far-infrared ray for treating chronic lower extremity lymphedema with dermatolymphangioadenitis: a postoperative complication of gynecological tumor resection. Arch Gynecol Obstet. 2017;295(6):1441–50. https://doi.org/10.1007/s00404-017-4371-3.
10. Li K, Liu N, Fu L. Therapeutic effect of heating and bandage treatment for chronic lymphedema of extremities accompanied with erysipelas: a report of 80 cases. Chin J Plast Surg. 2015;31(1):39–42.
11. Li K, Zhang Z, Liu NF, Sadigh P, Evans VJ, Zhou H, Gao W, Zhang YX. Far-infrared radiation thermotherapy improves tissue fibrosis in chronic extremity lymphedema. Lymphat Res Biol. 2018;16(3):248–57. https://doi.org/10.1089/lrb.2016.0057.
12. Li K, Zhang Z, Liu NF, Feng SQ, Tong Y, Zhang JF, Constantinides J, Lazzeri D, Grassetti L, Nicoli F, Zhang YX. Efficacy and safety of far infrared radiation in lymphedema treatment: clinical evaluation and laboratory analysis. Lasers Med Sci. 2017;32(3):485–94. https://doi.org/10.1007/s10103-016-2135-0.

Part VII

Treatment of Lymphedema: Surgical Treatment

Suction-Assisted Lipectomy with Simultaneous Skin Excision for Lymphedema - the "Flying Squirrel" Technique

26

Weifeng Zeng, Oksana Babchenko, and Wei F. Chen

Abstract

Liposuction is an effective bulk-reducing treatment for solid predominant extremity lymphedema. The skin excess created as a result of bulk removal is traditionally left behind due to theoretical wound healing concerns of immediate skin resection. The resulting skin excess is presumed to resolve by spontaneous skin contracture. Problems associated with this approach include contour irregularity, seroma, hematoma, and skin necrosis. Having experienced the above-mentioned complications, we modified the technique by excising excess skin immediately following liposuction. The senior author (WFC) reviewed his experience of immediate skin excision following liposuction for extremity lymphedema, and found it to be safe, associated with lower risks of postoperative complications, and resulting in a higher patient satisfaction. In this chapter, authors share their experience with this new approach. After reading this chapter, the reader will gain knowledge in patient selection, excess skin assessment, technical pearls of skin excision, and postoperative care for these complex patients.

Keywords

Lipectomy · Lymphedema · Liposuction · Skin excision
Extremity contour

W. Zeng · O. Babchenko
Division of Plastic and Reconstructive Surgery, Department of Surgery, University of Wisconsin-Madison, Madison, WI, USA

W. F. Chen (✉)
Center for Lymphedema Research and Reconstruction, Department of Plastic and Reconstructive Surgery, Cleveland Clinic, Cleveland, OH, USA

26.1 Introduction

Lymphedema has gone from being an untreatable condition to one that can now be surgically managed due to modern advancements in reconstructive microsurgery, supermicrosurgery, and optimization of debulking techniques [1–7]. The surgical techniques employed to treat lymphedema vary with the stage of lymphedema severity: early, fluid-predominant disease is amendable to physiologic reconstruction, while more severe, solid-predominant disease is amendable to bulk-reducing measures. Lymphedema was initially believed to be a condition of pathologic edema, however, the presence of the solid component of the disease with its characteristic features—such as subcutaneous fibrosis—distinguishes it from simple edema [8–10]. The solid disease component is only minimally present in early disease but becomes increasingly prominent as the pathology progresses. The solid disease component causes serious lymphedema-related morbidities in the intermediate to late stages of the disease [11, 12]. Physiologic reconstruction such as vascularized lymph node transfer (VLNT) and lymphaticovenular anastomosis (LVA) is ineffective in treating late stage, solid-predominant lymphedema [13]. Direct surgical debulking remains the only effective treatment for solid-predominant disease [14]. Debulking techniques include liposuction [15, 16], serial excision, [17], and the Charles procedure [18]. The Charles procedure is especially morbid and thus rarely utilized. In contrast, liposuction is particularly useful because of its technical simplicity and minimally invasive nature. Lymphedema liposuction is traditionally performed without concomitant skin excision despite the frequently large skin redundancy that results from liposuction debulking [13, 19]. Skin is traditionally not excised concurrently with liposuction due to theoretical wound healing and vascularity concerns. Instead, the large skin redundancy created following liposuction bulk reduction is presumed to resolve with spontaneous skin contracture [13, 19]. We performed simultaneous liposuction and skin excision in lymphedema patients and compared the outcome with that of the traditional technique, namely

N. Liu (ed.), *Peripheral Lymphedema*, https://doi.org/10.1007/978-981-16-3484-0_26

liposuction without skin excision. We found that concurrent skin excision after liposuction debulking is safe, associated with fewer complications, and results in higher patient satisfaction.

26.2 Concepts

Suction-assisted liposuction (SAL) for solid predominant lymphedema is traditionally performed without skin excision, but we have observed relatively high rates of complications with this practice, including contour irregularity, seroma and hematoma formation, and skin necrosis (Fig. 26.1). We attributed many of these complications to the skin redundancy created following SAL debulking. Mechanisms behind skin redundancy contributing to these complications may include formation of large dead spaces under redundant skin, which can promote seroma formation and contour irregularities, and skin folding onto itself when compression is applied, which can contribute to ischemia and skin necrosis (Fig. 26.2). We started excising excess skin immediately following SAL and saw substantial improvements in results, including reduction in complications, improvement of esthetic outcomes, and increased patient satisfaction. Our preference now is to perform immediate limb contouring by removing skin excess immediately after SAL (Fig. 26.3).

26.3 Patient Selection

It is important to accurately diagnose solid-predominant lymphedema and rule out conditions that can mimic this disease, such as lipedema and venous insufficiency. Patients should be screened for symptoms characteristically associated with lipedema such as painful lipodystrophy, easy bruising, distal parts (hands, feet) preservation, negative Stemmer sign, and only mild or normal lymphatic drainage seen on lymphatic imaging [20]. Venous color Doppler examination can be used to rule out patients with venous insufficiency. Imaging modalities, such as lymphoscintigraphy, indocyanine green lymphography, or magnetic resonance lymphangiography should be used to confirm the diagnosis of lymphedema [21–23]. In the senior author's practice, we prefer indocyanine green (ICG) lymphography as our study of choice for diagnosis and for tracking changes in lymphedema severity of our patients. The ICG lymphographic patterns visualize lymphatic flow and lymphatic dermal backflow, which are analogs for disease severity. In the ICG lymphography staging system, in stage 0 disease, no pathologic lymphatic pattern is seen. In stage I disease, a "splash" pattern is seen. In stages II–IV disease, a "stardust" pattern is seen, with a greater spread of the stardust pattern in more severe disease. In stage V disease, a "diffuse" pattern is seen (Fig. 26.4) [24].

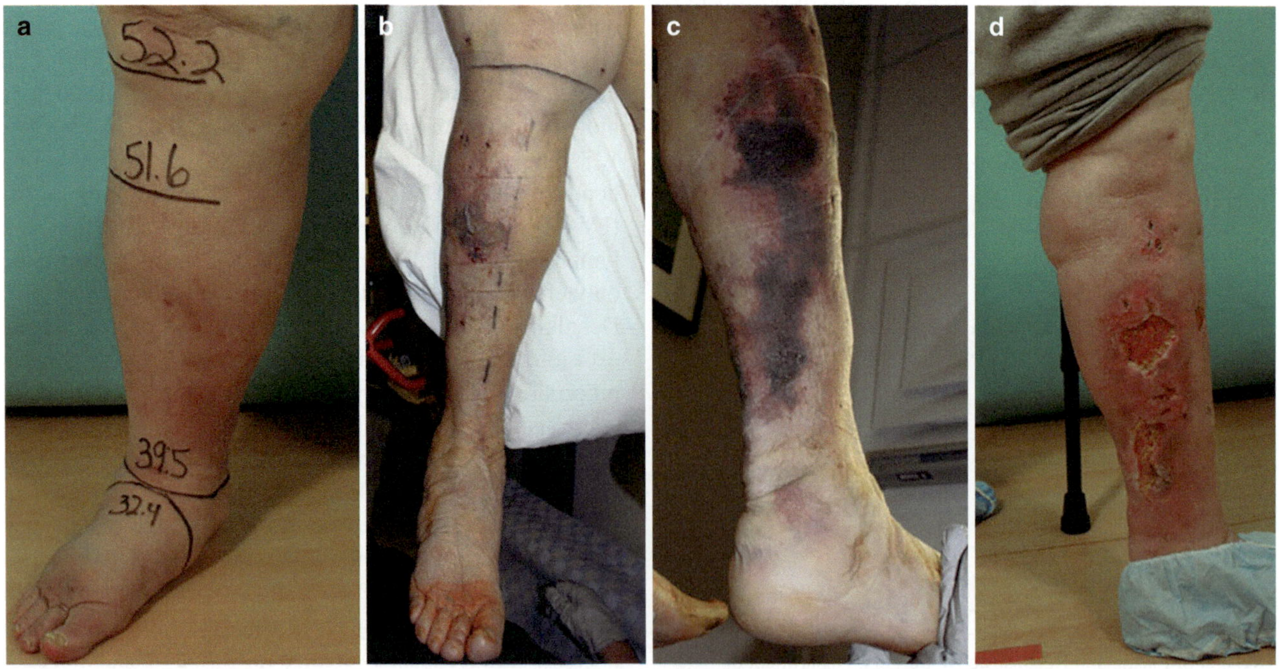

Fig. 26.1 (**a**) A patient who underwent SAL without skin excision. Contour irregularity and skin necrosis are seen (**b**, **c**). Skin ischemia became prominent on day 3 (**b**). One month postoperatively, skin necrosis and contour irregularity are seen (**c**). Several wounds developed due to skin necrosis (**d**). SAL, suction-assisted lipectomy (Chen WF, Zeng W-F, Hawkes PJ, Man J, Bowen M. Lymphedema Liposuction with Immediate Limb Contouring. Plastic and Reconstructive Surgery - Global Open. 2019 (reprinted with permission))

Patients with advanced lymphatic injury and solid-predominant limb lymphedema are suitable candidates for SAL debulking with concurrent skin excision. These patients typically have International Society of Lymphology (ISL) stage II and higher disease. The criteria for solid-predominant disease include (1) irreversible limb bulkiness, (2) limb bulkiness out of proportion to the volume suggested by quantitative bioimpedance spectroscopy (Fig. 26.5), and (3) magnetic resonance imaging (MRI) demonstrating abundant lipodystrophy [22].

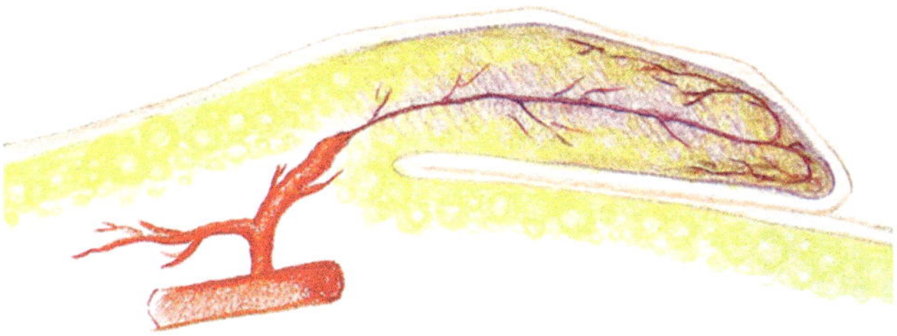

Fig. 26.2 The large amount of skin excess that results after SAL debulking is prone to folding onto itself, especially when compression bandages are applied, which contributes to ischemia and necrosis. SAL, suction-assisted lipectomy (Chen WF, Zeng W-F, Hawkes PJ, Man J, Bowen M. Lymphedema Liposuction with Immediate Limb Contouring. Plastic and Reconstructive Surgery - Global Open. 2019 (reprinted with permission))

26.4 Preoperative Preparation

A thorough patient history should be taken, with a focus on etiology, symptoms, functional impairment, disease progression, prior treatments, and response to prior treatments. Physical examination should begin with a visual inspection of the affected limb and the extent of limb swelling. It is important to note whether the swelling is fluid predominant, solid predominant, or a mixture of both. Early lymphedema is generally a fluid-predominant disease and on examination will present with pitting upon digital pressure. Late lymphedema is characterized by solid-predominant disease, lipodystrophy, fibrosis, and will not pit on examination.

Limb volumes should be measured. There are several ways to measure limb volumes: three-dimensional optoelectronic perometry, water displacement, and multilevel circumference measurements. The most commonly employed method is multilevel circumference measurements. It should

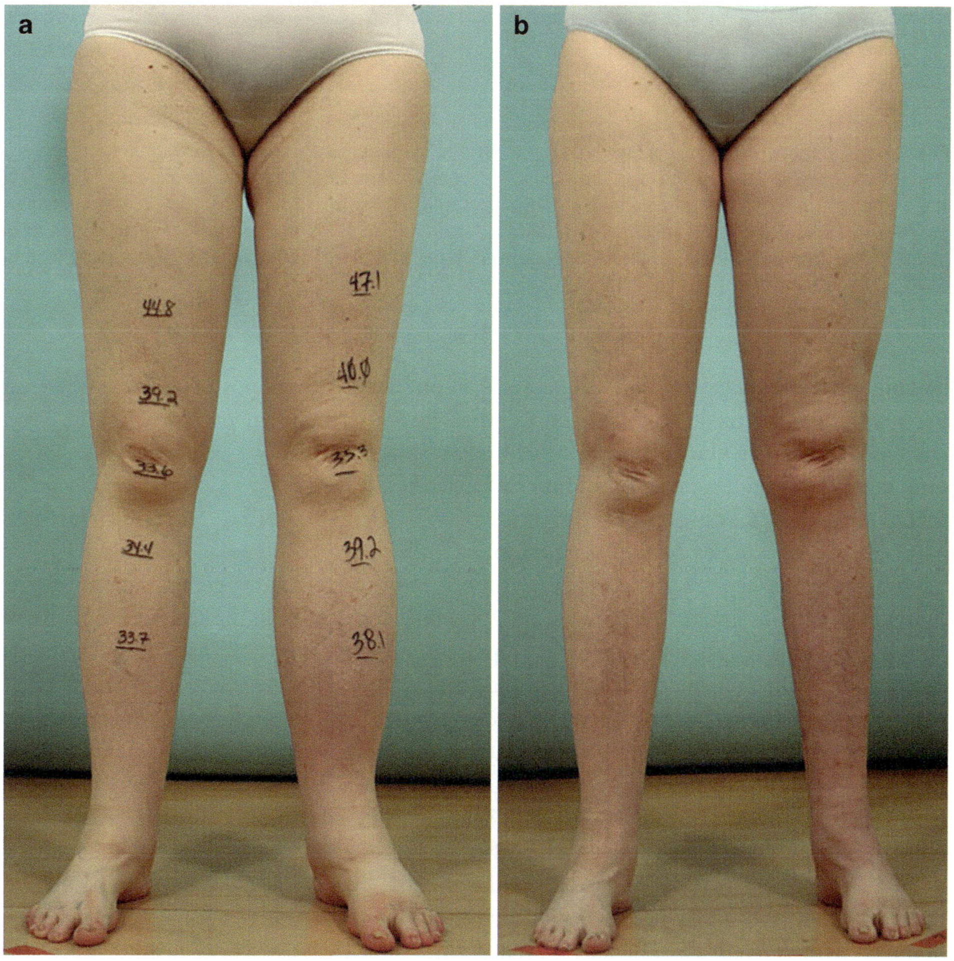

Fig. 26.3 A preoperative photo of a patient with left leg lymphedema (**a**). A 1-month postoperative photo after the patient underwent SAL with concurrent skin excision from the medial leg (**b**). Like the vast majority of these patients, her postoperative course was uneventful and no contour irregularity or ischemia was observed (Chen WF, Zeng W-F, Hawkes PJ, Man J, Bowen M. Lymphedema Liposuction with Immediate Limb Contouring. Plastic and Reconstructive Surgery - Global Open. 2019 (reprinted with permission))

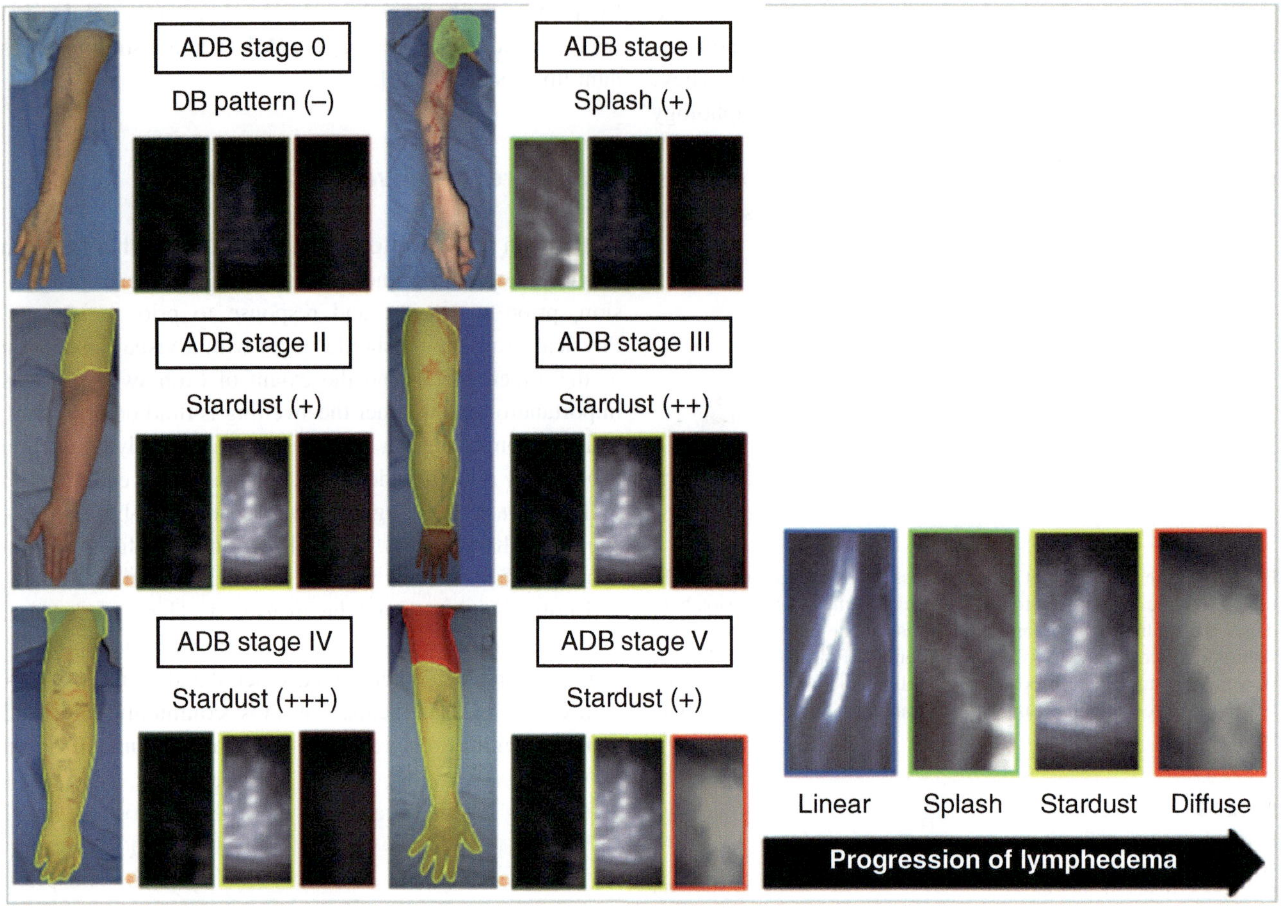

Fig. 26.4 Lymphographic staging system for the arm. In stage 0, no pathological pattern is seen. In stage I, a "splash" pattern is seen. In stage II, a "stardust" pattern is seen. In stage III, the "stardust" pattern progresses to the forearm. In stage IV, the "stardust" pattern encompasses the entire limb, including hand and forearm. In stage V, a "diffuse" pattern is seen. The lymphographic staging system for the leg (not pictured) is analogous to the system for the arm. ADB, arm dermal backflow (Yamamoto T, Iida T, Matsuda N, Kikuchi K, Yoshimatsu H, Mihara M, et al. Indocyanine green (ICG)-enhanced lymphography for evaluation of facial lymphoedema. J Plast Reconstr Aesthet Surg. 2011;64(11):1541–4 (reprinted with permission))

be noted that all volume-based measurements are influenced by a variety of extrinsic factors, such as weather, activity level, pressure garment use, and even time of day. Thus, volume measurements are inherently imprecise and should be thought of as rough estimates of the disease.

Confirmatory studies should be performed. ICG lymphography has shown to have a higher sensitivity and specificity than lymphoscintigraphy [13, 14, 25, 26]. In the senior author's practice, ICG lymphography has replaced lymphoscintigraphy as the imaging modality of choice for diagnosis, preoperative planning, and postoperative tracking.

A common practice is using the contralateral uninvolved limb as a template to preoperatively prepare compression garments prior to SAL [13, 14, 25, 26]. This is not feasible in patients with elevated body mass indexes (BMI), as liposuction of the lymphedematous limb results in the affected limb becoming smaller than the healthy limb (Fig. 26.6). We recommend using compression bandaging during the immediate postoperative period and transitioning to compression garments 4 weeks after surgery.

26.5 Surgical Techniques

Under general anesthesia, the circumferential affected limb is infiltrated with tumescent solution consisting of 1 mL of 1:1000 epinephrine mixed with 1 L of normal saline. The tumescent solution is instilled until a tight tissue turgor is appreciated. After waiting for 10 min for vasoconstriction to take effect, the limb is exsanguinated, a tourniquet is inflated, and SAL begins. We recommend utilizing power-assisted lipectomy to decrease operative time and reduce surgeon fatigue. The treatment area depends on whether the upper or lower extremity is being treated. For the upper extremity, the entire limb is debulked in a single procedure. For the lower extremity, however, the leg and thigh are sequentially deb-

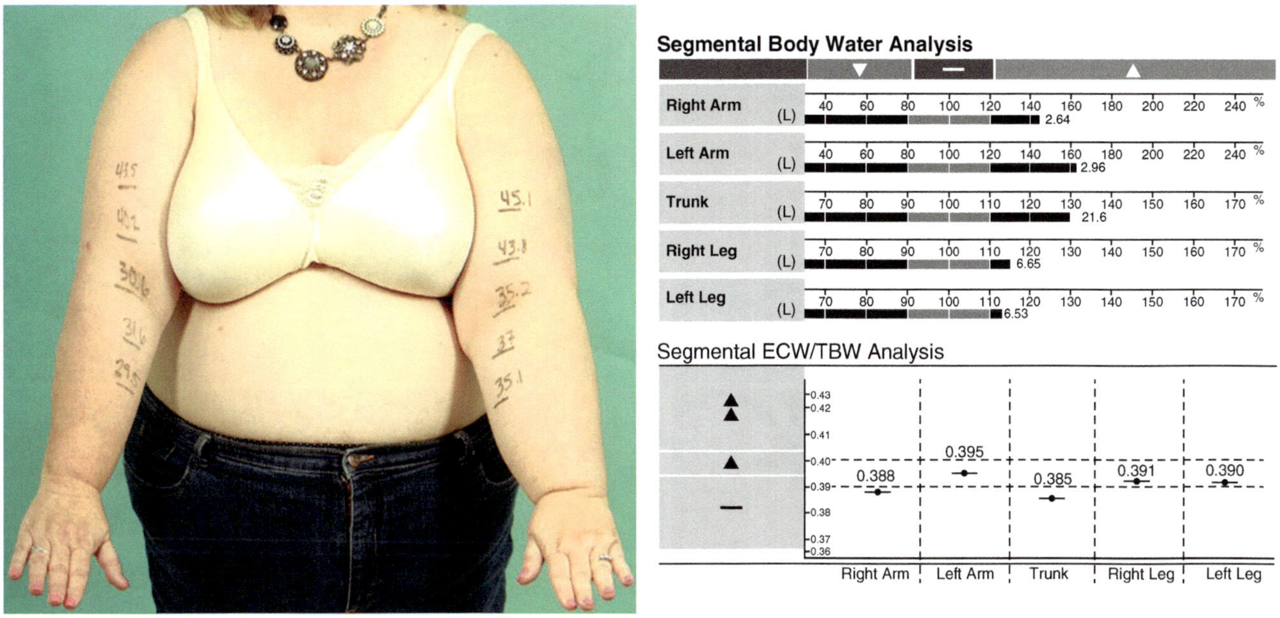

Fig. 26.5 BIS in this patient with left arm solid-predominant lymphedema showed a water discrepancy between her arms of only 0.32 L (2.96–2.64 L). This small amount of discrepancy does not explain the observed left arm bulk, confirming that her left arm lymphedema is solid predominant, not fluid predominant. BIS, bioimpedance spectroscopy (Chen WF, Zeng W-F, Hawkes PJ, Man J, Bowen M. Lymphedema Liposuction with Immediate Limb Contouring. Plastic and Reconstructive Surgery - Global Open. 2019 (reprinted with permission))

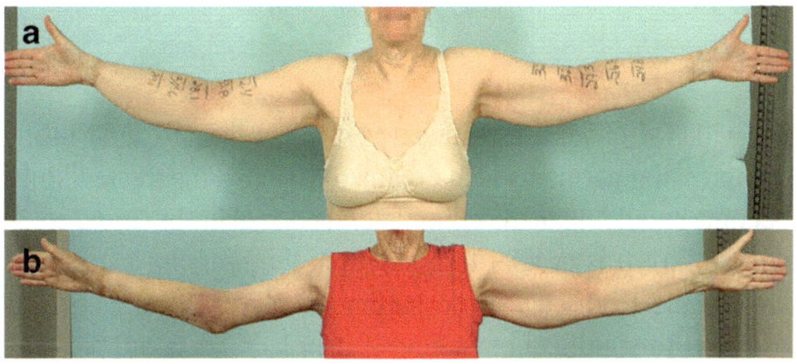

Fig. 26.6 A patient with right arm lymphedema preoperatively (**a**) and at 3 months postoperatively after SAL with immediate skin excision (**b**). As many patients have elevated BMIs, the treated lymphedematous limbs frequently become smaller than the contralateral healthy limbs after SAL with immediate skin excision. As such, the contralateral limb cannot serve as a template for preoperative pressure garment preparation. SAL, suction-assisted lipectomy; BMI, body mass index (Chen WF, Zeng W-F, Hawkes PJ, Man J, Bowen M. Lymphedema Liposuction with Immediate Limb Contouring. Plastic and Reconstructive Surgery - Global Open. 2019 (reprinted with permission))

ulked in separate procedures due to high liposuction volumes and for ease of recovery.

SAL is performed using 3–5 mm cannulae via 4–6 stab incisions. The endpoint of SAL is the achievement of a uniform subcutaneous tissue thickness of 0.5–1 cm, depending on the anatomic region. For example, more aggressive liposuction is performed to achieve a 0.5-cm thickness in naturally thinner subcutaneous regions, such as the pretibial area, whereas in naturally thicker subcutaneous regions, such as the thigh, a 1-cm thickness is used as the treatment endpoint. In order to optimize vascularity and preserve the dermal plexus, liposuction is performed in a deep to superficial plane. As the tourniquet obscures treatment of the most proximal portion of the limb, care must be taken to also debulk the concealed proximal region. To do this, once the limb distal to the tourniquet is fully treated, compression bandage is applied, and the tourniquet is released to allow treatment of the proximal segment, which was previously covered by the tourniquet.

Once liposuction is complete and desired subcutaneous thickness of 0.5–1 cm is reached, the degree of skin excess is assessed. Specifically, the ability to lift skin away from the deep fascia by 4 cm or more, as well as the undulating mobility of the skin excess, constitutes a positive "flying squirrel" sign (FSS) [27]. A positive FSS is an indication for excess skin removal, as leaving such an excessive amount of skin behind may cause increased risks of seroma, hematoma, contour deformity, difficulty with postoperative compression, and skin necrosis. Removing the large skin excess improves limb contour and decreases risks of all the aforementioned complications. The use of the 4-cm threshold as indication for skin excision was empirically derived. We nicknamed this sign "flying squirrel" due to the post-liposuction appearance of the limb with skin excess resembling this animal in flight. The skin excess is evaluated with the "double ellipse" technique [28] and is removed with a tailor-tack approach.

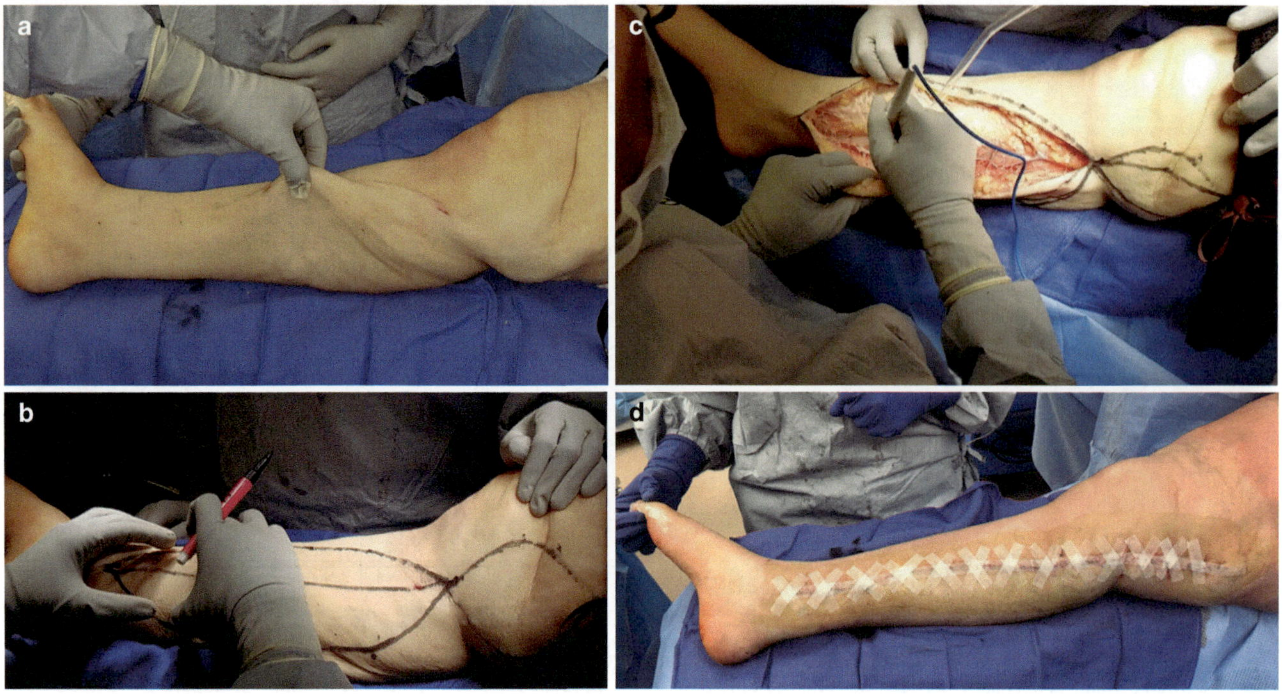

Fig. 26.7 After removal of 3300 mL of lipoaspirate from this patient's right leg, substantial skin excess is present (**a**). The amount of skin that can be safely excised is determined by a pinch test (**b**). As the skin flap has already been undermined by liposuction, skin excision is fast and simple (**c**). Immediate postoperative results following SAL with concomitant skin excision (**d**). SAL, suction-assisted lipectomy (Jones G., et al. Bostwick's Plastic and Reconstructive Breast Surgery. Thieme NY. 2019. Copyright holder, www.thieme.com (reprinted with permission))

The long axis of the excised skin is along the posterior/ulnar aspect of the arm and ulnar aspect of the forearm. In the lower extremity, the long axis of the excision is placed along the medial aspect of the leg and thigh (Fig. 26.7). No drains are used. Immediately following completion of surgery, compression with stretch bandages is applied.

26.6 Postoperative Care

After SAL, patients are admitted for 1–3 days for pain management. On postoperative day 1, therapy visits the patients to teach them proper bandaging techniques. Compression bandages are used for 4 weeks following surgery until edema subsides, and then 30–40 mmHg compression garments are used indefinitely. Patients are instructed to keep the treated limb elevated and only engage in light use for 4 weeks. Patients are seen at 1 week, 4 weeks, 3 months, 6 months, and 12 months following surgery, and then they are seen annually.

26.7 Expected Outcomes

The most notable changes in the volume of the affected extremity will happen in the first 4 weeks, as surgical edema subsides. After surgical edema fully resolves, the volume of the extremity will not change significantly if adherence to well-fitting compression garments is maintained. Usually, the treated limbs become smaller than the contralateral normal limbs (Figs. 26.3b and 26.7b). It is crucial to assure that the pressure garment is well-fitting to the latest measurements, as ill-fitting garments can lead to significant swelling if they lack adequate pressure or to extreme pain if they exert too much pressure.

26.8 Eligibility for Lymphatic Reconstruction with LVA or VLVT

Following lymphedema liposuction, all patients became eligible for physiologic lymphatic reconstruction with either vascularized lymph vessel transfer (VLVT) or lymphaticovenular anastomosis (LVA) in the senior author's practice [29, 30]. This is termed hybrid reconstruction. VLVT or LVA is only offered to those who are not confident in lifelong adherence to compression therapy. The choice of which physiologic reconstruction is most suitable for which patient, specifically VLVT versus LVA, depends on the degree of lymphatic regeneration following liposuction, as observed on postoperative ICG lymphography. LVA is only offered to those with the most rigorous lymphatic regeneration. Lymphatic regeneration can be seen 6 months after liposuction on ICG lymphography (Fig. 26.8) [30].

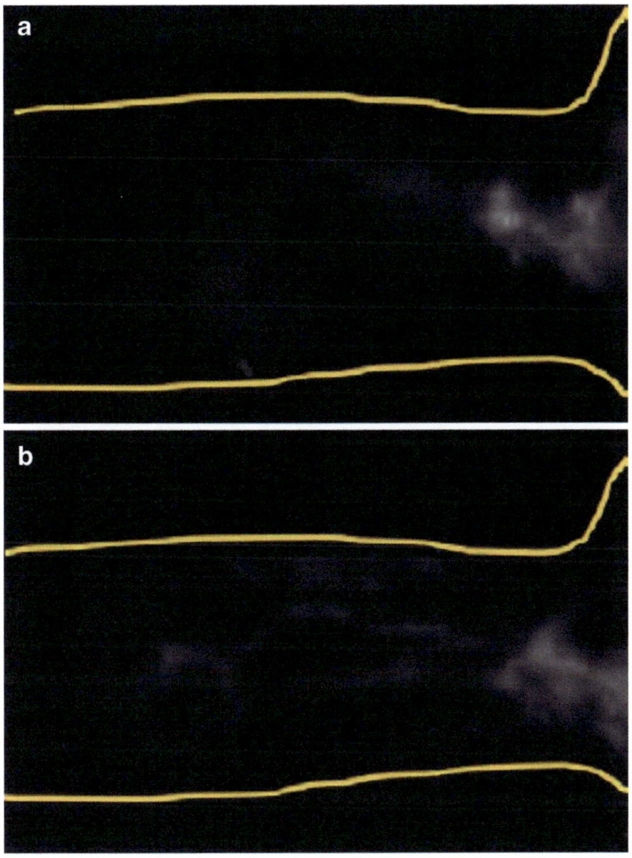

Fig. 26.8 An ICG lymphography of a preoperative, distal leg prior to undergoing SAL with skin excision. The peripheral outline of the leg is marked with yellow lines. Dermal backflow is evident, signifying lymphatic vessel dysfunction (**a**). ICG lymphography of a postoperative, distal leg, 6 months after SAL with skin excision. Although the pathologic dermal backflow pattern persists, there is also evidence of lymphangiogenesis, as demonstrated by the new linear lymphatic patterns of the mid-leg (**b**) [30]

26.9 Summary

Skin excision following liposuction for solid predominant lymphedema is safe, decreases postoperative complications, and improves surgical outcomes.

References

1. Koshima I, Inagawa K, Etoh K, Moriguchi T. [Supramicrosurgical lymphaticovenular anastomosis for the treatment of lymphedema in the extremities]. Nihon Geka Gakkai Zasshi. 1999;100(9):551–6.
2. Chang DW, Suami H, Skoracki R. A prospective analysis of 100 consecutive lymphovenous bypass cases for treatment of extremity lymphedema. Plast Reconstr Surg. 2013;132(5):1305–14.
3. Mardonado AA, Chen R, Chang DW. The use of supraclavicular free flap with vascularized lymph node transfer for treatment of lymphedema: A prospective study of 100 consecutive cases. J Surg Oncol. 2017;115(1):68–71.
4. Chen WF. How to get started performing supermicrosurgical lymphaticovenular anastomosis to treat lymphedema. Ann Plast Surg. 2018;81(6S Suppl 1):S15–20.
5. Koshima I, Narushima M, Mihara M, Yamamoto T, Hara H, Ohshima A, et al. Lymphadiposal flaps and lymphaticovenular anastomoses for severe leg edema: functional reconstruction for lymph drainage system. J Reconstr Microsurg. 2016;32(1):50–5.
6. Cheng MH, Huang JJ, Nguyen DH, Saint-Cyr M, Zenn MR, Tan BK, et al. A novel approach to the treatment of lower extremity lymphedema by transferring a vascularized submental lymph node flap to the ankle. Gynecol Oncol. 2012;126(1):93–8.
7. Lin CH, Ali R, Chen SC, Wallace C, Chang YC, Chen HC, et al. Vascularized groin lymph node transfer using the wrist as a recipient site for management of postmastectomy upper extremity lymphedema. Plast Reconstr Surg. 2009;123(4):1265–75.
8. Granzow JW. Lymphedema surgery: the current state of the art. Clin Exp Metastasis. 2018;35(5-6):553–8.
9. Greene AK, Goss JA. Diagnosis and staging of lymphedema. Semin Plast Surg. 2018;32(1):12–6.
10. Brorson H, Ohlin K, Olsson G, Nilsson M. Adipose tissue dominates chronic arm lymphedema following breast cancer: an analysis using volume rendered CT images. Lymphat Res Biol. 2006;4(4):199–210.
11. Rockson SG. Lymphedema. Vasc Med. 2016;21(1):77–81.
12. Grada AA, Phillips TJ. Lymphedema: Pathophysiology and clinical manifestations. J Am Acad Dermatol. 2017;77(6):1009–20.
13. Schaverien MV, Munnoch DA, Brorson H. Liposuction treatment of lymphedema. Semin Plast Surg. 2018;32(1):42–7.
14. Brorson H. Adipose tissue in lymphedema: the ignorance of adipose tissue in lymphedema. Lymphology. 2004;37(4):175–7.
15. Damstra RJ, Voesten HG, Klinkert P, Brorson H. Circumferential suction-assisted lipectomy for lymphoedema after surgery for breast cancer. Br J Surg. 2009;96(8):859–64.
16. Lamprou DA, Voesten HG, Damstra RJ, Wikkeling OR. Circumferential suction-assisted lipectomy in the treatment of primary and secondary end-stage lymphoedema of the leg. Br J Surg. 2017;104(1):84–9.
17. Salgado CJ, Mardini S, Spanio S, Tang WR, Sassu P, Chen HC. Radical reduction of lymphedema with preservation of perforators. Ann Plast Surg. 2007;59(2):173–9.
18. Dumanian GA, Futrell JW. The Charles procedure: misquoted and misunderstood since 1950. Plast Reconstr Surg. 1996;98(7):1258–63.
19. Hoffner M, Ohlin K, Svensson B, Manjer J, Hansson E, Troeng T, et al. Liposuction gives complete reduction of arm lymphedema following breast cancer treatment—a 5-year prospective study in 105 patients without recurrence. Plast Reconstr Surg Glob Open. 2018;6(8):e1912.
20. Wollina U. Lipedema—an update. Dermatol Ther. 2018;e12805.
21. Pecking AP, Alberini JL, Wartski M, Edeline V, Cluzan RV. Relationship between lymphoscintigraphy and clinical findings in lower limb lymphedema (LO): toward a comprehensive staging. Lymphology. 2008;41(1):1–10.
22. Trinh L, Peterson P, Brorson H, Mansson S. Assessment of subfascial muscle/water and fat accumulation in lymphedema patients using magnetic resonance imaging. Lymphat Res Biol. 2019;17(3):340–6.
23. Mihara M, Hara H, Araki J, Kikuchi K, Narushima M, Yamamoto T, et al. Indocyanine green (ICG) lymphography is superior to lymphoscintigraphy for diagnostic imaging of early lymphedema of the upper limbs. PLoS One. 2012;7(6):e38182.
24. Yamamoto T, Yamamoto N, Doi K, Oshima A, Yoshimatsu H, Todokoro T, et al. Indocyanine green-enhanced lymphography for upper extremity lymphedema: a novel severity staging system using dermal backflow patterns. Plast Reconstr Surg. 2011;128(4):941–7.
25. Yamamoto T, Iida T, Matsuda N, Kikuchi K, Yoshimatsu H, Mihara M, et al. Indocyanine green (ICG)-enhanced lymphography for

evaluation of facial lymphoedema. J Plast Reconstr Aesthet Surg. 2011;64(11):1541–4.
26. Mihara M, Hara H, Narushima M, Todokoro T, Iida T, Ohtsu H, et al. Indocyanine green lymphography is superior to lymphoscintigraphy in imaging diagnosis of secondary lymphedema of the lower limbs. J Vasc Surg Venous Lymphat Disord. 2013;1(2):194–201.
27. Chen WF, Zeng W-F, Hawkes PJ, Man J, Bowen M. Lymphedema liposuction with immediate limb contouring. Plast Reconstr Surg Glob Open. 2019;7(11):e2513.
28. Aly A, Pace D, Cram A. Brachioplasty in the patient with massive weight loss. Aesthet Surg J. 2006;26(1):76–84.
29. Chen WF, Bowen M, McNurlen M, Ding J. Vascularized lymph vessel transfer with supermicrosurgical ultra-thin superficial circumflex iliac artery flap for treatment of advanced lymphedema not treatable with supermicrosurgical lymphaticovenular anastomosis. Ann Plast Surg. 2018;80(supp 3):1.
30. Chen WF. Is it possible to perform lymphaticovenular after liposuction for lymphedema? J Surg. 2016;12(4):2.

Microsurgery: Vascularized Lymph Vessel Transfer

27

Weifeng Zeng, Oksana Babchenko, and Wei F. Chen

Abstract

Lymphaticovenular anastomosis (LVA) and vascularized lymph node transfer (VLNT) are the main established reconstructive treatments for fluid-predominant lymphedema. Both, however, have limitations. LVA is most effective for early disease with preserved functionality of lymphatic vessels, and VLNT carries a risk of donor site lymphedema as well as contour deformity. Vascularized lymph vessel transfer (VLVT) is a novel technique that can be utilized in more advanced, fluid-predominant lymphedema, does not have the risk of donor site lymphedema, and does not have associated contour deformity. In this chapter, the senior author (WFC) describes this novel technique, including patient selection, surgical planning, surgical technique, surgical outcomes, and postoperative care. After reading this chapter, the reader should gain both clinical and technical knowledge to begin incorporating VLVT into their lymphedema practice.

Keywords

Lymphedema · Vascularized lymph vessel transfer
Supermicrosurgery · Indocyanine green lymphography
Vascularized lymph node transfer

W. Zeng · O. Babchenko
Division of Plastic and Reconstructive Surgery, Department of Surgery, University of Wisconsin-Madison, Madison, WI, USA

W. F. Chen (✉)
Center for Lymphedema Research and Reconstruction, Department of Plastic and Reconstructive Surgery, Cleveland Clinic, Cleveland, OH, USA

27.1 Introduction

Surgical treatment of lymphedema is broadly divided into two approaches: debulking procedures for more severe, solid-predominant disease, such as liposuction [1, 2] and the Charles procedure [3], and physiologic reconstructive procedures for less severe, fluid-predominant disease. The two physiologic reconstructive procedures that are currently most utilized for fluid-predominant disease are vascularized lymph node transfer (VLNT) [4, 5] and lymphaticovenular anastomosis (LVA) [6, 7]. Generally, LVA is the preferred method for reconstruction in less advanced diseases. Specifically, LVA is the preferred method when lymphatic vessel functionality is still preserved, as is confirmed by indocyanine green (ICG) lymphography exhibiting healthy, linear lymphatic vessel patterns. Please see Chapter 28 for further technical details of LVA. In contrast, VLNT is performed in more advanced diseases. Specifically, VLNT is performed when lymphatic vessels are showing signs of dysfunction, as exhibited by stardust or diffuse ICG lymphography patterns.

During VLNT, the surgeon harvests lymph nodes from an unaffected part of the body on a dominant vascular supply and re-vascularizes them at the affected limb. The mechanism of action behind VLNT is not well understood and thought to be due to drainage of the edematous limb via direct nodal "pumping" mechanisms [8–10] and lymphangiogenesis [8, 11, 12]. Originally described in the 1980s, VLNT was traditionally based on the superficial circumflex iliac vessels and nodes. No serious complications were initially described and outcomes were favorable [8, 13–16]. However, in 2013, donor site lymphedema was first reported in a patient's leg following nodal harvest from the groin of that leg [17, 18]. Due to the recognized risk of donor site lymphedema in the lower extremity with groin node harvest, exploration of other, less vulnerable anatomical regions for lymph node harvest was initiated. Currently, other utilized lymph node harvest sites include submental [19–21], supraclavicular [5, 22, 23], lateral thoracic [12, 24–26], and most

N. Liu (ed.), *Peripheral Lymphedema*, https://doi.org/10.1007/978-981-16-3484-0_27

recently, omental [27–29], and jejunal mesenteric [30] lymph node basins. While LVA does not have the risk of donor site lymphedema, it is most effective in patients with early disease with more preserved lymphatic vessel functionality, and thus cannot substitute for VLNT.

Koshima et al. unveiled a new reconstructive technique for fluid-predominant lymphedema that parallels VLNT in patient selection criteria (i.e., patients can have advanced, fluid-predominant lymphedema with evidence of lymphatic vessel damage on ICG lymphography), likely mechanism of action, and outcomes [31]. Koshima et al. proposed transferring not lymph nodes themselves but rather healthy lymphatic vessels to the affected limb. This technique, called vascularized lymph vessel transfer (VLVT), was originally described based on the first dorsal metatarsal artery for patients with advanced lymphedema; outcomes were very favorable [31]. The flap is transferred as a free flap with only vascular anastomoses performed; no lymphatico-lymphatic anastomoses are done. The mechanism of action is thought to be similar to that of VLNT, specifically the peristaltic, pumping mechanism of healthy lymphatic vessels that mediates the therapeutic effect [9]. Benefits of VLVT over VLNT are an absence of donor site lymphedema risk and a much thinner, more esthetically inconspicuous flap at the recipient site that lacks the usual tissue bulk associated with VLNT flaps.

27.2 Patient Selection

Surgical intervention is offered when patients fail complex decongestive therapy (CDT). To be eligible for physiologic reconstructive procedures for lymphedema, specifically LVA, VLNT, or VLVT, patients should have fluid-predominant disease. If a patient has solid-predominant disease, debulking surgery—such as suction-assisted lipectomy (SAL)—is more suitable. Fluid predominant states can be confirmed by clinical examination and imaging modalities. On clinical examination, the presence of prominent pitting with manual pressure suggests fluid-predominant lymphedema, as solid predominant, fibrous lymphedema will not pit. Bioimpedance spectroscopy (BIS) and magnetic resonance imaging (MRI) can confirm a fluid-predominant state. In fluid-predominate disease, BIS will show significant limb fluid excess and MRI will show limb fluid with minimal lipodystrophy and minimal fibrosis.

To decide which reconstructive procedures to perform, lymphatic vessel functionality should be assessed with ICG lymphography. In ICG lymphography a nonradioactive contrast agent is injected peripherally and taken up by the lymphatic system. The contrast agent, fluorophore, fluoresces when optically excited at 800 nm. The visual patterns that emerge visualize lymphatic flow and lymphatic dermal backflow in the extremity, which are analogs for disease severity [32]. In progression from normal lymphatic function to severe disease, the lymphographic patterns are "linear," "splash," "stardust," and "diffuse." For patients with early disease who have preserved lymphatic vessel function, as indicated by "linear" lymphographic patterns, LVA should be offered. For patients with evidence of lymphatic vessel dysfunction and injury, such as absence of "linear" and/or presence of "diffuse" lymphographic patterns, VLVT or VLNT can be offered. As this chapter focuses on VLVT, we will not elaborate on VLNT, except in how it compares to VLVT. To summarize, the inclusion criteria for VLVT are fluid-predominant disease and advanced lymphatic injury. The exclusion criteria for VLVT are solid-predominant disease, which should be treated with debulking procedures, and early lymphatic injury, which should be treated with LVA.

Interestingly, after aggressive lymphedema liposuction, even patients with advanced, solid-predominant disease can become eligible for physiologic lymphatic reconstruction, specifically VLVT or LVA [33]. This is termed hybrid reconstruction and is offered only to patients who are not confident in lifelong adherence to compression therapy. The choice of which physiologic reconstruction is most suitable, specifically VLVT versus LVA, depends on the degree of lymphatic regeneration following liposuction. LVA is only offered to those with the most rigorous lymphatic regeneration on ICG lymphography, while VLVT can be offered to all others [33].

27.3 Preoperative Preparation

A thorough history and physical examination should be performed. The history should focus on etiology, symptoms, functional impairment, rate of disease progression, prior treatments, and response to prior treatments. The following questions should be answered: is the lymphedema primary or secondary? When did symptoms first start? How quickly is the disease progressing? When deciding on a treatment plan, it is important to understand the speed of disease progression. Those with rapid disease progression are preferentially considered for surgery, for delaying surgery in them could result in their rapidly progressing disease becoming too advanced for some or all of the reconstructive surgical options. Interestingly, disease duration does not always correlate with disease severity. For example, patients with severe lymphatic injury (e.g., iatrogenic surgical causes) may have only recent disease development, while patients with years of symptomatic disease may have only mild lymphatic injury.

Physical examination should focus on whether the disease is fluid predominant, solid predominant, or a mixture of both. The degree of swelling should be noted. The surgeon should evaluate skin and tissue quality. Most importantly, the surgeon should examine whether the lymphedematous extremity pits with digital pressure. Fluid-predominant lymphedema will pit with digital pressure, while solid-predominant lymphedema has lipodystrophy and fibrosis and thus will not pit with digital pressure. Imaging modalities, such as BIS and MRI, can also be utilized to confirm fluid predominance.

Limb volumes should be measured. There are many ways to estimate limb volumes, however, all volume-based measurements have flaws and can be influenced by extrinsic factors (e.g., activity level, pressure garment use, and even time of day). Thus, volume measurements are inherently imprecise and should be thought of as only rough estimates of the disease. Methods of volume measurements include direct measurements: three-dimensional (3D) optoelectronic perometry and water displacement, and indirect measurements: multilevel circumference measurements.

Some conditions, such as lipedema and venous insufficiency, can mimic lymphedema. Prior to surgical intervention, confirmatory studies should be done for both diagnosis and surgical planning. We recommend performing ICG lymphography, as it has been shown to have a more precise spatial resolution, higher sensitivity, and higher specificity than lymphoscintigraphy [34–36]. The degree of lymphatic dysfunction will guide the surgeon toward different treatment options. Specifically, if lymphatic vessel function is largely preserved, as evidenced by linear ICG lymphographic patterns, LVA should be offered. Conversely, if lymphatic function is severely compromised, as evidenced by diffuse ICG lymphographic patterns, VLVT can be offered.

VLVT is a free flap procedure. However because the pedicle is frequently very small (<0.8 mm), supermicrosurgical techniques are often required. Once a patient is selected for VLVT, a computed tomography angiography (CTA) scan is done to assess the superficial circumflex iliac vascular perforator anatomy. For upper extremity disease, the donor side is selected based on the more robust vascular anatomy, while for lower extremity disease—the contralateral groin is selected. For bilateral lower extremity disease, a superthin thoracodorsal artery perforator (TDAP) flap is used.

27.4 Surgical Technique

Instead of using the lymphatic vessels at the first dorsal metatarsal space as Koshima et al. described [31], we use the superficial circumflex iliac artery perforator (SCIP) flap due to its more favorable donor site and abundant lymphatic vessels. At the start of the procedure, lymphatic vessels should be visualized, vascular perforators should be identified, and the flap should be designed strategically over the perforators and lymphatic vessels. To visualize the lymphatic vessels, ICG lymphography is used: four 0.05 mL intradermal injections of 0.25% ICG solution are injected laterally to the anterior superior iliac spine (ASIS). The vascular perforators are then identified with Doppler ultrasound. The SCIP flap is designed with dimensions of ~10 × 6 cm over the perforators and lymphatic vessels (Fig. 27.1). A pinch test is done to assure the donor site can be closed primarily.

The inferior skin incision is made first and a depth of 3–5 mm is attained to include subcutaneous fat and superficial lymphatic vessels. In thin patients and those of average BMI, the dissection plane is just superficial to Scarpa's fascia. In obese patients, the dissection is along a nonanatomic plane to maintain a flap thickness of 3–5 mm and far superficial to Scarpa's fascia. Scarpa's fascia is not violated to assure that groin lymph nodes remain undisturbed, as the lymph nodes are deep to Scarpa's fascia. Scarpa's fascia is identified as a thin, fibrous plane between the superficial and deep fat layers. This plane is especially prominent laterally, adjacent to the ASIS. The fat layers can be distinguished based on their fat characteristics: superficial fat globules are smaller and more densely packed, while deeper fat globules are larger. This dissection can be done under ICG lymphographic guidance (Fig. 27.2) to assure that lymph nodes are not inadvertently taken. Lateral-to-medial, cephalad-directed dissection is performed until the superficial branch perforator and the superficial circumflex iliac vein of the superficial circumflex iliac system are identified (Figs. 27.3 and 27.4).

Once the perforator is identified as entering the flap, the superior skin incision is made. Pedicle length is increased by retrograde pedicle dissection. Lymph vessel presence in the SCIP flap can be confirmed by scanning the undersurface of

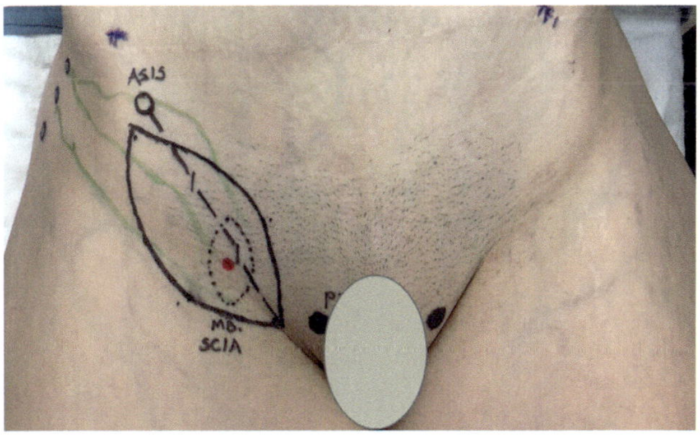

Fig. 27.1 The lymphatic vessels are visualized with ICG lymphography via intradermal injection of 0.25% ICG lateral to the ASIS, and their location is marked on the skin (green lines). SCIA perforator is identified with Doppler along a line extending from the groin crease to ASIS, and its location is marked on the skin (red dot). The SCIP-based VLVT flap is designed in approximately 10 × 6 cm dimensions to encompass the perforator and lymphatic vessels; the width is dictated by a pinch test to assure primary closure. ICG, indocyanine green; SCIA, superficial circumflex iliac artery; ASIS, anterior superior iliac spine; SCIP, superficial circumflex iliac artery perforator; VLVT, vascularized lymph vessel transfer [39]

the flap with Spy ELITE (Kalamazoo, Michigan) (Fig. 27.2). Recipient vessels are dissected and readied for anastomosis. For upper extremity lymphedema, the radial artery serves as the recipient site just proximal to the wrist. For lower extremity lymphedema, the posterior tibial artery is the recipient, just above the medial malleolus. Perforator-to-perforator anastomosis is preformed when the anatomy allows, and if no recipient perforators are identified, an end-to-side anastomosis is performed for the arteries due to a size mismatch. The flap's vein, the superficial circumflex iliac vein, is usually sizable and can be anastomosed end-to-end to the recipient vein (Fig. 27.5). Suture size is dictated by vessel size: for vessels <0.5 mm a 12-0 nylon is used and for vessels 0.5–0.8 mm an 11-0 nylon is used. No lymphaticovenular or lymphatico-lymphatic anastomoses are done; only vascular anastomoses are performed. For ease of flap inset, a full-thickness skin excision is performed, equal in shape and size to the flap dimensions (Fig. 27.6). The direction of lymphatic flow in the VLVT flap should align with the lymphatic flow orientation of the recipient site, to maximize spontaneous lymphatico-lymphatic anastomoses [37]. The donor site is primarily closed.

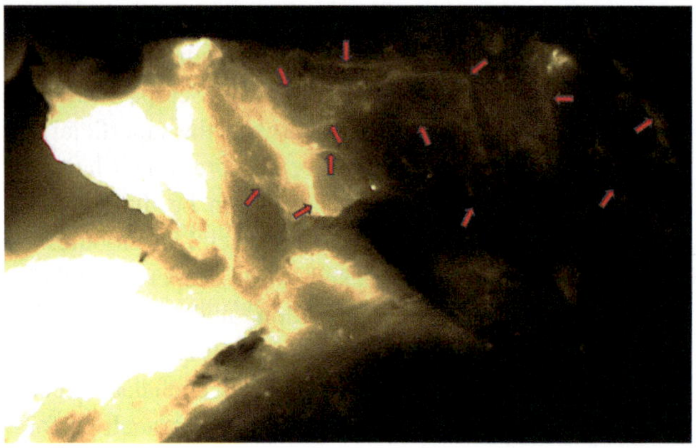

Fig. 27.2 Abundant lymphatic vessels are seen in the SCIP-based VLVT flap (red arrows), as captured by this image of the underside (adiposal side) of the flap. The ICG injection sites are the bright areas on the left. Lymph nodes are not visible in the flap; they are not at risk of being included if Scarpa's fascia is not violated. SCIP, superficial circumflex iliac artery perforator; VLVT, vascularized lymph vessel transfer; ICG, indocyanine green [39]

27.5 Postoperative Care

Flap monitoring is done over the first 4 postoperative days, and patients are discharged home on postoperative days 4–5. The affected extremity is elevated for 1 week. Compression bandages of the extremity are initiated on the 2nd postoperative week. For lower extremity lymphedema patients, ambulation is initiated on the 2nd postoperative week. Complex decongestive therapy (CDT) and newly fitted compression garments (30–40 mmHg) are resumed on the 4th postoperative week. Initially, compression garments are worn for 16 hours a day. Compression garment weaning can be initiated 6 months after surgery, with close supervision from the patients' therapists. If recurrence of extremity swelling is seen during the weaning process, garments should continue to be worn and another weaning process can be initiated at 12 months from surgery.

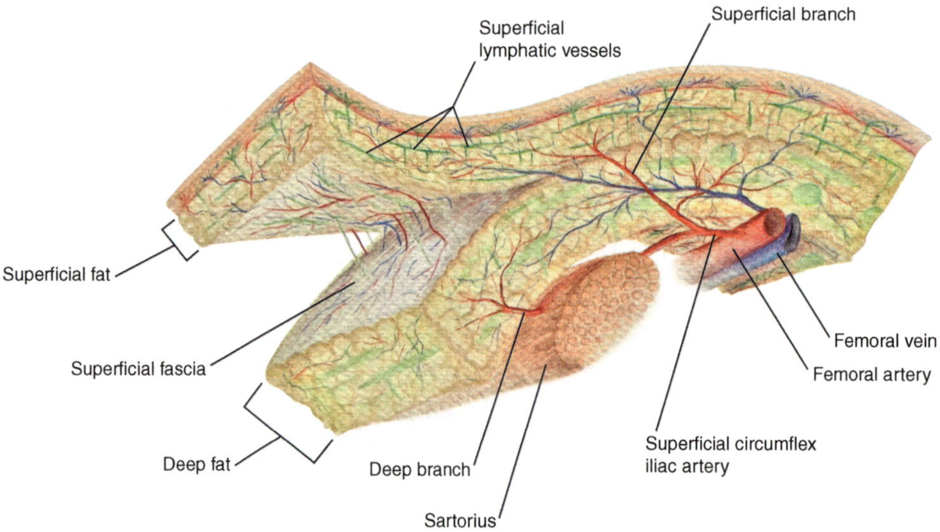

Fig. 27.3 In thin patients and those of average BMI, the SCIP-based VLVT flap is harvested immediately superficial to Scarpa's fascia, keeping the lymph nodes undisturbed as they are just deep to Scarpa's fascia. In obese patients, harvesting the flap immediately superficial to Scarpa's fascia would result in a thick flap and thus the flap is harvested along a nonanatomic plane 3–5 mm under the dermis. In all patients, the SCIP-based VLVT flap should be a thin (3–5 mm) flap, which allows for easy inset and esthetic discreetness. BMI, body mass index; SCIP, superficial circumflex iliac artery perforator; VLVT, vascularized lymph vessel transfer [39]

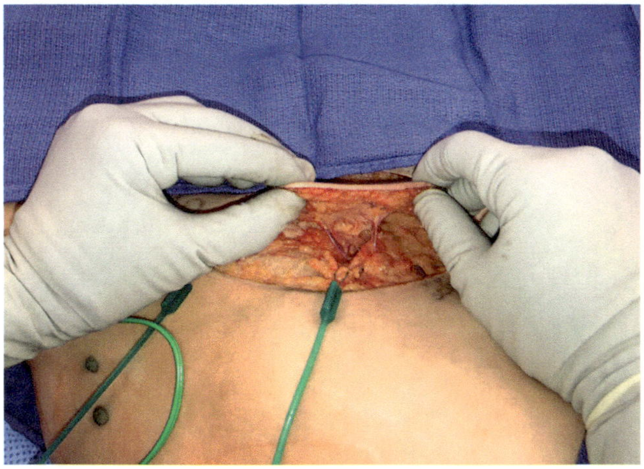

Fig. 27.4 SCIP-based VLVT flap is seen; the superficial circumflex iliac artery superficial branch perforator is on the right and the superficial circumflex iliac vein is on the left. Maintaining a thin (3–5 mm) SCIP-based VLVT flap allows inclusion of subdermal lymphatic vessels while minimizing tissue bulk. The thin flap allows for easy inset at the recipient site and relatively low metabolic demand, which allows it to survive on the small perforator. Furthermore, the thin flap assures that there is no contour deformity at the recipient site, which is an unfavorable result frequently seen in vascularized lymph node transfer. SCIP, superficial circumflex iliac artery perforator; VLVT, vascularized lymph vessel transfer [39]

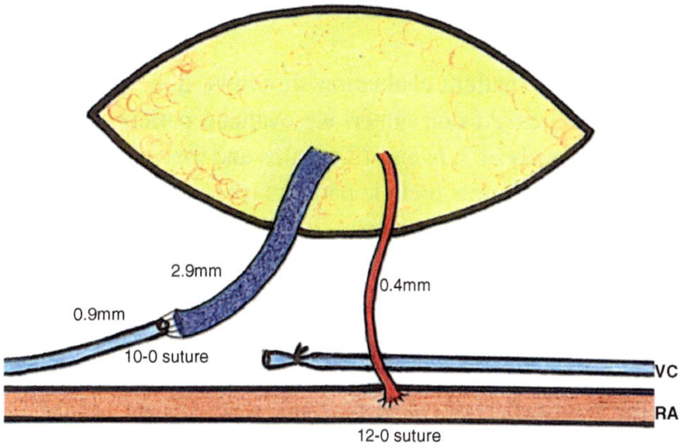

Fig. 27.5 Schematic depicting an example of an anastomotic configuration of the SCIP-based VLVT flap to an upper extremity recipient site. The arterial pedicle perfusing the flap is frequently small (in this case 0.4 mm) especially if it is not dissected to its origin and thus often requires supermicrosurgical anastomosis (<0.8 mm). It is usually anastomosed end-to-side to the recipient vessel, or end-to-end to a recipient perforator. A 12-0 suture is used for vessels <0.05 mm and an 11-0 suture is used for vessels 0.5–0.8 mm. Despite the pedicle's small size, we found it sufficient to perfuse the thin flap. The venous pedicle of the flap is usually large (in this case 2.9 mm) and can be anastomosed end-to-end to the recipient's vessels. The venous pedicle is smaller when the vena comitans is used instead of the superficial circumflex iliac vein. A 10-0 suture is typically used for the vein. SCIP, superficial circumflex iliac artery perforator; VLVT, vascularized lymph vessel transfer; RA, radial artery; VC, vena comitans [39]

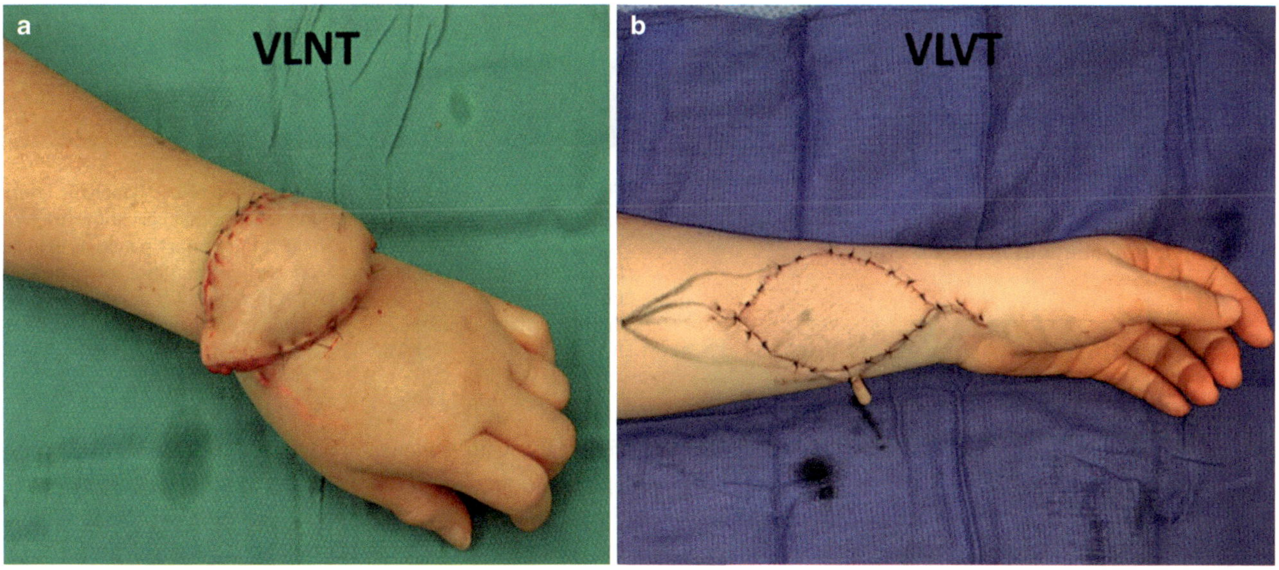

Fig. 27.6 Postoperative appearance of VLNT and VLVT. Contour deformity is a frequent occurrence in VLNT due to the bulkiness of the flap. In the current example, the flap inset was not fully completed due to venous congestion that resulted from full inset (**a**). The VLVT flap is thin (3–5 mm), and its inset (**b**) maintains the recipient site's esthetic contour [39]

27.6 Expected Outcomes

Postoperative patient evaluation should be done with multiple modalities. At our center, we evaluate patients pre- and postoperatively at 3, 6, and 12 months and then annually. Our evaluation measures include patient reports, physical examination, standardized circumference measurements, and ICG lymphography. For the upper extremity, circumference measurements are performed at the elbow crease and two levels above and below the elbow crease, at 5 cm intervals. For the lower extremity, circumference measurements are performed at the popliteal crease and two levels above and below the popliteal crease, at 10 cm intervals. For each measured extremity there is a total of five circumference measurements. ICG lymphography is performed using a standard technique as previously described [38]. Patients are asked about extremity pain, stiffness, subjective weight, garment use, and activity/exercise tolerance.

Despite the small pedicle of SCIP-based VLVT flaps, we have found that flap survival is excellent. There have been infrequent instances of partial (<5% of flap area) flap loss, which were managed with wound care. The majority of patients begin to experience edema reduction and relief of symptoms—such as decreased pain, paresthesias, stiffness, and improved range of motion—within 1–3 weeks after surgery [39]. Compression garment use can be decreased in about half the patients at 6 or at 12 months postoperatively, though full discontinuations of garment wear are often not attained. Virtually all patients demonstrate continued improvements at 1 year, including improved ICG lymphography patterns (Figs. 27.7 and 27.8) and statistically significant reduction in circumference measurements (Figs. 27.9 and 27.10). No patient has developed donor site lymphedema, either clinically or when the donor leg was screened with ICG lymphography postoperatively (Fig. 27.11). Patient satisfaction has been near unanimous in our experience.

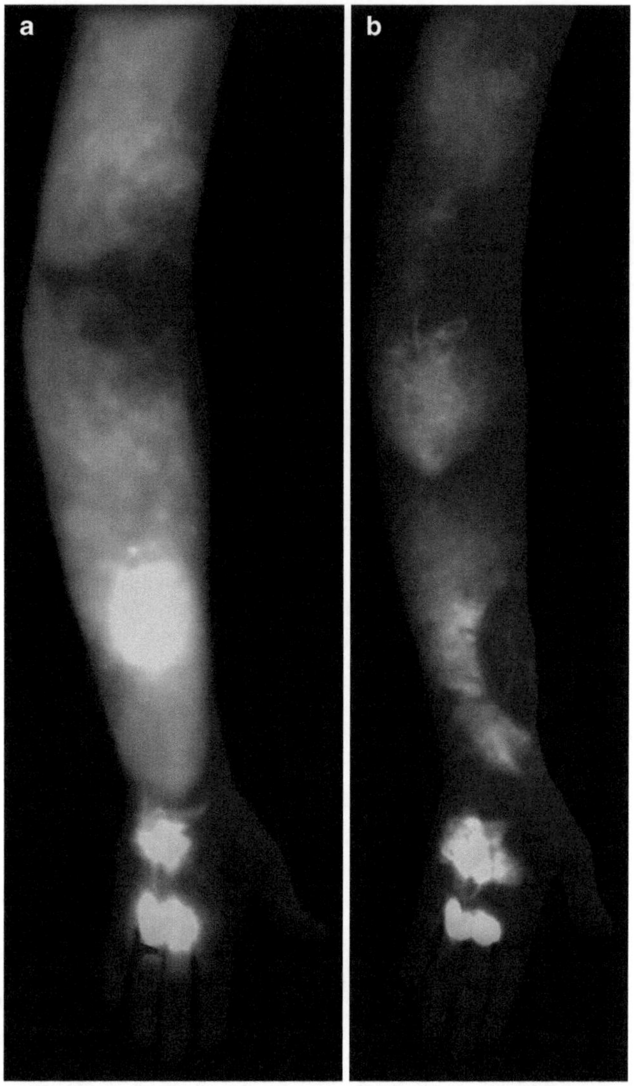

Fig. 27.7 ICG lymphography demonstrates a diffuse lymphatic injury pattern seen preoperatively, signifying severe dermal backflow (**a**). One year postoperatively, a reduction in the diffuse injury pattern is evident throughout the arm, indicating decreased extravasation of lymphatic fluid. Linear lymphatic patterns are seen in the VLVT flap, signifying the formation of spontaneous lymphatico-lymphatic anastomosis (**b**). ICG, indocyanine green; VLVT, vascularized lymph vessel transfer [39]

27.7 Transfer of Lymph Vessels Versus Lymph Nodes

Vascularized lymph node transfer is generally considered the procedure of choice for advanced, fluid-predominant lymphedema [40–45]. The main drawback of VLNT is the small but real risk of donor site lymphedema [17, 18, 46–49], which is a devastating, dreaded complication for both the patient and the surgeon. Recently, some have proposed using intraabdominal lymph nodes to eliminate the risk of donor site lymphedema. However, intraabdominal lymph node harvesting exposes patients to complications associated with abdominal surgery [30, 49].

Our group has previously offered VLNT for patients with fluid-predominant disease who were not LVA candidates (i.e., those with evidence of advanced lymphatic vessel damage). Although we did not observe donor-site lymphedema, the possibility of it remained prominent in the minds of both the patients and the surgeons, causing apprehension for both. Some patients declined surgery altogether after learning of the potential risk of donor-site lymphedema. While the surgical outcomes of VLNT were favorable in lymphedema improvement, patients frequently complained about the bulky contour deformity that the flaps caused (Fig. 27.6). Due to these drawbacks of VLNT, namely the risk of donor site lymphedema and flap bulkiness causing contour deformity, we began to seek alternatives.

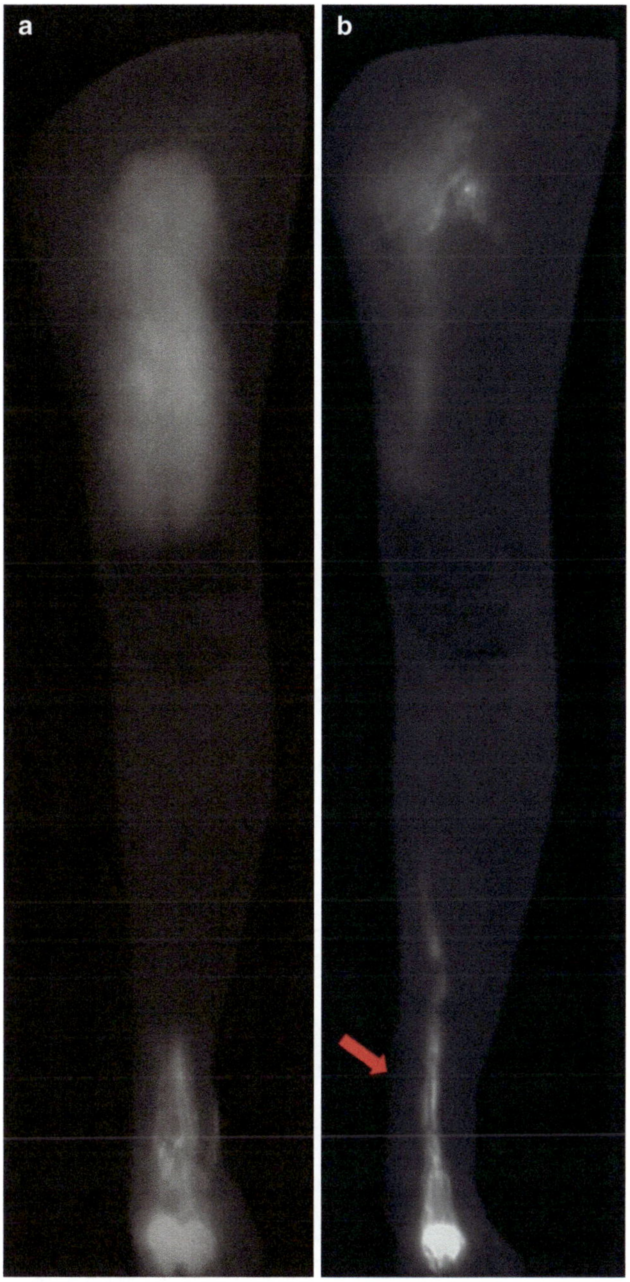

Fig. 27.8 ICG lymphography demonstrates a diffuse lymphatic injury pattern visible in the thigh, and a linear pattern in the foot (**a**). One year postoperatively, a reduction in the diffuse injury pattern is evident in the thigh, signifying decreased extravasation of lymphatic fluid. The healthy, linear lymphatic pattern in the foot now extends further proximally up the leg (**b**). The flap location is indicated by the red arrow; its lymphatic vessels are not visible due to their belonging to a different lymphosome than those draining the injection sites [39]

Koshima et al. introduced a new concept in the surgical treatment of lymphedema: transfer of healthy lymphatic vessels to lymphedema affected extremities. The lymphatic vessel transfer was based on the first dorsal metatarsal artery (FDMA) and their team reported favorable outcomes with this technique [31]. Their team hypothesized that the mechanism of action behind the surgery's success is in the peristaltic, pumping actions of the functional lymphatic vessels. They hypothesized these healthy, smooth muscle-lined lymphatic vessels transport lymphatic fluid into the venous system. Our group also had favorable outcomes with FDMA-based VLVT, consistent with Koshima et al. However, we encountered frequent donor site wound breakdown (Fig. 27.12). Seeking an alternative donor site, we investigated the SCIP-based VLVT, which proved favorable both in lymphedema improvement and in elimination of donor site complications [39]. We believe SCIP is a superior donor site to FDMA because it has a higher lymph vessel density, is familiar anatomy for plastic surgeons, and has a record of safety as shown by Hong et al. among others [48, 50–55]. The FDMA-based VLVT was effective in about 80% of patients from those who had previously failed LVA [31]. As the SCIP-based VLVT has a higher lymphatic vessel density, it may deliver higher therapeutic efficacy; this has been true in our experience [39].

The mechanism of action behind VLVT remains uncertain at this time, as does the mechanism behind VLNT. Preliminary evidence suggests that VLNT mediates its therapeutic effects via nodal pump mechanisms and lymphangiogenesis [9, 11, 12]. Pump mechanisms and lymphangiogenesis may also mediate the therapeutic effects of VLVT. VLVT transfers healthy, peristaltic lymph vessels lined with functional smooth muscles [31], and thus lymphatic fluid transport via pumping mechanism is likely present in VLVT. Furthermore, on postoperative ICG lymphography studies, lymphatic vessels within the VLVT flap are enhanced, indicating spontaneous formation of lymphatico-lymphatic anastomosis (LLA) (Fig. 27.7b). This is not surprising, given that spontaneous LLA has been previously reported following traditional free tissue transfer [37]. Spontaneous LLA, like angiogenesis, occurs organically during tissue healing [37].

There is another possibility of a therapeutic mechanism behind VLNT that warrants consideration and further study. Since transferring lymphatic vessels alone treats lymphedema [31, 39, 56], could the therapeutic potential of VLNT be in the inclusion of nearby lymphatic vessels into the flap and not in the inclusion of the lymph nodes themselves? Several pieces of evidence point to this possibility.

1. A generally accepted hypothesis of the mechanism behind VLNT is in the "pump" function of the lymph node. However, anatomical studies confirm that lymph nodes do not contain smooth muscle, which is necessary for contractile pumping. There is a minimal amount of smooth muscle in the small arteries and veins inside the lymph nodes, but none in the lymph node parenchyma itself [57].

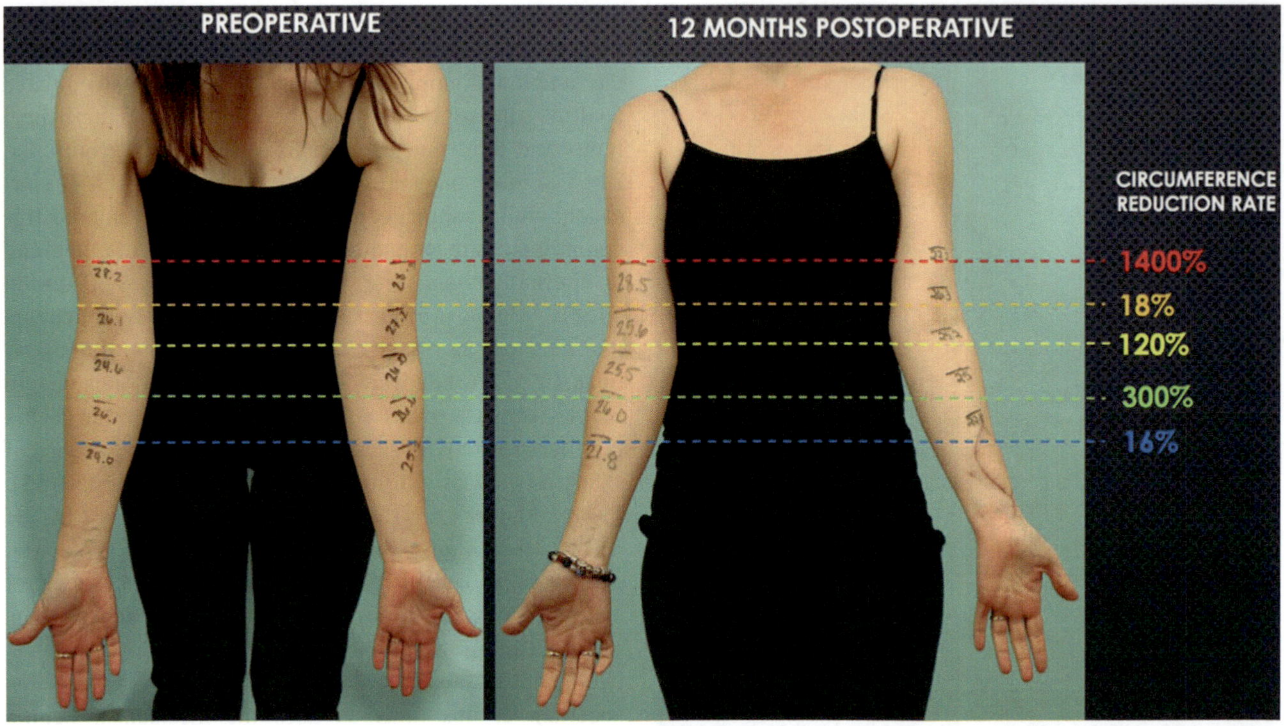

Fig. 27.9 The patient's left arm demonstrates a reduction in circumference when comparing preoperative (**a**) to 1-year postoperative (**b**) measurements. The percentage of circumference reduction varies with arm levels. Interestingly, the uppermost measurements tend to exhibit the greatest amount of reduction, despite being the furthest from the VLVT flap. Circumference reduction rate = $[(a - b) - (c - d)] / (c - d)$, where a = postoperative affected arm, b = postoperative healthy arm, c = preoperative affected arm, d = preoperative healthy arm [39]

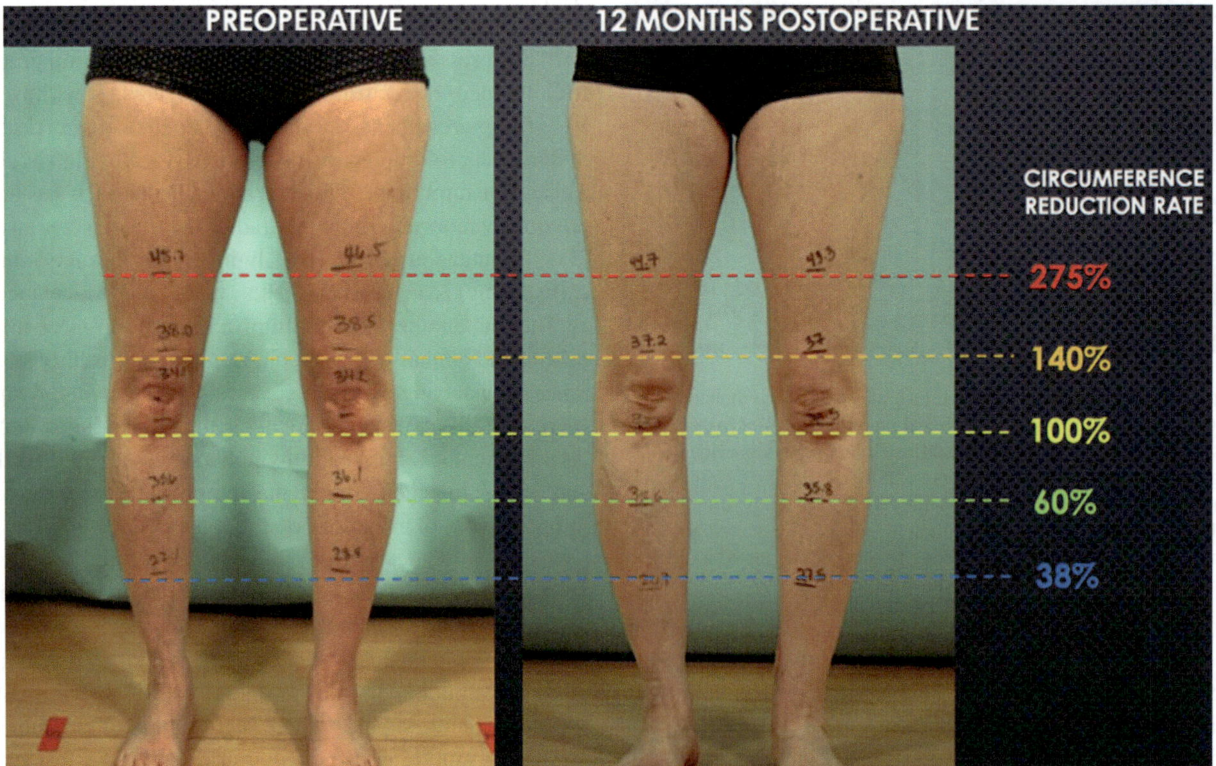

Fig. 27.10 The patient's left leg demonstrates a reduction in circumference when comparing preoperative (**a**) to 1-year postoperative (**b**) measurements. The percentage of circumference reduction varies with leg levels, as in the arm. Again, the uppermost measurements tend to exhibit the greatest amount of reduction, despite being the furthest from the VLVT flap. Circumference reduction rate = $[(a - b) - (c - d)] / (c - d)$, where a = postoperative affected leg, b = postoperative healthy leg, c = preoperative affected leg, d = preoperative healthy leg [39]

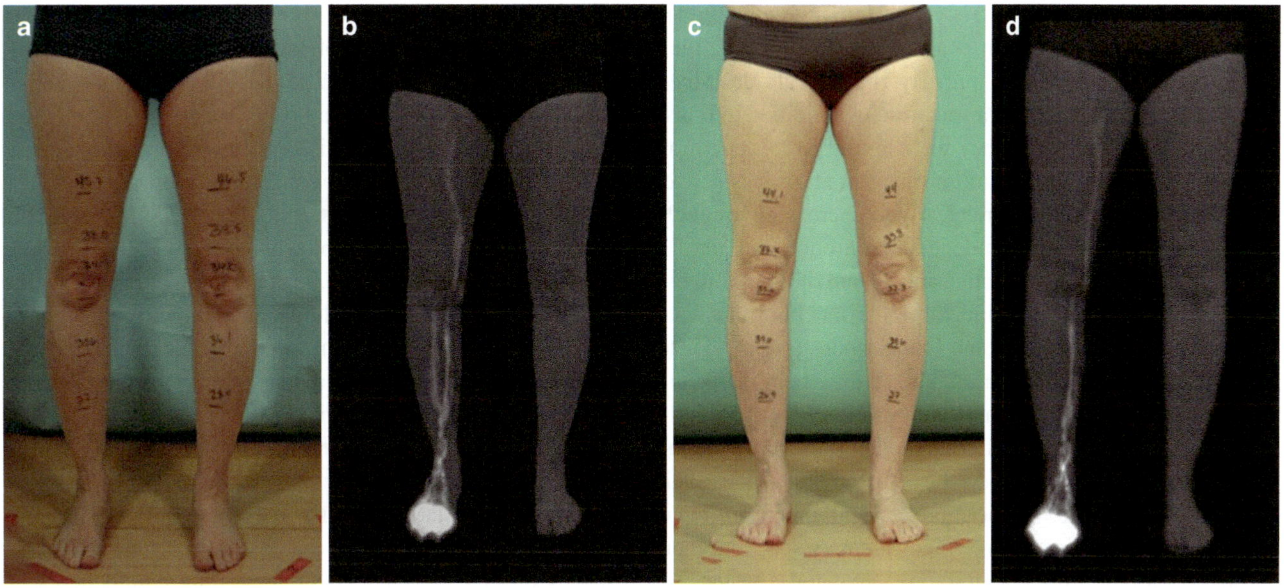

Fig. 27.11 This patient underwent a right SCIP-based VLVT flap transferred to her affected arm. Her preoperative clinical photo (**a**) and lymphatic vessel pattern (**b**) are shown next to her postoperative clinical photo (**c**) and lymphatic vessel pattern (**d**). In the postoperative photo there is no swelling (**c**), and in the postoperative lymphographic images there is no evidence of lymphatic injury (**d**). SCIP, superficial circumflex iliac artery perforator; VLVT, vascularized lymph vessel transfer; ICG, indocyanine green

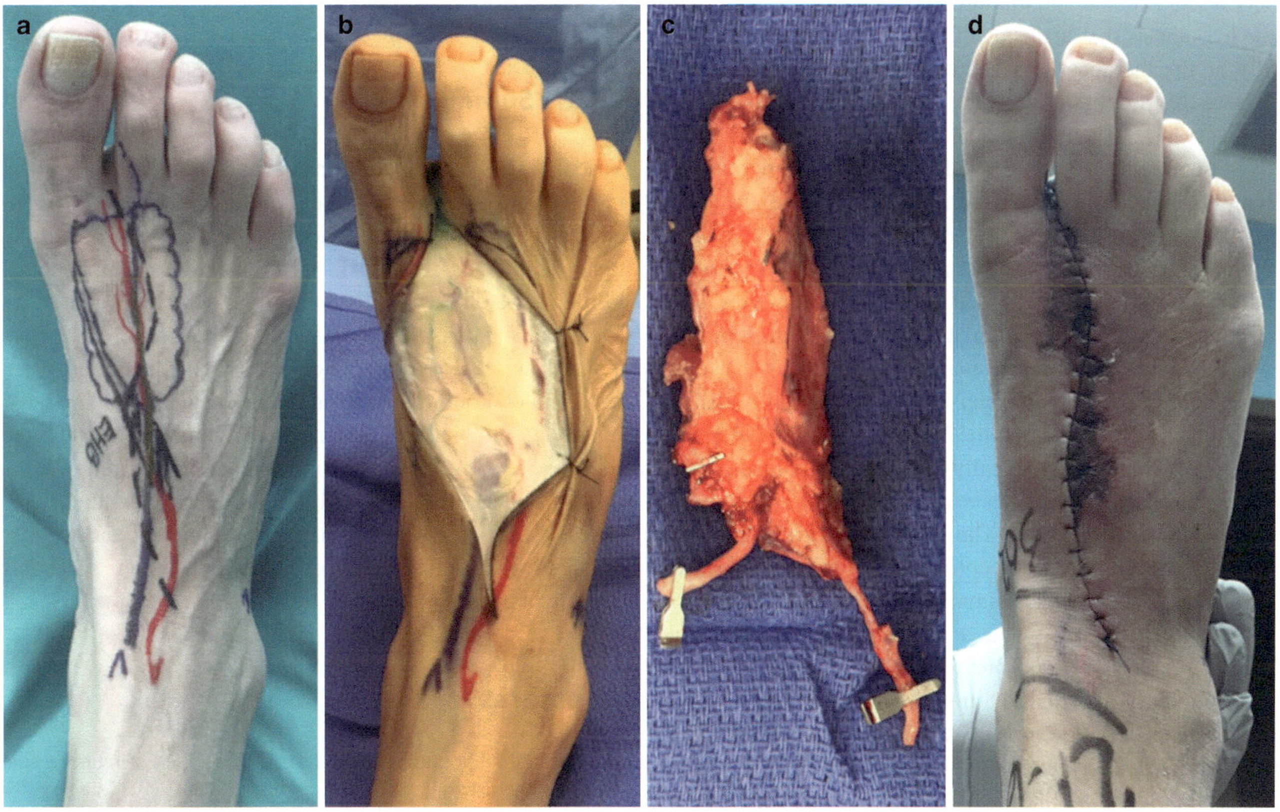

Fig. 27.12 FDMA-based VLVT flap. Flap markings are depicted (**a**). This flap had 3–4 lymphatic vessels, one of which can be seen on the left (**b**). Harvested FDMA-based VLVT flap is depicted (**c**). Donor wound breakdown after marginal skin necrosis often occurred in our experience (**d**). FDMA, first dorsal metatarsal artery; VLVT, vascularized lymph vessel transfer [39]

2. Lymph nodes have a life cycle. Human lymph nodes develop and reach their peak in childhood, and then slowly degenerate after puberty. Pan et al. described lymph nodes as being on a spectrum of solidified to transparent, based on where they were in this cycle. As lymph nodes age, they become more transparent, or less active, which histologically correlates with decreasing amounts of lymphoid tissue. This degeneration continues until a lymph node becomes inactive and devoid of lymphoid tissue [57]. It is not possible to predict at this time what stage of the lymph cycle the lymph nodes are in prior to their transfer. In some cases, VLNT may be transferring transparent, inactive lymph nodes, especially in elderly patients. Theoretically, lymph nodes will continue the degeneration process once they are transferred to their new recipient site. Furthermore, the inflammatory environment of the diseased recipient site may speed up their degeneration, turning them into inactive nodes faster.

In discussions with fellow lymphedema surgeons, surgeons frequently report that including larger volumes of skin and subcutaneous tissue in their VLNT flaps seems to result in better outcomes, while over-dissection of the VLNT flaps tends to result in worse outcomes. Since the subcutaneous tissue surrounding lymphatic nodes is where lymphatic vessels are most abundant, this anecdotal evidence also supports the hypothesis that inclusion of lymphatic vessels may actually be the therapeutic mechanism behind VLNT flaps. We believe this possibility warrants discussion and further study.

Vascularized lymph node transfer remains an effective treatment option for advanced, fluid-predominant lymphedema. However, its drawbacks include the small but devastating possibility of donor site lymphedema and the common occurrence of contour deformity due to flap bulk. We believe SCIP-based VLVT is a superior technique to VLNT due to elimination of the risk of donor site lymphedema. As the SCIP-based VLVT flap is harvested superficial to Scarpa's fascia, donor site lymph nodes are undisturbed. Furthermore, the SCIP-based VLVT flap produces a favorable, esthetically inconspicuous inset, eliminating the need for secondary debulking that is commonly needed with VLNT [58]. The challenge with SCIP-based VLVT is that anastomotic configuration is not straightforward due to vessel size mismatch, necessitating perforator-to-perforator or end-to-side anastomoses, as well as hand sown vein anastomoses. Due to small arterial pedicles that are frequently less than 0.8 mm, supermicrosurgical skills are often needed. The surgeon should be prepared and confident in their supermicrosurgical skills. Supermicrosurgical skills should be attained and refined through practice on simulation models prior to operations on patients, for patent, functional anastomoses are a prerequisite to surgical success [59].

Over the last 3 years, we have performed VLVT in 36 patients with secondary lymphedema, 34 of which had excellent outcomes. Two of the 36 patients had vascular pedicles that were exceedingly small and recurrent spasm was encountered during pedicle dissection, which prompted us to stop the flap harvest due to concern for flap survival. The number of upper to lower extremity lymphedema was about equal in our group of VLVT patients. For the 34 patients who underwent completed VLVT, all patients had objective and subjective improvements in lymphedema and lymphedema-associated symptoms within weeks of surgery. Objective improvements included improved ICG lymphography patterns and decreased volumetric measurements, both of which improved in all patients. Some patients' symptoms continued to improve up to 1 year postoperatively. Five patients have completely stopped using compression garments and others have weaned garment use. We have not compared the efficacy of VLVT versus VLNT in treating lymphedema. In the senior author's opinion, both of these procedures are effective. At our center, VLVT has replaced VLNT as the treatment of choice for patients with fluid-predominant disease and advanced lymphatic injury and for patients who did not improve significantly after LVA. VLVT has demonstrated consistently positive results for our group. Further study is needed in long-term outcomes and the mechanism of action of VLVT.

27.8 Summary

Vascularized lymph vessel transfer is a promising technique in the treatment of advanced, fluid-predominant lymphedema. This technique does not include lymphatic nodes and thus eliminates the risk of donor-site lymphedema. Furthermore, the VLVT flap is thin, which results in an esthetically inconspicuous inset. In contrast, VLNT harbors a small but real risk of donor site lymphedema and often results in contour deformity at the inset site due to flap bulk. Finally, due to its higher density of lymphatic vessels, the SCIP-based VLVT flap may offer higher therapeutic benefits over the FDMA-based VLVT. In our experience, the SCIP-based VLVT is an effective and safe technique, and we recommend its inclusion in every lymphedema surgeon's armamentarium.

References

1. Damstra R, Voesten H, Klinkert P, Brorson H. Circumferential suction-assisted lipectomy for lymphoedema after surgery for breast cancer. Br J Surg Inc Eur J Surg Swiss Surg. 2009;96:859–64.
2. Lamprou D, Voesten H, Damstra R, Wikkeling O. Circumferential suction-assisted lipectomy in the treatment of primary and secondary end-stage lymphoedema of the leg. Br J Surg. 2017;104:84–9.

3. Dumanian GA, Futrell JW. The Charles procedure: misquoted and misunderstood since 1950. Plast Reconstr Surg. 1996;98(7):1258–63.
4. Dayan E, Smith ML, Sultan M, Samson W, Dayan JH. Performing vascularized groin lymph node transfer with confidence: the use of four anatomic and physiologic modalities for safe and effective flap harvest. Plast Reconstr Surg. 2013;132:60.
5. Althubaiti GA, Crosby MA, Chang DW. Vascularized supraclavicular lymph node transfer for lower extremity lymphedema treatment. Plast Reconstr Surg. 2013;131:133e–5e.
6. Koshima I, Inagawa K, Urushibara K, Moriguchi T. Supermicrosurgical lymphaticovenular anastomosis for the treatment of lymphedema in the upper extremities. J Reconstr Microsurg. 2000;16:437–42.
7. Nagase T, Gonda K, Inoue K, Higashino T, Fukuda N, Gorai K, et al. Treatment of lymphedema with lymphaticovenular anastomoses. Int J Clin Oncol. 2005;10:304–10.
8. Lin C-H, Ali R, Chen S-C, Wallace C, Chang Y-C, Chen H-C, et al. Vascularized groin lymph node transfer using the wrist as a recipient site for management of postmastectomy upper extremity lymphedema. Plast Reconstr Surg. 2009;123:1265–75.
9. Cheng M-H, Huang J-J, Wu C-W, Yang C-Y, Lin C-Y, Henry SL, et al. The mechanism of vascularized lymph node transfer for lymphedema: natural lymphaticovenous drainage. Plast Reconstr Surg. 2014;133:192e–8e.
10. Becker C, Vasile JV, Levine JL, Batista BN, Studinger RM, Chen CM, et al. Microlymphatic surgery for the treatment of iatrogenic lymphedema. Clin Plast Surg. 2012;39:385–98.
11. Can J, Cai R, Li S, Zhang D. Experimental study of lymph node auto-transplantation in rats. Chin Med J (Engl). 1998;111:239–41.
12. Shesol BF, Nakashima R, Alavi A, Hamilton RW. Successful lymph node transplantation in rats, with restoration of lymphatic function. Plast Reconstr Surg. 1979;63:817–23.
13. Becker C, Assouad J, Riquet M, Hidden G. Postmastectomy lymphedema: long-term results following microsurgical lymph node transplantation. Ann Surg. 2006;243:313.
14. O'Brien BM, Hickey MJ, Hurley JV, Dvir E, Khazanchi RK, Pederson WC, et al. Microsurgical transfer of the greater omentum in the treatment of canine obstructive lymphoedema. Br J Plast Surg. 1990;43:440–6.
15. Chen H-C, O'Brien BM, Rogers I, Pribaz J, Eaton C. Lymph node transfer for the treatment of obstructive lymphoedema in the canine model. Br J Plast Surg. 1990;43:578–86.
16. Cheng M-H, Chen S-C, Henry SL, Tan BK, Lin MC-Y, Huang J-J. Vascularized groin lymph node flap transfer for postmastectomy upper limb lymphedema: flap anatomy, recipient sites, and outcomes. Plast Reconstr Surg. 2013;131:1286–98.
17. Azuma S, Yamamoto T, Koshima I. Donor-site lymphatic function after microvascular lymph node transfer should be followed using indocyanine green lymphography. Plast Reconstr Surg. 2013;131:443e–4e.
18. Vignes S, Blanchard M, Yannoutsos A, Arrault M. Complications of autologous lymph-node transplantation for limb lymphoedema. Eur J Vasc Endovasc Surg. 2013;45:516–20.
19. Cheng M, Lin C, Patel KM. A prospective clinical assessment of anatomic variability of the submental vascularized lymph node flap. J Surg Oncol. 2017;115:43–7.
20. Cheng M-H, Huang J-J, Nguyen DH, Saint-Cyr M, Zenn MR, Tan BK, et al. A novel approach to the treatment of lower extremity lymphedema by transferring a vascularized submental lymph node flap to the ankle. Gynecol Oncol. 2012;126:93–8.
21. Tzou CH, Meng S, Ines T, Reissig L, Pichler U, Steinbacher J, et al. Surgical anatomy of the vascularized submental lymph node flap: anatomic study of correlation of submental artery perforators and quantity of submental lymph node. J Surg Oncol. 2017;115:54–9.
22. Mardonado AA, Chen R, Chang DW. The use of supraclavicular free flap with vascularized lymph node transfer for treatment of lymphedema: a prospective study of 100 consecutive cases. J Surg Oncol. 2017;115:68–71.
23. Constantinescu T, Patel KM, Visconti G, Nicoli F, Chen H-C. Supraclavicular lymph node flap for lymphedema: early experience and technical refinements. Plast Reconstr Surg. 2015;136:108.
24. Barreiro GC, Baptista RR, Kasai KE, dos Anjos DM, de Freitas BF, Modolin M, et al. Lymph fasciocutaneous lateral thoracic artery flap: anatomical study and clinical use. J Reconstr Microsurg. 2014;30:389–96.
25. McCulley SJ, Schaverien MV, Tan VK, Macmillan RD. Lateral thoracic artery perforator (LTAP) flap in partial breast reconstruction. J Plast Reconstr Aesthet Surg. 2015;68:686–91.
26. Kim JT, Kim SW. Another option of perforator flap in the lateral thoracic area: lateral thoracic perforator flap. J Reconstr Microsurg. 2014;30:443–50.
27. Chu Y-Y, Allen RJ Jr, Wu T-J, Cheng M-H. Greater omental lymph node flap for upper limb lymphedema with lymph nodes–depleted patient. Plast Reconstr Surg Glob Open. 2017;5
28. Attash SM, Al-Sheikh MY. Omental flap for treatment of long standing lymphoedema of the lower limb: can it end the suffering? Report of four cases with review of literatures. Case Rep. 2013;2013:bcr2012008463.
29. Nguyen AT, Suami H. Laparoscopic free omental lymphatic flap for the treatment of lymphedema. Plast Reconstr Surg. 2015;136:114–8.
30. Coriddi M, Skoracki R, Eiferman D. Vascularized jejunal mesenteric lymph node transfer for treatment of extremity lymphedema. Microsurgery. 2017;37:177–8.
31. Koshima I, Narushima M, Mihara M, Yamamoto T, Hara H, Ohshima A, et al. Lymphadiposal flaps and lymphaticovenular anastomoses for severe leg edema: functional reconstruction for lymph drainage system. J Reconstr Microsurg. 2016;32:050–5.
32. Yamamoto T, Yamamoto N, Doi K, Oshima A, Yoshimatsu H, Todokoro T, et al. Indocyanine green–enhanced lymphography for upper extremity lymphedema: a novel severity staging system using dermal backflow patterns. Plast Reconstr Surg. 2011;128:941–7.
33. Chen WF. Is it possible to perform lymphaticovenular anastomosis after liposuction for lymphedema? J Surg. 2016;12:2.
34. Greene AK, Goss JA. Diagnosis and staging of lymphedema. New York: Thieme; 2018. p. 012–6.
35. Rockson SG, Miller LT, Senie R, Brennan MJ, Casley-Smith JR, Földi E, et al. Workgroup III: diagnosis and management of lymphedema. Cancer Interdiscip Int J Am Cancer Soc. 1998;83:2882–5.
36. Narushima M, Yamamoto T, Ogata F, Yoshimatsu H, Mihara M, Koshima I. Indocyanine green lymphography findings in limb lymphedema. J Reconstr Microsurg. 2016;32:072–9.
37. Yamamoto T, Iida T, Yoshimatsu H, Fuse Y, Hayashi A, Yamamoto N. Lymph flow restoration after tissue replantation and transfer: importance of lymph axiality and possibility of lymph flow reconstruction without lymph node transfer or lymphatic anastomosis. Plast Reconstr Surg. 2018;142:796–804.
38. Chen WF, Zhao H, Yamamoto T, Hara H, Ding J. Indocyanine green lymphographic evidence of surgical efficacy following microsurgical and supermicrosurgical lymphedema reconstructions. J Reconstr Microsurg. 2016;32:688–98.
39. Chen WF, McNurlen M, Ding J, Bowen M. Vascularized lymph vessel transfer for extremity lymphedema—is transfer of lymph node still necessary? Int Microsurg J IMJ. 2019;3(3):1.
40. Raju A, Chang DW. Vascularized lymph node transfer for treatment of lymphedema: a comprehensive literature review. Ann Surg. 2015;261:1013–23.
41. Ozturk CN, Ozturk C, Glasgow M, Platek M, Ashary Z, Kuhn J, et al. Free vascularized lymph node transfer for treatment of

lymphedema: a systematic evidence based review. J Plast Reconstr Aesthet Surg. 2016;69:1234–47.
42. Tourani SS, Taylor GI, Ashton MW. Vascularized lymph node transfer: a review of the current evidence. Plast Reconstr Surg. 2016;137:985–93.
43. Allen RJ Jr, Cheng M. Lymphedema surgery: patient selection and an overview of surgical techniques. J Surg Oncol. 2016;113:923–31.
44. Scaglioni MF, Arvanitakis M, Chen Y, Giovanoli P, Chia-Shen Yang J, Chang EI. Comprehensive review of vascularized lymph node transfers for lymphedema: outcomes and complications. Microsurgery. 2018;38:222–9.
45. Kung TA, Champaneria MC, Maki JH, Neligan PC. Current concepts in the surgical management of lymphedema. Plast Reconstr Surg. 2017;139:1003e–13e.
46. Pons G, Masia J, Loschi P, Nardulli ML, Duch J. A case of donor-site lymphoedema after lymph node–superficial circumflex iliac artery perforator flap transfer. J Plast Reconstr Aesthet Surg. 2014;67:119–23.
47. Dayan JH, Dayan E, Smith ML. Reverse lymphatic mapping: a new technique for maximizing safety in vascularized lymph node transfer. Plast Reconstr Surg. 2015;135:277–85.
48. Goh TL, Park SW, Cho JY, Choi JW, Hong JP. The search for the ideal thin skin flap: superficial circumflex iliac artery perforator flap—a review of 210 cases. Plast Reconstr Surg. 2015;135:592–601.
49. Coriddi M, Wee C, Meyerson J, Eiferman D, Skoracki R. Vascularized jejunal mesenteric lymph node transfer: a novel surgical treatment for extremity lymphedema. J Am Coll Surg. 2017;225:650–7.
50. Hong JP, Sun SH, Ben-Nakhi M. Modified superficial circumflex iliac artery perforator flap and supermicrosurgery technique for lower extremity reconstruction: a new approach for moderate-sized defects. Ann Plast Surg. 2013;71:380–3.
51. Kim JH, Kim KN, Yoon CS. Reconstruction of moderate-sized distal limb defects using a superthin superficial circumflex iliac artery perforator flap. J Reconstr Microsurg. 2015;31:631–5.
52. Yoshimatsu H, Yamamoto T, Hayashi A, Iida T. Proximal-to-distally elevated superficial circumflex iliac artery perforator flap enabling hybrid reconstruction. Plast Reconstr Surg. 2016;138:910–22.
53. Feng S, Xi W, Zhang Z, Tremp M, Schaefer DJ, Sadigh PL, et al. A reappraisal of the surgical planning of the superficial circumflex iliac artery perforator flap. J Plast Reconstr Aesthet Surg. 2017;70:469–77.
54. Lee K-T, Park BY, Kim E-J, Kim J-H, Jang K-T, Choi S-H, et al. Superthin SCIP flap for reconstruction of subungual melanoma: aesthetic functional surgery. Plast Reconstr Surg. 2017;140:1278–89.
55. Myung Y, Yim S, Kim B. A comparison of axial circumference between superficial circumflex iliac artery perforator flap and other workhorse flaps in dorsal foot reconstruction. J Plast Surg Hand Surg. 2017;51:381–6.
56. Chen WF, Bowen M, McNurlen M, Ding J. Vascularized lymph vessel transfer with supermicrosurgical ultra-thin superficial circumflex iliac artery flap for treatment of advanced lymphedema not treatable with supermicrosurgical lymphaticovenular anastomosis. Ann Plast Surg. 2018;80
57. Pan W-R. Atlas of lymphatic anatomy in the head, neck, chest and limbs. Singapore: Springer; 2017.
58. Wei F-C, Celik N, Chen H-C, Cheng M-H, Huang W-C. Combined anterolateral thigh flap and vascularized fibula osteoseptocutaneous flap in reconstruction of extensive composite mandibular defects. Plast Reconstr Surg. 2002;109:45–52.
59. Koshima I, Yamamoto T, Narushima M, Mihara M, Iida T. Perforator flaps and supermicrosurgery. Clin Plast Surg. 2010;37:683–9.

Microsurgery: Lymphaticovenular Anastomosis for the Treatment of Lymphedema

28

Weifeng Zeng, Oksana Babchenko, and Wei F. Chen

Abstract

Recent advancements in microsurgery and supermicrosurgery have made lymphedema a surgically manageable condition. Lymphaticovenular anastomosis (LVA) is an established supermicrosurgical treatment of lymphedema. LVA is minimally invasive and conceptually simple: lymphatic vessels are anastomosed directly into superficial veins, allowing lymphatic outflow to drain into veins and thus bypass obstructed lymphatic drainage pathways. However, LVA is not widely practiced due to perceived technical complexity, lack of technique standardization, and some reports of inconsistent outcomes. However, many surgical groups, including ours, have reported reliably favorable outcomes with LVA. We believe the inconsistency in some reported outcomes is likely related to variability in patient selection, surgical plan and technique, and postoperative care. In this chapter, the senior author (WFC) shares his experience with LVA, reviewing patient selection, surgical planning, surgical technique, advanced technical pearls, and postoperative care. After reading this chapter, the readers should have sufficient clinical and technical knowledge to begin performing LVA and achieving favorable outcomes.

Keywords

Lymphedema · Supermicrosurgery · Indocyanine green lymphography · Lymphaticovenular anastomosis · Lymphatic mapping · Venotomy · Microsurgery training · Postoperative care

W. Zeng · O. Babchenko
Division of Plastic and Reconstructive Surgery, Department of Surgery, University of Wisconsin-Madison, Madison, WI, USA

W. F. Chen (✉)
Center for Lymphedema Research and Reconstruction, Department of Plastic and Reconstructive Surgery, Cleveland Clinic, Cleveland, OH, USA

28.1 Introduction

Surgical innovation has transformed the treatment of lymphedema from a progressive, poorly treatable disease to one that can be surgically managed and in some patients even clinically cured. Surgical treatment of lymphedema varies with disease severity. More severe, solid-predominant disease requires debulking surgical treatments, such as suction-assisted lipectomy (SAL) [1, 2] surgical excision, and the Charles procedure [3]. Less severe, fluid-predominant lymphedema is amendable to physiologic reconstructive procedures, such as lymphaticovenular anastomosis (LVA) [4, 5], vascularized lymph node transfer (VLNT) [6, 7], and more recently, vascularized lymph vessel transfer (VLVT) [8, 9]. The goal of reconstructive procedures is to restore lymphatic drainage, while the goal of debulking procedures is to remove pathologic tissue. After both debulking and reconstructive procedures, adherence to compression therapy is important, however, with successful reconstructive procedures, compression can often be discontinued at a later time.

LVA requires performing anastomoses of very small vessels, in the size range 0.2–0.8 mm, to allow lymphatic drainage to flow from lymphatic vessels directly into veins, to bypass obstructed lymphatic drainage pathways [4, 10, 11]. Performing anastomoses of very small vessels (0.2–0.8 mm) is a specialized microsurgical technique that is termed supermicrosurgery. Supermicrosurgery was first introduced by Koshima et al. [12, 13] 20 years ago, and this technique has allowed for the creation of LVA [4]. The concept of LVA was not new. Lympho-venous bypass (LVB) was reported prior to Koshima's supermicrosurgical LVA [14]. The differences were that LVBs were microsurgical (frequently involving vessels >0.8 mm) and were usually performed in the proximal limb segments [15]. The reported outcomes of LVBs were inconsistent and therefore the technique was mostly abandoned [14, 16].

Although LVA is an established supermicrosurgical treatment for lymphedema that is minimally invasive and that has

N. Liu (ed.), *Peripheral Lymphedema*, https://doi.org/10.1007/978-981-16-3484-0_28

favorable outcomes [4, 12, 17–20], it is not frequently performed in the United States. Instead, VLNT is the favored lymphedema reconstruction procedure in the United States despite it being more invasive and carrying a small but real risk of donor site lymphedema [21, 22]. Underutilization of LVA may be due to surgeons' unfamiliarity with supermicrosurgery and LVA-related techniques, uncertainty in patient selection, and uncertainty in surgical outcomes. At the time of writing this chapter, the senior author (WFC) has performed over 250 cases of supermicrosurgical LVAs with reliably favorable outcomes for his patients [11, 23–25]. In this chapter the senior author shares his approach to LVA, detailing patient selection, supermicrosurgery technique, strategies for surmounting the supermicrosurgery learning curve using a simulation model, LVA technical pearls, postoperative cares, outcome assessment, and other considerations for building a surgical lymphedema program.

28.2 Concepts

Lymphedema surgery is categorized into reconstructive procedures that aim to restore lymphatic drainage and debulking procedures that aim to remove the disease-compromised tissue. Reconstructive procedures are performed for less severe, fluid-predominant lymphedema, or, as has been recently shown, after extensive liposuction debulking in some cases of more advanced disease [26]. Reconstructive procedures include LVA [4, 12, 20, 27], VLNT [6, 7, 28–34], and more recently, VLVT [8, 9, 35]. Debulking procedures are performed for more severe, solid-predominant lymphedema and include SAL [1, 2, 36, 37], direct surgical excision, and the Charles procedure [3, 38].

LVA is a supermicrosurgical procedure that reestablishes a flow pathway for lymph to return to cardiovascular circulation by anastomosing superficial lymphatic vessels to subdermal veins. Interestingly, there have been reports of natural lymphaticovenular anastomoses occurring in pathologic conditions of the lymphatic system, such as lymphedema and lymph outflow obstruction, as well as in the natural healing process after tissue trauma [39]. These findings suggest that LVA may be a natural compensatory response to obstructed and regenerating lymphatic systems.

LVA requires supermicrosurgery techniques, as the vessels are usually 0.2–0.8 mm in diameter. The choice of anastomotic configuration can vary depending on local anatomy, but the goal is to recruit all of the available lymphatic vessels to maximize lymphatic drainage. There are several types of LVA, each named in the lymphatic vessel-to-vein convention. These LVA variations include the following anastomoses: end-to-end, side-to-side, side-to-end, lambda, doubled end-to-side, and the "Octopus," which was developed by the senior author (Fig. 28.1) [25].

The choice of anastomotic configuration depends on the relative caliber and proximity of vessels, flow direction, and the functionality of the lymphatic vessel and vein. The senior author recommends that microsurgeons who want to offer LVA to their patients should be trained in and familiar with all of these configurations, so that s/he can decide which one is most appropriate for each anastomosis.

28.3 Patient Selection

LVA is the treatment of choice for early, fluid-predominant disease with functionally preserved lymphatic vessels. Patients who are good candidates are characterized by fully reversible, pitting edema, signifying fluid-predominant disease. MRI and/or bioimpedance spectroscopy (BIS) can be useful to confirm fluid predominance. On MRI the adiposity vs. fluid signals are easily differentiated [40–45], while BIS provides segmental quantitative measurements of tissue fluid content [46–48] (Fig. 28.2).

Once fluid predominance is confirmed, either through physical examination, or in conjunction with MRI and/or BIS, then indocyanine green (ICG) lymphography should be done to assess lymph vessel functionality [49–51]. On ICG lymphography, preservation of a "linear" lymphographic pattern indicates healthy, functioning lymph vessels (Fig. 28.3). In early lymphedema where functional lymph vessels are still abundant, LVA is the preferred choice for surgical intervention. Furthermore, in early disease the technical execution of LVA is straightforward, as the surgeon can easily map the linear lymph vessels and plan anastomotic sites precisely; highly favorable results can be expected.

While both upper and lower extremities can greatly benefit from LVA, it is the senior author's experience that arm lymphedema improves to a greater degree than leg lymphedema following LVA [11, 18]. This difference is likely mediated by differences in venous pressures in the upper versus lower extremities. As arms are more anatomically elevated than legs, arms have lower venous pressures than legs. Lower venous pressures facilitate favorable lymph-to-vein pressure gradients. In other words, lymph is more likely to flow forward—from the lymph vessel to the vein—if the vein has a relatively lower pressure. In contrast, higher venous pressure is more likely to obstruct forward lymph flow, or to cause unfavorable backflow, which is flow from the vein back to the lymph vessel.

It is commonly believed that LVA is contraindicated when no "linear" lymph flow pattern is present on ICG lymphography. This has not been the senior author's experience. While it is true that LVA works best in limbs with relatively preserved lymphatic function (i.e., evidence of linear patterns on ICG lymphography), LVA can still result in favorable outcomes in fluid-predominant lymphedematous limbs with

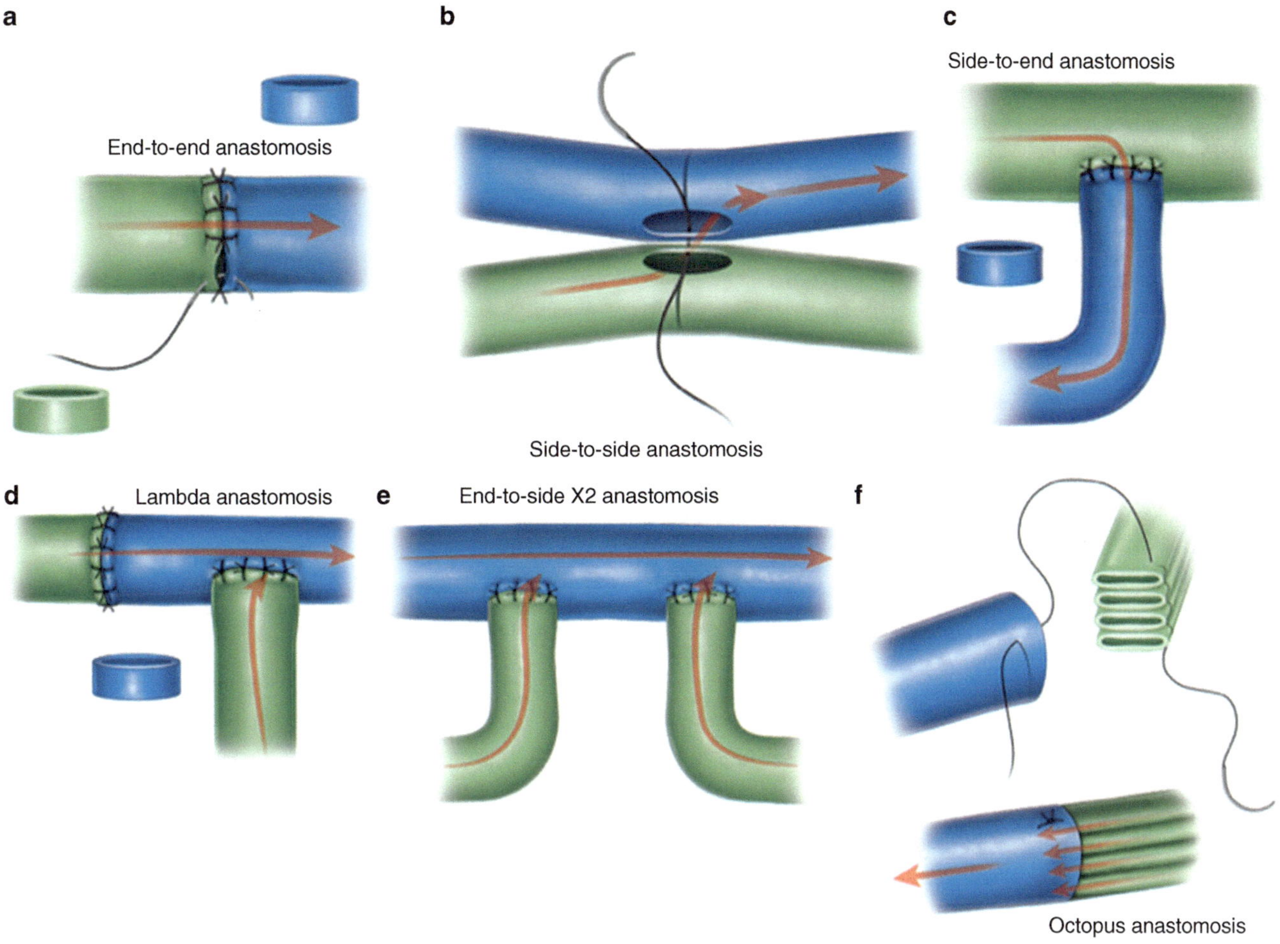

Fig. 28.1 Common configurations of lymphaticovenular anastomoses. Lymphatic vessels are represented in green, and veins are represented in blue. Flow direction is depicted with red arrows (Jones G., et al. Bostwick's Plastic and Reconstructive Breast Surgery. Thieme NY. 2019. Copyright holder, www.thieme.com (reprinted with permission))

compromised lymphatic function (i.e., limbs with splash, stardust, and even diffuse lymphographic patterns). While this is true for both upper and lower extremities, the lower extremity should be evaluated more cautiously due to the less favorable, higher venous pressures of the lower extremity. If the lower extremity has evidence of compromised lymphatic function based on ICG lymphography, it may still be in the patient's favor to perform LVA, as the procedure is minimally invasive and some improvement is likely. If there is a lack of improvement or insufficient improvement, the surgeon can proceed to more invasive operations, such as VLVT or VLNT. However, the patient should be cautioned that when LVA is performed on extremities with severely compromised lymphatic function (i.e., splash, stardust, and diffuse lymphographic patterns), longer extremity elevation, and longer and stricter use of compression garments may be needed to optimize the outcomes [18].

Mihara et al. described how lymphedema severity changes the structure of lymphatic vessels due to increasing vessel injury. In order of increasing lymphedema severity, Mihara described lymphatic vessels as normal, ectatic, contracted, and sclerotic [52, 53]. In the senior author's experience, only sclerotic vessels cannot effectively transport lymph; all other degrees of injury—normal, ectatic, and, to a lesser degree, contracted lymph vessels—can transport lymph and thus can be used to build LVA. Applying this to ICG lymphographic patterns yields the following guideline: if a surgeon is using normal, ectatic, and contracted vessels for LVA, there is about a 100%, 70%, and 53% probability of finding adequate vessels for LVA when operating on "linear," "stardust," and "diffuse" lymphographic patterns, respectively [53]. Thus, even when a patient displays only "stardust" or "diffuse" ICG lymphographic patterns, LVA continues to be a viable, minimally invasive option for fluid-predominant disease. Often, patients with advanced lymphatic injury (e.g., "diffuse" ICG lymphographic pattern) prefer to try LVA first, as it is minimally invasive, can still produce good outcomes, and does not preclude them from more invasive techniques in the future, such as VLVT or VLNT. It is the senior author's opinion that for fluid-predominant disease with signs of

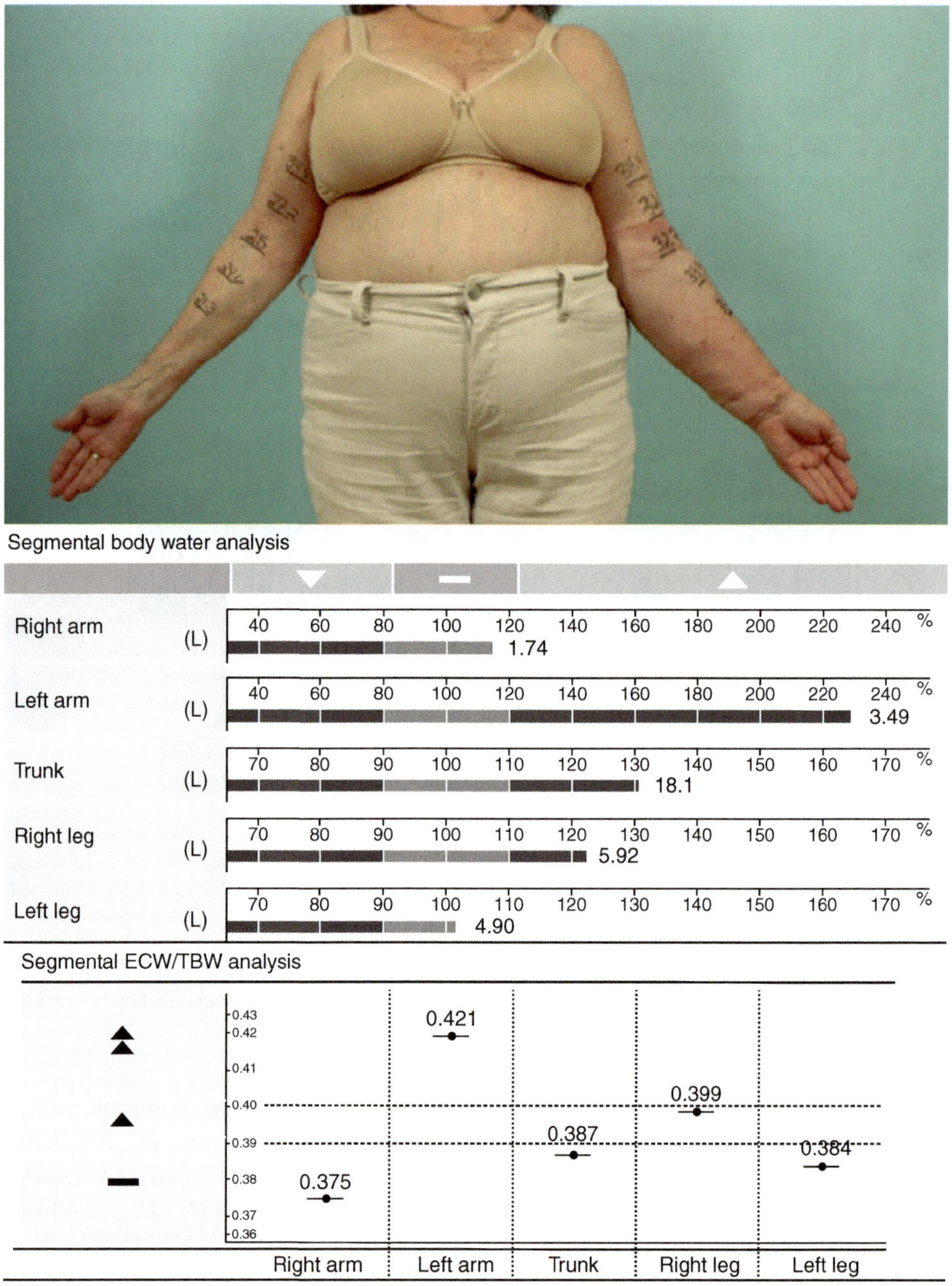

Fig. 28.2 BIS can be used to confirm a fluid-predominant state. This result demonstrates a fluid predominant state of the left arm, as seen by the highly elevated values. BIS, Bioimpedance spectroscopy (Jones G., et al. Bostwick's Plastic and Reconstructive Breast Surgery. Thieme NY. 2019. Copyright holder, www.thieme.com (reprinted with permission))

advanced lymphatic injury, it is a safe and reasonable option to try LVA first in select cases.

At times, ICG signal may be entirely absent on ICG lymphography. This can occur in both congenital and acquired lymphedema and may be due to several reasons. (1) The penetration depth of the scanning device may be insufficient to detect deeper ICG signals. (2) There may be sluggish lymphatic transport. (3) The injection sites may not be drained by the relevant lymphosomes. (4) It may be due to individual anatomy variations. In situations where there are no visible ICG signals, we recommend mapping the veins using near-infrared technology, and planning the exploratory incisions at the location of the veins. This is termed the "follow-the-vein" (FTV) approach, and its premise is based on the fact that lymphatic vessels closely parallel vein trajectories, especially in the superficial fat layer [4, 12, 14, 20, 54]. In the senior author's experience, lymph vessel(s) can usually be found within a 3-cm radius from a vein (Figs. 28.4 and 28.5) [11]. When there is no linear ICG lymphographic pattern, the FTV approach is a viable, safe option for planning LVA.

28.4 Preoperative Preparation

A thorough history and physical examination should be performed. The history should focus on etiology, symptoms, functional impairment, rate of disease progression, prior treatments, and response to prior treatments. It should be

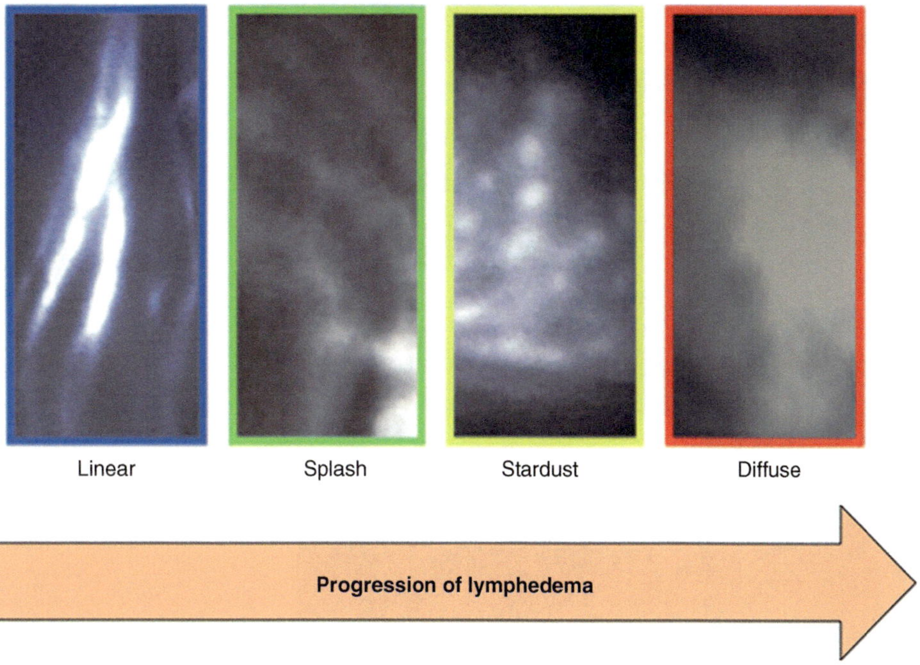

Fig. 28.3 ICG lymphography showing lymphatic flow patterns. A linear pattern is the normal pattern of lymph flow. Splash, stardust, and diffuse are lymph flow patterns in order of progressive severity of lymphedema. ICG, indocyanine green (Yamamoto T, Iida T, Matsuda N, Kikuchi K, Yoshimatsu H, Mihara M, et al. Indocyanine green (ICG)-enhanced lymphography for evaluation of facial lymphoedema. J Plast Reconstr Aesthet Surg. 2011;64(11):1541–4 (reprinted with permission))

noted whether the lymphedema is primary or secondary [55]. It is important to note that although disease duration often correlates with symptom severity, it does not always correlate. For example, sometimes patients with years of symptomatic disease may have only mild lymphatic injury. Conversely, patients with severe lymphatic injury (e.g., surgical causes) may have only recent disease development [53, 56]. When formulating a treatment plan, it is essential to note the speed of disease progression. Patients with rapid disease progression are preferentially considered for surgery, for delaying surgery in them could result in their rapidly progressing disease becoming advanced enough to contraindicate them from some surgical treatments. There is also a lowered threshold to surgical intervention in the pediatric patient population, for lymphedema progression has a high probability in their lifetimes [57].

Physical examination should focus on whether the disease is fluid predominant, solid predominant, or a mixture of both. During the visual inspection of the affected limb it is important to note the degree of swelling. Palpation and digital pressure are important for assessing skin and tissue quality and for evaluating ease of pitting. Early, less severe lymphedema is usually fluid predominant and demonstrates pitting with digital pressure. Late, more severe lymphedema tends to be solid predominant, with abundant lipodystrophy and fibrosis; solid-predominant disease will not pit with digital pressure.

Measurement of limb volume should also be done. There are many ways to estimate limb volumes, however, all have flaws and are easily influenced by extrinsic factors (e.g., activity level, pressure garment use, and even time of day). Thus, volume measurements are inherently imprecise and should be thought of as only rough estimates of the disease. Methods of volume measurements include direct measurements: three-dimensional (3D) optoelectronic perometry and water displacement, and indirect measurements: multilevel circumference measurements. For direct measurements, 3D perometry is far easier and more efficient than water displacement. However, 3D volume scanning lacks precision, as changes in patient posture during measurement can affect the measurement. We recommend using 3D scanning as a patient tracking modality, for it effectively demonstrates limb volume progression over time. We do not recommend its use as a diagnostic modality.

Although lymphedema is considered by some to be a clinical diagnosis, confirmatory studies should be done when surgical intervention is considered. Many conditions can mimic lymphedema, such as lipedema and venous insufficiency. Traditionally, lymphoscintigraphy has been the gold standard in diagnosing extremity lymphedema; it uses technetium-99m-sulfur colloid as a tracer of lymphatic transit. However, due to lymphoscintigraphy's poor spatial resolution and radiation exposure, we prefer to utilize ICG lymphography. ICG lymphography has also been shown to have a higher sensitivity and specificity than lymphoscintigraphy [58–60]. In ICG lymphography, a nonradioactive contrast agent is injected peripherally and taken up by the lymphatic system. ICG uses fluorophore, which fluoresces when optically excited at 800 nm. The visual patterns that emerge are correlates of lymphatic flow and lymphatic dermal backflow in the extremity, which are analogs for disease severity [50]. In progression from normal-to-severe disease, the dermal backflow patterns are "linear," "splash," "stardust," and "diffuse" (Fig. 28.3).

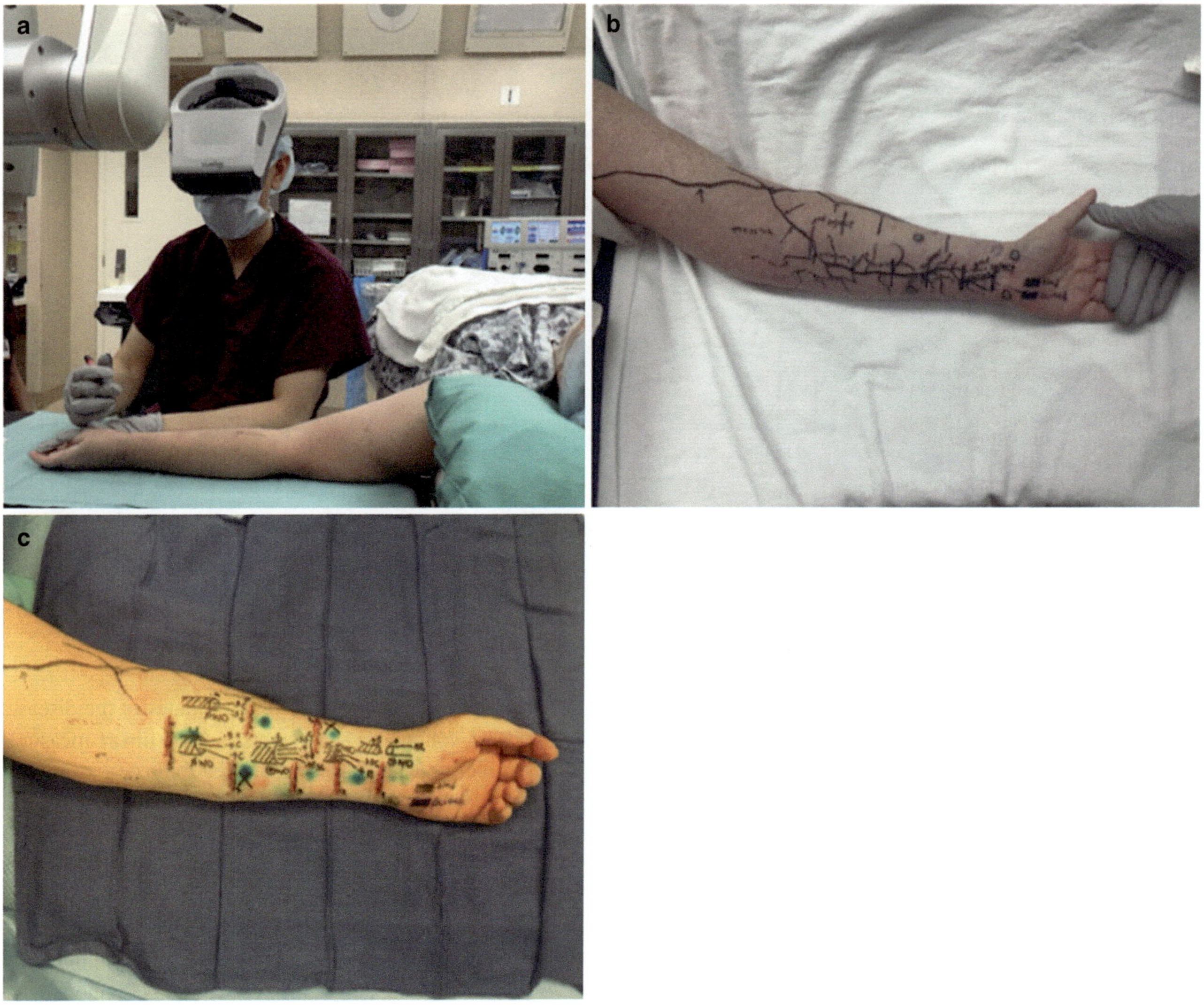

Fig. 28.4 The solid blue and red lines show lymphatic vessels mapped with ICG lymphography. Dotted lines represent superficial veins mapped with near-infrared technology. Incisions (short, black lines) are planned at intersecting points of the veins and lymphatic vessels (**a**). Postoperative skin markings depict the LVA anastomotic techniques that were performed (**b**). ICG, indocyanine green; LVA, lymphaticovenular anastomosis [24]

In our practice, ICG lymphography has replaced lymphoscintigraphy as the imaging modality of choice for diagnosis, preoperative planning, and postoperative outcome tracking [61, 62]. It should be noted that when using ICG lymphography for diagnostic purposes only, a precise protocol is not necessary. However, when using ICG lymphography for assessment of lymphedema severity (i.e., lymph vessel function) and outcome tracking, a standardized protocol is of otmost importance to assure reliable, comparable measurements between patients and patient encounters. Specifically, ICG dose, injection sites, background lighting, patient position, sequence of scanning, exposure time, working distance, study duration, and even person performing the study should be kept constant.

28.5 Surgical Techniques: Lymphaticovenular Anastomosis

Lymphaticovenular Anastomosis (LVA) is most effective when performed on functioning lymphatic vessels, but as previously described, can also be performed on lymphatic vessels with mild to moderate damage. To assess lymphatic vessel functionality, ICG lymphography is used. Linear patterns on ICG lymphography indicate preservation of a functional lymphatic system, and when linear patterns are present, LVA is the procedure of choice. However, more advanced ICG lymphographic patterns, such as splash, stardust, and even diffuse, may be considered for LVA, as long as the disease is fluid predominant.

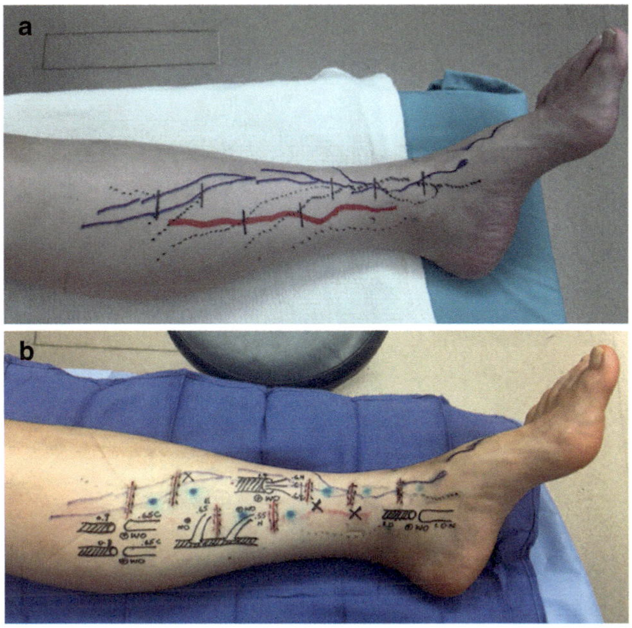

Fig. 28.5 A near-infrared vein finder headpiece is used to localize superficial veins close to the lymphatic vessels (**a**). Superficial veins and lymphatic vessels mapped out on the patient's arm. Solid lines represent lymphatic vessels identified using ICG lymphography. Dotted lines represent superficial veins identified using near-infrared vein finder (**b**). Postoperative skin markings depict the LVA anastomotic techniques that were performed. Incisions were placed at the locations where lymphatic vessels and veins were in close proximity (**c**). ICG, indocyanine green (Chen WF. How to Get Started Performing Supermicrosurgical Lymphaticovenular Anastomosis to Treat Lymphedema. Ann Plast Surg. 2018;81(6S Suppl 1):S15–S20 (reprinted with permission))

Although LVA can be performed under local anesthesia, it is generally performed under general anesthesia for patient comfort [63]. A preoperative ICG lymphography is done in the operating room (OR) to map out all the available lymphatic vessels of the extremity [11, 23, 64]. Then, infrared vein localization is utilized to map out superficial veins (Figs. 28.4a and 28.5a, b). After both the lymphatic vessels and the superficial veins are mapped out, incisions are planned at the points where the lymphatic vessels and veins are intersecting or lie in closest proximity (Figs. 28.4a and 28.5b).

The microscope should be set at an initial magnification level of 10–15×; needle electrocautery should be set at 8 W. Half a milliliter of isosulfan blue is injected about 2 cm distal to each planned incision site to help with lymphatic vessel identification. Each incision should be about 1–1.5 cm. As the surgeon begins the skin incision, s/he must be especially careful when dividing the last strands of dermis, for the superficial veins that are appropriate for LVA are often found just deep into the dermis. Following the careful division of the dermis, the magnification level should be increased to 18–25× and a micro-dissector utilized to carefully skeletonize and preserve all lymphatic vessels and veins that are encountered while dissecting through the superficial and deep fat layers. Lymphatic vessels are often located just deep to the superficial fascia, although can be found anywhere between the skin and deep fascia. Once the surgeon exposes the underlying deep fascia, dissection is complete, as deep fascia should not be entered.

When deciding on the anastomotic configuration of each LVA, the surgeon's goal should be to recruit all available lymphatic vessels to maximize lymph drainage into the venous system [11, 23]. To remind the reader, the LVA anastomotic configuration nomenclature is in the lymph-to-vein direction. Side-to-end and side-to-side anastomoses allow the most potential drainage, and should be performed whenever feasible. These configurations result in the most drainage because they allow both antegrade and retrograde drainage from the lymph vessel, which then empties into the venous system [19, 65, 66]. The anastomotic configuration is generally dictated by the calibers and positions of vessels. When the lumen of the lymphatic vessel equals or exceeds the lumen of the vein, side-to-end anastomoses can be performed. However, if the lumen of the lymphatic vessel is smaller than the lumen of the vein, end-to-side anastomosis should be performed (Fig. 28.7b). If the lymphatic vessel and vein are comparable in size, either side-to-side or end-to-end configuration can be performed (Fig. 28.6a) [19, 65, 66]. While side-to-side is advantageous due to potential bidirectional lymphatic drainage, it is a difficult anastomosis to perform, and we do not advise attempting it on vessels that are less than 0.3 mm. If there are multiple, small lymphatic vessels, they can be anastomosed to a single vein using the "octopus" technique (Fig. 28.6c, d) [25]. To be successful in LVA, the surgeon should be comfortable and skilled in all anastomotic techniques and maneuvers, for this will allow the greatest flexibility, creativity, and efficacy when encountering various anatomical variations of vessel position, size, and location.

When the surgeon decides on the anastomotic configuration plan and is ready to perform the anastomoses, the microscope magnification should be increased. As the vessels of interest are generally in the 0.2–0.6 mm range, optimal visualization is achieved at 25–35× magnification. Higher magnification beyond 35× is not advised due to the extreme narrowing of the operative field. The selection of suture depends on vessel size. For vessels less than 0.5 mm, a 12-0 suture on a 50-μm needle is advised, and for vessels equal to or larger than 0.5 mm, an 11-0 can be utilized. The surgeon will quickly realize that the 50-μm needle of the 12-0 suture is prone to bending; care must be taken to prevent it from bending and to bend it back into a suture needle shape if bending occurs.

Prior to operating on humans, we strongly advise new LVA surgeons to hone supermicrosurgical skills on a

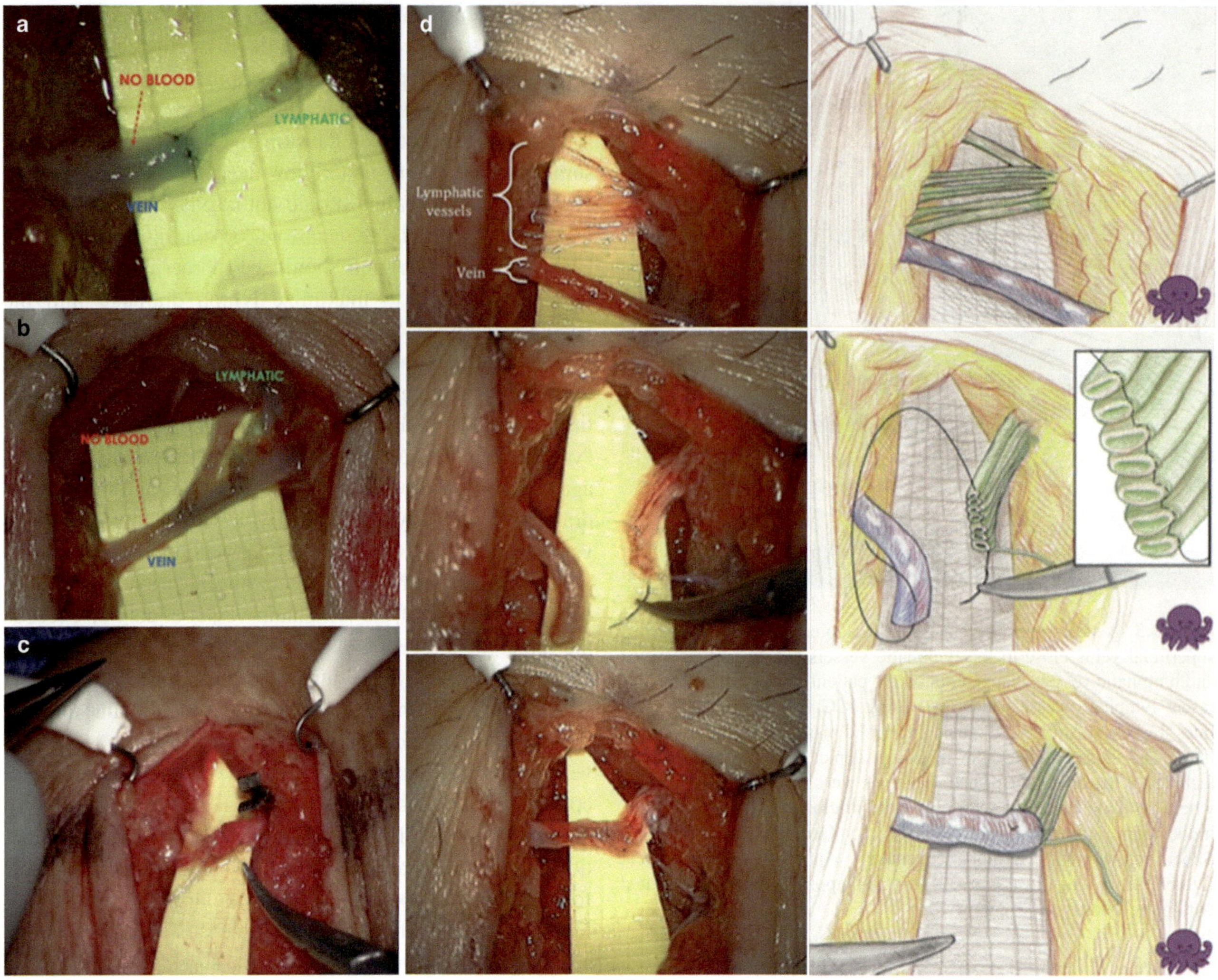

Fig. 28.6 End-to-end anastomosis (**a**), double end-to-side anastomosis (**b**), and the octopus anastomosis (**c**, **d**). The "washout" sign can be easily seen from the absence of blood in the vein and the presence of the green/blue-tinted lymphatic fluid in the vein, indicating forward flow of lymphatic fluid into the venous system (**a**, **b**). Four-to-one octopus LVA with a U-stitch that "intussuscepts" all four lymphatic vessels into one vein (**c**). Cartoon illustration of the octopus technique that uses transadventitial suturing to gather the lymphatic vessels together (**d**) (Chen WF. How to Get Started Performing Supermicrosurgical Lymphaticovenular Anastomosis to Treat Lymphedema. Ann Plast Surg. 2018;81(6S Suppl 1):S15–S20; Chen WF, Yamamoto T, Fisher M, Liao J, Carr J. The "octopus" lymphaticovenular anastomosis: evolving beyond the standard supermicrosurgical technique. J Reconstr Microsurg. 2015;31:450–7 (reprinted with permission))

chicken thigh simulation model. The techniques and skills required for supermicrosurgery are unique and even excellent skills in microsurgery will not readily translate due to the variation of technique in supermicrosurgery. As such, practice and proficiency on a simulation model are warranted prior to operating on patients, for this will assure that favorable outcomes will be possible and probable from the first clinical LVA. Without proficient skills in supermicrosurgery that reliably produce patent, leak-free anastomoses, LVA will not be effective. We have developed the chicken thigh model as a biologic and humane simulation model on which to train in supermicrosurgery (Fig. 28.7) [67, 68].

Achieving a leakproof anastomosis requires placing an adequate amount of sutures. Although the vessels are quite small and the relative pressure of LVA is far less than in arterial circulation, we still find that for a ~0.4 mm diameter vessel anastomosis, about six stitches are usually required. Achieving a leakproof anastomosis is important because as lymphatic pressure increases in a leak-free vessel, is can then overcome the venous pressure and thus lymphatic fluid will be "washed-out" into the venous circulation (Fig. 28.8a) [11, 23]. It should be noted that more damaged lymphatic vessels can have compromised peristalses and may demonstrate a delayed "washout" sign. Thus, they may need to be reassessed several minutes after the anastomosis is done. If the

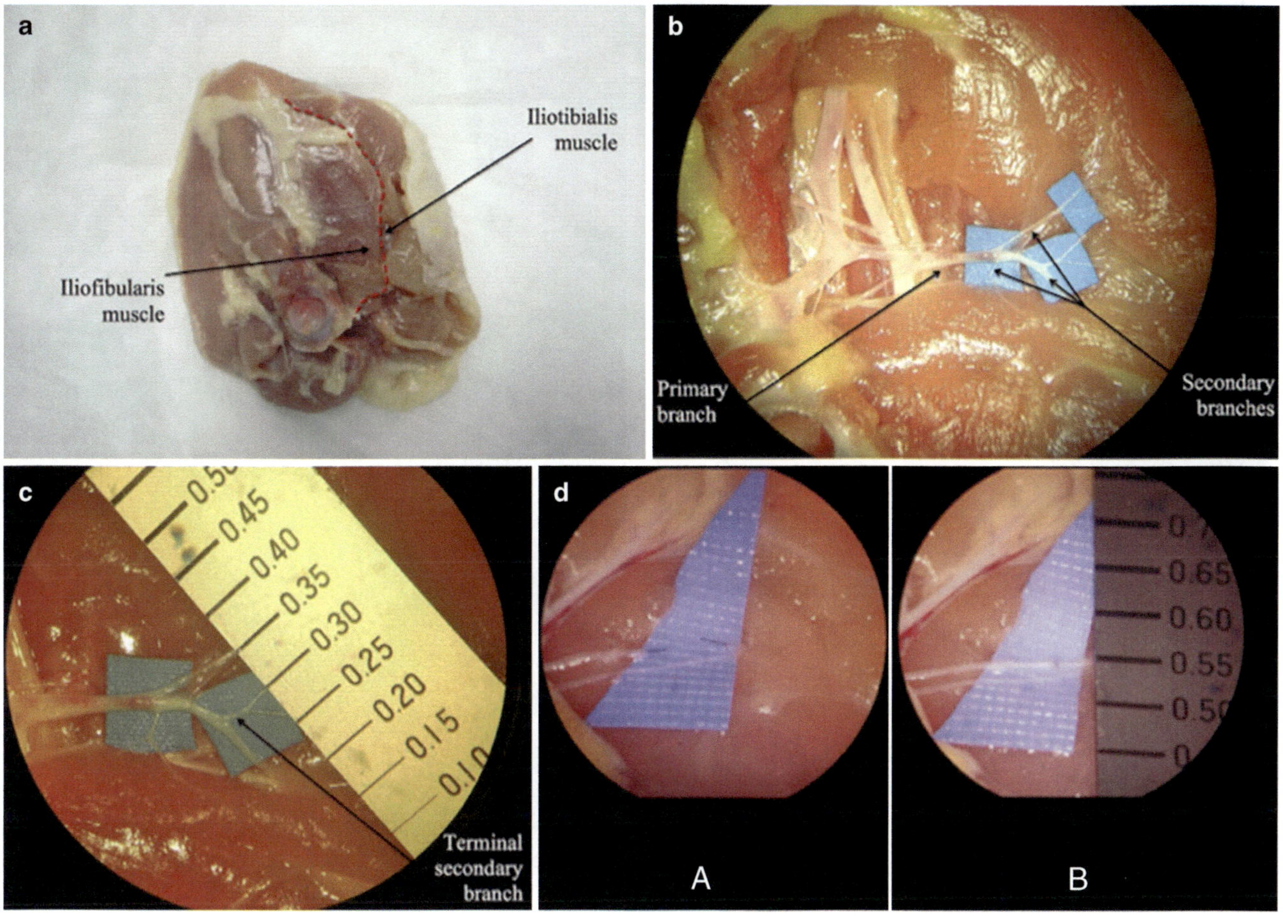

Fig. 28.7 Simple, store-bought chicken thighs can be utilized to train in supermicrosurgery in a realistic and highly effective simulation model. The chicken thighs obtained should be the bone intact variety, as the ischiatic neurovascular bundle is closely associated with the bone, and boneless chicken thighs will have damaged neurovascular anatomy. The red, dotted line indicates the intramuscular areolar plane where the neurovascular bundle can easily be found with minimal dissection (**a**). The ischiatic neurovascular bundle and its branches are seen here, under 10× magnification. The main trunk and primary branches can be used for regular microsurgical training, while the secondary and tertiary branches can be used for supermicrosurgical training (**b**). Vessels as small as 0.2–0.3 mm can usually be found in all chicken thighs (**c**). Here, a 0.55-mm vessel is anastomosed with a 12-0 nylon; a 7-0 nylon can be used as a temporary luminal stent to prevent the lumen from collapsing (**d**) (Chen WF, Eid A, Yamamoto T, Keith J, Nimmons GL, Lawrence WT. A novel supermicrosurgery training model: the chicken thigh. J Plast Reconstr Aesthet Surg. 2014;67:973–8 (reprinted with permission))

anastomosis continues to have a "back-flow" sign—signifying that venous pressure is greater than lymphatic pressure (Fig. 28.8b), the LVA is at risk of thrombosis. We found that external compression helps convert some of the unfavorable "back-flow" anastomoses to favorable "washout" anastomoses (i.e., lymph-to-vein flow direction) [24], and thus external limb compression should be applied in the OR if a "back-flow" sign continues to be observed (Figs. 28.9 and 28.10). The mechanism behind this phenomenon is likely that compression increases lymphatic pressure to a greater degree than vein pressure due to lymphatic outflow obstruction. The increased lymphatic pressure then facilitates lymphatic fluid to be emptied into the venous circulation, achieving the "washout" sign of the favorable lymph-to-vein flow direction (Fig. 28.9b) [24]. Once the operation is finished, the entire extremity should be compressed with compression bandages.

The ideal number of anastomoses per extremity is not known. In our experience [11, 23, 25] the more lymph drainage pathways that are formed the better the outcome, but beyond a certain number of anastomoses there is a diminishing return. Furthermore, the quality and functionality of lymphatic vessels are more important than the number of LVAs: more functional, healthier lymphatic vessels can generate more lymphatic drainage with less LVAs. Additional research is needed to delineate the optimal number of LVAs per affected limb, although such a study is difficult to undertake due to variations in anatomy, disease, anastomotic technique, and surgeon skill. The senior author averages between 8 and 15 anastomoses per extremity over the five-hour surgery.

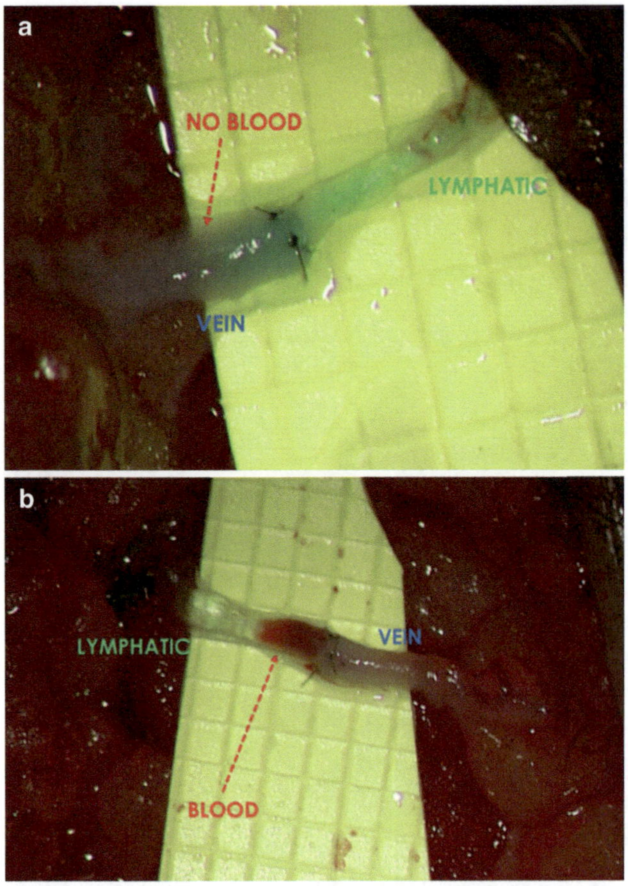

Fig. 28.8 When the lymphatic pressure exceeds the venous pressure, there is a dilution of blood in the vein as blue/green-tinted lymphatic fluid washes its way into the venous circulation; this is termed a "washout" sign and is a favorable sign demonstrating lymph-to-vein lymphatic flow (**a**). When venous pressure exceeds the lymphatic pressure, an unfavorable gradient occurs that causes venous blood to flow backward into the lymphatic system; this is termed the "back-flow" sign (**b**). Post-operative compression helps to turn some "back-flow" anastomoses to the correct, antegrade (lymph-to-vein flow) directions [24]

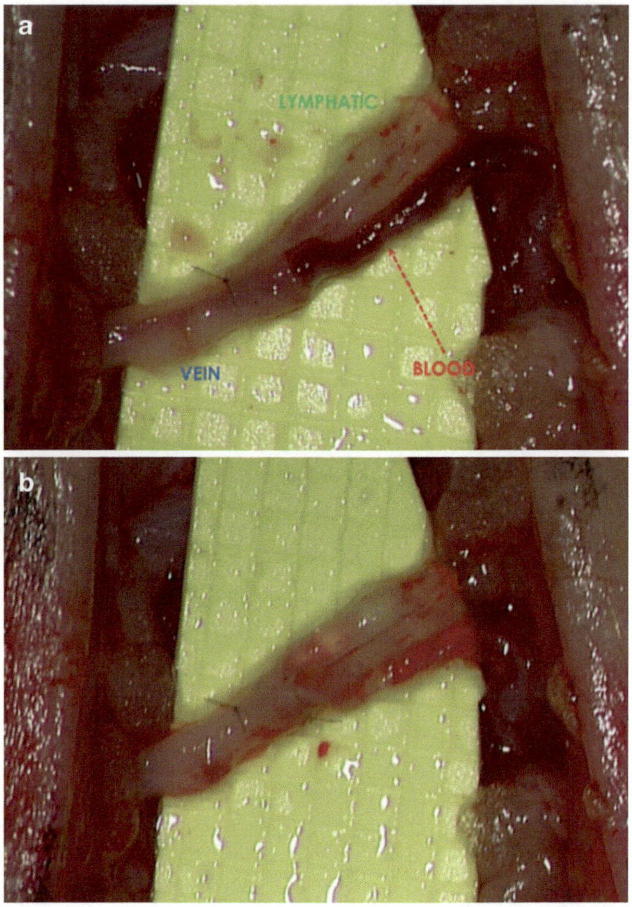

Fig. 28.9 An "octopus" anastomotic configuration with three lymphatic vessels-to-one vein LVA is seen showing "back-flow" sign in all three lymphatic vessels, which is most prominent in the inferior lymphatic vessel (**a**). After external limb compression, conversion to "washout" pattern is seen in the three lymphatic vessels, signifying forward flow (lymph-to-vein direction). Engorgement of lymph vessels can also be appreciated, especially in the top vessel (**b**). LVA, lymphaticovenular anastomosis [24]

Surgical pearls from the senior author:

1. **Using both lymph and vein mapping for strategic incision placement increases LVA success.** Although LVA can be performed when mapping either lymphatic or venous anatomy alone and finding the other vessel usually in close (~3 cm) proximity, mapping both the lymphatic and venous vessels simultaneously increases LVA success. Mapping both allows for the surgeon to make incisions precisely at the places where lymphatic and venous channels are closest together, including where one passes over the other or intersection points. In a prospective study where incision location was determined by both ICG lymphography for lymphatic mapping and near-infrared venography for venous mapping, our team saw a higher number of LVAs per incision, a higher success rate in creating LVA per incision, and smaller incisions (Figs. 28.4 and 28.5) [11, 23, 24].
2. **The number and quality of lymph drainage pathways are more important than the number of LVAs.** Healthier lymphatic vessels are more effective at transporting lymphatic fluid than damaged vessels. Ectatic vessels maybe even more efficient transporters of lymph than normal lymphatic vessels, for their peristaltic function is preserved while their diameter is enlarged. To optimize LVA quality, we recommend choosing ectatic and normal over contracted lymphatic vessels. Although the ideal number of LVAs per affected extremity is not known, it is generally agreed upon that more is better. We recommend thinking of the number of drainage pathways preferentially to the number of LVAs. For example, a side-to-end LVA has two drainage pathways: the antegrade lymph-to-vein drainage and the retrograde lymph-to-vein drainage [19, 65, 69]. Thus, a side-to-end LVA is more favorable than an end-to-end LVA, for the latter pro-

vides only one drainage pathway. If multiple lymph vessels are available but only one vein is found, the "octopus" technique can be employed to maximize the drainage pathways (Fig. 28.6c, d) [25].

3. **Immediate compression can help convert pressure gradients from unfavorable to favorable.** As the surgeon prepares a lymph vessel for LVA by either cutting it for end-to-end anastomosis or by creating a lymphotomy for side-to-end anastomosis, s/he is able to visualize lymphatic egress from the vessel. If the lymphatic egress is brisk and powerful, this is a prognostic factor for a favorable LVA pressure gradient. A swift, brisk lymphatic egress indicates a higher lymphatic pressure that is likely to easily overcome the venous pressure, allowing for lymph-to-vein drainage. When multiple LVAs are created from such lymph vessels, a prompt postoperative improvement can be expected. Conversely, when lymph vessels lack swift, spontaneous lymph egress and require distal-to-proximal massage to "milk out" the lymphatic fluid, it is indicative of poor lymph vessel peristaltic function. When LVAs are created from these poorly functioning lymphatic vessels, a "back-flow" sign is common, which demonstrates unfavorable vein-to-lymph flow direction (Figs. 28.8b and 28.9a). External compression can convert some of these unfavorable gradients to favorable ones by increasing lymphatic pressure to a greater degree than venous pressure and thus reversing the flow toward the favorable, lymph-to-vein, flow direction (Figs. 28.9b and 28.10). Our team has previously demonstrated that immediate postoperative limb compression helps to increase procedural efficacy of LVA [24].
4. **Correct instruments are crucial.** As LVAs require anastomoses with vessels in the 0.2–0.6 mm range, standard microsurgical instruments do not suffice. For example, standard microsurgical #3 and #5 jeweler's forceps have a 0.3 mm tip; this is not practical when using them to handle a 0.3 mm lymph vessel. We strongly recommend using titanium supermicrosurgical instruments with forceps tips sharpened to 0.05 mm [70]. As suture needles become important instruments in microsurgery for positioning and maneuvering the vessels and as large sutures can easily injury the small vessels, the correct size of suture and needle are also very important. Recommended sutures are 11-0 nylon with 70-μm needle for 0.5–0.8 mm vessels, and 12-0 nylon with 50-μm needle for 0.2–0.4 vessels. Larger sutures, such as 10-0 and 9-0 and their needles are simply too thick for LVA.
5. **Airborne suture tying technique will increase efficiency and decrease vessel trauma.** Originally described by Chen et al. [71], the airborne suture technique is a way to tie anastomotic sutures more efficiently. This technique keeps the short end of the suture "airborne" while the surgeon is tying the knots [72]. Keeping the suture end in the air is advantageous because when the suture end is not kept in the air—as is the case with regular tying—the short suture end usually lands and sticks to vessel adventitia, from which it needs to be grasped away. The act of grasping the suture end off of a delicate, 0.3 mm vessel runs the risk of injuring the vessel. As such, it is advantageous to keep the short suture end in the air. This technique also increases efficiency in tying. Once this technique is understood and practiced, it will soon become second nature. We believe this technique is a valuable skill and should be mastered by any surgeon who performs supermicrosurgical LVA [73].
6. **Use the "ripping" and "needle-guided" techniques for venotomy/lymphotomy creation.** Creating a venotomy or lymphotomy (i.e., side-opening in a vessel) of a precise size is challenging, especially when vessels are less than 0.5 mm. We recommend becoming familiar with two useful techniques to facilitate venotomy/lymphotomy creation: the ripping and the needle-guided technique. In the ripping technique, the surgeon gently and with control rips the vessel sidewall, layer by layer, until a side opening of the desired size is created. This technique is both simple and provides the surgeon with excellent control over the size of the opening. The needle-guided technique [74] relies on the mathematical proof that a vessel diameter is 2/3 of its flattened width (Fig. 28.11). This principle is used to precisely cut a correctly sized venotomy/lymphotomy. First, a single knot is tied in the center of the desired side-window position and a long tail is kept that will be used to gently tension the vessel sidewall up as the side window is created. Then, the flattened width of the vessel that will be anastomosed to the venotomy/lymphotomy is mentally noted against the length of a suture needle (e.g., "the flattened

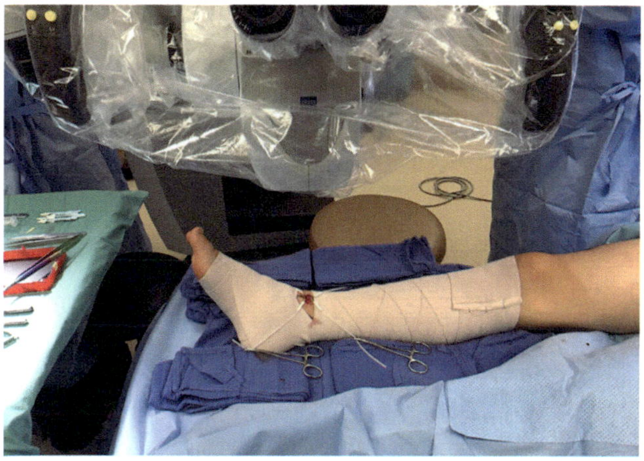

Fig. 28.10 When LVA showed a "back-flow" pattern, compression bandaging was applied both proximally and distally to the incision to promote "washout" sign, or forward (lymph-to-vein direction) lymphatic flow. LVA, lymphaticovenular anastomosis [24]

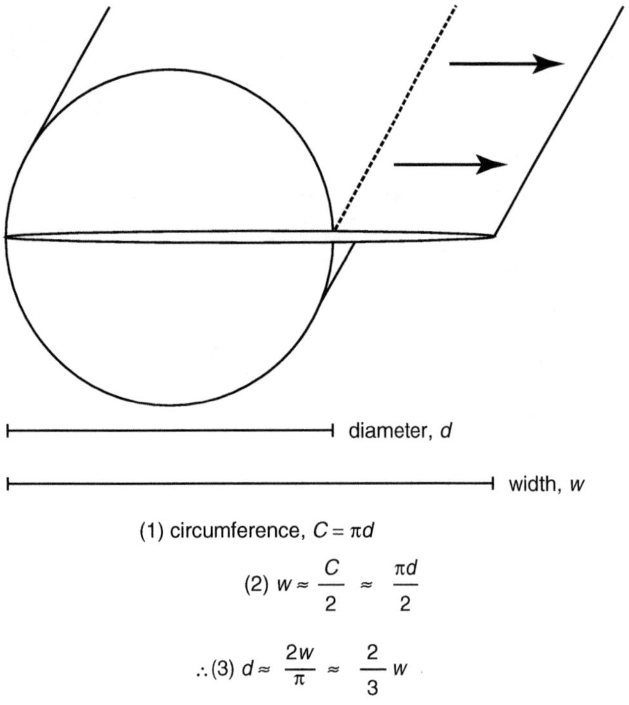

Fig. 28.11 Explanation of the mathematical basis for the measurements employed in venotomy/lymphotomy creation. The diameter of an inflated vessel is equal to two-third of its flattened width. This measurement is useful as the intraoperative flattened vessel is what a surgeon sees prior to venotomy/lymphotomy creation, while the inflated vessel with its true diameter is seen only after the anastomosis is complete and fluid flows through the anastomosis (Zeng W, Shulzhenko NO, Dingle AM, Poore SO. Precise One-Suture Needle-Guided Technique for Window Creation in Supermicrosurgical End-to-Side Anastomosis. J Reconstr Microsurg. 2018;34:e1–2 (reprinted with permission))

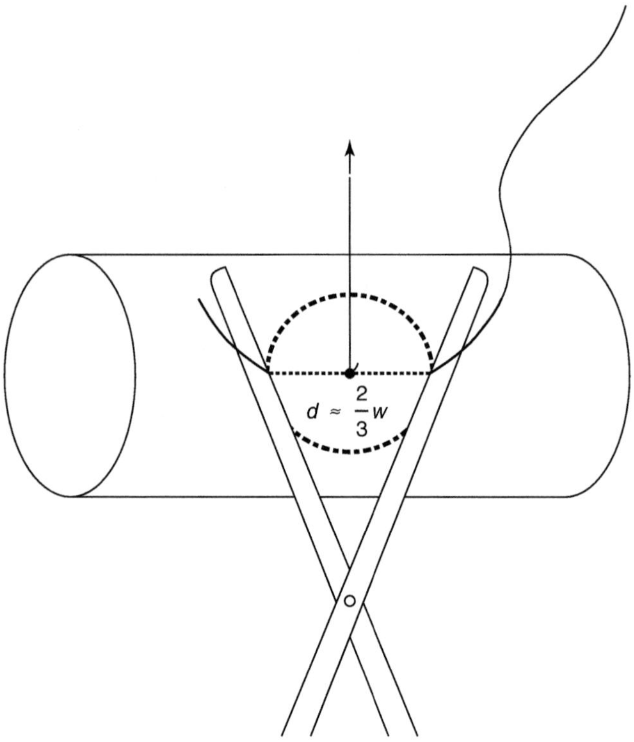

Fig. 28.12 Illustration of the venotomy/lymphotomy (side-window) creation. A single knot has been tied in the center of the desired side-window position and a long tail is kept on it, so that it can be used to gently tension the vessel sidewall up as the side-window is created. A needle is passed with entry and exit points spaced 2/3 w (2/3 of the flattened width of the vessel that will be anastomosed there). The center knot is gently tugged and the scissors are ready to cut along the curvature of the needle. This maneuver creates a side-window with a diameter equal to the diameter of the vessel that will be anastomosed there (Zeng W, Shulzhenko NO, Dingle AM, Poore SO. Precise One-Suture Needle-Guided Technique for Window Creation in Supermicrosurgical End-to-Side Anastomosis. J Reconstr Microsurg. 2018;34:e1–2 (reprinted with permission))

vessel width is about 1/2 the length of the needle"). Then, the needle is placed through the future venotomy/lymphotomy site with 2/3 of the mentally noted length buried in the vessel sidewall. Supermicrosurgical scissors are used to cut immediately underneath the partially buried suture needle as the center knot is gently pulled up; this creates a venotomy/lymphotomy with the diameter of the soon-to-be anastomosed vessel (Fig. 28.12). This technique is simple and very useful for both supermicrosurgery and microsurgery.

7. **Use a 6-0 to 8-0 suture to "stent" open the lumen of a vessel during anastomosis.** Originally described by Narushima et al. [75, 76], this technique is now widely practiced among supermicrosurgeons, especially for vessels under 0.5 mm and for end-to-side and side-to-end anastomotic configurations [19, 77]. It is helpful in preventing the lumen from collapsing, which often happens in supermicrosurgery. It is also a helpful technique for newer supermicrosurgeons. Depending on the vessel size, a suitable suture is selected and a short end is cut to function as a stent (Fig. 28.8d). Prior to inserting the suture stent, examine it under the microscope to assure that it is smooth and thus will not injure vessel intima.
8. **Overcoming the learning curve on a simulation model is imperative prior to operating on patients.** Supermicrosurgery is technically challenging and distinct in technique from regular microsurgery. It has a steep learning curve. We do not recommend even highly experienced microsurgeons to offer LVA to patients without simulation training, for the quality of LVA anastomoses predicts LVA success. Many simulation models are described, with biologic simulation models being superior to synthetic models [78, 79]. We recommend the chicken thigh simulation model, which is simple and humane (Fig. 28.8) [67, 68]. This model uses grocery store bought, bone-intact chicken thighs. The ischiatic neurovascular bundle is easily found after dissecting along the fat plane between iliotibialis and iliofibularis on the medial side of the chicken thigh. Primary, secondary,

and tertiary branches can be easily dissected from the main vessel trunks. The secondary and tertiary branches can be used for supermicrosurgical practice for all anastomotic configurations, with vessels ranging from 0.2 to 0.8 mm. In our experience, about 50 patent supermicrosurgical anastomoses are necessary prior to achieving competency in supermicrosurgery [67].

28.6 Postoperative Care

LVA is minimally invasive and can be performed as an outpatient procedure. General diet is resumed immediately. Showers are permitted on postoperative day 3; patients are instructed to avoid scrubbing the incisions and to gently pat themselves dry. Newly constructed LVAs remain delicate for about 4 weeks.

Compression (ACE) bandages are placed on the limb immediately following surgery [24]. ACE bandage application is started at the distal most part of the extremity (fingers/toes) where more pressure is applied, and pressure is gradually decreased as the bandage moves proximally up the extremity. For the first 3 weeks after surgery, patients are instructed to stand for at least 10 min every hour (and more if pain/swelling allows) and to elevate the limb above the level of the heart while resting. Patients should be provided with a sling for arms and an elevating foam block for the leg and arm. After 3 weeks, light activity is advised between periods of continued limb elevation [11, 23].

The patient is released to resume normal activities 4 weeks after surgery. Also at this time sutures are removed and patients begin seeing lymphedema therapists. Lymphedema therapists should provide home exercises for the patient and new compression garments. The compression garments should be worn daily at 30–40 mmHg; a compression regimen will help improve pain and discomfort [80, 81] as well as prevent recurrence of swelling. Lymphedema precautions should be continued even after surgical intervention [82], including compression garment use with physical activity and air travel, and caution with minor trauma (cuts and scratches). Usually, postoperative improvement is seen within 1 month, and improvement can continue to progress over a year [11].

To assess the results and efficacy of LVA at the 3 months follow up, SPY fluorescence imaging is used for visualizing ICG lymphography [83]. This is again repeated at 6 and 12 months, and then patients are imaged yearly. Compression garments can begin to be weaned off at 6 months post surgery. To wean the garments, patients can either reduce the compression strength of the garment or reduce the number of hours a day they are wearing them. If swelling recurs, weaning should be stopped and garments should be worn again; weaning can again be attempted at 12 months postoperatively.

28.7 Expected Outcomes

LVA is the surgical treatment of choice for early lymphedema, but can also be used in later stages, as long as the disease remains fluid predominant. LVA is efficacious for not only volume reduction, but also a significant improvement in symptoms including swelling, tightness, heaviness, restricted range of motion, fibrosis, and recurrent infections. Outcome measures are tracked with multiple modalities including circumference measurements, bioimpedance spectroscopy (BIS) [84], ICG lymphography [83], patient self-assessment, and quality of life assessment (LYMQOL) [85–87]. These modalities are used both preoperatively and at postoperative visits at 3-, 6-, and 12-months.

In patients who have healthy, linear patterns on ICG lymphography, lymphedema improvement can be expected soon after surgery. In general, the healthier and the more functional the lymphatic vessels are in a patient, the more effective the LVA procedure is likely to be. However, even patients who appear to have advanced disease on ICG lymphography may have excellent outcomes, as long as they have fluid-predominant disease. For example, in patients with a diffuse lymphatic pattern of Campisi stage III disease who still have a fluid-predominant status (as confirmed by BIS or MRI), there will likely be a significant improvement in symptoms after surgery (Fig. 28.13). In fluid predominant disease and concurrent diffuse lymphatic pattern, the apparent non-functionality of the lymphatic vessels (as indicated by the "diffuse" ICG pattern) may be due to high pressure in the lymphatic system from downstream blockage. After creation of LVAs, the high lymphatic pressures enable profound drainage of lymph fluid into the venous channels (Fig. 28.13). Furthermore, as lymphatic pressure is released, the non-sclerotic lymphatic vessels return to a functional status, allowing symptoms to continue to improve [11]. In congenital lymphedema patients who lack a lymphatic ICG signal [51], LVA incisions are planned along veins. In this patient population, LVA also produces improvement in lymphedema symptoms, which suggests that the lymphatic vessels that these patients have are at least somewhat functional, for they are able to move lymphatic fluid into the venous system [88].

Volume reductions after LVA vary with disease severity. For fluid-predominant disease (generally patients with Campisi stage 1 and 2 lymphedema) extremity volume will decrease significantly over the first 3–6 months after LVA and will continue to decrease up to 12 months or longer [4, 14]. For disease that has a larger solid component (generally patients with Campisi stage 3 and 4 lymphedema), extremity volume will still decrease but not as much as for fluid-predominant disease [11]. The most favorable LVA outcomes are generally seen in cases of early surgical intervention for earlier stages of lymphedema, where lymphatic vessels remain functional and fibrosis has not yet occurred.

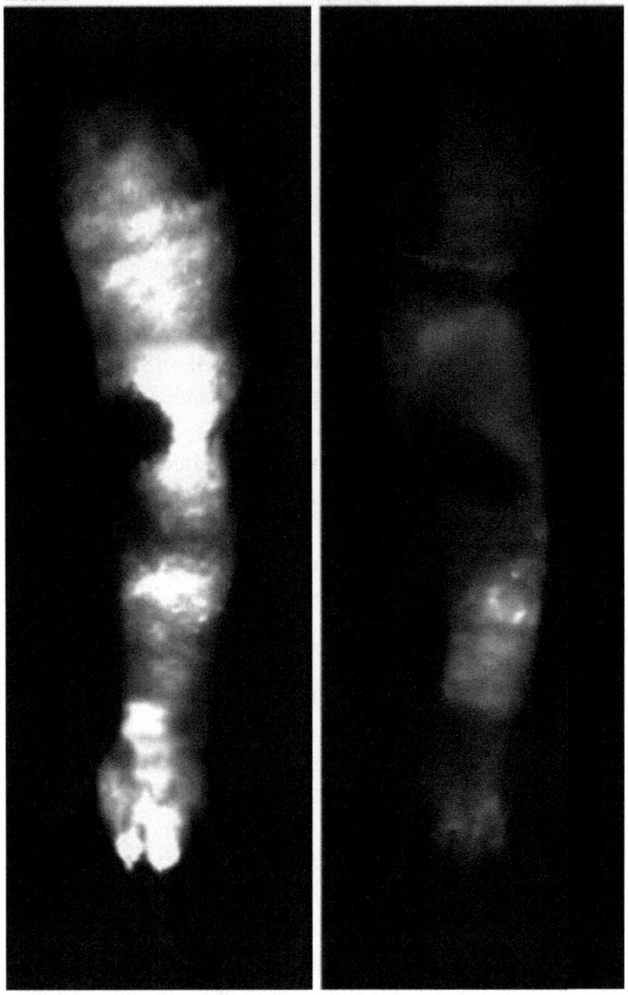

Fig. 28.13 This demonstrates a preoperative and 1-year postoperative ICG lymphography study of a patient with postmastectomy Campisi stage III lymphedema of the left arm who underwent LVA. The preoperative image shows severe dermal backflow on the hand dorsum, elbow, and upper arm. The postoperative image shows global improvement of the entire limb with a profound improvement and near resolution of the dermal backflow of the hand dorsum. ICG, indocyanine green; LVA, lymphaticovenular anastomosis (Chen WF. How to Get Started Performing Supermicrosurgical Lymphaticovenular Anastomosis to Treat Lymphedema. Ann Plast Surg. 2018;81(6S Suppl 1):S15–S20 (reprinted with permission))

Measuring outcomes is an important part of any lymphedema practice. Volume-based measurements are the most commonly used outcome measures. Volume can be measured by various ways, which were discussed previously. At our center we prefer using circumference-based lymphedema indices [89–92]; indices can reduce potential confounding variables such as changes in weight, as BMI is taken into account. Other outcome measurements include water displacement, tissue tonometry, perometer, bioimpedance spectroscopy, contrast-enhanced magnetic resonance lymphangiography, among others. We recommend that outcomes should be measured and monitored via multiple assessment methods due to limitations of each method [11].

28.8 Summary

LVA creates drainage pathways for lymphatic fluid from the lymphatic system to the venous circulation. It is an effective surgical method for lymphedema treatment. Earlier surgical interventions in earlier stages of disease correlate with faster and greater reductions of lymphedema symptoms. LVA can still be considered in later stages of disease and outcomes will still be favorable as long as the disease remains fluid predominant. Microsurgeons should not undertake LVA until they become skilled in supermicrosurgery on a simulation system, as supermicrosurgery techniques differ from microsurgery, and the quality of LVA anastomoses predict LVA success. Careful patient selection, precise surgical plan, thoughtful choice of anastomotic configuration, excellent supermicrosurgical technique, and dedicated postoperative care are crucial for successful outcomes.

References

1. Damstra R, Voesten H, Klinkert P, Brorson H. Circumferential suction-assisted lipectomy for lymphoedema after surgery for breast cancer. Br J Surg Inc Eur J Surg Swiss Surg. 2009;96:859–64.
2. Lamprou D, Voesten H, Damstra R, Wikkeling O. Circumferential suction-assisted lipectomy in the treatment of primary and secondary end-stage lymphoedema of the leg. Br J Surg. 2017;104:84–9.
3. Dumanian GA, Futrell JW. The Charles procedure: misquoted and misunderstood since 1950. Plast Reconstr Surg. 1996;98(7):1258–63.
4. Koshima I, Inagawa K, Urushibara K, Moriguchi T. Supermicrosurgical lymphaticovenular anastomosis for the treatment of lymphedema in the upper extremities. J Reconstr Microsurg. 2000;16:437–42.
5. Nagase T, Gonda K, Inoue K, Higashino T, Fukuda N, Gorai K, et al. Treatment of lymphedema with lymphaticovenular anastomoses. Int J Clin Oncol. 2005;10:304–10.
6. Dayan E, Smith ML, Sultan M, Samson W, Dayan JH. Performing vascularized groin lymph node transfer with confidence: the use of four anatomic and physiologic modalities for safe and effective flap harvest. Plast Reconstr Surg. 2013;132:60.
7. Althubaiti GA, Crosby MA, Chang DW. Vascularized supraclavicular lymph node transfer for lower extremity lymphedema treatment. Plast Reconstr Surg. 2013;131:133e–5e.
8. Koshima I, Narushima M, Mihara M, Yamamoto T, Hara H, Ohshima A, et al. Lymphadiposal flaps and lymphaticovenular anastomoses for severe leg edema: functional reconstruction for lymph drainage system. J Reconstr Microsurg. 2016;32:050–5.
9. Chen WF, Bowen M, McNurlen M, Ding J. Vascularized lymph vessel transfer with supermicrosurgical ultra-thin superficial circumflex iliac artery flap for treatment of advanced lymphedema not treatable with supermicrosurgical lymphaticovenular anastomosis. Ann Plast Surg. 2018;80.
10. Koshima I, Nanba Y, Tsutsui T, Takahashi Y, Itoh S, Fujitsu M. Minimal invasive lymphaticovenular anastomosis under local

anesthesia for leg lymphedema: is it effective for stage III and IV? Ann Plast Surg. 2004;53:261–6.
11. Chen WF, Bowen M, Ding J. Lessons learned after 100 cases supermicrosurgical lymphaticovenular anastomosis—a single surgeons' experience. Ann Plast Surg. 2018;80(suppl 3).
12. Koshima I, Inagawa K, Etoh K, Moriguchi T. Supramicrosurgical lymphaticovenular anastomosis for the treatment of lymphedema in the extremities. Nihon Geka Gakkai Zasshi. 1999;100:551–6.
13. Masia J, Olivares L, Koshima I, Teo T, Suominen S, Van Landuyt K, et al. Barcelona consensus on supermicrosurgery. J Reconstr Microsurg. 2014;30:053–8.
14. Huang G-K, Hu R-Q, Liu Z-Z, Shen Y-L, Lan T-D, Pan G-P. Microlymphaticovenous anastomosis in the treatment of lower limb obstructive lymphedema: analysis of 91 cases. Plast Reconstr Surg. 1985;76:671–85.
15. Campisi C, Tosatti E, Casaccia M, Ieracitano V, Cordaro S, Padula P, et al. Microsurgery of the lymphatic vessels. Minerva Chir. 1986;41:469.
16. Campisi C, Boccardo F. Vein graft interposition in treating peripheral lymphoedemas. Handchir Mikrochir Plast Chir. 2003;35:221–4.
17. Basta MN, Gao LL, Wu LC. Operative treatment of peripheral lymphedema: a systematic meta-analysis of the efficacy and safety of lymphovenous microsurgery and tissue transplantation. Plast Reconstr Surg. 2014;133:905–13.
18. Chang DW, Suami H, Skoracki R. A prospective analysis of 100 consecutive lymphovenous bypass cases for treatment of extremity lymphedema. Plast Reconstr Surg. 2013;132:1305–14.
19. Yamamoto T, Narushima M, Kikuchi K, Yoshimatsu H, Todokoro T, Mihara M, et al. Lambda-shaped anastomosis with intravascular stenting method for safe and effective lymphaticovenular anastomosis. Plast Reconstr Surg. 2011;127:1987–92.
20. Koshima I, Nanba Y, Tsutsui T, Takahashi Y, Itoh S. Long-term follow-up after lymphaticovenular anastomosis for lymphedema in the leg. J Reconstr Microsurg. 2003;19:209–16.
21. Dayan JH, Dayan E, Smith ML. Reverse lymphatic mapping: a new technique for maximizing safety in vascularized lymph node transfer. Plast Reconstr Surg. 2015;135:277–85.
22. Scaglioni MF, Arvanitakis M, Chen Y, Giovanoli P, Chia-Shen Yang J, Chang EI. Comprehensive review of vascularized lymph node transfers for lymphedema: outcomes and complications. Microsurgery. 2018;38:222–9.
23. Chen WF. How to get started performing supermicrosurgical lymphaticovenular anastomosis to treat lymphedema. Ann Plast Surg. 2018;81:S15–20.
24. Chen WF, Bowen M, Ding J. Immediate limb compression following supermicrosurgical lymphaticovenular anastomosis—is it helpful or harmful? Int Microsurg J IMJ. 2018;2(1):1.
25. Chen WF, Yamamoto T, Fisher M, Liao J, Carr J. The "octopus" lymphaticovenular anastomosis: evolving beyond the standard supermicrosurgical technique. J Reconstr Microsurg. 2015;31:450–7.
26. Chen WF. Is it possible to perform lymphaticovenular anastomosis after liposuction for lymphedema? J Surg. 2016;12:2.
27. Giacalone G, Yamamoto T, Hayashi A, Belva F, Gysen M, Hayashi N, et al. Lymphatic supermicrosurgery for the treatment of recurrent lymphocele and severe lymphorrhea. Microsurgery. 2019;39:326–31.
28. Lin C-H, Ali R, Chen S-C, Wallace C, Chang Y-C, Chen H-C, et al. Vascularized groin lymph node transfer using the wrist as a recipient site for management of postmastectomy upper extremity lymphedema. Plast Reconstr Surg. 2009;123:1265–75.
29. Cheng M-H, Huang J-J, Nguyen DH, Saint-Cyr M, Zenn MR, Tan BK, et al. A novel approach to the treatment of lower extremity lymphedema by transferring a vascularized submental lymph node flap to the ankle. Gynecol Oncol. 2012;126:93–8.
30. Chen H-C, O'Brien BM, Rogers I, Pribaz J, Eaton C. Lymph node transfer for the treatment of obstructive lymphoedema in the canine model. Br J Plast Surg. 1990;43:578–86.
31. Batista BN, Germain M, Faria JCM, Becker C. Lymph node flap transfer for patients with secondary lower limb lymphedema. Microsurgery. 2017;37:29–33.
32. Mardonado AA, Chen R, Chang DW. The use of supraclavicular free flap with vascularized lymph node transfer for treatment of lymphedema: a prospective study of 100 consecutive cases. J Surg Oncol. 2017;115:68–71.
33. Gould DJ, Mehrara BJ, Neligan P, Cheng M, Patel KM. Lymph node transplantation for the treatment of lymphedema. J Surg Oncol. 2018;118:736–42.
34. Cheng M-H, Chen S-C, Henry SL, Tan BK, Lin MC-Y, Huang J-J. Vascularized groin lymph node flap transfer for postmastectomy upper limb lymphedema: flap anatomy, recipient sites, and outcomes. Plast Reconstr Surg. 2013;131:1286–98.
35. Chen WF, McNurlen M, Ding J, Bowen M. Vascularized lymph vessel transfer for extremity lymphedema—is transfer of lymph node still necessary? Int Microsurg J IMJ. 2019;3(3):1.
36. Boyages J, Kastanias K, Koelmeyer LA, Winch CJ, Lam TC, Sherman KA, et al. Liposuction for advanced lymphedema: a multidisciplinary approach for complete reduction of arm and leg swelling. Ann Surg Oncol. 2015;22:1263–70.
37. Chen WF, Zeng W-F, Hawkes PJ, Man J, Bowen M. Lymphedema liposuction with immediate limb contouring. Plast Reconstr Surg Glob Open. 2019;7.
38. Sapountzis S, Ciudad P, Lim SY, Chilgar RM, Kiranantawat K, Nicoli F, et al. Modified Charles procedure and lymph node flap transfer for advanced lower extremity lymphedema. Microsurgery. 2014;34:439–47.
39. Edwards J, Kinmonth J. Lymphovenous shunts in man. Br Med J. 1969;4:579–86.
40. Case TC, Witte CL, Witte MH, Unger EC, Williams WH. Magnetic resonance imaging in human lymphedema: comparison with lymphangioscintigraphy. Magn Reson Imaging. 1992;10:549–58.
41. Werner G, Scheck R, Kaiserling E. Magnetic resonance imaging of peripheral lymphedema. Lymphology. 1998;31:34–6.
42. Tassenoy A, Vermeiren K, van der Veen P, Stadnik T, De Ridder F, Peeters E, et al. Demonstration of tissue alterations by ultrasonography, magnetic resonance imaging and spectroscopy, and histology in breast cancer patients without lymphedema after axillary node dissection. Lymphology. 2006;39:118–26.
43. Li Y, Lu Q, Chen T, Yao Y, Zhao Z, Li Y, et al. Thickness of soft tissue of lower extremities measured with magnetic resonance imaging as a new indicator for staging unilateral secondary lower extremity lymphedema. Acta Radiol. 2015;56:1016–24.
44. Wang L, Wu X, Wu M, Zhao Z, Tang H, Li S, et al. Edema areas of calves measured with magnetic resonance imaging as a novel indicator for early staging of lower extremity lymphedema. Lymphat Res Biol. 2018;16:240–7.
45. Trinh L, Peterson P, Brorson H, Månsson S. Assessment of subfascial muscle/water and fat accumulation in lymphedema patients using magnetic resonance imaging. Lymphat Res Biol. 2019;17:340–6.
46. Seward C, Skolny M, Brunelle C, Asdourian M, Salama L, Taghian AG. A comprehensive review of bioimpedance spectroscopy as a diagnostic tool for the detection and measurement of breast cancer-related lymphedema. J Surg Oncol. 2016;114:537–42.
47. Steele ML, Janda M, Vagenas D, Ward LC, Cornish BH, Box R, et al. A bioimpedance spectroscopy-based method for diagnosis of lower-limb lymphedema. Lymphat Res Biol. 2020;18(2):101–9.
48. Qin ES, Bowen MJ, James SL, Chen WF. Multi-segment bioimpedance can assess patients with bilateral lymphedema. J Plast Reconstr Aesthet Surg. 2020;73:328–36.

49. Yamamoto T, Narushima M, Doi K, Oshima A, Ogata F, Mihara M, et al. Characteristic indocyanine green lymphography findings in lower extremity lymphedema: the generation of a novel lymphedema severity staging system using dermal backflow patterns. Plast Reconstr Surg. 2011;127:1979–86.
50. Yamamoto T, Yamamoto N, Doi K, Oshima A, Yoshimatsu H, Todokoro T, et al. Indocyanine green-enhanced lymphography for upper extremity lymphedema: a novel severity staging system using dermal backflow patterns. Plast Reconstr Surg. 2011;128:941–7.
51. Yamamoto T, Yoshimatsu H, Narushima M, Yamamoto N, Hayashi A, Koshima I. Indocyanine green lymphography findings in primary leg lymphedema. Eur J Vasc Endovasc Surg. 2015;49:95–102.
52. Hara H, Mihara M, Seki Y, Todokoro T, Iida T, Koshima I. Comparison of indocyanine green lymphographic findings with the conditions of collecting lymphatic vessels of limbs in patients with lymphedema. Plast Reconstr Surg. 2013;132:1612–8.
53. Mihara M, Hara H, Hayashi Y, Narushima M, Yamamoto T, Todokoro T, et al. Pathological steps of cancer-related lymphedema: histological changes in the collecting lymphatic vessels after lymphadenectomy. PLoS One. 2012;7.
54. Hara H, Mihara M, Ohtsu H, Narushima M, Iida T, Koshima I. Indication of lymphaticovenous anastomosis for lower limb primary lymphedema. Plast Reconstr Surg. 2015;136:883–93.
55. Lee B, Andrade M, Bergan J, Boccardo F, Campisi C, Damstra R, et al. Diagnosis and treatment of primary lymphedema. Consensus document of the International Union of Phlebology (IUP)-2009. Int Angiol. 2010;29:454–70.
56. Hara H, Mihara M, Anan T, Fukumoto T, Narushima M, Iida T, et al. Pathological investigation of acquired lymphangiectasia accompanied by lower limb lymphedema: lymphocyte infiltration in the dermis and epidermis. Lymphat Res Biol. 2016;14:172–80.
57. Campisi C, Da Rin E, Bellini C, Bonioli E, Boccardo F. Pediatric lymphedema and correlated syndromes: role of microsurgery. Microsurg Off J Int Microsurg Soc Eur Fed Soc Microsurg. 2008;28:138–42.
58. Greene AK, Goss JA. Diagnosis and staging of lymphedema. New York: Thieme; 2018. p. 012–6.
59. Rockson SG, Miller LT, Senie R, Brennan MJ, Casley-Smith JR, Földi E, et al. Workgroup III: diagnosis and management of lymphedema. Cancer Interdiscip Int J Am Cancer Soc. 1998;83:2882–5.
60. Narushima M, Yamamoto T, Ogata F, Yoshimatsu H, Mihara M, Koshima I. Indocyanine green lymphography findings in limb lymphedema. J Reconstr Microsurg. 2016;32:072–9.
61. Mihara M, Hara H, Narushima M, Todokoro T, Iida T, Ohtsu H, et al. Indocyanine green lymphography is superior to lymphoscintigraphy in imaging diagnosis of secondary lymphedema of the lower limbs. J Vasc Surg Venous Lymphat Disord. 2013;1:194–201.
62. Yamamoto T, Iida T, Matsuda N, Kikuchi K, Yoshimatsu H, Mihara M, et al. Indocyanine green (ICG)-enhanced lymphography for evaluation of facial lymphoedema. J Plast Reconstr Aesthet Surg. 2011;64:1541–4.
63. Chan VS, Narushima M, Hara H, Yamamoto T, Mihara M, Iida T, et al. Local anesthesia for lymphaticovenular anastomosis. Ann Plast Surg. 2014;72:180–3.
64. Hara H, Mihara M. Multi-area lymphaticovenous anastomosis with multi-lymphosome injection in indocyanine green lymphography: a prospective study. Microsurgery. 2019;39:167–73.
65. Yamamoto T, Yoshimatsu H, Narushima M, Yamamoto N, Koshima I. Split intravascular stents for side-to-end lymphaticovenular anastomosis. Ann Plast Surg. 2013;71:538–40.
66. Yamamoto T, Kikuchi K, Yoshimatsu H, Koshima I. Ladder-shaped lymphaticovenular anastomosis using multiple side-to-side lymphatic anastomoses for a leg lymphedema patient. Microsurgery. 2014;34:404–8.
67. Chen WF, Eid A, Yamamoto T, Keith J, Nimmons GL, Lawrence WT. A novel supermicrosurgery training model: the chicken thigh. J Plast Reconstr Aesthet Surg. 2014;67:973–8.
68. Zeng W, Shulzhenko NO, Feldman CC, Dingle AM, Poore SO. "Blue-blood"-infused chicken thigh training model for microsurgery and supermicrosurgery. Plast Reconstr Surg Glob Open. 2018;6.
69. Yamamoto T, Yoshimatsu H, Yamamoto N, Narushima M, Iida T, Koshima I. Side-to-end lymphaticovenular anastomosis through temporary lymphatic expansion. PLoS One. 2013;8.
70. Mihara M, Hayashi Y, Iida T, Narushima M, Koshima I. Instruments for supermicrosurgery in Japan. Plast Reconstr Surg. 2012;129:404e–6e.
71. Chen H-C, Mardini S, Tsai F-C. "Airborne" suture tying technique for the microvascular anastomosis. Plast Reconstr Surg. 2004;113:1225–8.
72. Agko M, Ciudad P, Chen H. "Airborne" suture tying technique: simple steps to make it easy. Head Neck. 2017;39:2558–61.
73. Onoda S, Masahito K. The utility of the airborne technique for lymphaticovenular anastomosis. Plast Reconstr Surg. 2019;143:459e–60e.
74. Zeng W, Shulzhenko NO, Dingle AM, Poore SO. Precise one-suture needle-guided technique for window creation in supermicrosurgical end-to-side anastomosis. J Reconstr Microsurg. 2018;34:e1–2.
75. Narushima M, Koshima I, Mihara M, Uchida G, Gonda K. Intravascular stenting (IVaS) for safe and precise supermicrosurgery. Ann Plast Surg. 2008;60:41–4.
76. Nuri T, Ueda K, Yamada A, Hara M. Preparatory intravascular stenting technique: an easier method of supermicrosurgical lymphaticovenular anastomosis. Ann Plast Surg. 2013;71:541–3.
77. Ayestaray B, Andreoletti J-B. The hemi-stenting technique in lymphaticovenular anastomosis. J Plast Reconstr Aesthet Surg. 2013;66:438–9.
78. Malagón-López P, Carrasco-López C, Vilà J, Pi-Folguera J, Higueras-Suñe C. Supermicrosurgery training model for lymphaticovenous anastomosis in advanced lymphedema by iliolumbar vein and ureter anastomosis in the rat. Microsurgery. 2019;39:480–1.
79. Yamashita S, Sugiyama N, Hasegawa K, Namba Y, Kimata Y. A novel model for supermicrosurgery training: the superficial inferior epigastric artery flap in rats. J Reconstr Microsurg. 2008;24:537–43.
80. Brorson H, Ohlin K, Olsson G, Svensson B, Svensson H. Controlled compression and liposuction treatment for lower extremity lymphedema. Lymphology. 2008;41:52–63.
81. Brorson H, Svensson H. Liposuction combined with controlled compression therapy reduces arm lymphedema more effectively than controlled compression therapy alone. Plast Reconstr Surg. 1998;1058–67.
82. Chang DW, Masia J, Garza R III, Skoracki R, Neligan PC. Lymphedema: surgical and medical therapy. Plast Reconstr Surg. 2016;138:209S–18S.
83. Chen WF, Zhao H, Yamamoto T, Hara H, Ding J. Indocyanine green lymphographic evidence of surgical efficacy following microsurgical and supermicrosurgical lymphedema reconstructions. J Reconstr Microsurg. 2016;32:688–98.
84. Qin ES, Bowen MJ, Chen WF. Diagnostic accuracy of bioimpedance spectroscopy in patients with lymphedema: a retrospective cohort analysis. J Plast Reconstr Aesthet Surg. 2018;71:1041–50.
85. Patel KM, Lin C-Y, Cheng M-H. A prospective evaluation of lymphedema-specific quality-of-life outcomes following vascularized lymph node transfer. Ann Surg Oncol. 2015;22:2424–30.
86. Phillips GS, Gore S, Ramsden A, Furniss D. Lymphaticovenular anastomosis improves quality of life and limb volume in patients with secondary lymphedema after breast cancer treatment. Breast J. 2019;25:859–64.

87. Salgarello M, Mangialardi ML, Pino V, Gentileschi S, Visconti G. A prospective evaluation of health-related quality of life following lymphaticovenular anastomosis for upper and lower extremities lymphedema. J Reconstr Microsurg. 2018;34:701–7.
88. Yamamoto T, Koshima I, Yoshimatsu H, Narushima M, Miahara M, Iida T. Simultaneous multi-site lymphaticovenular anastomoses for primary lower extremity and genital lymphoedema complicated with severe lymphorrhea. J Plast Reconstr Aesthet Surg. 2011;64:812–5.
89. Yamamoto T, Matsuda N, Todokoro T, Yoshimatsu H, Narushima M, Mihara M, et al. Lower extremity lymphedema index: a simple method for severity evaluation of lower extremity lymphedema. Ann Plast Surg. 2011;67:637–40.
90. Yamamoto T, Yamamoto N, Hara H, Mihara M, Narushima M, Koshima I. Upper extremity lymphedema index: a simple method for severity evaluation of upper extremity lymphedema. Ann Plast Surg. 2013;70:47–9.
91. Yamamoto N, Yamamoto T, Hayashi N, Hayashi A, Iida T, Koshima I. Arm volumetry versus upper extremity lymphedema index: validity of upper extremity lymphedema index for body-type corrected arm volume evaluation. Ann Plast Surg. 2016;76:697–9.
92. Yamamoto T, Yamamoto N, Hayashi N, Hayashi A, Koshima I. Practicality of the lower extremity lymphedema index: lymphedema index versus volumetry-based evaluations for body-type–corrected lower extremity volume evaluation. Ann Plast Surg. 2016;77:115–8.

Microsurgery: Lymph Node/Flap Transplantation

29

Li Ping

Abstract

Vascularized supraclavicular lymph node flap and vascularized inguinal lymph node flap transplantation are two surgical options for lymphedema. These operations include the microvascular transplantation of functional lymph nodes into an affected extremity to restore physiological lymphatic function. The lymph nodes are distributed around the flap vascular pedicle. The donor site of the flap is concealed, and there is little surgical trauma as harvesting the donor flap. Only the anastomosis of artery and vein is needed, while no lymphatic-venous anastomosis is needed. It is suitable for progressive lymphedema in which the lymphatic-venous cannot be found for anastomosis. The mechanism of these operations is not fully clear. Complications include iatrogenic lymphedema and chronic pain at the donor site.

Keywords

Lymphedema · Microsurgery · Free flap · Vascularized lymph node transfer · Supraclavicular lymph node flap · Vascularized groin lymph node flap

As one of the surgical methods to reconstruct the lymphokinesis, the vascularized lymph node flap transplantation is to freely transplant a group of normal functioning lymph nodes and blood vessels in the form of tissue flap through microsurgical technique to the limb subject to lymphedema, thus realizing the purpose of reconstructing the lymphatic return pathways. This surgical method has been widely applied clinically since its first report in 1982 and satisfied clinical effects have been achieved [1, 2]. The traditional lymphatic venous anastomosis requires sufficient functioning lymphatic vessels to reconstruct lymphokinesis with veins, which is applicable to early lymphedema. For the advanced fibrotic lymphedema or congenital lymphedema, the vascularized lymph nodes flap transplantation is more suitable with longer curative effects and higher proportion of suspending postoperative pressure therapy [3, 4]. Literatures report that the donor sites of the vascularized lymph node flaps that are usually adopted include the submandibular lymph node flap, the inguinal lymph node flap, the supraclavicular lymph node flap, and the omentum majus lymph node flap. The recipient sites of the vascularized lymph node flaps can be selected at the proximal or distal end of the limb, both of which can achieve therapeutic purposes [5]. For the action mechanism of vascularized lymph node flap in reconstructing the limb lymphokinesis, it is still unclear yet. Generally, it is believed that there may be two mechanisms. One is the "pump" hypothesis of lymph nodes, that is, the transplanted lymph nodes can absorb the lymph fluid from the surrounding tissues, and the backflow lymph fluid is directly pumped to the flap veins and back to the blood through the inherent lymph-venous structure in the lymph nodes, functioning similar to a "pump" in the lymphatic return pathway. Another hypothesis believes that the transplanted vascularized lymph nodes can secrete cytokines, mainly the vascular endothelial growth factor-C (VEGF-C) that can promote lymphatic regeneration in tissues surrounding the transplanted lymph nodes to reconstruct the lymphatic return [6, 7]. The complications of vascularized lymph node flap transplantation may include flap necrosis due to vascular crisis, delayed wound healing, wound infection, and wound pains. There are also reports of iatrogenic lymphedema at donor sites in a few cases [8].

L. Ping (✉)
Department of Microsurgery, Trauma and Hand Surgery, The First Affiliated Hospital Sun Yat-sen University, Guangzhou, P.R. China

N. Liu (ed.), *Peripheral Lymphedema*, https://doi.org/10.1007/978-981-16-3484-0_29

29.1 Vascularized Supraclavicular Lymph Node Flap

The supraclavicular flap was originally applied to repair soft tissues in the head and neck. The supraclavicular lymph nodes are distributed around the vascular pedicle mainly for draining lymph fluid from the lungs, the esophagus, and the thyroid gland. As its excision will seldomly affect the lymphatic return at the donor site, it has been recently applied to the treatment of lymphedema [9–11].

The arterial supply of the flap: from the perforating branch of the transverse cervical artery, which originates from the thyroid neck stem. The length of the vascular pedicle is 4.72 ± 1.03 cm on the right and 4.86 ± 0.99 cm on the left; the number of lymph nodes in the flap is 1.5 ± 1.85 on the right and 3 ± 2.26 on the left; the distance of the lymph nodes to the jugular vein incision is 8.29 ± 2.15 cm on the right and 6.10 ± 1.21 cm on the left. The venous return of the flap: the accompanying veins of the transverse cervical artery and the branch of the external jugular vein.

29.1.1 Surgical Incision Design and Surgical Techniques

The flap is located in the posterior cervical triangle. The flap is designed oval in shape and about 10 × 4 cm in size. The inferior margin is 1.5 cm above the collarbone with the anterior margin to the sternocleidomastoid and the posterior margin to the trapezius and the external jugular vein. First, incise the anterior margin and dissect layer by layer. The transverse carotid artery is located on the deep omohyoid and the shallow anterior scalene muscle. Following the transverse cervical blood vessels (from the sternocleidomastoid to the trapezius), do not separate the vessels from the fibrofatty tissue on the surface. The lymph nodes are located in this layer. During the surgery, there is no need of exposing the lymph nodes and the omohyoid passes through the flap. Incise the omohyoid from the inside or outside of the flap, and extract it from the flap, then repair the omohyoid as incised before the flap donor site is sutured. Incise the posterior margin of the flap and dissect the complete flap. Keep the branches of the external jugular vein and the superficial jugular vein in the flap, suture the donor site of the supraclavicular flap directly to close the incision. If the recipient site of the vascularized lymph node flap is chosen on the foot back, dissect the dorsal pedal artery and the accompanying vein for end-to-end anastomosis with the flap's nutrient vessels respectively to reconstruct the flap's blood supply, and finally place the drainage tube. Observe the flap's blood supply closely after surgery.

Advantages of the supraclavicular lymph node flap: the concealed position of the flap, very small risk of iatrogenic lymphedema at the donor site, fewer subcutaneous soft tissues of the flap; disadvantages of the flap: relatively great anatomical variation of the vascular pedicle, complex structure of the supraclavicular fossa, involving many important tissue structures such as the carotid artery, the brachial plexus, the accessory nerves, and the thoracic ducts, which require careful dissection to avoid damaging these tissues.

Case 1: Female, 59 years old, who was subject to stage II lymphedema of both lower limbs after radical treatment and pelvic lymph node dissection because of cervical cancer, more severe for the right side and no response to conservative treatment for 6 months (Fig. 29.1). The right supraclavicular lymph node flap was transplanted after hospitalization to treat the right lower limb lymphedema (Figs. 29.2, 29.3, 29.4, 29.5, 29.6, 29.7, 29.8, and 29.9).

Case 2: Male, 29 years old, who has been subject to the secondary lymphedema of both lower limbs for 3 years after inguinal lymphadenectomy because of testicular cancer, more severe for the left lower limb and no obvious response

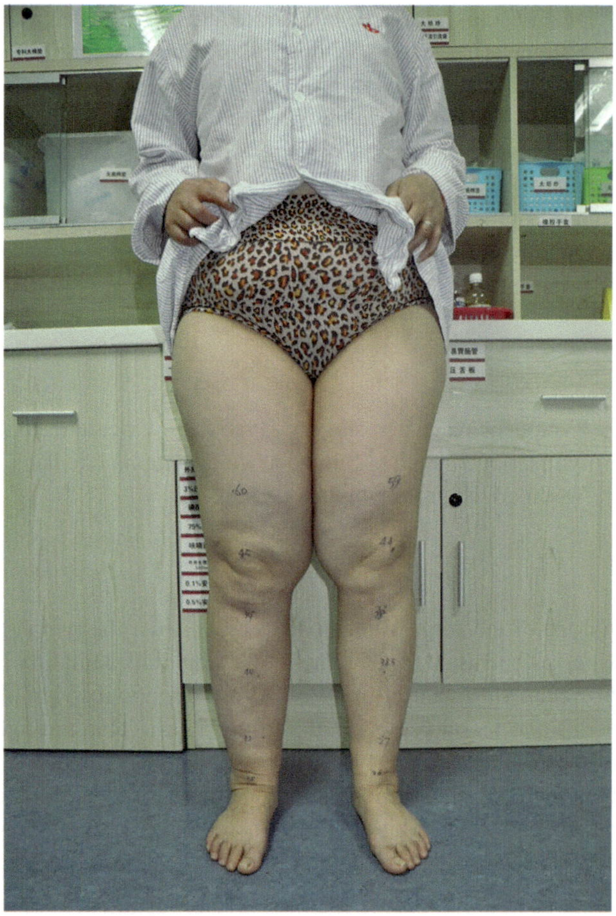

Fig. 29.1 Stage II lymphedema of both lower limbs before surgery, more severe for the right side

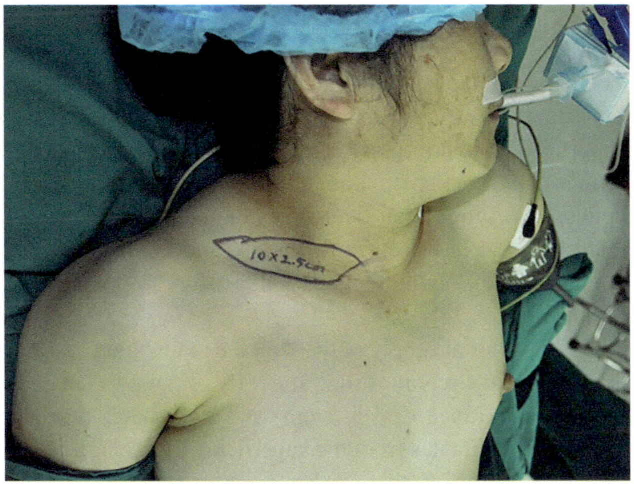

Fig. 29.2 Design of right supraclavicular lymph node flap, 10 × 2.5 cm

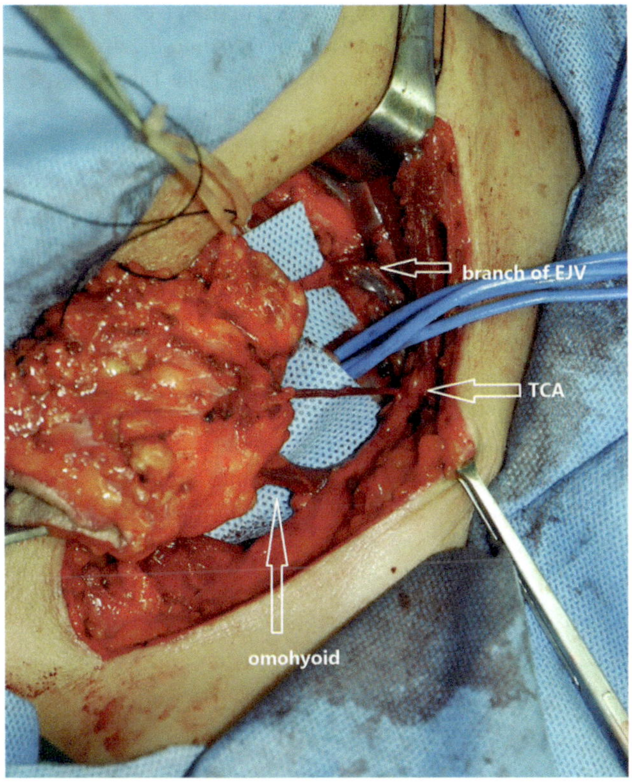

Fig. 29.3 Vascular dissection of the flap

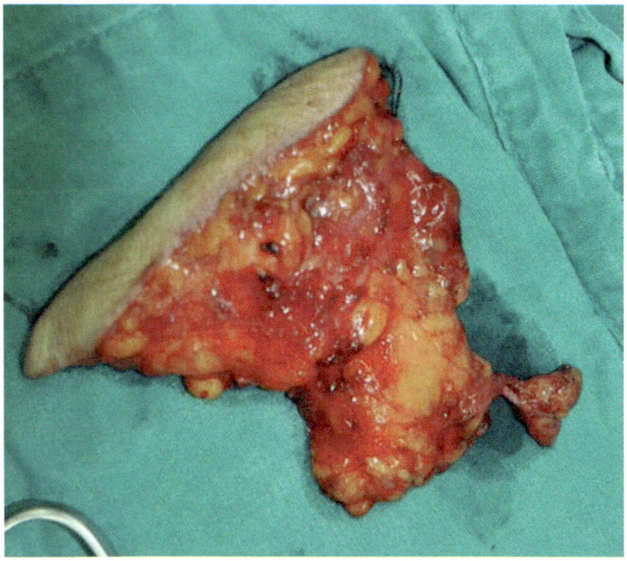

Fig. 29.4 Completion of the flap dissection

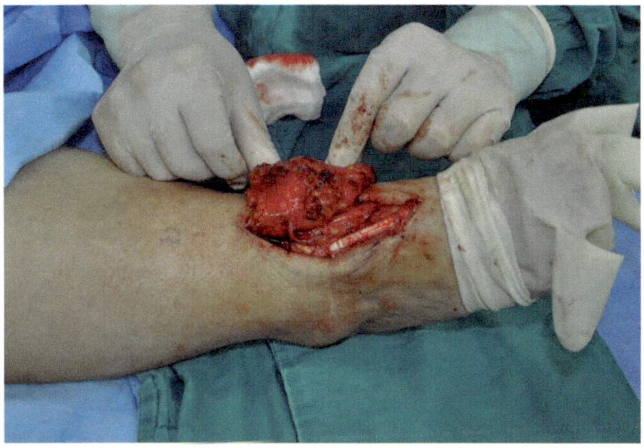

Fig. 29.5 Transplantation of the flap to the foot and completion of the vascular anastomosis

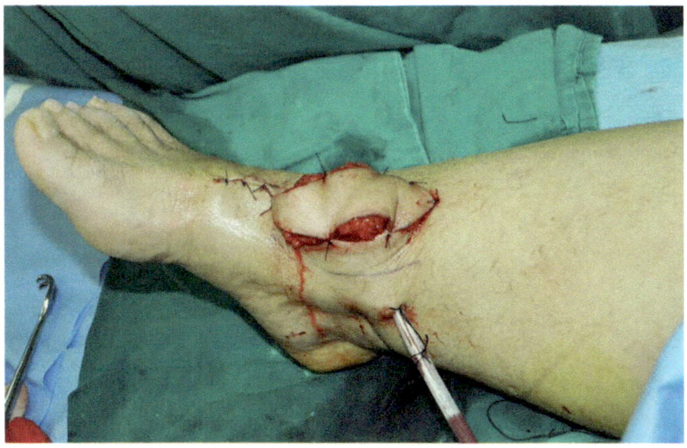

Fig. 29.6 Completion of the flap transplantation

to conservative treatment for 1 year (Fig. 29.10). The right supraclavicular lymph node flap was transplanted to treat the left lower limb lymphedema (Figs. 29.11, 29.12, 29.13, 29.14, 29.15, 29.16, and 29.17).

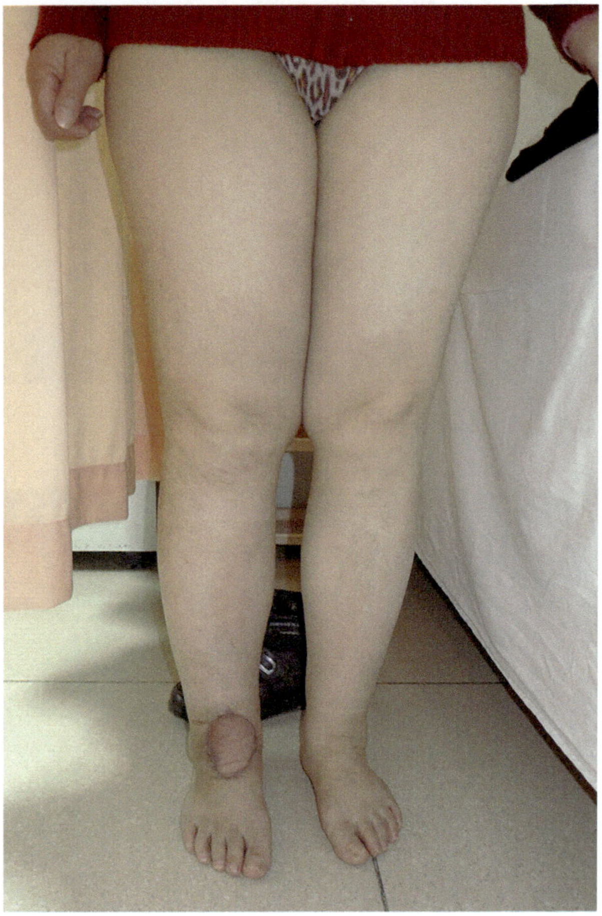

Fig. 29.7 The circumference of the right thigh and the right shank was reduced by 2 cm and 1.5 cm respectively 10 months after surgery

29.2 Inguinal Lymph Node Flap

The inguinal flap is the first free flap used clinically mainly for repairing wounds and soft tissues. This flap uses the superficial iliac artery as the vascular pedicle. It has been found that the flap contains superficial inguinal lymph nodes, therefore, it can be used as the vascularized lymph node flap and has been most widely applied in the transplantation of lymph node flap for treatment of lymphedema.

For the arterial supply of the flap: the main blood vessel is the superficial circumflex iliac artery (SCIA) with a length of about 2 cm (range of 1.5–3 cm) and a diameter of about 1.5 mm. It originates from the superficial femoral artery and functions upward to the anterior superior spine; or it originates from the same trunk with the superficial inferior epigastric artery (SIEA). For the venous return of the flap: the superficial iliac vein functions subcutaneously in the inguinal region with a length of about 3 cm (range of 2–4 cm) and a diameter of about 1.8 mm, then flows into the great saphenous vein [12]. The number of lymph nodes ranges between 3.6 ± 2.5 on the left and 3.0 ± 1.6 on the right.

The surgical method: mark the pubic tubercle, the anterior superior spine, the inguinal ligament, and the femoral artery before surgery. The medial margin of the flap should not exceed the femoral artery with the lateral margin along the medial margin of the sartorius muscle, the superior margin of 2 cm above the inguinal ligament, the inferior margin at the position where the superficial circumflex vein meets the great saphenous vein. The flap is designed oval, generally 10×5 cm in size. The surgical approach from "the pedicle to the flap's outer margin" can be adopted. First of all, incise the skin on the surface of the femoral artery pulsation to expose the superficial condylar vein and trace it to the great saphenous vein. If the superficial iliac circumflex artery is

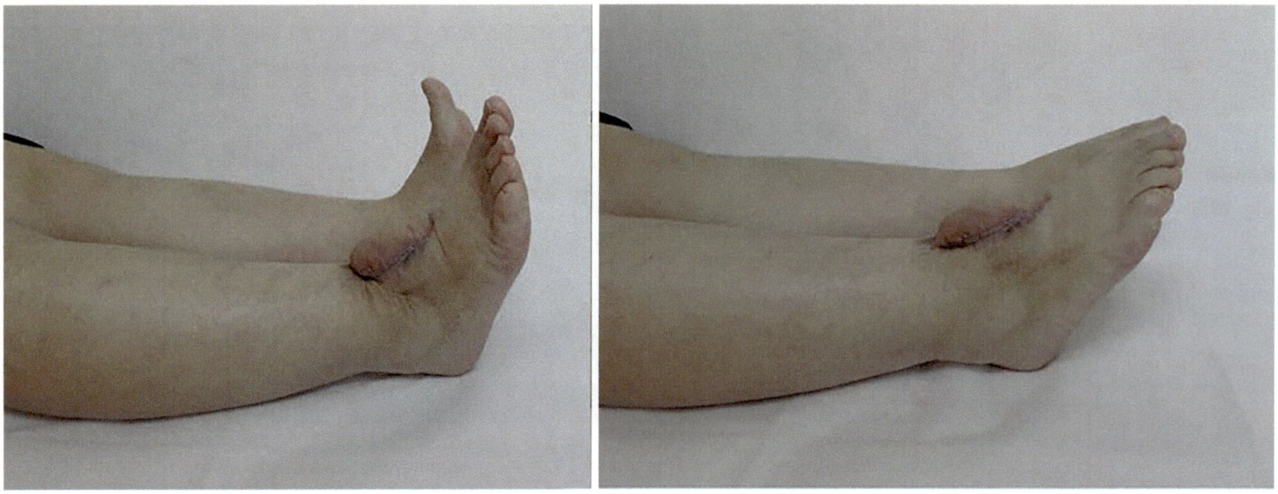

Fig. 29.8 The ankle functioned normally 10 months after surgery

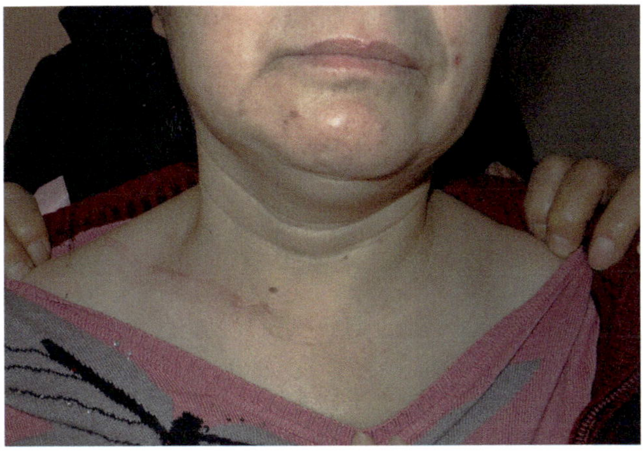

Fig. 29.9 No iatrogenic lymphedema at the flap's donor site

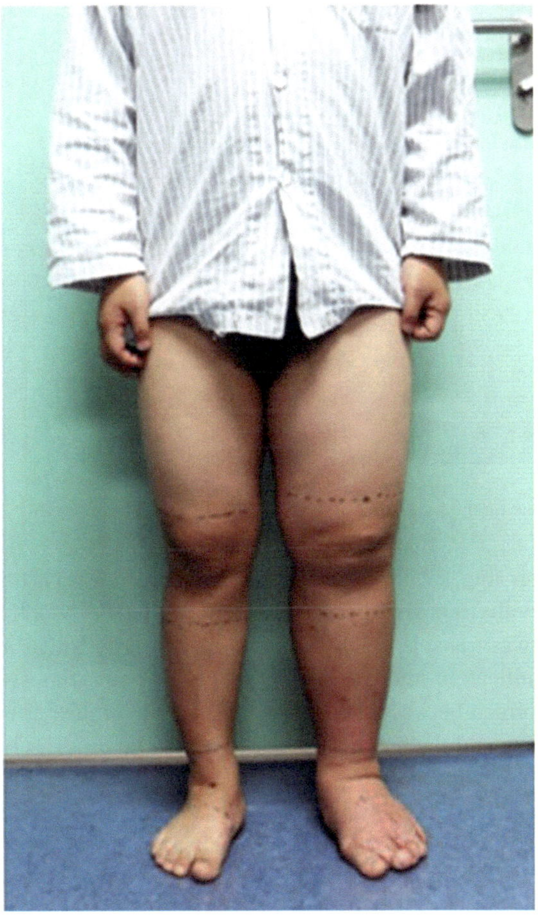

Fig. 29.10 Stage II secondary lymphedema of both lower limbs before surgery, more severe to the left side

found in the surgical field, the femoral artery is traced until its origin; if no superficial iliac circumflex artery is found, seek the origin of superficial iliac circumflex artery from the femoral artery. Open the deep fascia and the femoral artery sheath meanwhile for avoiding damaging the superficial iliac circumflex artery. When the superficial iliac circumflex artery is found, this artery is generally divided into superficial and deep branches after 1 cm course. The superficial branch and the lymph nodes are contained in the adipose tissue, and have many small blood vessels. Carefully dissect and retain the superficial branch. If the superficial branch is thin, the deep branch has to be kept at the same time and ligated to enter the branch of the lower muscle. Carefully observe the course of the vascular pedicle to ensure that it is in the center of the flap and then design the flap range. Alternatively, the surgical approach from the "outer margin of the flap to the pedicle" can be adopted. First of all, separate from the anterior superior spine and the inguinal ligament. If no superficial iliac artery is found, incise from the outer margin of the sartorius muscle and strip on the muscle fascia surface toward the pedicle. When the deep branch of the superficial iliac circumflex artery is found on the underside of the flap, ligate the artery to enter the branch of the lower muscle, continue the separation toward the pedicle until the femoral artery is found. Incise the skin above the pedicle and separate the subcutaneous tissue to find the superficial iliac circumflex vein and trace it to the great saphenous vein. After excision of the venous pedicle, the flap excision process is finally completed. When treating the upper limb lymphedema, the flap recipient site can be selected on the medial arm with the artery selected on the lateral arm and the vein selected from the cephalic vein or the basilic vein for end-to-end anastomosis, respectively. The flap recipient site can be selected on the medial arm, opposed to the wrist. As the medial arm is concealed, generally, no surgery has been performed here before and it is earlier to dissect local tissues. Moreover, the artery on the lateral arm is the anastomotic vessel, which will not affect the main artery (brachial artery).

Advantages of the inguinal lymph node flap: concealed donor site of the flap, the venous return as a big cutaneous vein, reliable arterial blood supply. The lymph nodes in the lateral group mainly drain the low abdominal wall, the back and the upper gluteal region, and will generally not cause lymphatic return disorders at the donor site. The draining lymph nodes to the lower limbs are categorized in the medial and the intermediate groups [13]. Disadvantages of the flap: the vascular pedicle of the flap is short and the blood vessels are thin, which are prone to have anatomical variation. Therefore, microsurgical techniques are required to separate and anastomose the pedicle blood vessels, and the microsurgery training is necessitated.

Case 3: Female, 45 years old, who was subject to stage II lymphedema of the right upper limb after radical treatment and axillary lymph node dissection because of right breast cancer without obvious response to conservative treatment for 6 months (Fig. 29.18). The left inguinal lymph node flap was transplanted to the inner side of the right arm. Under an

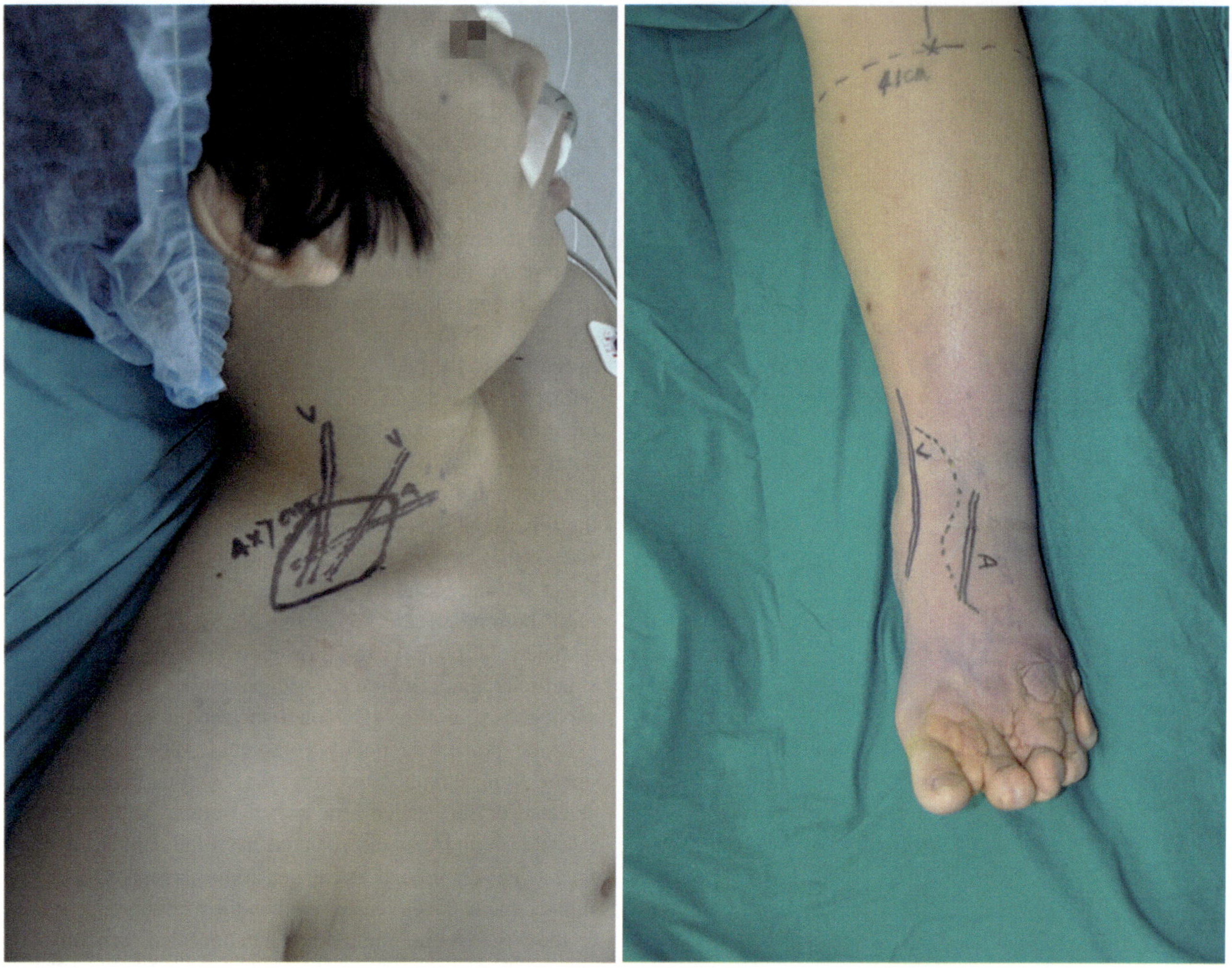

Fig. 29.11 Design of right supraclavicular lymph node flap and the recipient site on the foot back

8× magnification microscope, the end-to-end anastomosis was performed between the superficial iliac circumflex artery of the flap and the brachial artery of the lateral arm (branch of the brachial artery), the superficial iliac circumflex vein with the cephalic vein, respectively (Figs. 29.19, 29.20, 29.21, 29.22, 29.23, 29.24, and 29.25).

Case 4: Female, 58 years old, who was subject to stage II lymphedema of the right upper limb after radical treatment and axillary lymph node dissection because of right breast cancer (Fig. 29.26). The lymph fat aspiration was performed 3 months ago. In this surgery, the left inguinal lymph node flap was transplanted to the right medial arm. Under an 8× magnification microscope, the end-to-end anastomosis was performed between the superficial iliac circumflex artery of the flap and the brachial artery of the lateral arm (branch of the brachial artery), the superficial iliac circumflex vein with the cephalic vein, respectively (Figs. 29.27, 29.28, 29.29, 29.30, 29.31, 29.32, and 29.33).

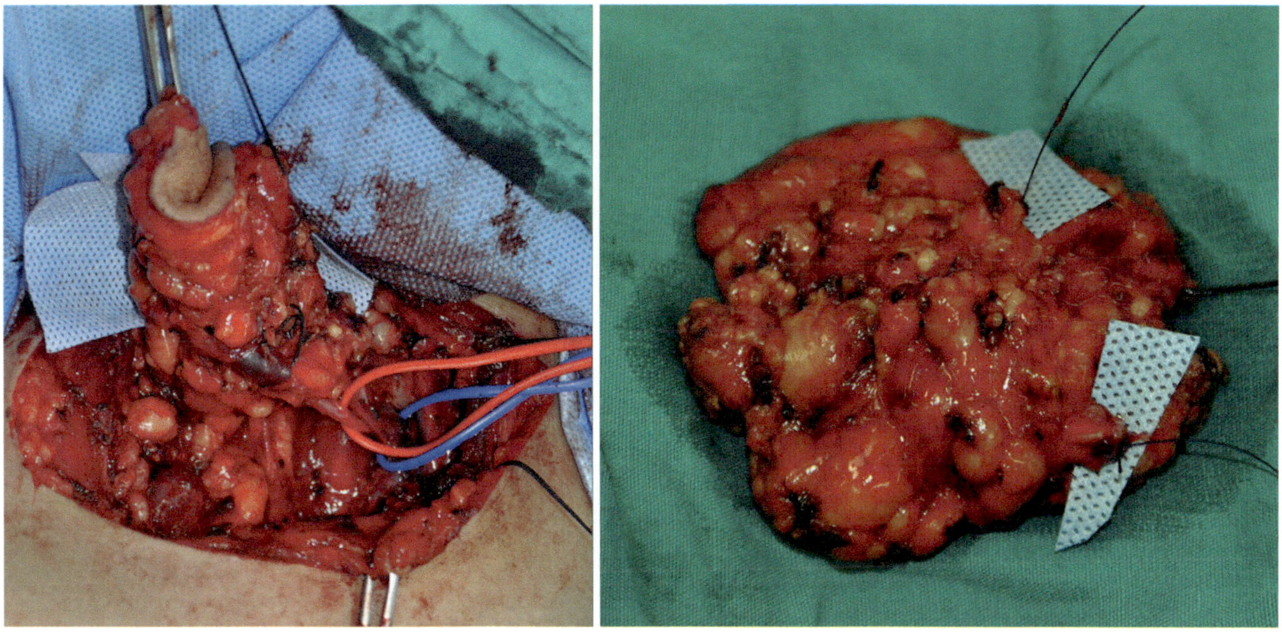

Fig. 29.12 Dissection of the flap blood vessels and excision of the flap

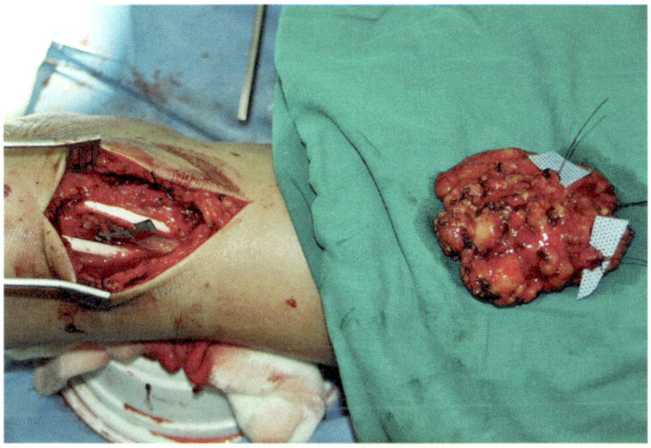

Fig. 29.13 Dissection of the dorsal artery of the flap recipient site

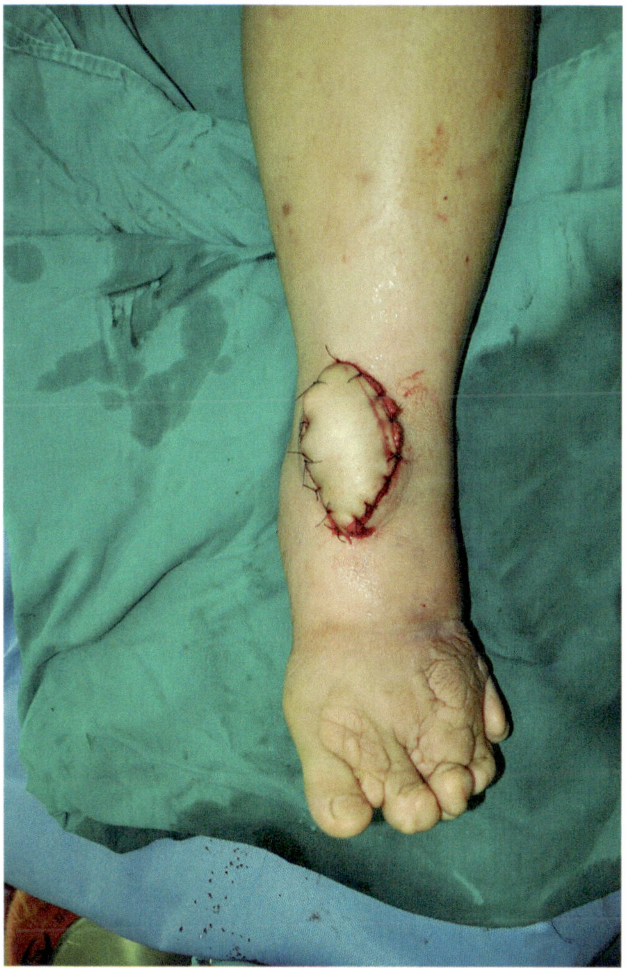

Fig. 29.14 Completion of the flap's vascular anastomosis

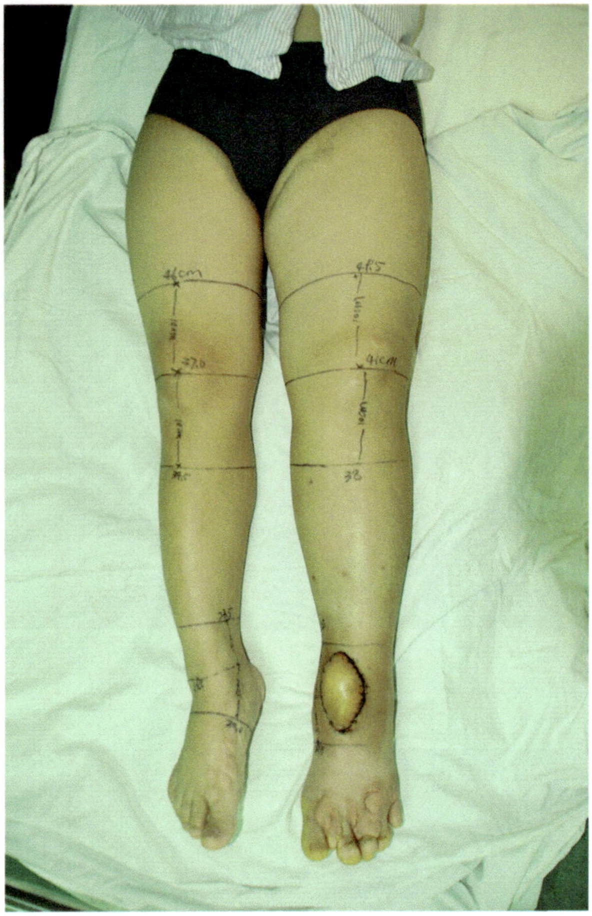

Fig. 29.15 The flap survived 7 days after surgery

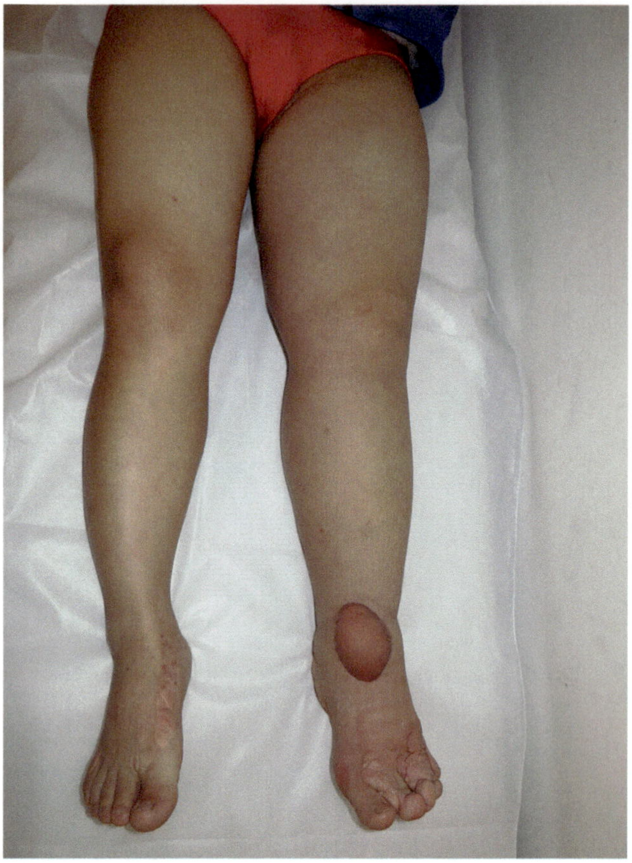

Fig. 29.16 The circumference of the left thigh and the left shank was reduced by 2.2 and 1.5 cm 1 year after surgery

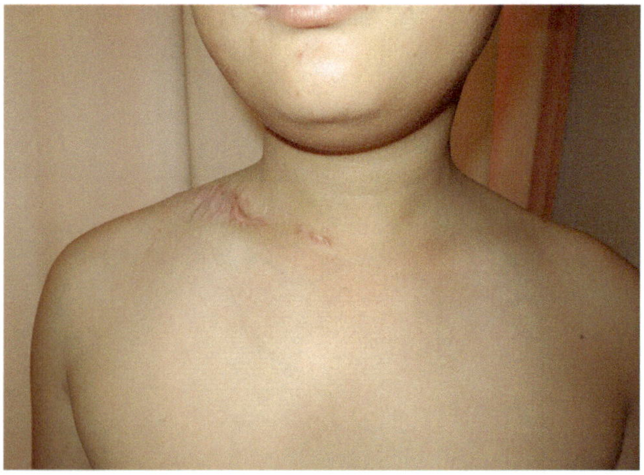

Fig. 29.17 No iatrogenic lymphedema at the flap's donor site 1 year after surgery

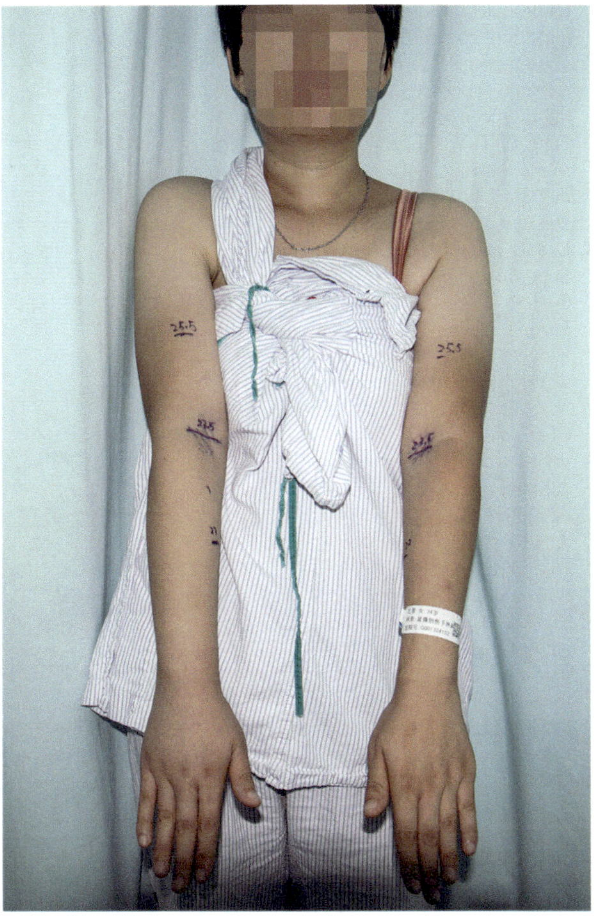

Fig. 29.18 Stage II secondary lymphedema of the right upper limb

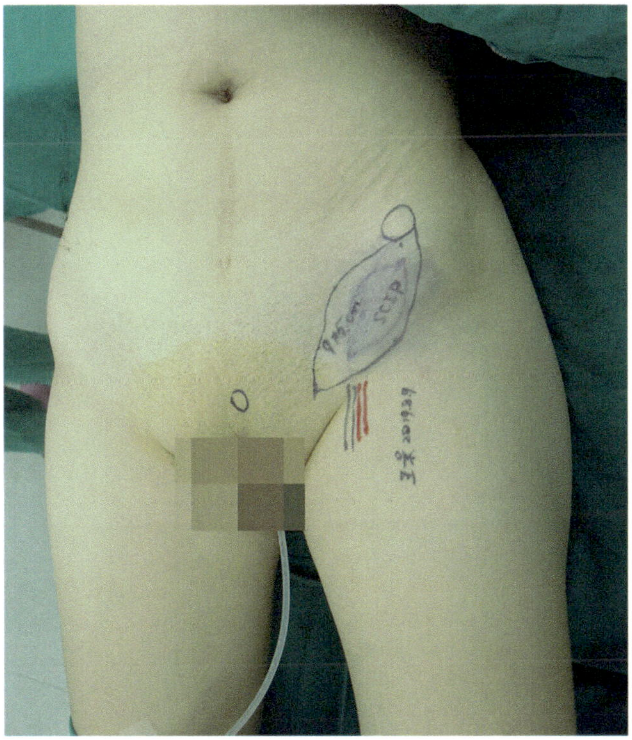

Fig. 29.19 Design of left inguinal lymph node flap, 9 × 5 cm

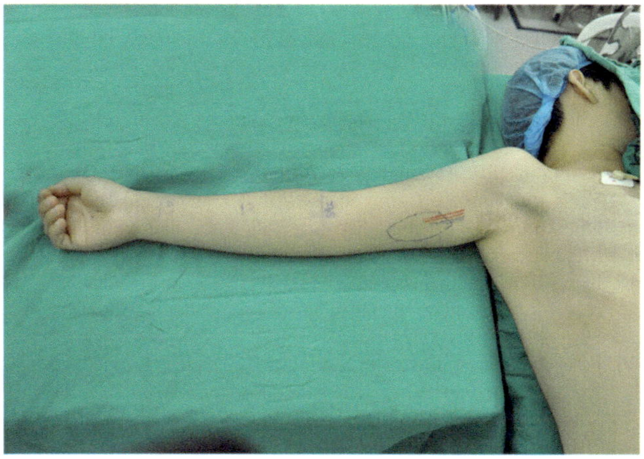

Fig. 29.20 The right medial arm as the recipient site of the flap

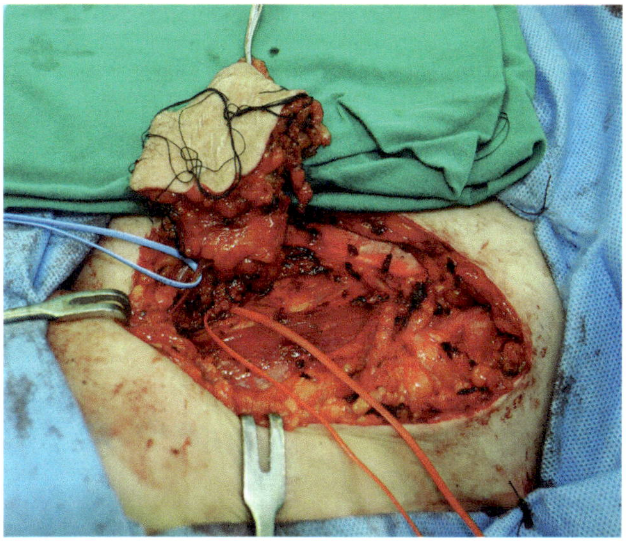

Fig. 29.21 Completion of the flap dissection without breaking the vascular pedicle

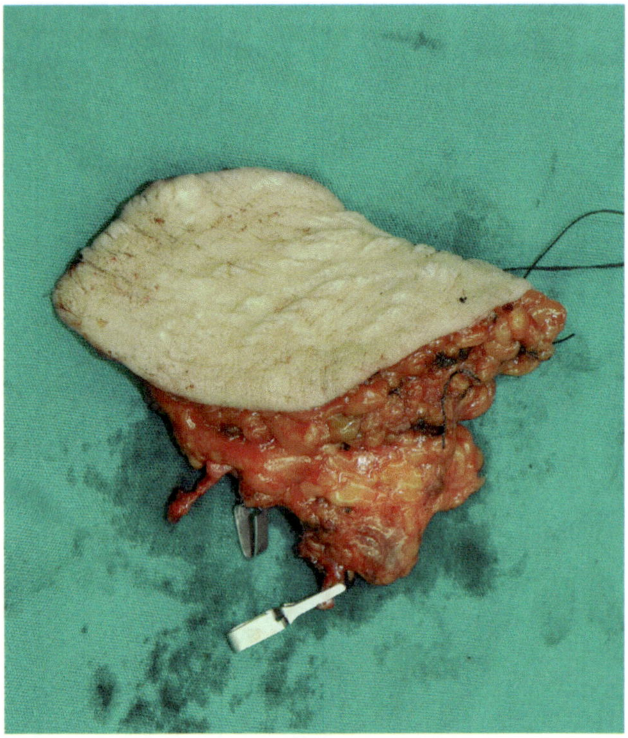

Fig. 29.22 Excision of the inguinal lymph node flap

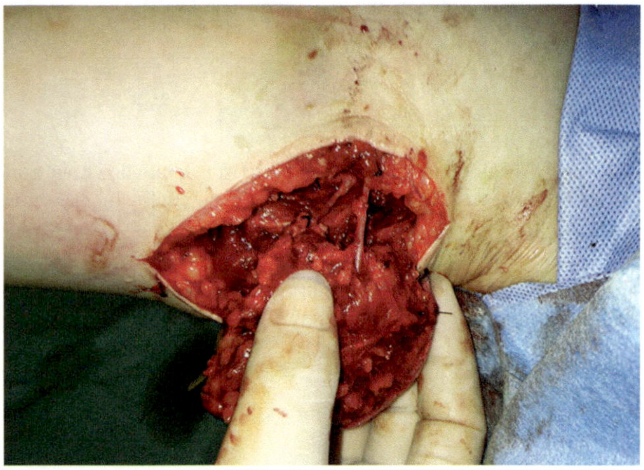

Fig. 29.23 Anastomosis of the flap vessels with the artery and the cephalic vein respectively on the lateral arm

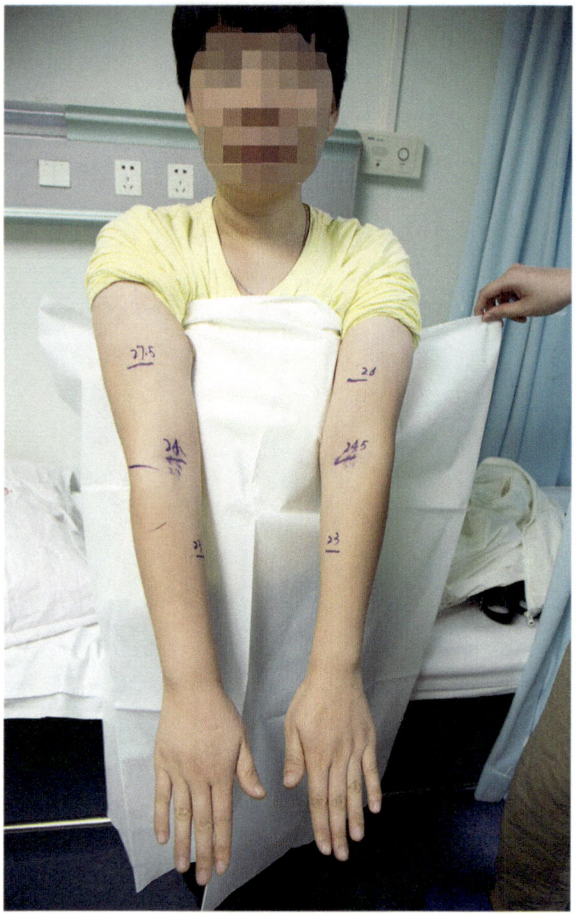

Fig. 29.24 The edema of the right wrist and the forearm was alleviated half a year after surgery

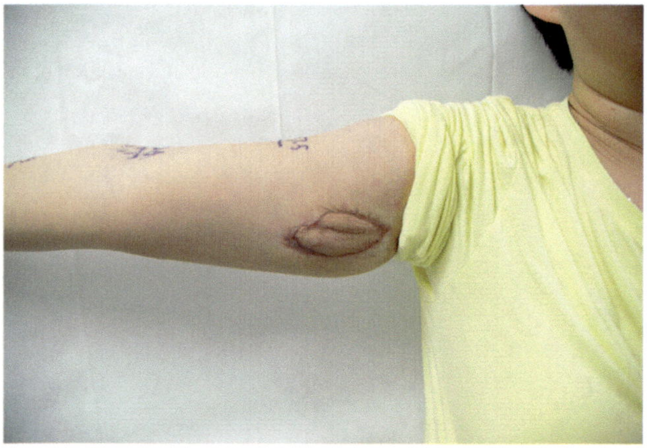

Fig. 29.25 The flap appearance half a year after surgery

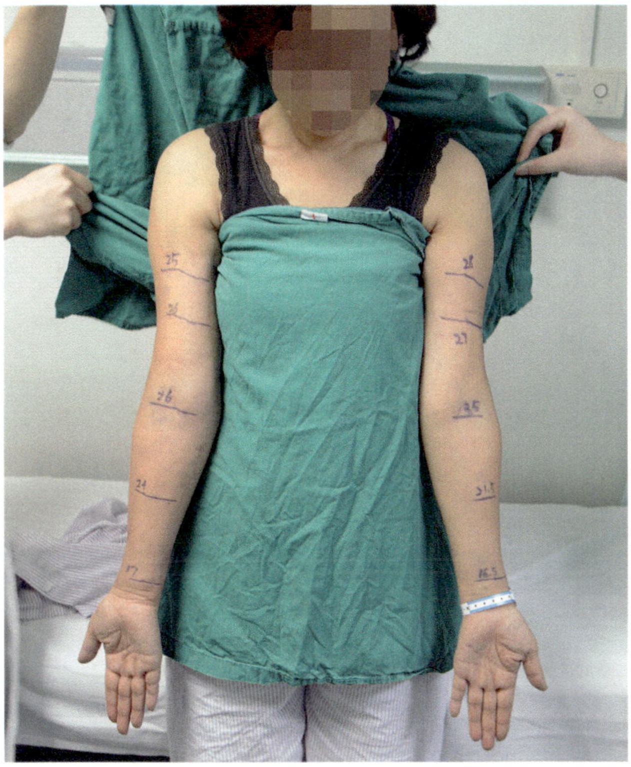

Fig. 29.26 Secondary lymphedema of the right upper limb before surgery, aspiration surgery was performed 3 months ago

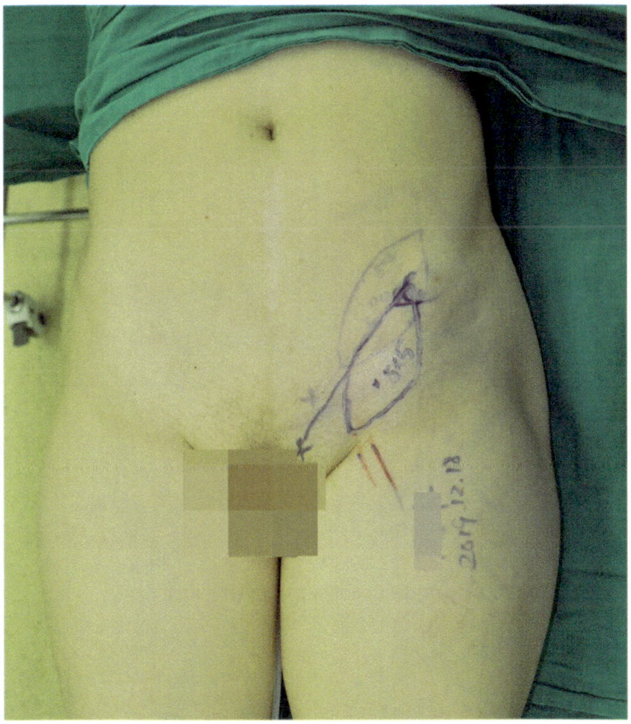

Fig. 29.27 Design of left inguinal lymph node flap, 8 × 5 cm

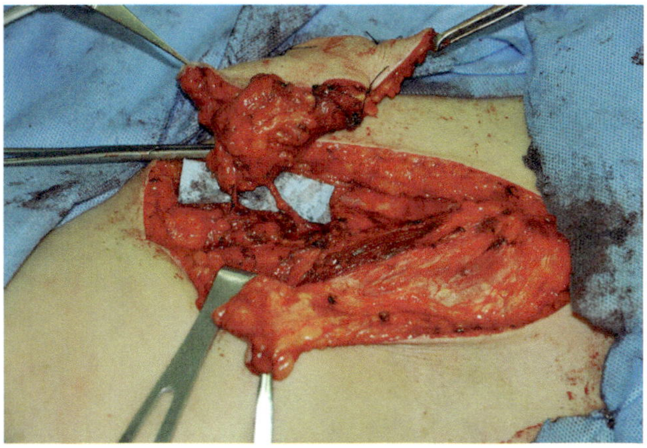

Fig. 29.28 Dissection of the flap vessels during surgery (superficial iliac circumflex artery and superficial iliac circumflex vein)

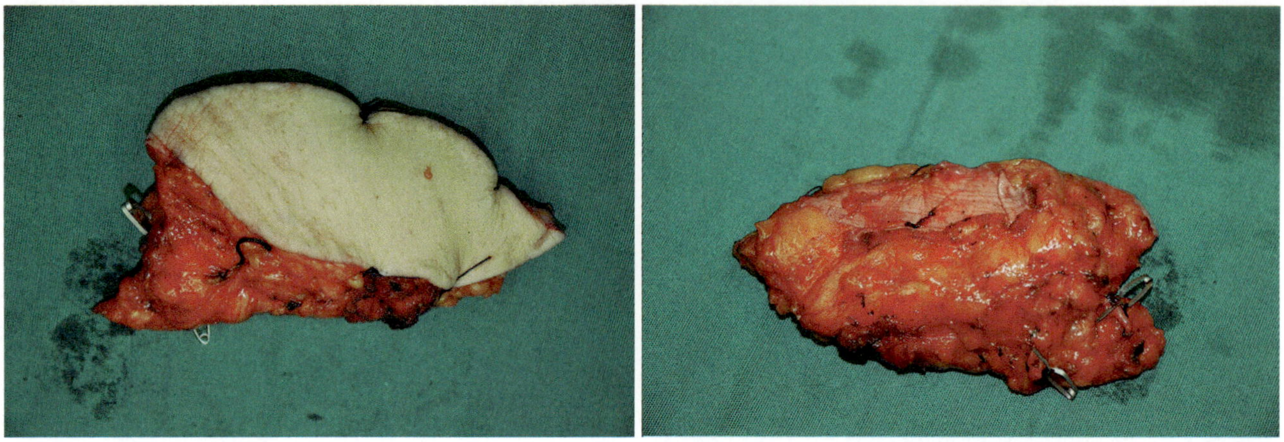

Fig. 29.29 Excision of the inguinal lymph node flap

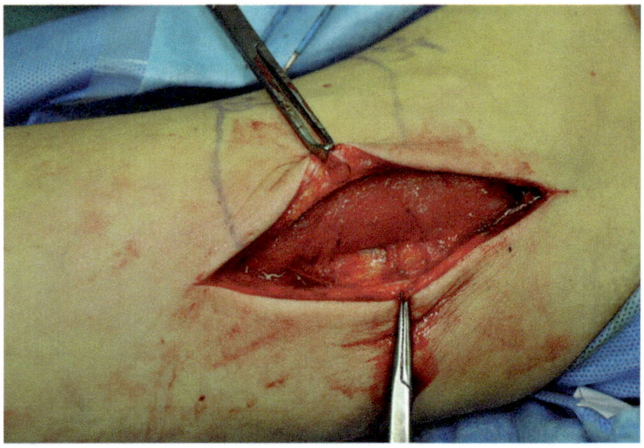

Fig. 29.30 Artery of the flap recipient site—artery of the lateral arm

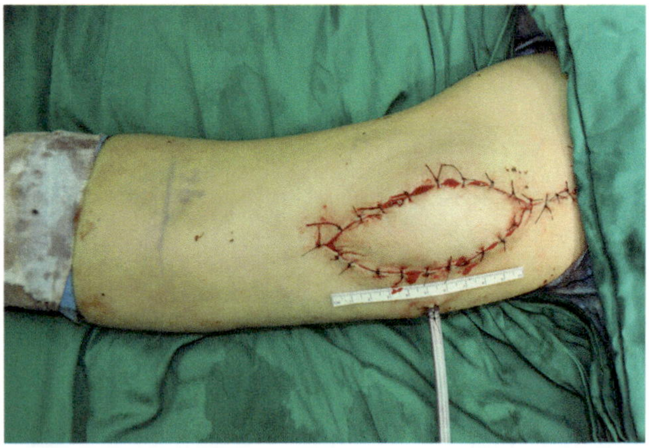

Fig. 29.31 Completion of the anastomosis between the flap vessels and the recipient site

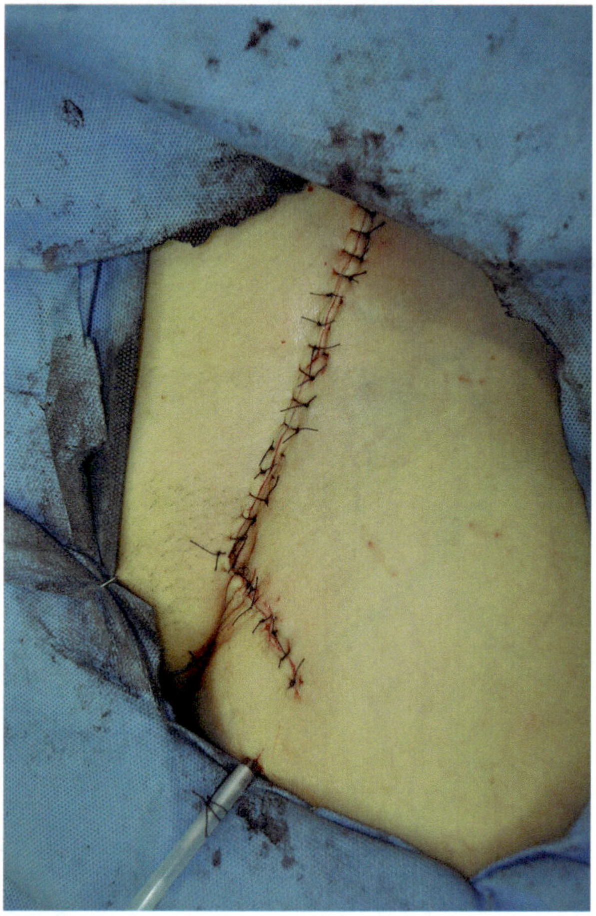

Fig. 29.32 Closure of the donor site of the inguinal flap

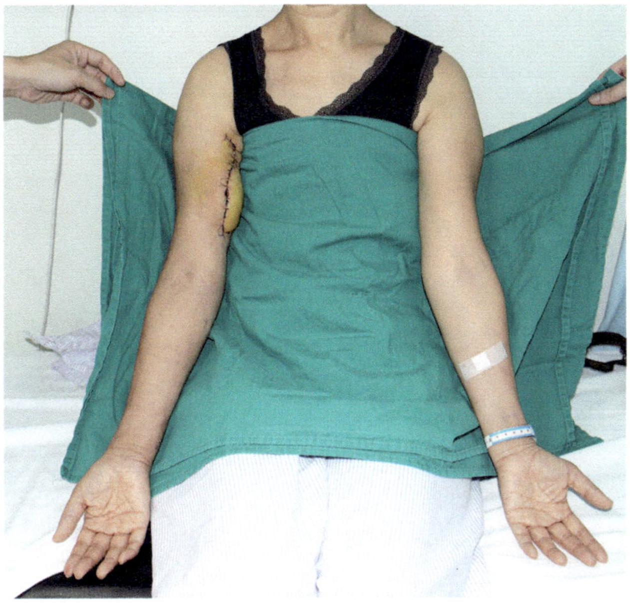

Fig. 29.33 The flap survived on the 8th day after surgery

References

1. Clodius L, Smith PJ, Bruna J, Serafin D. The lymphatics of the groin flap. Ann Plast Surg. 1982;9(6):447–58.
2. Koide S, Lin CY, Chen C, Cheng MH. Long-term outcome of lower extremity lymphedema treated with vascularized lymph node flap transfer with or without venous complications. J Surg Oncol. 2020;121(1):129–37.
3. Engel H, Lin CY, Huang JJ, Cheng MH. Outcomes of lymphedema microsurgery for breast cancer-related lymphedema with or without microvascular breast reconstruction. Ann Surg. 2017;268(6):1076–83.
4. Becker C. Autologous lymph node transfers. J Reconstr Microsurg. 2016;32(1):28–33.
5. Schaverien MV, Badash I, Patel KM, et al. Vascularized lymph node transfer for lymphedema. Semin Plast Surg. 2018;32(1):28–35.
6. Cheng MH, Huang JJ, Wu CW, et al. The mechanism of vascularized lymph node transfer for lymphedema: natural lymphaticovenous drainage. Plast Reconstr Surg. 2014; 133(2):192e–8e.
7. Ito R, Zelken J, Yang CY, et al. Proposed pathway and mechanism of vascularized lymph node flaps. Gynecol Oncol. 2016;141(1):182–8.
8. Scaglioni MF, Arvanitakis M, Chen YC, et al. Comprehensive review of vascularized lymph node transfers for lymphedema: outcomes and complications. Microsurgery. 2018;38(2):222–9.
9. Pallua N, Machens HG, Rennekampff O, et al. The fasciocutaneous supraclavicular artery island flap for releasing postburn mentosternal contractures. Plast Reconstr Surg. 1997;99(07):1878–84.
10. Mardonado AA, Chen R, Chang DW. The use of supraclavicular free flap with vascularized lymph node transfer for treatment of lymphedema: a prospective study of 100 consecutive cases. J Surg Oncol. 2017;115(1):68–71.
11. Steinbacher J, Tinhofer IE, Meng S, et al. The surgical anatomy of the supraclavicular lymph node flap: a basis for the free vascularized lymph node transfer. J Surg Oncol. 2017;115(1):60–2.
12. Cheng MH, Chen SC, Henry SL, et al. Vascularized groin lymph node flap transfer for postmastectomy upper limb lymphedema: flap anatomy, recipient sites, and outcomes. Plast Reconstr Surg. 2013;131(6):1286–98.
13. Viitanen TP, Mäki MT, Seppänen MP, et al. Donor-site lymphatic function after microvascular lymph node transfer. Plast Reconstr Surg. 2012;130:1246–53.

Lymphatic Tissue Transfer for the Treatment of Axillary Dissection Related Lymphedema

30

Lan Mu, Ru Chen, Xiaojie Zhong, and Peng Tang

Abstract

Breast cancer-related upper-arm lymphedema is one of the most common postoperative complications of Breast cancer [Sisman et al. J BUON, 17(3):565–569, 2012], having an incidence of 20% [Suami and Chang, Plast Reconstr Surg 126:1853–1863, 2010; Mclaughlin et al. J Clin Oncol 26(32):5220–5226, 2008; Clark et al. QJM 98:343–348, 2005]. There are multiple possible reasons such as operation, radiotherapy, et al. [Yen et al. Ann Surg Oncol 16(4):979–988, 2009]. The most severe complications include paramorphia and dysfunction, which impair the quality of life of patients [Pusic et al. J Cancer Surviv 2012]. There has been no clear and effective cure method reported. In our research, we simultaneously performed breast reconstruction and treatment of breast cancer-related upper-arm lymphedema with Lymphatic TRAM/DIEP flap, modifying the method introduced by Dr. Corinne Becker [Becker et al. Ann Surg. 243:313–315, 2006] and Dr. Anne M. Saaristo [Saaristo et al. Ann Surg 255(3):468–473, 2012], and have been following up with mid-upper-arm circumference measurement, clinical symptoms, and lymphoscintigraphy, looking forward to making the effective evaluation of the method of breasts restoration, breast reconstruction and lymphatic transplantation aimed to treat upper limb lymphedema after breast cancer surgery.

Keywords

Vascularized lymphatic deep inferior epigastric artery perforator flap · Super iliac artery lymphatic nodes · Axillary dissection related lymphedema treatment · Breast reconstruction

L. Mu (✉)
Plastic & Aesthetic Surgery Department of Hainan Cancer Hospital, Hainan Medical College, Haikou, Hainan, China

R. Chen · X. Zhong · P. Tang
Breast Cancer Department, Hainan Cancer Hospital, Hainan Medical College, Haikou, Hainan, China

Lymphedema is a chronic progressive disease, the first manifestation is lymphatic drainage obstruction because of the lymphatic system congenital structural abnormalities, trauma and parasites. Protein-rich lymphatic fluid accumulates abnormally in the tissue, resulting in complex inflammatory responses, thickening of surrounding tissues and fibrosis, eventually lead to thickening of the skin and increased limb circumference, which affects limb appearance and function [1]. Until now, the treatment of lymphedema is still in the exploration stage, and various treatment measures are still controversial. As a new treatment for lymphedema, vascularized lymph node transplantation is to transfer lymph nodes and their nourishing vessels to the limb with lymphedema in the form of tissue flap, so as to reconstruct the lymphatic drainage pathway. Current studies have shown that vascularized lymph node transplantation can effectively relieve the symptoms of lymphedema, but the mechanism remains controversial. The progress of animal experiments and clinical studies on the treatment of vascularized lymph node transplantation is summarized as follows.

30.1 Animal Studies of Vascularized Lymph Node Transplantation

In 1928, Jaffe and Richter began the transplantation of non-anastomotic lymph nodes in a Dutch mouse model [2], and since then, animal studies have been conducted on the transplantation of non-anastomotic lymph nodes or fragments of lymph nodes in multiple centers. In these studies, only a few lymph nodes can survive completely, and most of them would gradually lose their original tissue structure after lymph node transplantation, but they can also play a role in promoting lymphatic drainage [3–6]. More than half a century later, with the popularity of free tissue transplantation with anastomotic blood vessels, Shesol et al. [7] successfully carried out lymph node transplantation with anastomotic blood vessels in the rat model. All lymph nodes survived the

N. Liu (ed.), *Peripheral Lymphedema*, https://doi.org/10.1007/978-981-16-3484-0_30

operation, and the original tissue structure and function were retained, revealing the importance of preserving and anastomosing transplanted lymph nodes with nourishing blood vessels. At the same time, they also found that regional microenvironment changes can significantly affect the survival of lymph nodes. The survival rate of lymph node transplantation 2–7 days after lymph node dissection is significantly lower than that of immediate postoperative transplantation. Therefore, the researchers suggest that an open lymphatic system may be another important factor in promoting the survival of transplanted lymph nodes, but this conclusion needs further verification.

Chen et al. [8] observed the therapeutic effect of hematic lymph node transplantation on chronic lymphedema of the hind limb of dogs. The peripheral diameter of the hind limb after 3–6 months of postoperative edema decreased significantly compared with that before surgery, but it did not return to the normal peripheral diameter. Meanwhile, the transplanted lymph nodes survived and maintained the original tissue morphology. Postoperative lymphangiography revealed spontaneous lymphangitic recanalization in the surgical area, and lymphatic development indicated that the lymph nodes and the liver had been ingestion of the developer. These results preliminarily confirmed the possibility of reconstructing the lymphatic pathway from the self-sufficient part to the venous system by transplanting hematic lymph nodes. Tobbia et al. [9], based on the model of lymphedema in sheep, compared the lymphatic reflux function of lymph node transplantation with non-anastomotic vessels and lymph node transplantation with blood vessels and found that the lymphatic reflux function of lymph node transplantation group with blood vessels was significantly better than that of non-anastomotic vessels group 8–12 weeks after surgery. VEGF-c is the main regulator of lymphangiogenesis [10], and its role in the treatment of lymphedema has attracted extensive attention from scholars.

Animal experiments have confirmed that the combination of the blood transport lymph node transplantation combination VEGF-c can promote the new lymph nodes around the lymph nodes, thus enhancing the drainage function of the lymph nodes. The proliferation and formation of the endothelial cells in vitro and lymphocyte cells in vitro can promote the production of lymphatic cells, and the secretion of lymphatic factors is promoted. According to the study of the model of the lymphocytic edema of the posterior limb of the mice, the study showed that the transplantation of the combined fat stem cells with the blood node of the lymph node was significantly reduced by the transplantation of the blood flow lymph nodes, and the lymphatic reflux was greatly reduced. But the combined therapy used in the above studies has the potential risk of promoting the proliferation of tumor cells, so it is careful to use the "15-1616" in the tumor patients.

30.2 Mechanism of Lymph Node Transplantation with Blood Circulation

At present, there are two main hypotheses about the mechanism of hematic lymph node transplantation in the treatment of lymphedema, namely the siphon hypothesis and the lymph node pump Hypothesis [11].

30.2.1 The Lymphatic Wick Hypothesis

The Lymphatic wick hypothesis was proposed by Honkonen et al. [12], who believed that the transplanted lymph nodes connected the lymphatic vessels at the near and far end of the destroyed lymphatic pathway and played the role of siphon and drainage. This hypothesis is based on the premise that the transplanted lymph node and the recipient lymphatic vessels can spontaneously recanalize the connection, reshaping the input and output lymphatic vessels of the transplanted lymph node. Suami et al. [11] took the forelimb of the dog as a model and observed that after the transplantation of the axillary vascularized lymph nodes, a new collateral traffic was formed between the transplanted lymph nodes and the ipsilateral intromammary lymph nodes, but they also found that the new lymphatic pathway was different from the original lymphatic loop structure of the axilla. They believe that lymphatic vessels can "sense" the location of surrounding lymph nodes and grow toward them, but how the lymph nodes affect the growth of lymph vessels remains controversial. Some scholars believe that lymph nodes can secrete endogenous vegf-c to promote the growth of lymphatic vessels, but this has not been confirmed [10, 13]. Another controversial aspect of the siphon hypothesis is that in advanced lymphedema, where capillaries dilate and the function of collecting lymphatics is degraded, it is difficult to establish effective lymphatic reflux even if the lymphatic-lymph node pathway is reconstructed, which is inconsistent with clinical observation.

30.2.2 Lymph Node Pump Hypothesis

The lymph node pump hypothesis refers to that the transplanted lymph nodes can absorb lymph fluid from the surrounding tissues and "pump" the reflux lymph fluid into the venous pathway through the inherent lymph-venous traffic structure in the lymph nodes, playing a similar role in the lymphatic reflux pathway [14–16]. Cheng, etc. [14] on the edge of the lymph node flap injection of indocyanine green (indocyanine green, ICG) immediately for fluorescence enhancement after contrast agent, observed developer appeared in the transplanted vein lymph node, then appeared in the anastomosis of the vein, and accordingly puts forward the theory of lymph node pump, but failed to explain how to absorb the ICG, lymph node and how to contrast agents "pump" into the veins. Since then, Aschen [13] in mice with acute lymphedema model to transplant the observed a lot of the lymphatic vessels in lymph nodes grows, the area between lymphatic vessels and graft lymphatic spontaneous lymphatic anastomosis, and lymph nodes in the newborn after lymphatic vessels and capillaries close micro vein, this finding further confirms the presence of lymph node lymphatic and venous traffic. In [17] such as Ito experiments, in order to eliminate the impact of injection pressure to the ICG absorption, will contain the inguinal lymph node flap and does not contain a groin abdominal flap immersed in ICG and mixed solution in different concentrations of protein found in the appropriate protein concentrations, contains lymph nodes in the groin flap vein appear ICG enhancement, and do not include the abdominal lymph node flap is no enhancement. This suggests that the presence of lymph nodes is crucial for lymphatic reflux, and they believe that Starling forces are driving the transfer of proteins and water molecules between the ends of the lymphatic capillaries in the lymph nodes and the venules behind the capillaries, which carry the lymph back into the vein. In recent years, the research on the lymph node pump theory is constantly improving, but at present, there is still a lack of exact evidence, and further research is needed.

30.3 Clinical Study of Lymph Node Transplantation Vascularized

30.3.1 Clinical Efficacy Analysis

In 1982, Coldius et al. [18] first reported the clinical application of lymph node transplantation with blood transport., Becker, etc. [19] with the surgical treatment of the 24 patients with refractory secondary upper limb lymphedema after breast cancer, their lymph nodes of patients with inguinal zone vessels taking, separation and in the form of vascular anastomosis of tissue flap transplantation to side armpit, ten cases of postoperative patients with upper limb week diameter returned to normal, 12 patients with upper limb diameter weeks, though not back to normal, but the pre-operative declined significantly, the remaining two cases of patients with upper limb week diameter compared with pre-operative no improvement. Lin et al. [16] transferred the inguinal flap with lymph nodes to the wrist to treat 13 cases of upper limb shower

In patients with lymphedema, the peri-diameter of the upper limb decreased significantly in 92% of patients after surgery, and the development speed of the lymph imaging tracer increased faster than that before surgery, suggesting that the function of lymph reflux in the upper limb was improved. Based on the anatomical study on the distribution of human inguinal lymph nodes, Mu Lan et al. applied abdominal skin flap with lymph node transplantation to repair the chest wall after breast cancer surgery, treated upper limb lymphedema with autologous tissue breast reconstruction, and filled the pits with malformations, achieving good clinical results [20–26]. On the basis of Lin et al., Saaristo et al. [27] proposed that for patients with secondary lymphedema of the upper limb after breast cancer surgery, lymph node transplantation with blood circulation could be combined with second-stage autologous tissue breast reconstruction, and two groups of vascular pedicles could be anastomosed simultaneously. Saaristo et al. performed the above operations on nine patients. 6 months after the operation, seven patients had lower upper limb circumference than before, and three patients could stop physical therapy. Subsequently, Nguyen et al. [28] proposed a systematic flap design process to guide the selection of recipient vessels and flap incisions during breast reconstruction with abdominal free flap combined with lymph node transplantation. Nguyen et al. applied this design process to 29 patients and found that 79% experienced significant improvement in postoperative lymphedema. However, the follow-up time of the above clinical studies was short, only 6–11 months. In theory, lymphedema may occur when the load of lymphatic reflux is greater than the capacity of lymphatic vessels, so lymphedema recurrence is possible in the long term. Recently, Ciudad [29] reported one case of application of mandible with blood transplantation to treat cervical cancer lymph node cases of postoperative lower limb lymphedema, postoperative week 6 months in patients with upper limb diameter greatly reduce the pre-operative, cellulitis progress is under control, but the postoperative edema 1 year again, prompt early postoperative relieve lymphedema still has the possibility of future recurrence. Therefore, the results of long-term follow-up are of more reference value when evaluating the therapeutic effect of lymph node with blood circulation.

30.3.2 Donor Site Selection

The inguinal region is relatively fixed anatomically, with the concealed postoperative scar, and can also be combined with an abdominal skin flap for breast reconstruction. Therefore, it has become the most commonly used donor area for lymph node transplantation with blood supply. Clinically, superficial inguinal lymph nodes on the upper lateral surface pedicled by a superficial circumflex iliac artery or inferior abdominal wall artery are mainly selected. It is generally believed that the drainage of superficial inguinal lymph nodes in the upper lateral inguinal region is mainly lymphatic fluid in the lower abdominal wall, lower back and buttocks, while the lymph nodes in the recurred lower extremities are mainly located below the femoral artery and great saphenous vein junction [30, 31], but there are variations or individual differences in the anatomical structure of the inguinal region. Vignes et al. [32] reported two cases of secondary lymphedema of the lower extremity caused by inguinal lymph node transplantation. Sulo et al. As far as possible in order to protect the donor lymphatic system functions, such as Dayan [33] proposed to reverse the lymphatic mapping is applied to the area for the taking, lymph nodes through the abdominal wall injection ICG angiography, lower limb technetium injection of the radioactive element, intraoperative double lymphatic imaging to distinguish for transplantation of lymph nodes and lymph nodes should be preserved, but still, need to further explore the effectiveness of this technique. In addition to the inguinal area, the lower jaw, supraclavicular, axillary are also common with the blood supply of lymph nodes. One of the disadvantages of axillary lymph node resection is the risk of secondary lymphedema. On the other hand, the recurrence and metastasis probability of contralateral axillary lymph node in breast cancer patients is up to 3.6–6% [34], so the selection of contralateral axillary lymph node as the donor area should be cautious. Although the mandibular lymph node transplantation avoids iatrogenic lymphedema in the donor area, it has the risk of damaging the mandibular marginal nerve, and the scar of the surgical incision is obvious, which has a great influence on the aesthetics [35] Chang [36] conducted a prospective study on the transplantation of 100 cases of supraclavicular lymph node flap for the treatment of limb lymphedema, but no secondary lymphedema was found in the donor area, and complications related to donor area and flap were rare. At the same time, the supraclavicular scar is relatively concealed, which is an ideal lymph node donor area at present. As early as 1990, O 'brien et al. [37] attempted to use retinal lymph node transplantation to treat lymphedema, but it has not been widely used clinically due to the problems such as the need for laparotomy and the loss of function of postoperative fibrosis of transplanted lymph nodes. In recent years, after scholars found that superficial lymph node transplantation was prone to bring about the problem of lymphedema in the donor area, retinal lymph node transplantation was paid more attention again. With laparoscopy, Nguyen et al. [38, 39] proposed minimally invasive free hematogenous retinal lymph node transplantation for the treatment of limb lymphedema, avoiding the donor complications caused by laparotomy. In addition, 42 patients were treated clinically, and symptoms improved in 83% of them, but pancreatitis occurred in 1 patient. In theory, there is no risk of secondary lymphedema in the donor area, but there are still risks of serious complications such as intestinal obstruction and pancreatitis in intraperitoneal surgery, so its application value and safety still need to be further explored.

30.3.3 Recipient Site Selection

The most common recipient of lymph node transplantation is the proximal limb, the armpit or the groin. Transplantation of lymph nodes in the proximal limb can restore the lymphatic reflux pathway anatomically, but for patients receiving local radiotherapy after tumor resection, the tissues of the proximal limb are scarred, and it is more difficult to find suitable vessels for anastomosis, while the tissue damage of the distal limb, namely the wrist or ankle, is relatively small and the anastomosis difficulty is relatively low. According to existing studies [16, 29], both distal and proximal lymph node transplantation can improve lymphedema, but there are no studies comparing the efficacy of the two.

30.4 Indication

30.4.1 Middle or Serious Degree Lymphedema

30.4.2 No Function After One Year Physician Treatment

30.5 Contraindication

30.5.1 Distant Metastases

30.5.2 Local Recurrence

30.5.3 General Anesthesia Contraindication

30.6 Pre-Operation Preparing

30.6.1 MDCTA

MDCTA is needed to evaluate not only donor site: pre-operation, the pedicle vessels of abdominal flap , position and numbers of super iliac artery lymphatic nodes.

But recipient site, pre-operation , the thoracodorsal vessels or internal mammary artery and vein.

30.6.2 The Isotope Radiography Before the Operation Shows Obstruction of Lymphatic Return

30.6.3 Pre-Operation Planning with Stand-Up Position

The chest incision and abdominal flap were designed according to the size of the opposite side, patients' expectations, the defect of the affected side and available tissue of the abdomen. Sometimes we may reduce the incision, even making an additional incision parallel to the groin in order to give consideration to lymph nodes around the superficial circumflex iliac vessel.

30.7 Operation Techniques

30.7.1 General in Tube Anesthesia

30.7.2 Patients Were Layed on Back Position, Make Sure the Table Can Make the Patient "Sit Down" Position During the Procedure When the Abdominal Wall Need to be Closed with Arm Exposure in Field

30.7.3 Procedures

30.7.3.1 Chest Wall Incision and Vessels Dissection and Axilla Scar Contracture Release

We decided the transplantation middle of the lower abdominal flap according to pre-operative MDCT to make sure that lymph nodes can be located in the axilla after transferring. During the operation, the scar contracture of the axilla is completely relaxed and disclosure the axillary vein. Then exploration of the thoracodorsal vessel (and, if necessary) the internal mammary vessel would be decided to be the anastomosis site. Both distal and proximal ends of the internal mammary artery and vein can be used as recipient site vessels [40].

30.7.3.2 Lymphatic Abdominal Flap Dissection

Pay much more attention to that, and the incision is superfacial on the side of super iliac artery lymphatic flap dissection. Not only to guarantee the lymphatic nodes were included inside the flap, but the local flap above survived well.

30.7.3.3 Vessels Anastomosis

If the vascular pedicle was on the same side as the lymph nodes, only the pedicle vessel needed anastomosis, if not, the anastomosis must take place in the two groups of vessels.

Proximal and distal ends of the internal mammary artery and vein were used at the same time when it is necessary.

30.7.3.4 Position of the Lymphatic Tissue

Lymph nodes were placed along the axillary vein.

30.7.3.5 Shaping of the Reconstructive Breast

To set how big the new breast is before operation with the patient. Usually, the inferior mammary fold position will be similar to the opposite breast.

30.7.3.6 Donor Site Closure

Donor site closure included dissociation of abdominal incision from cartilage ensiformis to symphysis ossium pubis and umbilical plasty. Then drainage was placed, and the incision was close by each layer.

30.8 Postoperative Treatment and Follow-Up

After the operation, the elastic bandages are applied for one year as an physical treatment. The follow-up visits are conducted one month, three months, six months, twelve months and twenty-four months away from the operation. The measurement indexes include mid-upper-arm circumference, clinical symptoms and lymphoscintigraphy.

Typical Case

Female, 55 years old, 11 years after left mastectomy and axillary dissection, 3 months radiation therapy, left arm lymphedema 8 years postoperation, 1-year non-surgical treatment but no function. 5 cm larger of the left arm circle than the right side (Fig. 30.1). Procedure was performed: bilateral

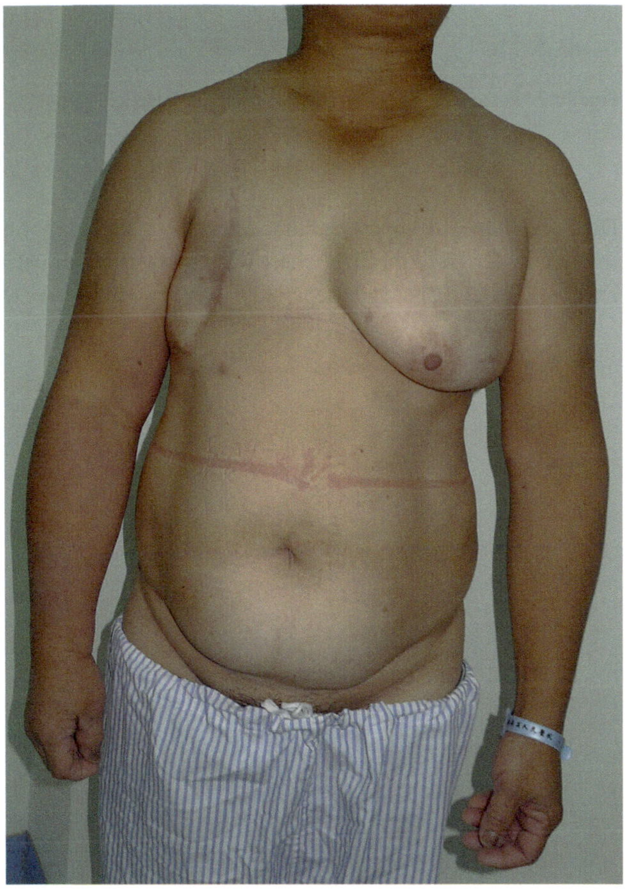

Fig. 30.1 Pre-operation (front view)

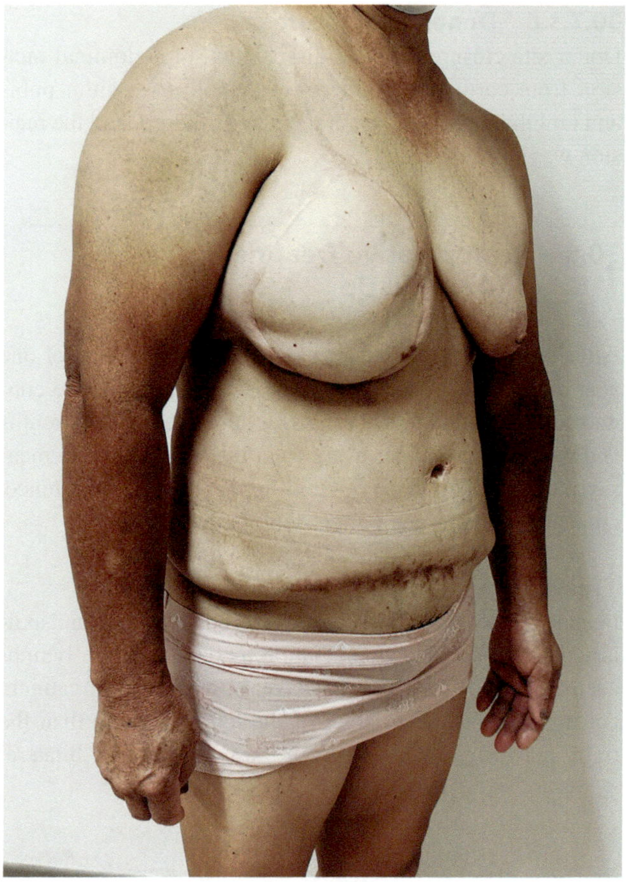

Fig. 30.2 Postoperation, 7th year's follow-up (oblique left view)

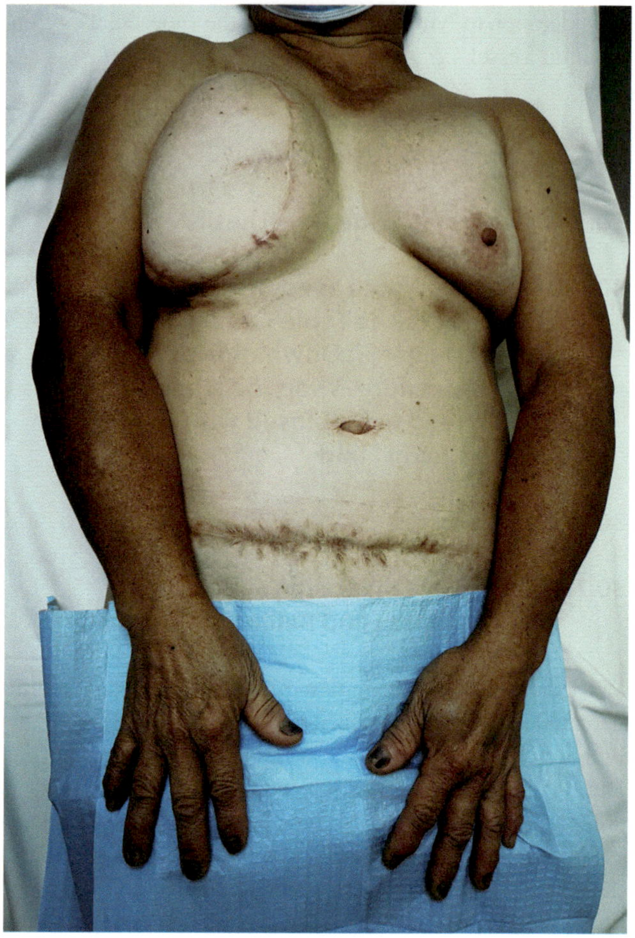

Fig. 30.3 Postoperation, 7th year's follow-up (lay on back view)

DIEP free flap with superficial iliac artery lymphatic flap was freely transferred to the right chest wall, two groups of deep epigastric artery and vein separately were anastomosed to thoracodorsal vessels and internal mammary vessels (end-end). The seventh year's follow-up result is very satisfied (Figs. 30.1, 30.2, 30.3, 30.4, 30.5 and 30.6).

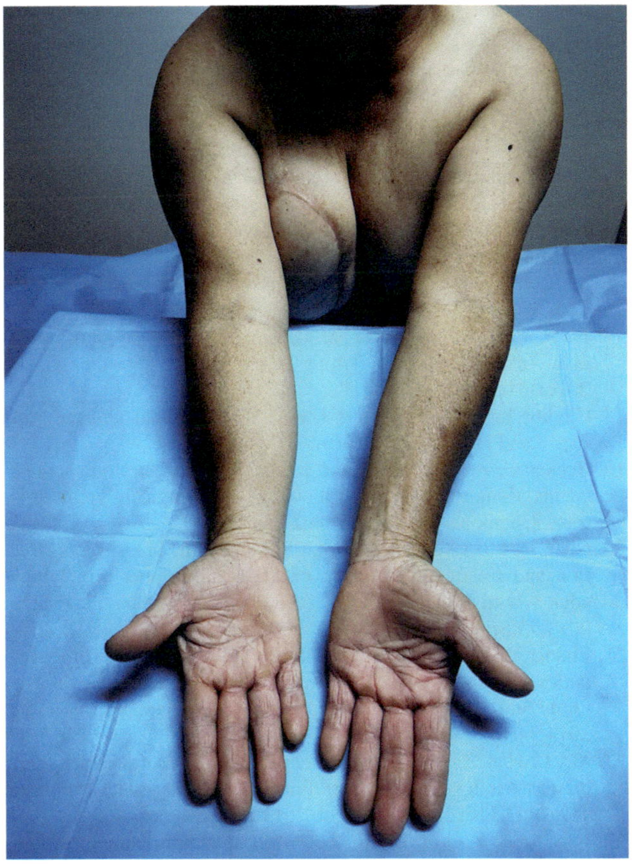

Fig. 30.4 Postoperation, 7th year's follow-up (bilateral arms front view)

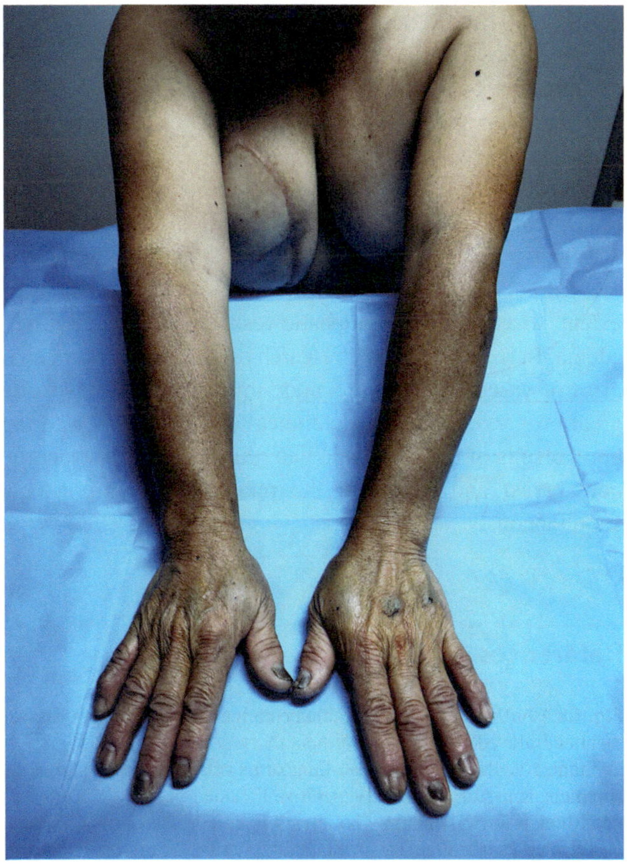

Fig. 30.5 Postoperation, 7th year's follow-up (bilateral arms back view)

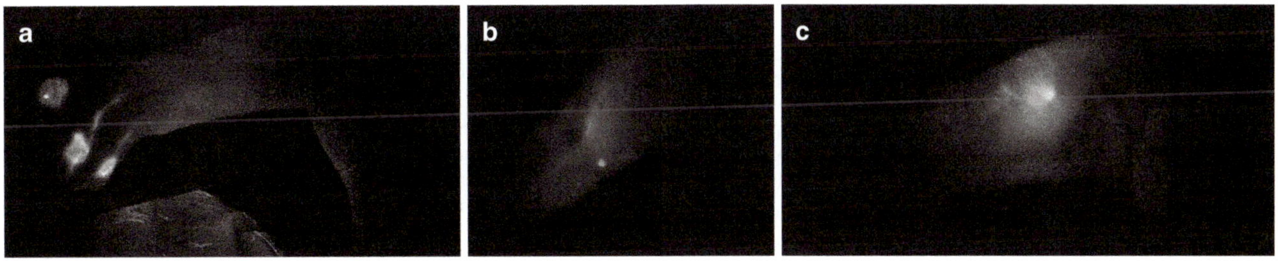

Fig. 30.6 Postoperation, 7th year's follow-up, non-invasion vivo near-infrared imaging function in methylene blue for lymphatic flow system of the right arm to the axillary area. (**a**) (back view of right hand and fore arm), (**b**) (front view of elbow), (**c**) (front view of upper arm and axillary area)

30.9 Summarizes

Lymphedema, as a common chronic disease, not only brings pain and other uncomfortable symptoms to patients but also seriously affects the function of the affected limb. Traditional treatment methods include comprehensive anti-lymphatic stasis treatment, liposuction, and removal of diseased tissue. As a new treatment, hematic lymph node transplantation can reconstruct the physiologic lymphatic network to a large extent, so as to dredge lymphatic vessels and relieve lymphedema. In recent years, the research on the treatment mechanism of vascularized lymph node transplantation has made great progress. Our primary clinical experience showed the good results of the lymphatic flap transfer to reconstruct the new breast and treatment the related arm lymphedema simultaneously.

References

1. Rockson SG. The unique biology of lymphatic edema. Lymphat Res Biol. 2009;7(2):97–100.
2. Jaffe HL, Richter MN. The regeneration of autoplastic lymph node transplants. J Exp Med. 1928;47(6):977–80.
3. Blum KS, Hadamitzky C, Gratz KF, et al. Effects of autotransplanted lymph node fragments on the lymphatic system in the pig model. Breast Cancer Res Treat. 2010;120(1):59–66.
4. Fu K, Izquierdo R, Vandevender D, et al. Transplantation of lymph node fragments in a rabbit ear lymphedema model: a new method for restoring the lymphatic pathway. Plast Reconstr Surg. 1998;101(1):134–41.
5. Pabst R, Rothkötter HJ. Regeneration of autotransplanted lymph node fragments. Cell Tissue Res. 1988;251(3):597–601.
6. Piller NB, Clodius L. Lymphoedema of the rabbit ear following partial and complete lymphatic blockade; its effects on fibrotic development, enzyme types and their activity levels. Br J Exp Pathol. 1978;59(3):319–26.
7. Shesol BF, Nakashima R, Alavi A, et al. Successful lymph node transplantation in rats, with restoration of lymphatic function. Plast Reconstr Surg. 1979;63(6):817–23.
8. Chen HC, O'Brien BM, Rogers IW, et al. Lymph node transfer for the treatment of obstructive lymphoedema in the canine model. Br J Plast Surg. 1990;43(5):578–86.
9. Tobbia D, Semple J, Baker A, et al. Experimental assessment of autologous lymph node transplantation as treatment of postsurgical lymphedema. Plast Reconstr Surg. 2009;124(3):777–86.
10. Jeltsch M, Kaipainen A, Joukov V, et al. Hyperplasia of lymphatic vessels in VEGF-C transgenic mice. Science. 1997;276(5317):1423–5.
11. Tourani SS, Taylor GI, Ashton MW. Vascularized lymph node transfer: a review of the current evidence. Plast Reconstr Surg. 2016;137(3):985–93.
12. Honkonen KM, Visuri MT, Tervala TV, et al. Lymph node transfer and perinodal lymphatic growth factor treatment for lymphedema. Ann Surg. 2013;257(5):961–7.
13. Aschen SZ, Farias-Eisner G, Cuzzone DA, et al. Lymph node transplantation results in spontaneous lymphatic reconnection and restoration of lymphatic flow. Plast Reconstr Surg. 2014;133(2):301–10.
14. Cheng MH, Chen SC, Henry SL, et al. Vascularized groin lymph node flap transfer for postmastectomy upper limb lymphedema: flap anatomy, recipient sites, and outcomes. Plast Reconstr Surg. 2013;131(6):1286–98.
15. Cheng MH, Huang JJ, Nguyen DH, et al. A novel approach to the treatment of lower extremity lymphedema by transferring a vascularized submental lymph node flap to the ankle. Gynecol Oncol. 2012;126(1):93–8.
16. Lin CH, Ali R, Chen SC, et al. Vascularized groin lymph node transfer using the wrist as a recipient site for management of postmastectomy upper extremity lymphedema. Plast Reconstr Surg. 2009;123(4):1265–75.
17. Ito R, Zelken J, Yang CY, et al. Proposed pathway and mechanism of vascularized lymph node flaps. Gynecol Oncol. 2016;141(1):182–8.
18. Clodius L, Smith PJ, Bruna J, et al. The lymphatics of the groin flap. Ann Plast Surg. 1982;9(6):447–58.
19. Becker C, Assouad J, Riquet M, et al. Postmastectomy lymphedema: long-term results following microsurgical lymph node transplantation. Ann Surg. 2006;243(3):313–5.
20. Chen R, Mu L, Zhang H, et al. Simultaneous breast reconstruction and treatment of breast cancer-related upper arm lymphedema with lymphatic lower abdominal flap. Ann Plast Surg. 2014;73(Suppl 1):S12–7.
21. Zhang H, Chen W, Mu L, et al. The distribution of lymph nodes and their nutrient vessels in the groin region: an anatomic study for design of the lymph node flap. Microsurgery. 2014;34(7):558–61.
22. Mu L, Han Z, Ru C, et al. Breast reconstruction and treatment of mastectomy related upper limb lymphedema with lymphatic TRAM/DIEP. Chin Clin Oncol. 2013;18(1):54–6.
23. Lan M, Be Y, et al. Breast reconstruction and treatment of mastectomy related upper limb lymphedema with lymphatic flap transfer and L-V anastomosis. Chin J Plast Surg. 2017;3(33): 161–7.
24. Lan M. Advancement of breast reconstruction and simultaneously treatment and prevention of mastectomy related upper limb lymphedema. Chin J Plast Surg. 2018;34(4):247–51.
25. Lan M, Yan L, Bi Y, Zang H, et al. 2 Clinical cases application of microsurgical arterial, venous and supermicrosurgical lymphovenous anastomoses performed using three-dimensional on-screen visualization. Chin J Microsurg. **2019**;42(**5**):**13**–6.
26. Lan M, Yan L, Bi Y, Zang H, et al. Primary clinical application of microsurgical arterial, venous and supermicrosurgical lymphovenous anastomoses performed using three-dimensional on-screen visualization. J Plast Reconstr Aesthet Surg. https://doi.org/10.1016/j.bjps.2019.08.013.
27. Nguyen AT, Chang EI, Suami H, et al. An algorithmic approach to simultaneous vascularized lymph node transfer with microvascular breast reconstruction. Ann Surg Oncol. 2015;22(9): 2919–24.
28. Ciudad P, Date S, Manrique OJ, et al. Recurrent advanced lower extremity lymphedema following initial successful vascularized lymph node transfer: a clinical and histopathological analysis. Arch Plast Surg. 2017;44(1):87–9.
29. Saaristo AM, Niemi TS, Viitanen TP, et al. Microvascular breast reconstruction and lymph node transfer for postmastectomy lymphedema patients. Ann Surg. 2012;255(3):468–73.
30. Scaglioni MF, Suami H. Lymphatic anatomy of the inguinal region in aid of vascularized lymph node flap harvesting. J Plast Reconstr Aesthet Surg. 2015;68(3):419–27.
31. Tourani SS, Taylor GI, Ashton MW. Anatomy of the superficial lymphatics of the abdominal wall and the upper thigh and its implications in lymphatic microsurgery. J Plast Reconstr Aesthet Surg. 2013;66(10):1390–5.

32. Vignes S, Blanchard M, Yannoutsos A, et al. Complications of autologous lymph-node transplantation for limb lymphoedema. Eur J Vasc Endovasc Surg. 2013;45(5):516–20.
33. Sulo E, Hartiala P, Viitanen T, et al. Risk of donor-site lymphatic vessel dysfunction after microvascular lymph node transfer. J Plast Reconstr Aesthet Surg. 2015;68(4):551–8.
34. Dayan JH, Dayan E, Smith ML. Reverse lymphatic mapping: a new technique for maximizing safety in vascularized lymph node transfer. Plast Reconstr Surg. 2015;135(1):277–85.
35. Finegold DN, Baty CJ, Knickelbein KZ, et al. Connexin 47 mutations increase risk for secondary lymphedema following breast cancer treatment. Clin Cancer Res. 2012;18(8):2382–90.
36. Poccia I, Lin CY, Cheng MH. Platysma-sparing vascularized submental lymph node flap transfer for extremity lymphedema. J Surg Oncol. 2017;115(1):48–53.
37. Chang DW. Lymphaticovenular bypass for lymphedema management in breast cancer patients: a prospective study. Plast Reconstr Surg. 2010;126(3):752–8.
38. O'Brien BM, Hickey MJ, Hurley JV, et al. Microsurgical transfer of the greater momentum in the treatment of canine obstructive lymphoedema. Br J Plast Surg. 1990;43(4):440–6.
39. Nguyen AT, Suami H, Hanasono MM, et al. Long-term outcomes of the minimally invasive free vascularized omental lymphatic flap for the treatment of lymphedema. J Surg Oncol. 2017;115(1):84–9.
40. Lanhua M, Jun X,Yuanbo L, et al. Breast reconstrction with the free bipedicled inferior TRAM or DIEP flaps by anastomosis to the proximal and distal ends of the internal mammmary vessels. Seminars. In Annuls of Plastic Surgery. 2002;16(1):61–7.

Silicone Tube Implantation

31

Waldemar L. Olszewski, Marzanna T. Zaleska, and Rajesh Hydrabadi

Abstract

Advanced cases of lymphedema are characterized by total obstruction of the main lymphatic collecting trunks. There are no lymphatics suitable for the lymphatico-venous anastomoses. The solution may be generating new pathways for edema fluid flow by bypassing the obstruction sites by implanting the silicone tubings. Silicone is hydrophobic, non-adherent for cells and microorganisms, does not evoke evident anti-foreign body reaction, it is pliable and easily adjusting to limb movement without twisting. It can be easily removed if necessary. The inguinal and axillary regions, where obstruction of edema fluid flow is seen, can easily be bypassed subcutaneously.

Keywords

Lymphedema · Lymph · Tissue fluid · Compression Silicone · Tubes

31.1 Introduction

A number of conservative and surgical methods for the treatment of limb lymphedema had been and is now practiced [1–18]. However, none of them proved to restore the shape and function of limbs to normal conditions and prevent recurrence of the chronic and acute DLA. The microsurgical operations can be performed if some fragments of the peripheral collecting lymphatics remain patent and partially drain the tissue edema fluid. However, in advanced cases of lymphedema, all main lymphatics are obstructed, and tissue fluid accumulates in the interstitial spaces, spontaneously forming "lakes" and blind or interconnected "channels" of irregular shape. In such cases, the only solution is constructing artificial pathways for edema fluid flow away to the non-obstructed regions where absorption of fluid can take place (Fig. 31.1). This can be done by implantation of silicone tubes placed along, what used to be, and at present non-functioning, collecting lymphatics (Figs. 31.2, 31.3, 31.4, 31.5).

In 2010, we performed the first operations of subcutaneous implantation of silicone tubes placed from the lower leg to the lumbar or hypogastric regions in a group of patients with obstructive lymphedema of lower limbs developed after lymphadenectomy and irradiation in the pelvis because of uterine cancer [19]. Subsequently, we implanted silicone tubes in a group of patients with postmastectomy lymphedema [20]. Implantation was followed by external compression as intermittent pneumatic compression and elastic support of tissues, and prophylactic administration of low-doses of benzathine penicillin.

We summarized the 3–6 years long-term evidence of the efficacy of silicone tubing drainage in 150 patients with lymphedema of lower and upper limbs treated by silicone tubes implant bypassing the lymph flow obstruction site [21].

31.2 Implant Characteristics

Sterile silicone tubing medical-grade o.d. 3 mm and i.d. 2 mm was used (New Age, Southhampton, PA, USA). The tubing material was hydrophobic, preventing ingrowth of connective tissue into the lumen and around them. Hydrophobic properties were tried previously on rats allowing to pull out the implanted tubing without resistance even months after implantation. The concentrity of tubings did not change, and there was no reduction of ovality. Three tubes of a length adjusted to that of the limb were tied together, and

W. L. Olszewski (✉)
Department of Vascular Surgery, Central Clinical Hospital, Ministry of Internal Affairs, Warsaw, Poland

M. T. Zaleska
Department of Vascular Surgery, Central Clinical Hospital, Ministry of Internal Affairs, Warsaw, Poland

Department of Applied Physiology, Mossakowski Medical Research Institute, Warsaw, Poland

R. Hydrabadi
Vein Clinic, Ahmedabad, India

N. Liu (ed.), *Peripheral Lymphedema*, https://doi.org/10.1007/978-981-16-3484-0_31

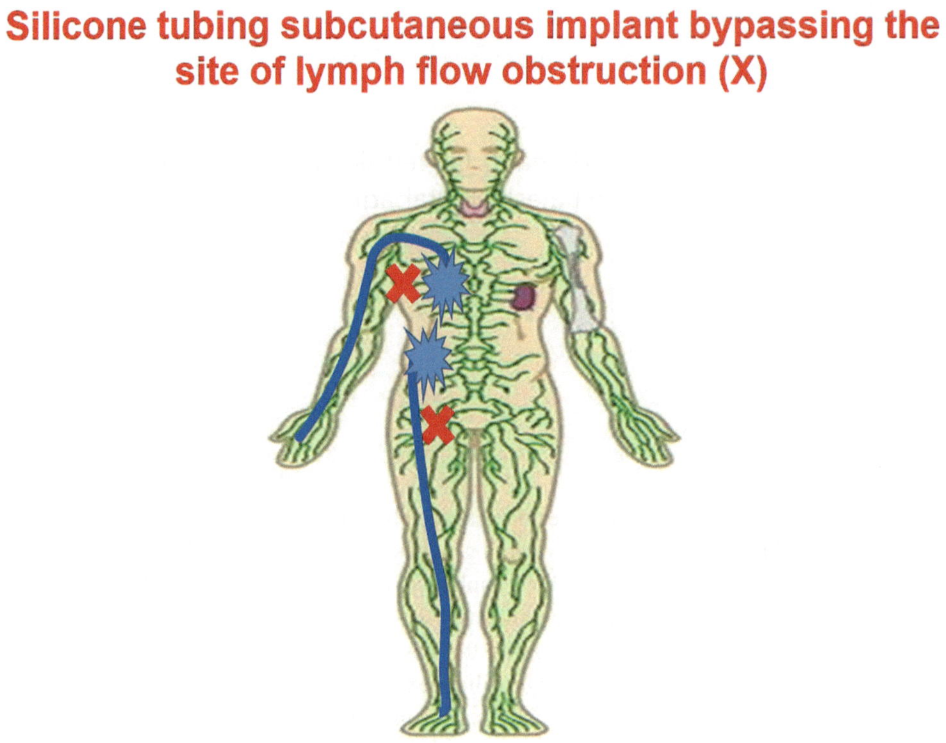

Fig. 31.1 Advanced cases of lymphedema are characterized by total obstruction of the main lymphatic collecting trunks. There are no lymphatics suitable for the lymphatico-venous anastomoses. The solution may be generating new pathways for edema fluid flow by bypassing the obstruction sites by implanting the silicone tubings. Silicone is hydrophobic, non-adherent for cells and microorganisms, does not evoke evident anti-foreign body reaction, it is pliable and easily adjusting to limb movement without twisting. It can be easily removed if necessary. The inguinal and axillary regions, where obstruction of edema fluid flow is seen, can easily be bypassed subcutaneously

SILICONE IMPLANTATION PROCEDURE

THREE-MODALITY PROCEDURE

1. Silicone tubing implantation
2. Intermittent pneumatic compression and elastic support
3. Prophylactic long term penicillin every 14 d to prevent bacterial colonization

Fig. 31.2 The principles of the silicone tubing bypassing procedure

multiple lateral holes of a 2 mm diameter were made at distances of 3 cm. On a cross-view they formed space between them for the accumulation of edema fluid after implantation.

31.3 Implantation Technique

Lower limb. A 2 cm long incision was made at the ankle level, another 3 cm long in the groin, and one 2 cm long in the hypogastrium or lumbar region 10 cm above the inguinal crease (Figs. 31.4, 31.5). A 1.5 cm wide and 100 cm long conductor metal tube, routinely used for insertion of arterial femoro-popliteal grafts, was introduced under the skin and bluntly moved in the subcutaneous tissue toward the thigh and internal aspect of the calf. Silicone tubing tubes were introduced into its lumen and moved upwards. The conductor tube was then removed. Upper limb. A 2 cm long incision was made 2 cm above the radial metacarpal joint and another at the scapular region (Fig. 31.4). The same technique as for the lower limb was applied. In cases with hand edema, the lower end of tubes tubings was placed in the hand dorsum. No fixing of tubes tubings to the surrounding tissues was made either in the lower or upper limb.

31.4 Clinical Aspects

31.4.1 Postoperative Treatment

Patients were put on daily 1 h intermittent pneumatic compression (IPC) of the treated limb for 14 days in our OPD. IPC was further carried out as home care. Elastic stockings second degree 26–32 mmHg of compression were used as before surgery. Oral 1 g of amoxicillin was given for one month. Long-lasting penicillin administration was administered as before the operations. Patients had the limb circumference measurements made at five levels daily for the first 14 days in the OPD, then weekly at home at the same time of the day and same limb position. We saw them monthly for the first 3 months followed by bimonthly control during the following years.

31.4.2 Results in Lower Limbs

31.4.2.1 Clinical Evaluation

First-fifty patients, out of the total of 150, who were followed-up for at least 36 months, were evaluated. Five patients carried implants for over 6 years. Inflammatory reaction along the implant was observed in the follow-up in five

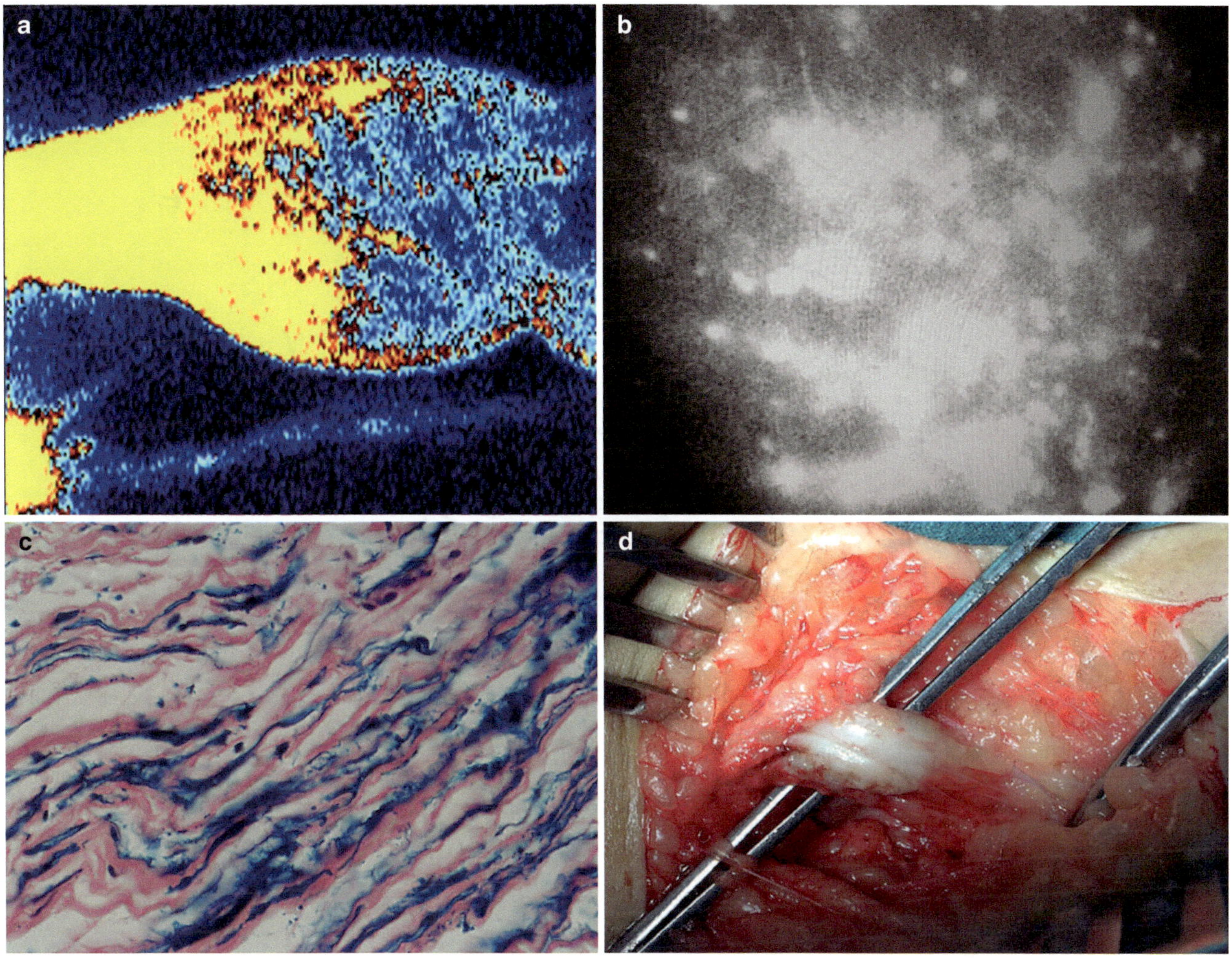

Fig. 31.3 Pictures illustrating where and why edema fluid accumulates in lymphedema as a rationale for searching methods of decompression. (**a**) Calf lymphoscintigram showing subepidermal lymphatic flow (previously called "dermal backflow) and no lymphatic collectors, (**b**) indocyanine green lymphography in concert with the lymphoscintigraphic picture, (**c**) soft tissue "channels" formed by the accumulating fluid, and (**d**) totally fibrotic inguinal lymph node obstructing lymph flow from the limb. Edema fluid accumulated in these no-lymphatics tissues needs a new flow pathway away

patients. In three inflammation limited to the upper end of the implant in the hypogastrium was observed, most likely as a reaction to microbes drained from the calf. Inflammation was controlled without recurrence by seven days of oral amoxicillin and three consecutive intra-tubing injections of augmentin. Evident decrease of limb girth and restriction of edematous limb movements, squatting, and kneeling was observed in all patients.

31.4.2.2 Lymphoscintigraphic Pre- and Post-Implantation Pictures

On lymphoscintigrams, patency of all implanted tubings was found preserved (Figs. 31.6, 31.7, 31.8, 31.9).

31.4.2.3 Circumference and Volume Changes

For clarity of presentation, the most important the mid-calf and mid-thigh circumferences are presented. Volume was calculated by the truncated cone formula. The circumference decreased in all patients within the first 2 weeks, differently at different levels of the limb. In the 3 years follow-up, it was in the mid-calf a mean −8.7% ($P < 0.05$) with a range of −3.2% to −31.0% and in the mid-thigh a mean −1.8% ($P < 0.05$) with a range of −9.3% to +3% equal to 0–900 ml (Fig. 31.10). Most decrease was observed in the calf. Wide range in the decrease of limb girth was the consequence of individual differences in edema fluid volume accumulating in the subcutaneous tissue.

31.4.2.4 Changes in Tissue Stiffness (Tonometry)

The tissue stiffness measured with a deep tonometer decreased in all patients within the first 2 weeks. In the mid-calf it decreased from a mean 2.1 kg/sq cm to mean 1.6 kg/sq cm ($p < 0.01$) with a range of 1.0–1.4 kg/sq cm. In the mid-thigh

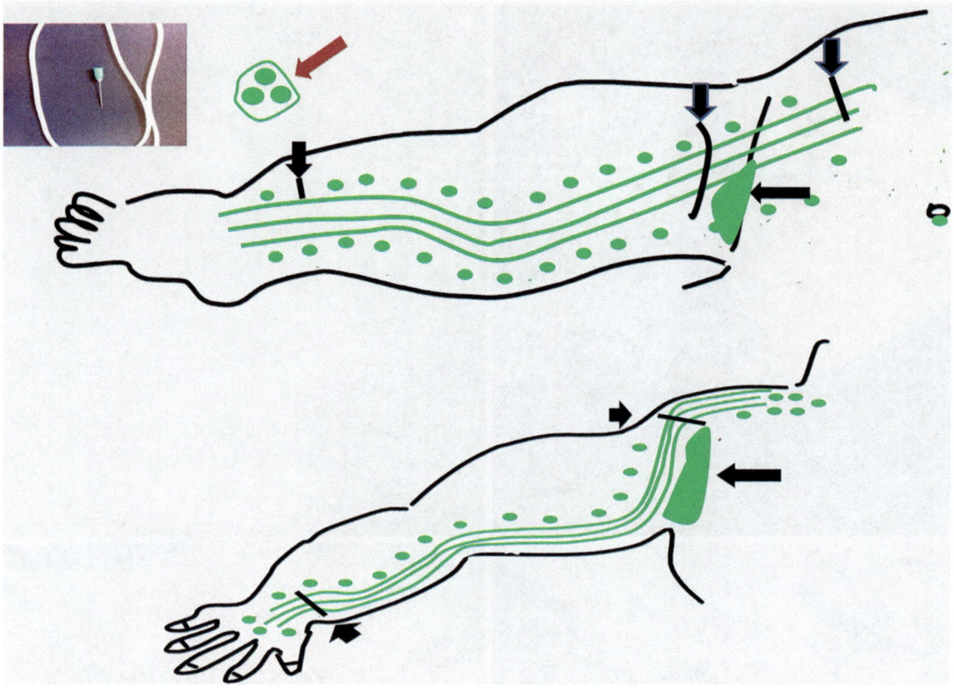

Fig. 31.4 Upper panel. A schematic design of the operation of the subcutaneous implantation of silicone tubes from the foot, along the limb, above the inguinal ligament, to the hypogastric or lumbar regions. Horizontal arrow points to the groin, site of lymph vessels, and lymph nodes obstruction. Implanted tubes bypass this region. Small vertical arrows show the sites of skin incisions for implantation. Dots around tubes symbolize fluid. In the upper part of the figure, an insert illustrating the size of tubes and a cross-section drawing of three tubes and fluid accumulating around them (arrow). Lower panel. A schematic design of the operation of implantation of silicone tubes from the hand to the scapula regions. Horizontal arrow points to the axilla, site of lymphadenectomy and radiotherapy. Implanted tubes bypass this region. Small vertical arrows show sites of skin incisions for implantation

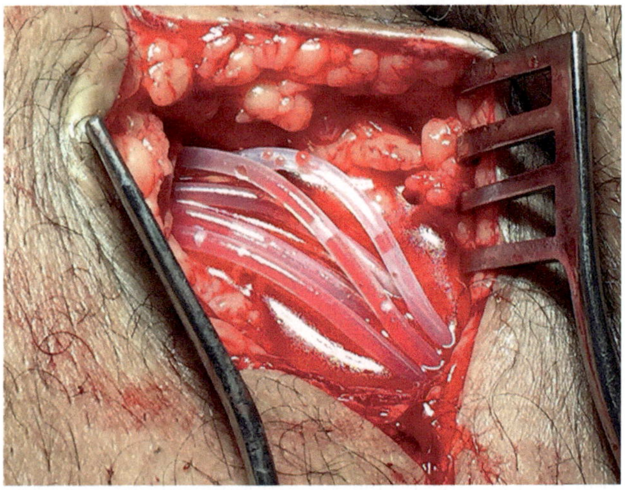

Fig. 31.5 Silicone tubings have been implanted subcutaneously from the lower calf through the inguinal region up to the hypogastrium. They fill up immediately with edema fluid. Usually, three tubes are inserted. In case of large thigh edema some three more tubings draining the upper thigh may be added

the mean decrease was 0.6 ((NS) with a range from 0.7 kg/sq cm to 0.5 kg/sq cm (Fig. 31.10). Stiffness remained at that low level throughout the entire follow-up period.

31.4.3 Results in Upper Limbs

31.4.3.1 Clinical Evaluation

Fifty patients were followed-up for at least 24 months. There were only two incidents of peri-tubing inflammation successfully controlled by oral antibiotics.

31.4.3.2 Lymphoscintigraphic Pre- and Post-Implantation Pictures

All tubings remained patent along the follow-up period and could easily be visualized (Figs. 31.11, 31.12).

31.4.3.3 Circumference and Volume Changes

The circumference decreased in all patients within the first 2 weeks with slight differences at different limb levels. In the two-year follow-up in the mid-forearm a mean decrease was −8.5% ($P < 0.01$) with a range of −3.0% to −22.0%, and in the mid-arm a mean −12% ($P < 0.05$) with a range of −7% to −22% (Fig. 31.13). That corresponded to 180–700 ml volume for the limb. The wide range in decrease of limb girth was the consequence of individual differences in edema fluid volume accumulating in the subcutaneous tissue.

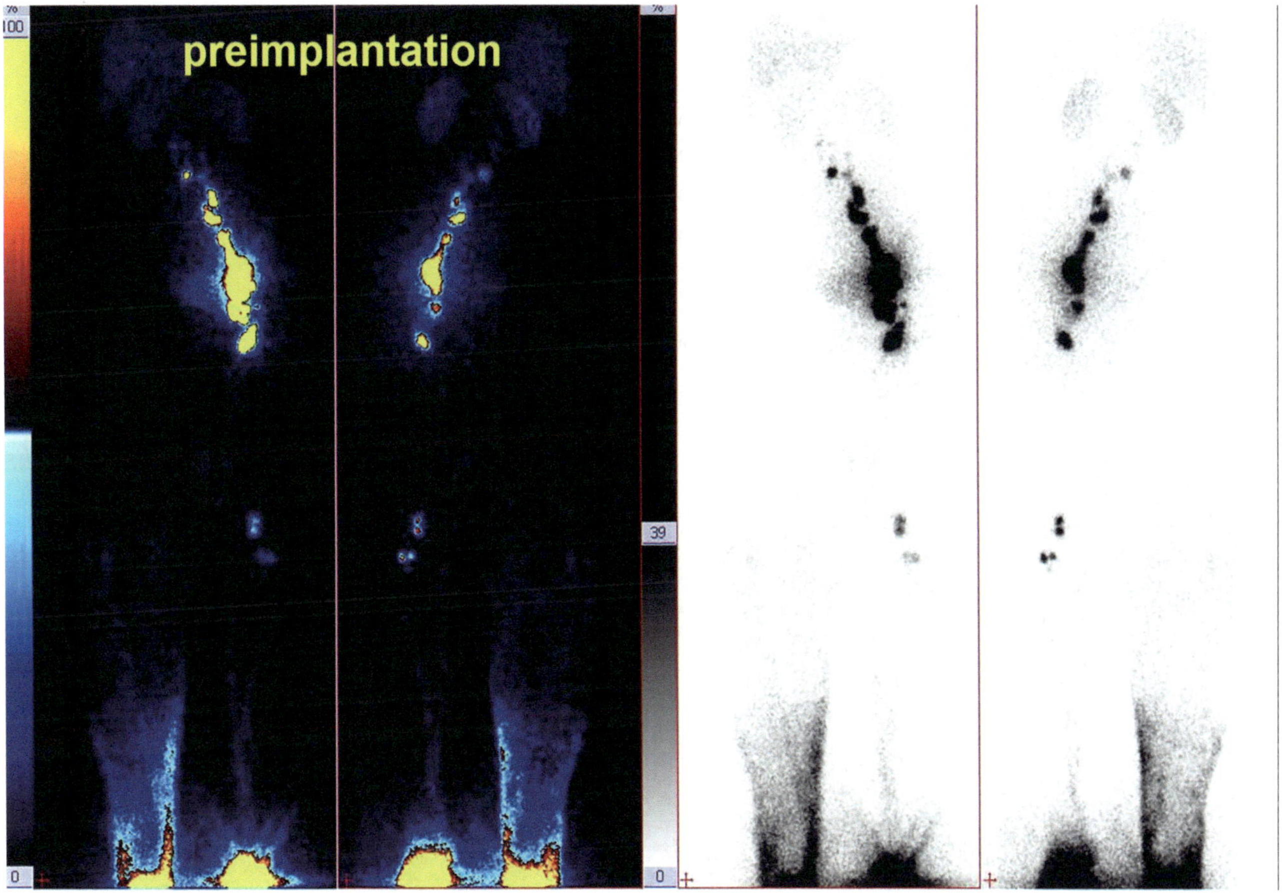

Fig. 31.6 Lymphoscintigram of the right lower limb with lymphedema before silicone implantation. No lymphatics are depicted

31.4.3.4 Changes in Stiffness (Tonometry)

The tissue stiffness measured with deep tonometer decreased in all patients within the first 2 weeks. In the mid-forearm it decreased in the two-year follow-up by a mean 56% ($P < 0.01$) with a range of 48% to 69% and from mean 1.24 kg/sq cm to 0.58 kg/sq cm. In the mid-arm the mean decrease was 40% ($P < 0.05$) in a range of 31% to 55% from 0.62 kg/sq cm to 0.29 kg/sq cm (Fig. 31.13). Stiffness remained at that low level throughout the entire follow-up period.

31.4.4 Visualization of the Implanted Tubings for Control of Their Patency

The non-ionic X-ray-contrast medium was injected around the lower pole or directly into the tubings at various time points after implantation. Patency and a large fluid-filled space around them was seen (Figs. 31.14, 31.15).

31.4.5 Force to Be Applied on the Lymphedema Limb to Propel Fluid in Implanted Tubings

In order to move tissue fluid in the tubings two force vectors are necessary, a vertical and longitudinal (Fig. 31.16).

31.4.6 Ultrasonography of Tubings

On ultrasonography of tubings in limbs, the implanted tubings were identified in all cases. Their position remained unchanged over the follow-up period, and the lumen was patent (Fig. 31.17). Accumulation of fluid around tubings was seen in all cases. With the decrease of limb circumference, less or no fluid was observed compared with the pre-implantation images.

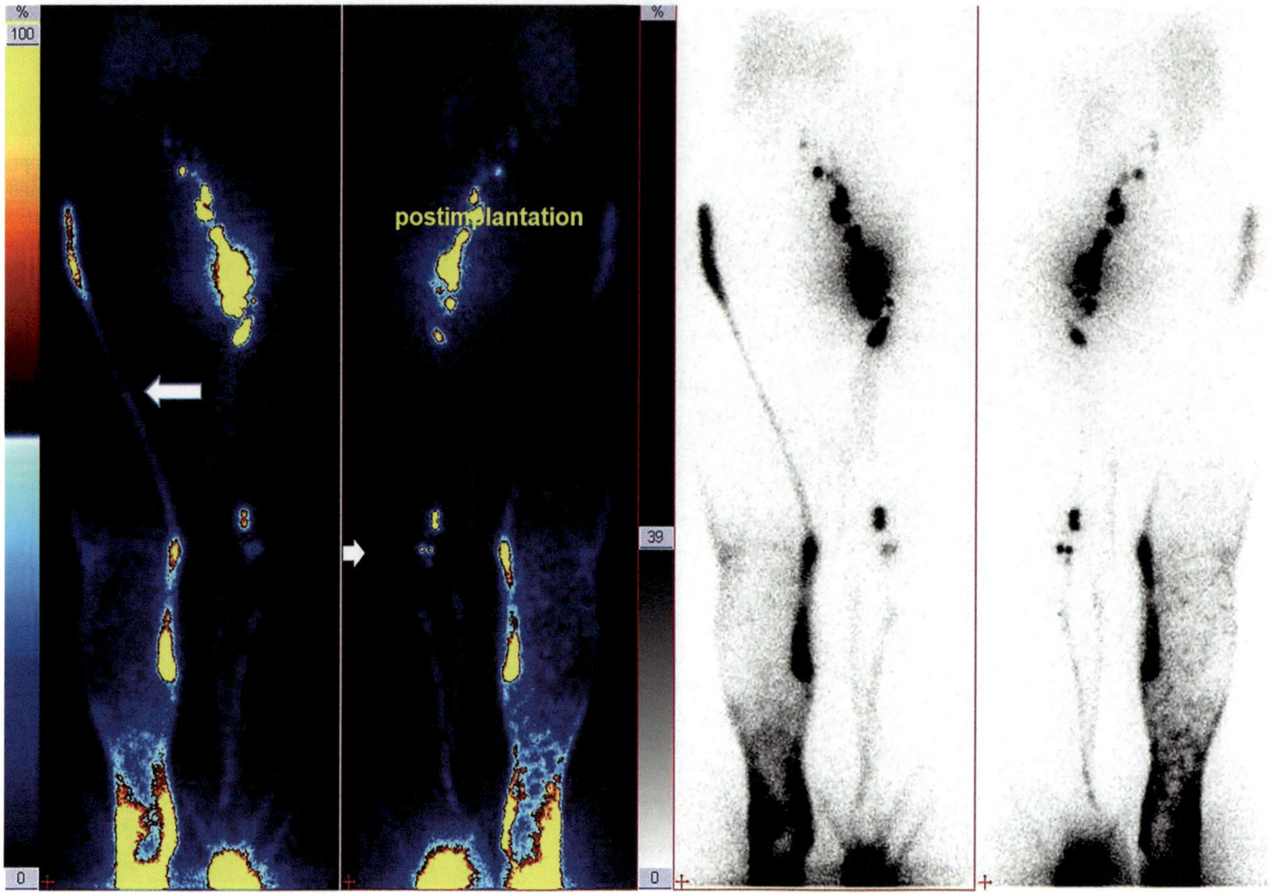

Fig. 31.7 Lymphoscintigram of the right lower limb one year after silicone tubing implantation. See the tubing filled with the tracer (arrow) and evident drainage of the distal parts of the calf (comparing with the before implantation picture)

31.5 General Comments

The presented method provided an immediate decrease of limb circumference within days after implantation and stabilization of size for years and a decrease of tissue stiffness, enabling easy limb movements. Tubes bypassing the lymph flow obstruction site were proved to remain patent. Interestingly, edema fluid flew into tubings upon external massage and its movement along tubings and around them to hypogastrium or scapular tissues.

The decrease in limb circumference was accompanied by less fluid around the implants on ultrasound and X-rays of opacified tubings. This could be accounted for by the effective evacuation of fluid to the hypogastrium or lumbar or shoulder tissues. External compression of edematous tissues brought about the flow of fluid into tubings at their length through lateral holes and to the upper ends of tubings to further be spread in normal tissues.

The implanted silicone tubings are passive channels. The accumulating tissue fluid cannot flow along the mechanically inert tubes by itself. It requires a propelling force. Massaging of tissues along the implanted tubes generated intra-tubing pressures of 30–60 mmHg. This could also be obtained by application of intermittent pneumatic compression as well as walking in short stretch bandages or stockings.

The silicone tissue fluid pathways were proved to be durably efficient in transporting away excess fluid. So far, no occlusion of tubes was observed in any patient. Interestingly, the obtained results were not dependent on the stage of lymphedema. It has been documented that the medical-grade silicone tubings are biologically inert and do not evoke clinically recognizable foreign body reactions. The polymer disintegration rate in minimal [22]. Any trace of it remains in tissues and may be phagocytized. Moreover, they are hydrophobic, thus preventing obstruction by ingrowing fibrous tissue. It is also important that bacteria generally do not adhere to silicone surfaces [23, 24].

There were no major inflammatory reactions to the implanted tubing in 95% of lower limbs and no episodes in upper limb lymphedema. In some patients with lower limb lymphedema, a several days lasting inflammation was seen at the upper end of implants. It was easily controlled by antibiotics.

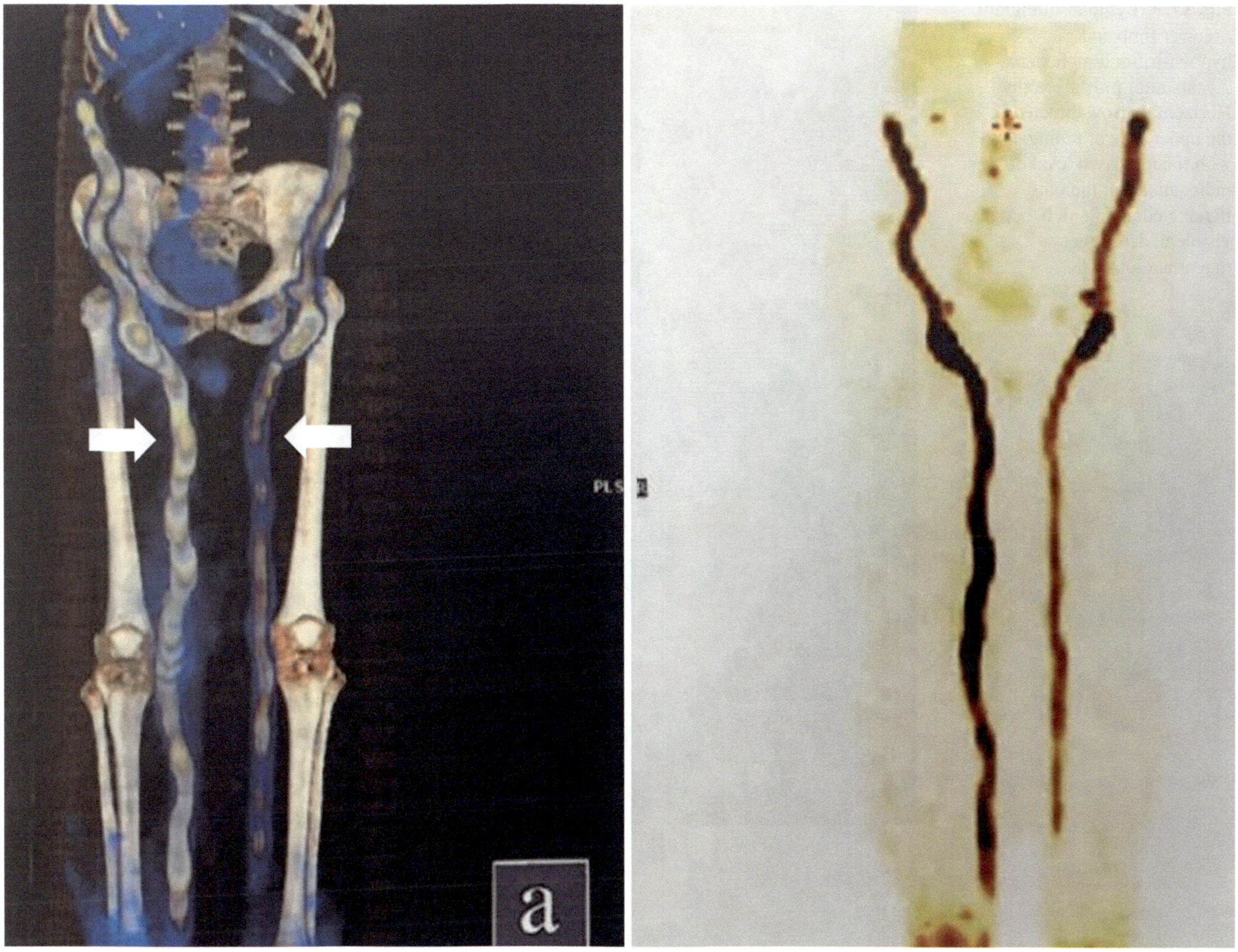

Fig. 31.8 The SPECT-CT hybrid lymphoscintigraphic picture of silicone tubes implanted in both limbs from the foot to the lumbar regions 3 years ago. Positioning of the implant is clearly visible. "Foggy" shadow in the lower part of limbs and around tubes is that of edema fluid accumulation. The diameter of the isotopic outline of tubes is larger than in reality due to the radiation scattering

An open question remains whether tubes should remain in tissues indefinitely or be removed, expecting that an encapsulated channel has been formed conducting fluid. This needs further studies. A thin capsule is being formed around tubes; however, it remains highly permeable. Removal of tubings can be carried out within 3 minutes through a 2 cm incision. Silicone does not adhere to tissues, and there is no penetration of fibroblasts into the lumen.

The question remains open about the absorption capacity of healthy tissues at the outlet of tubings. We observed a low degree edema developing in the lumbar and scapular regions during the day activities subsiding during the night rest. This could be accounted for by sufficient absorption capacity from these regions.

In conclusion, this three modality procedures composed of implantation of silicone tubings bypassing the lymph flow obstruction site, post-implant limb compression, and prophylactic low dose long-term penicillin administration proved to be very efficient in a long-term follow-up of over 3 years. The short-lasting (30 min) surgical procedure and lack of reaction to the implant made the method worth applying in advanced stages of lymphedema in large cohorts of patients by one surgeon.

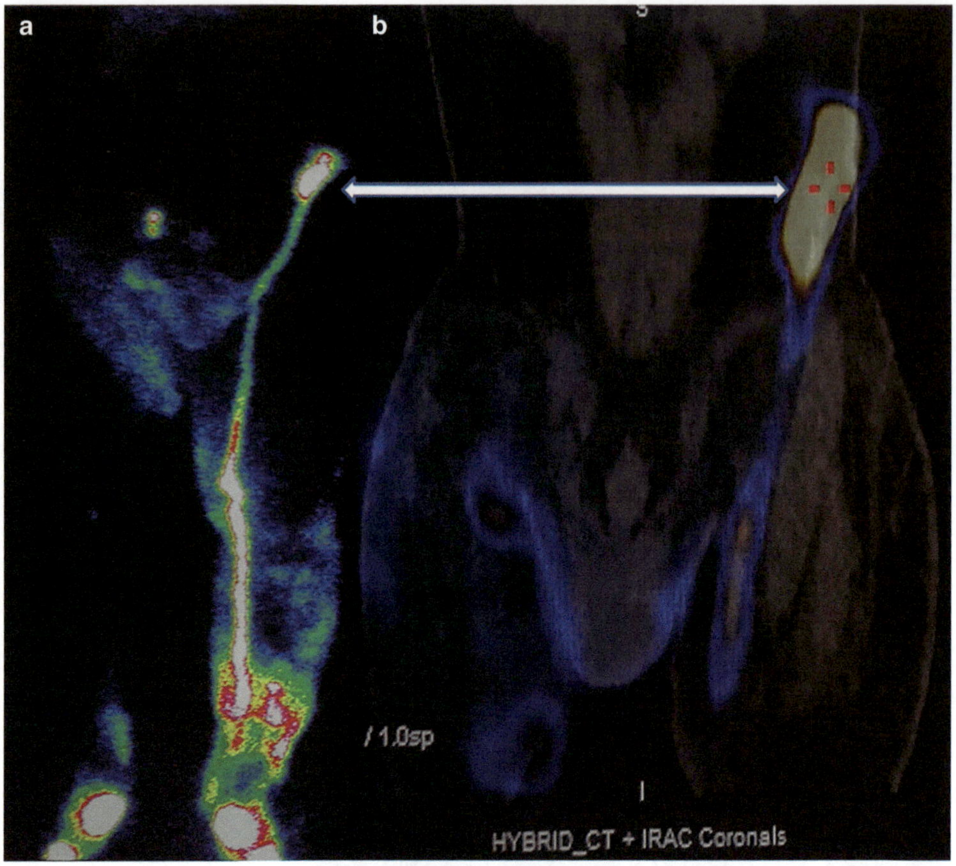

Fig. 31.9 Lymphoscintigram of lower limb and hypogastrium lymphedema 2 years after prostatectomy. Horizontal arrow directed at the upper pole of tubing a. with the increased level of radioactivity of the outflowing edema fluid, b. better visible under higher magnification

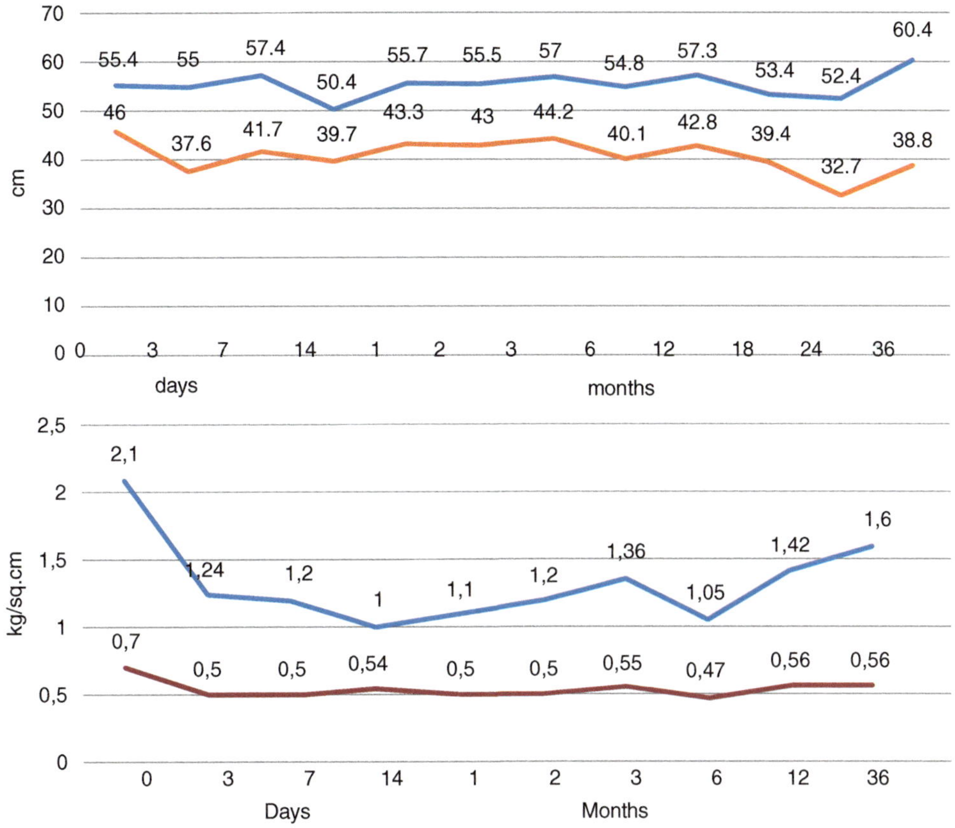

Fig. 31.10 Post-implantation results in 50 patients with lymphedema of lower limbs in a 3-years follow-up. Upper panel. Change in limb circumference in the mid-calf and mid-thigh. The values are cm, means, SD 5–23 cm. Note that there was an immediate decrease in calf circumference and its maintenance thereafter. Ultrasonography revealed no more mobile fluid. There were no significant changes in the thigh. Major individual differences in the effects of drainage are reflected by a large standard deviation. Lower panel. Change in the limb tissue stiffness (tonometry) in the mid-calf and mid-thigh. The values are kg/sq. cm, means, SD 0.16–1.5. Note rapid decrease in stiffness within the first two weeks and maintenance of the increased elasticity over the next 3 years, both in the calf and thigh. Major individual differences in the decrease of stiffness reflected by a large standard deviation

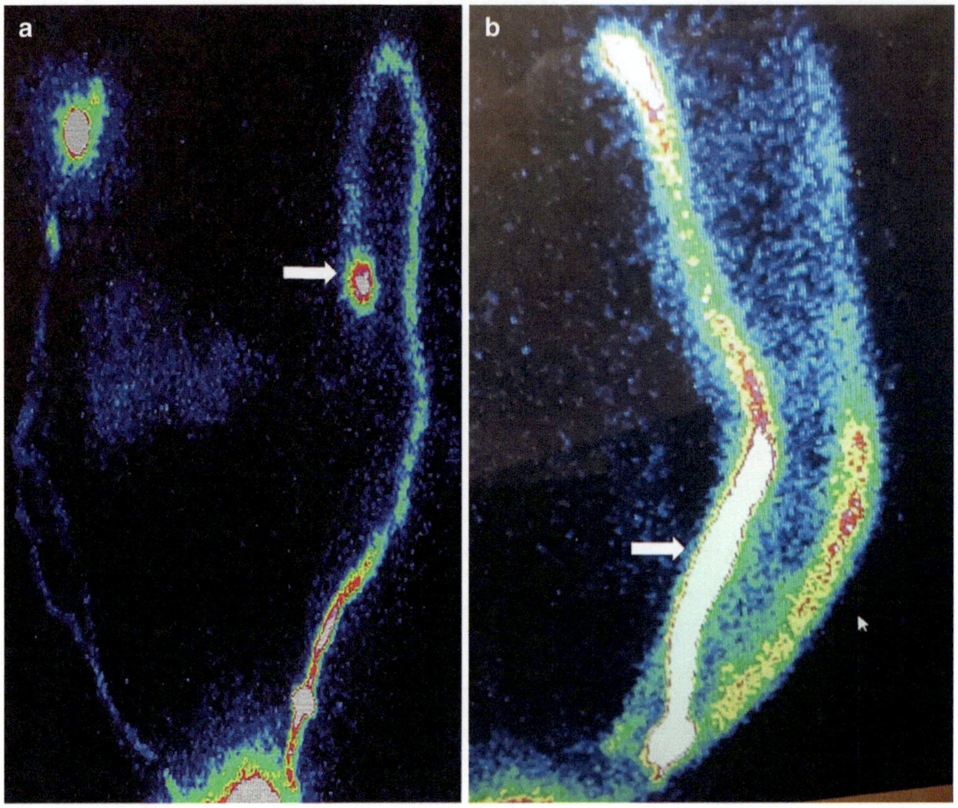

Fig. 31.11 Lymphoscintigram of the left upper limb with implanted silicone tubings 2–3 years back. (**a**) Upper pole of tubing at the scapula level with increased radioactivity proving tracer flow, (**b**) large accumulation of fluid around the tubings creating a reservoir that can be massaged away by compression

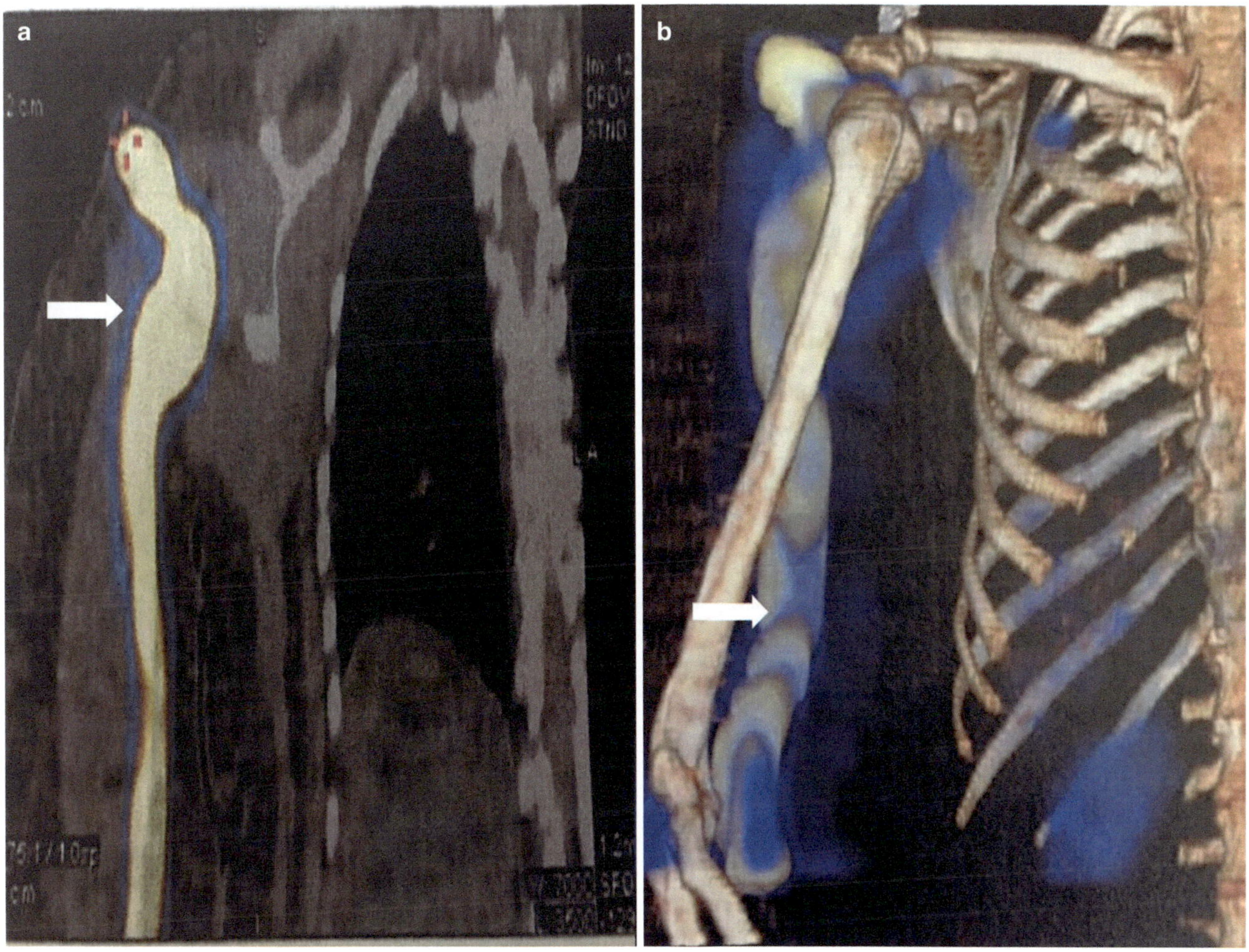

Fig. 31.12 Lymphoscintigraphic picture of the left lower limb with silicone tubes (arrow) bypassing the axillary region three years after implantation. Note that fluid accumulated not only in but also around the tubes, especially in the upper arm. (**b**) SPECT-CT hybrid lymphoscintigraphic picture of tubes. Positioning of implant clearly visible in the forearm and behind the arm reaching scapular region. The shadow in soft tissues and around tubes shows sites of edema fluid accumulation. The diameter of the isotopic outline of tubing is larger than in reality due to the radiation scattering

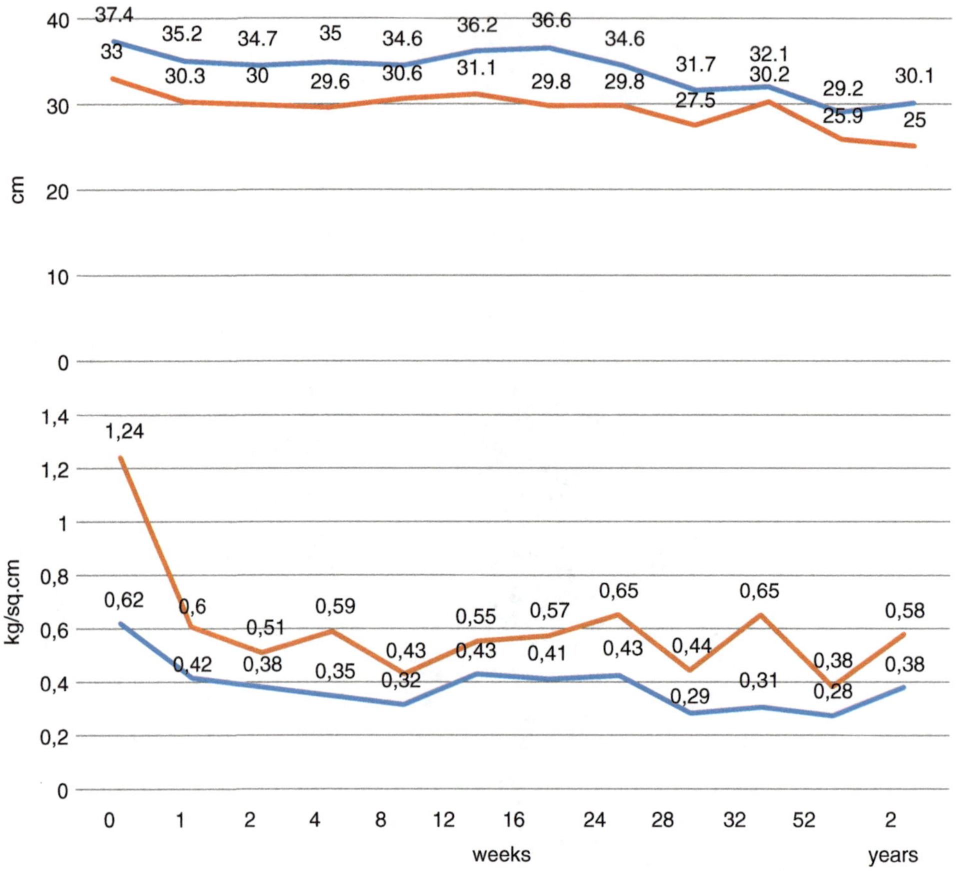

Fig. 31.13 Post-implantation results in 50 patients with lymphedema of upper limbs in a 2-years follow-up. Upper panel. Change of the limb circumference in the mid-forearm and mid-arm. The values are cm, means, SD 0.3 cm. Note that there was an immediate decrease in the limb circumference, and it proceeded thereafter. Lower panel. Limb tissue stiffness (tonometry) in the mid-forearm and mid-arm. The values are kg/sq cm, means, SD 0.2. Note rapid decrease in the stiffness within the first week and maintenance of increased elasticity over the next 2 years in the entire limb

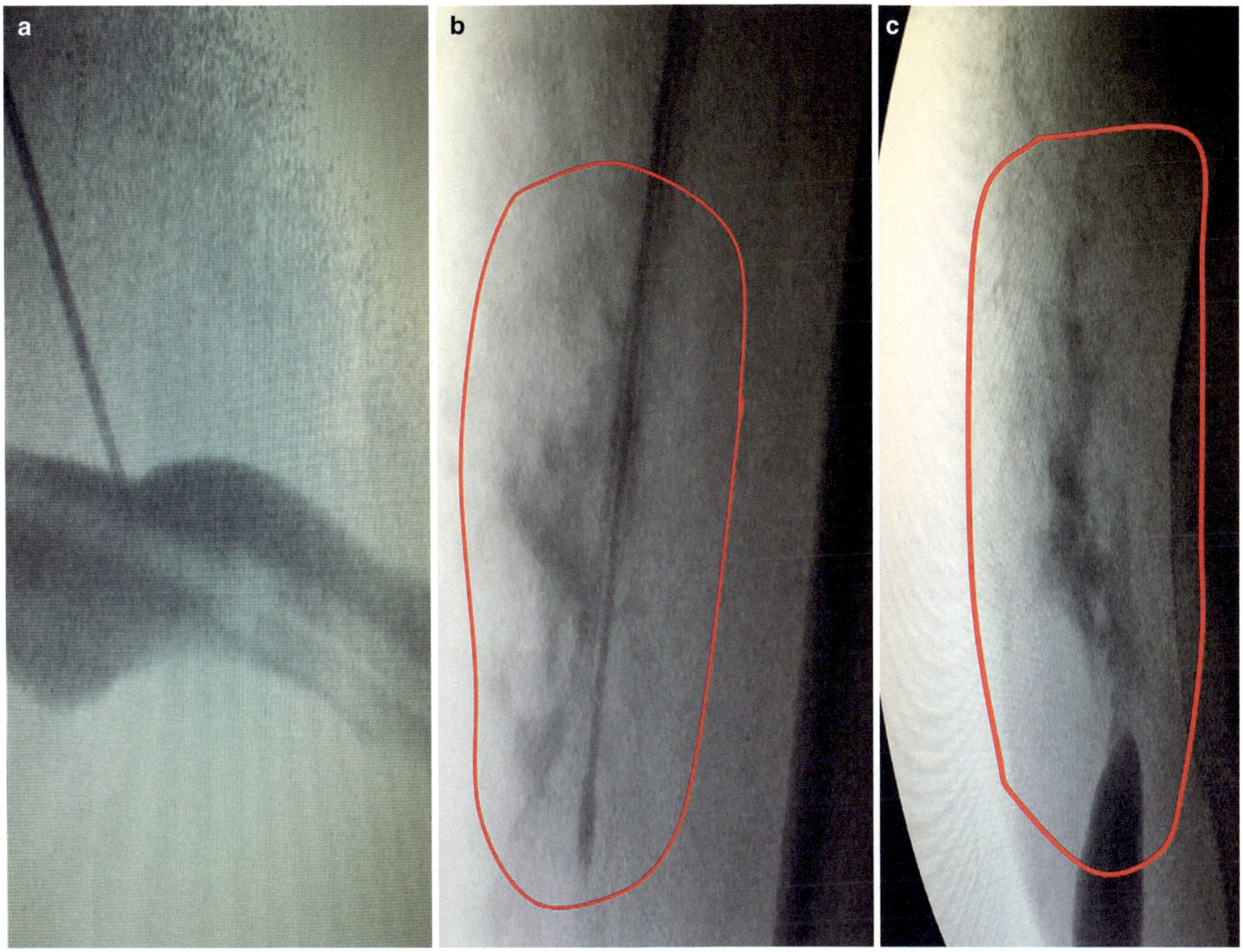

Fig. 31.14 Silicone tubes implanted into lower limb contrasted by the angiographic non-ionic medium to prove fluid flow in and out of the lumen, two years after operation, (**a**) transcutaneous injection into tubes, (**b**) injected contrast medium flows out from the lower end of the implant in the calf (circle), (**c**) injected contrast medium flows out from the upper end of the implant in the lumbar region (circle). Images prove free tissue space connection with implanted tubes

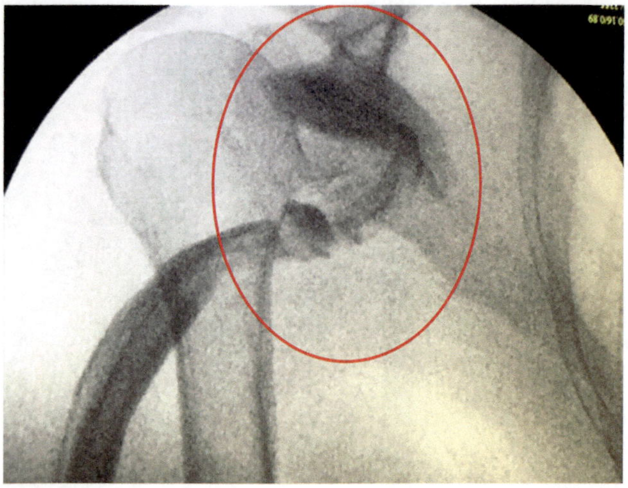

Fig. 31.15 Silicone tubes implanted into upper limb contrasted by the angiographic non-ionic medium to prove fluid flow in and out of the lumen, two years after the operation. The injected contrast medium flows out from the upper end of the implant in the scapula area (circle)

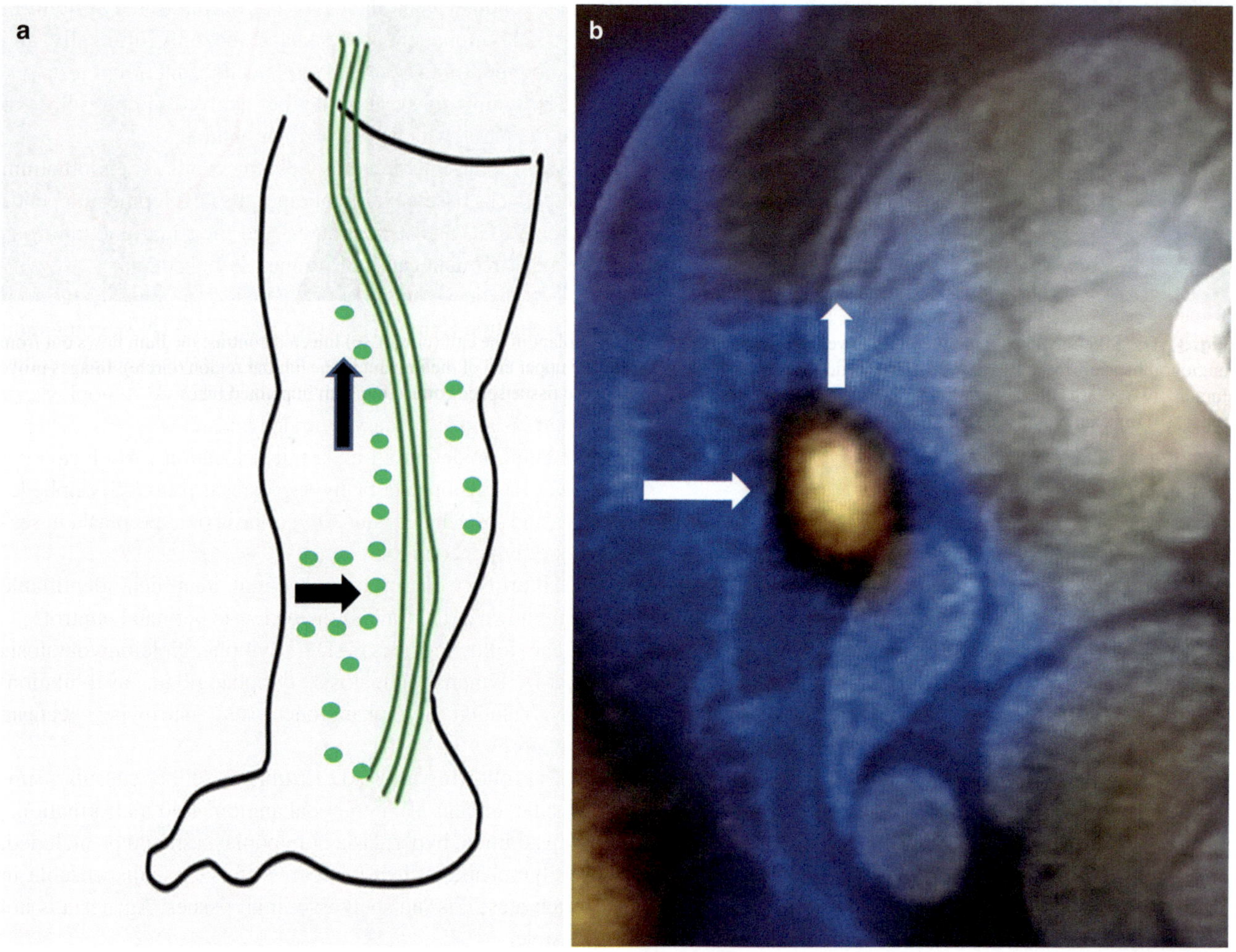

Fig. 31.16 Scheme and lymphoscintigram showing that two forces should be applied for compression treatment after silicone tubing implantation. A vertical is to drive fluid into tubings, and a horizontal along the limb axis is to propel fluid through and around the tubings to the hypogastrium

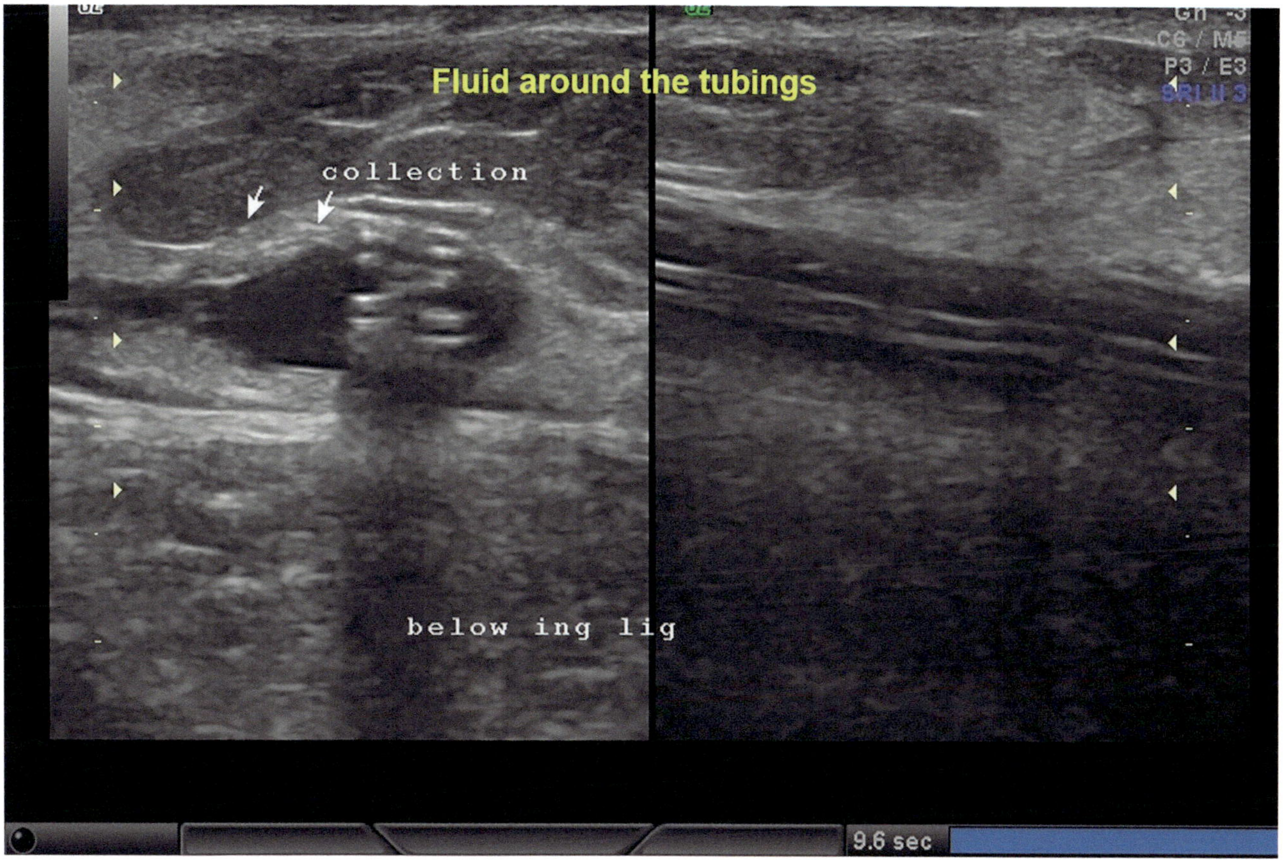

Fig. 31.17 Ultrasonography turned to be necessary and extremely useful in controlling the tubings position and accumulation, as well as, massaging away edema fluid from around them

References

1. Charles H. Elephantiasis of the leg. In: Latham A, English TC, editors. A system of treatment, vol. 3. London: Churchill; 1912.
2. Sistrunk WE. Contribution to plastic surgery: removal of scars by stages; the Kondoleon operation for elephantiasis. Ann Surg. 1927;85:185–93.
3. Thompson N. The surgical treatment of chronic lymphedema of the extremities. Surg Clin North Am. 1967;47:445–503.
4. Goldsmith HS, De los Santos L, Beattie EJ. Relief of chronic lymphedema by omental transposition. Ann Surg. 1967;166:573–85.
5. Jørgensen MG, Toyserkani NM, Sørensen JA. The effect of prophylactic lymphovenous anastomosis and shunts for preventing cancer-related lymphedema: a systematic review and meta-analysis. Microsurgery. 2017 Mar 28; https://doi.org/10.1002/micr.30180.
6. Olszewski WL. Experimental lympho-venous anastomoses. Proceedings of the congress, polish society of surgeons, Lodz; Dent Abstr 1966:62.
7. Nielubowicz J, Olszewski WL. Surgical lymphatico-venous anostomosis. (Preliminary note). Minerva Cardioangiol. 1967;15:254–6.
8. Nielubowicz J, Olszewski W. Experimental lymphovenous anastomosis. Br J Surg. 1968;55:449–51.
9. Nielubowicz J, Olszewski W. Surgical lympho-venous shunts in patients with secondary Lymphedema. Br J Surg. 1968;55:440.
10. Olszewski WL. The lymphovenous microsurgical shunts for treatment of lymphedema of lower limbs: indications in 2011. Int Angiol. 2011;30:499–503.
11. Olszewski WL. Lymphovenous microsurgical shunts in treatment of lymphedema of lower limbs: a 45-year experience of one surgeon/one center. Eur J Vasc Endovasc Surg. 2013;45:282–90.
12. Yamamoto T, Yamamoto N, Numahata T, Yokoyama A, Tashiro K, Yoshimatsu H, et al. Navigation lymphatic supermicrosurgery for the treatment of cancer-related peripheral lymphedema. J Vasc Endovascular Surg. 2014;48:139–43.
13. Lin CH, Ali R, Chen SC, Wallace C, Chang YC, Chen HC, et al. Vascularized groin lymph node transfer using the wrist as a recipient site for management of postmastectomy upper extremity lymphedema. Plast Reconstr Surg. 2009;123:1265–75.
14. Becker C, Vasile JV, Levine JL, Batista BN, Studinger RM, Chen CM, et al. Microlymphatic surgery for the treatment of iatrogenic lymphedema. Clin Plast Surg. 2012;39:385–98.
15. Cheng MH, Huang JJ, Nguyen DH, Saint-Cyr M, Zenn MR, Tan BK, et al. A novel approach to the treatment of lower extremity lymphedema by transferring a vascularized submental lymph node flap to the ankle. Gynecol Oncol. 2012;126:93–8.
16. Kim DI, Lee BB, Huh S, Lee SJ, Hwang JH, Kim YI. Excision of subcutaneous tissue and deep muscle fascia for advanced lymphedema. Lymphology. 1998;31:190–4.
17. Sando WC, Nahai F. Suction lipectomy in the management of limb lymphedema. Clin Plast Surg. 1989;16:369–73.
18. Brorson H, Svensson H. Complete reduction of lymphoedema of the arm by liposuction after breast cancer. Scand J Plast Reconstr Surg Hand Surg. 1997;31:137–43.
19. Olszewski WL, Zaleska M. A novel method of edema fluid drainage in obstructive lymphedema of limbs by implantation of hydro-

phobic silicone tubes. J Vasc Surg Venous Lymphat Disord. 2015 Oct;3(4):401–8.
20. Olszewski WL, Zaleska MT. Treatment of postmastectomy lymphedema by bypassing the armpit with implanted silicone tubings. Int Angiol. 2017 Feb;36(1):50–8.
21. Olszewski WL, Zaleska MT, Hydrabadi R, Banker M, Kurulkar P. Edema fluid can be successfully evacuated from the lymphedematous limbs by implantation of silicone tubings bypassing the site of flow obstruction long-term observations lymphat. Res Biol. 2019 Oct;17(5):557–64.
22. Mojsiewicz-Pieńkowska K, Szymkowska K, Krenczkowska D. Direct Human Contact with Siloxanes (Silicones) – Safety or Risk Part 1. Characteristics of Siloxanes (Silicones) Front. Pharmacol. 30 May 2016 | https://doi.org/10.3389/fphar.2016.00132
23. Gristina AG, Costerton JW. Bacterial adherence to biomaterials and tissue. J Bone Joint Surg. 2008;67:264–73.
24. Magennis EP, Hook AL, Williams P, Alexander MA. Making silicone rubber highly resistant to bacterial attachment using thiol-ene grafting. ACS Appl Mater Interfaces. 2016;8:30780–7.

Treatment of Lymphedema: Liposuction

32

Jianfeng Xin, Wenbin Shen, and Yiyin Li

Abstract

Since 2009, The Department of Lymphatic Surgery of Beijing Shijitan Hospital Affiliated with Capital Medical University has adopted liposuction to treat lymphedema, which has achieved good results. In our analysis of 30 patients with primary lymphedema of the lower extremities, the total volume of aspirated fat was 900–3900 mL, and the volume of blood loss was 160–1100 mL during liposuction. Regarding the comparison of objective parameters, (1) the volume of lower extremity significantly decreased immediately after surgery and at 3 month follow-up compared with that prior to operation (31.4 ± 16.4 Vs. 6.6 ± 10.0 vs. 12.2 ± 10.7, $P < 0.05$); (2) Female patients demonstrated greater volume of aspirated fat and higher liposuction rate than males during operation, whereas male patients showed greater volume of blood loss as well as greater percent volume difference prior to operation, immediately after operation and at 3 month follow-up; (3) Patients with history of erysipelas manifested higher volume of blood loss, lower volume of aspirated adipose tissue and lower liposuction rate; (4) Stage II patients demonstrated greater volume of aspirated adipose tissue and higher liposuction rate than Stage III patients during operation, in contrast to less blood loss and lower percent volume difference prior to operation, immediately after operation and at 3 month follow-up than Stage III patients. (5) Regarding subjective assessment, the experienced heaviness and fatigue were significantly alleviated, whereas tenderness and tightness were aggravated. Liposuction is an effective therapy for primary lymphedema of the lower extremities. It is necessary to combine liposuction with other therapeutic methods to improve lymphatic circulation. Patient's gender, stage of lymphedema, and history of recurrent erysipelas are major factors affecting the technical difficulty of the operation and prognosis.

Keywords

Lymphedema · Liposuction · Lympholiposuction · Lower extremity · Tumescent · Primary · Fat

32.1 Background

Liposuction refers to a surgical technique that uses various equipment to aspirate excess subcutaneous fat through small incisions made on the skin to improve body esthetics.

Since Illouz [1] first reported the usage of the negative pressure suction method for fat aspiration in 1980, liposuction has been widely applied in various therapeutic fields. Because lymphedema can cause abnormal proliferation of subcutaneous adipose tissue, many national and international scholars treat lymphedema with liposuction and have achieved good results in recent years. Brorson [2] and Boyages [3] have reported that liposuction combined with postoperative controlled compression therapy (CCT) is effective for the treatment of limb lymphedema. The results of Boyages' study showed that the percent volume difference decreased from preoperative 47.3% to 4.3% at 6 months after surgery. Kun Chang [4] also reported 49 cases of lower extremity lymphedema treated with liposuction followed by lymphaticovenous anastomosis (LVA). The mean volume difference was reduced from preoperative 2729 ml to 889 ml at 12 months postoperatively, demonstrating that liposuction combined with LVA is effective.

Since the lymphedematous limbs contain a large amount of pathologically proliferated adipose tissue and excessive lymphatic fluid, the volume reduction process by the aspiration for extremity lymphedema is similar to but different from liposuction. For this reason, we believe

J. Xin · W. Shen (✉) · Y. Li
Department of Lymphatic Surgery, Beijing Shijitan Hospital, Capital Medical University, Beijing, China

N. Liu (ed.), *Peripheral Lymphedema*, https://doi.org/10.1007/978-981-16-3484-0_32

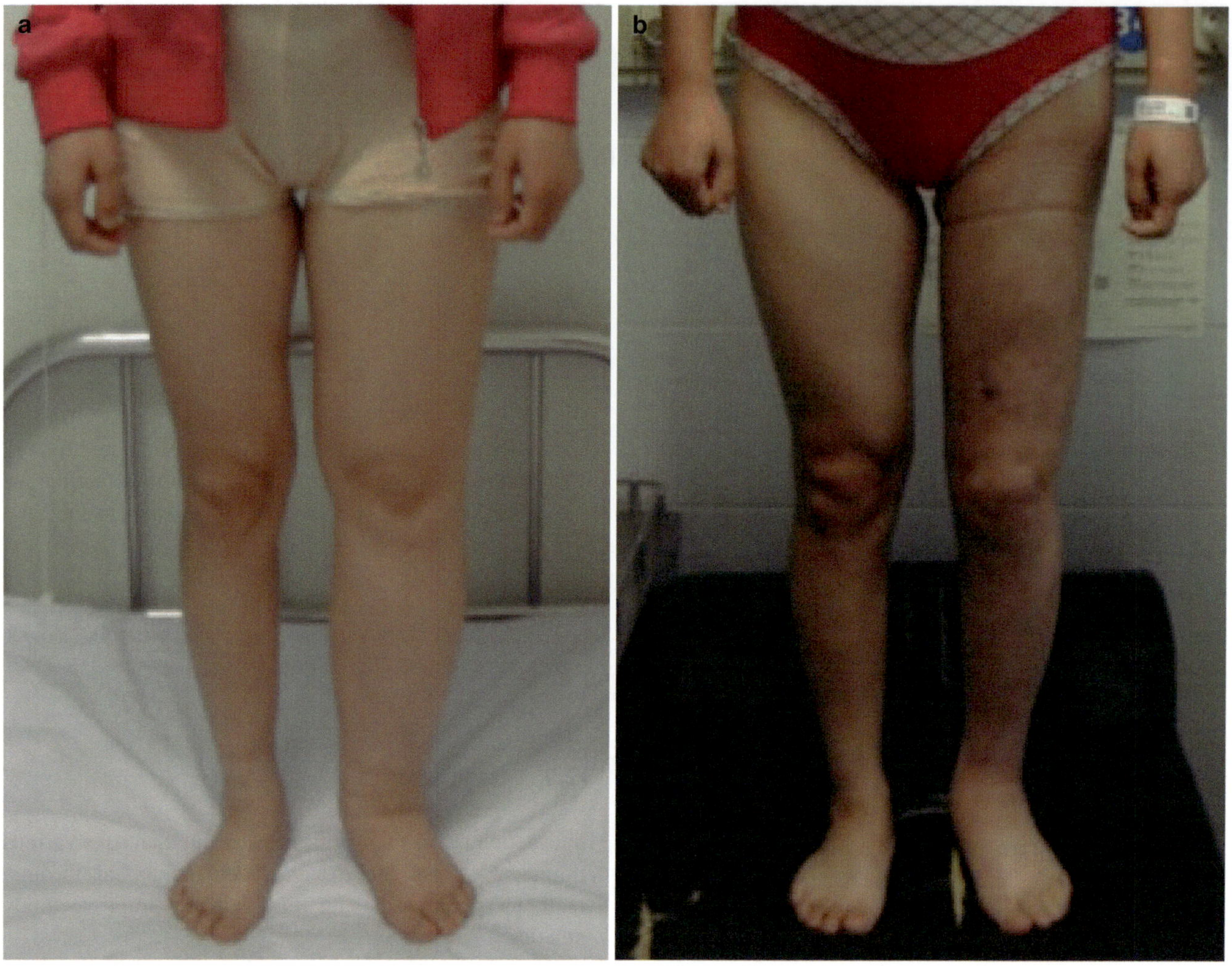

Fig. 32.1 The patient, female, 32 years old, primary lymphedema of the left lower extremity. A. Preoperative. B. 3 month after operation

that "lympholiposuction" is more appropriate to define this surgical technique [5]. (Fig. 32.1, 32.2 and 32.3).

We performed liposuction on 30 patients with primary lymphedema of unilateral lower limbs and analyzed the results to improve the treatment of the disease.

32.2 Materials and Methods

32.2.1 Patients

Two hundred and eighty-six patients with primary lymphedema admitted to Beijing Shijitan Hospital from July 2016 to August 2017 were screened, and the inclusion criteria were as follows: (1) Patients with primary lymphedema of the unilateral lower extremity; (2) according to the lymphedema staging established by International Society of Lymphology (ISL) in 2013 (Lymphology [6]), patients were classified as either stage II or stage III; (3) the first operation was liposuction; (4) compression stockings were mandatory after surgery; (5) patients were followed up for more than 3 months. Exclusion criteria: (1) patients with stage 0 and stage I lymphedema; (2) patients with a history of surgical treatment of lymphedema; (3) lower extremity lymphedema was treated by liposuction combined with other surgical methods at the same time.

A total of 30 patients were enrolled, including 13 males and 17 females, aged (36 ± 16.3) years (range 12–65). The mean course of the disease was 167 months (range 6–600). There were 14 cases in Stage II and 16 cases in stage III. There were 18 cases of left lower extremity lymphedema and 12 cases of right lower extremity lymphedema. Nine patients had a history of recurrent erysipelas, 1 with swelling of the right upper limb and right face, 1 with swelling of the scrotum, and 3 with hypertension and diabetes.

32.2.2 Preoperative Preparation

32.2.2.1 Limb Measurement

Conventional liposuction uses contour lines to mark liposuction sites. However, for extremity lymphedema, mostly occurs unilaterally, with some occurring bilaterally. For this reason, it is impossible to mark the limbs to be operated by

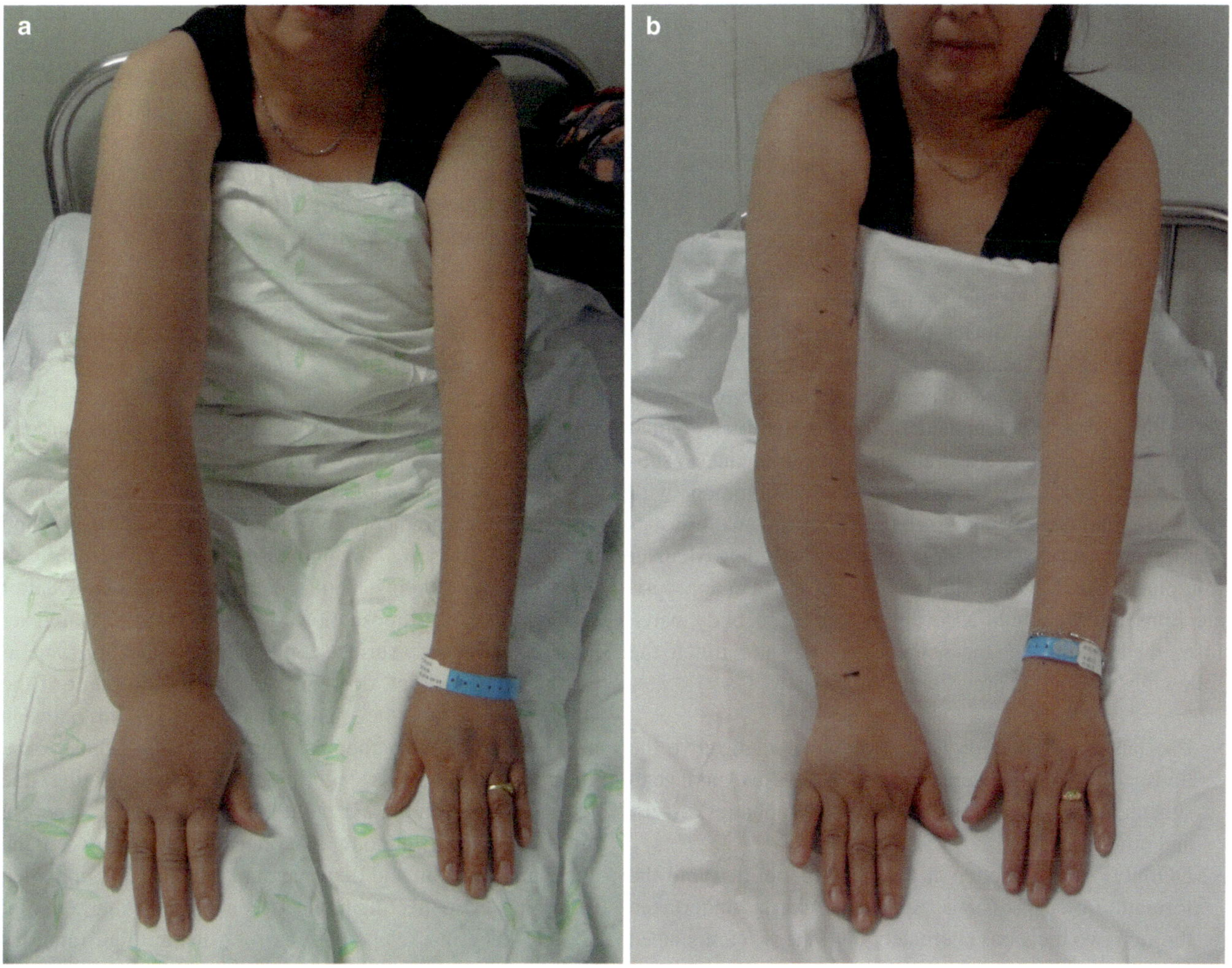

Fig. 32.2 The patient, female, 51 years old, secondary lymphedema of the right upper extremity. A: Preoperative.B: 3 month after operation

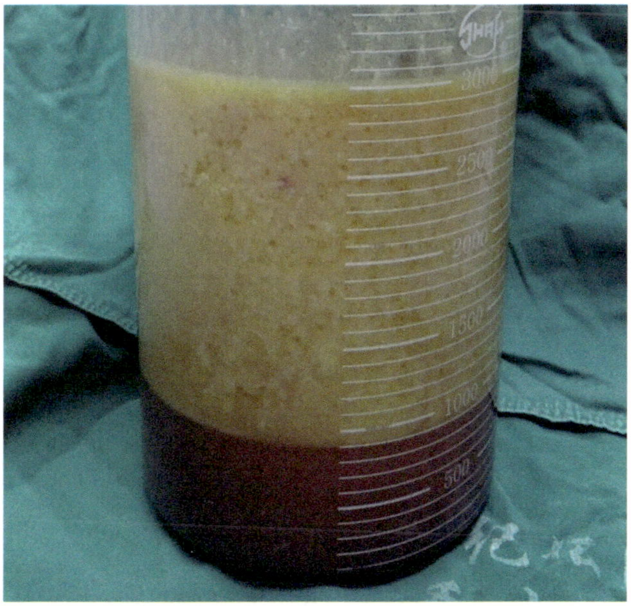

Fig. 32.3 This picture shows the aspirate collected from the lymphedematous extremity of the patient. The aspirate sediments into an upper adipose fraction and a lower fluid (lymph, blood, and tumescent solution) fraction

the aforementioned marking method. Therefore, before surgery, the circumferences of both limbs should be measured at the marks made symmetrically on the skin. For patients with unilateral limb lymphedema, the amount of fat aspirated is determined based on the circumference of the healthy limb. For patients with bilateral limb lymphedema, the postoperative appearance of both limbs should be designed according to the esthetics of the limbs.

32.2.3 Surgical Method

Anesthesia and Position Selection: General anesthesia with endotracheal intubation.

Incision Site Selection: Make a small incision of about 0.5 cm in length on the inner and outer thighs just above the knee and the inner and outer legs just below the knee as suction access points.

Infusion of Tumescent Solution: Use a fluid infuser to infuse the tumescent solution (formula: 0.9% normal saline 3000 ml, 0.1% epinephrine hydrochloride 3 ml, 2% lidocaine hydrochloride 30 ml, 5% sodium bicarbonate 30 ml)

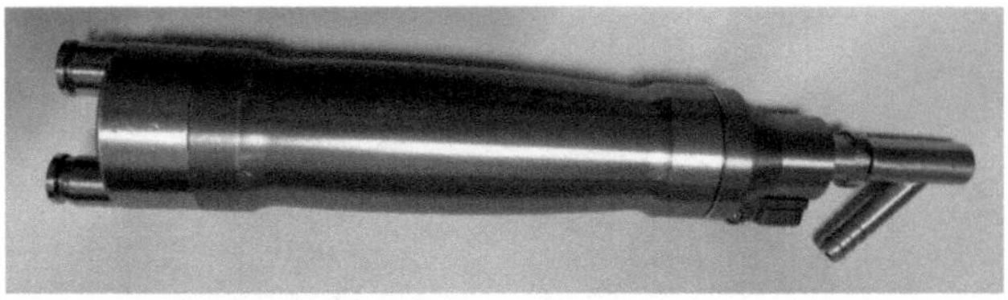

Fig. 32.4 This picture shows the liposuction handle

into the subcutaneous adipose tissue that needs to be aspirated. Continue this infusion process until the skin takes on an orange peel appearance.

Operation: Due to excessive adipose tissue proliferation and fibrosis in the lymphedematous extremities, which requires greater strength and energy to break up and to subsequently aspirate, we choose liposuction equipment with resonance and negative pressure (GZXZ resonance liposuction system, produced by Yangguang Zhongtian Medical Equipment Co., Ltd. in Shanxi). (Fig. 32.4). Select appropriate liposuction cannula according to different body parts. Insert the cannula from the incision sites. Pay attention to the followings during the procedure:

- Use fan-shaped suction technique rather than move the liposuction cannula laterally to avoid excessive damage to subcutaneous blood vessels, nerves, lymphatic vessels, and other tissue.
- DO NOT repeat suction at the same tunnel to avoid the formation of depressions. Aspiration can be undertaken through two incisions alternately until the two fan-shaped tunnels overlap each other.
- Try NOT to damage the dermis during the aspiration process so as not to cause postoperative skin necrosis.
- At the end of liposuction, remove excess blood and fluid in the subcutaneous space as much as possible. Measure the circumferences of the operated limb again at various points marked on its surface before the operation. The operative procedure is considered complete when the circumference measurements of the operated limb at the points marked preoperatively are close to those of the healthy limb or close to the preoperatively designed valued.
- Place a Jackson-Pratt (JP) drain subcutaneously to drain excess fluid. The operated limb is applied with compression bandaging.

Postoperative Management

- Routine application of antibiotics: Broad-spectrum antibiotics can be administered intravenously for 3 days.
- Hemostasis treatment: Hemostatic medication can be given, depending on the estimated blood loss, but the course of treatment generally does not exceed 3 days. Patients with a higher risk for thrombosis may not be given any hemostatic medication.
- The compression bandage is applied for 3 days. At postoperative Day 3, the dressing is changed, and the drainage tubes are removed.
- At postoperative Day 3, after dressing change and drain removal, the operated extremity can be applied with compression stocking. Patient is then allowed to start to exercise.

32.2.4 Measurement

BMI BMI was calculated before and 3 months after surgery. BMI = weight (kg)/height^2 (m^2).

Volume Difference and Percent Volume Difference: Based on limb measurement and volume calculation method devised by Brorson [7], volume difference and percent volume difference were calculated before, immediately after and 3 months after liposuction. (1) Points to be measured are marked on the body surface at the following locations: metatarsophalangeal joint, dorsum of the foot (mid point of the arch of the foot), the ankle (anterior midpoint between medial and lateral malleolus), the knee (mid point of the knee joint), the lower leg (lower 1/3 of connecting line between the ankle marker point and the knee marker point), the middle leg (midpoint of connecting line between the ankle marker point and the knee marker point), the upper leg (upper 1/3 of connecting line between the ankle marker point and the knee marker point), the root of the thigh (anterior midpoint of the horizontal line drawn from the medial side of the thigh root, i.e. at the level of the lower border of pubic symphysis), the lower thigh (lower 1/3 of connecting line between the knee marker point and the thigh root marker point), the midthigh (the midpoint of connecting line between the knee marker point and the thigh root marker point), the upper thigh (upper 1/3 of connecting line between the knee marker point and the thigh root marker point). (2) The circumferences of the lower limbs were measured at the aforementioned body surface marker points. (3) The length of the legs and the thighs of both lower limbs were measured. The length of the legs is the distance from the ankle marker point to the knee marker point; the length of the thighs is the distance from the knee marker point to the thigh root marker point. (4) The volume of the lower limbs was calculated according to the circumferences measured at each body surface marker point and the length of the legs and the thighs; (5) The volume difference and percent volume difference were calculated.

$$\text{Lower Limb volume} = 1/3\boldsymbol{\pi}\mathbf{h}(R_1^2 + r_1^2 + R_1 \times r_1) + 1/3\boldsymbol{\pi}\mathbf{h}(R_2^2 + r_2^2 + R_2 \times r_2) + \ldots + 1/3\boldsymbol{\pi}\mathbf{h}(R_n^2 + r_n^2 + R_n \times r_n),$$

where R is the radius of the cross-section at the lower marker point (R_1 is the radius of the cross-section at the ankle marker point), r is the radius of the cross-section at the adjacent upper marker point, and h is the distance between two adjacent marker points.

$$\text{Volume difference} = \text{affected limb volume} - \text{healthy limb volume};$$
$$\text{Percent volume difference} = \left[\left(\text{affected limb volume} - \text{healthy limb volume}\right) / \text{healthy limb volume}\right] \times 100\%.$$

Volume of Blood Loss: Preoperative hemoglobin, postoperative hemoglobin, and volume of intraoperative blood transfusion were recorded. Preoperative blood volume was obtained based on the formula derived by Nadler et al. [8]. Subsequently, the volume of blood loss was calculated according to the formula derived by Budny et al. [9].

$$\text{Pre-operative blood volume}(\text{ml})\text{ of men} = 0.0003669 \times height^3\left(\text{cm}^3\right) + \left[32.19 \times weight(\text{kg}) + 604\right]$$
$$\text{Pre-operative blood volume}(\text{ml})\text{ of women} = 0.0003561 \times height^3\left(\text{cm}^3\right) + \left[33.08 \times weight(\text{kg}) + 183\right]$$
$$\begin{aligned}\text{Actual volume of blood loss}(\text{ml}) = {} & \text{pre-operative blood volume} \\ & \times \begin{bmatrix}\left(\text{pre-operative hemoglobin} - \text{post-operative hemoglobin}\right) \\ /\text{pre-operative hemoglobin}\end{bmatrix} \\ & + \text{volume of intra-operative blood transfusion}\end{aligned}$$

Others: Record duration of operation, volume of aspirated fat and liposuction rate.

32.2.5 Subjective Evaluation

At preoperation and 3 months follow-up, the patients filled out the questionnaire to evaluate their subjective feelings, which encompass stiffness, tension, heaviness, tenderness, pain, numbness, fatigue, and weakness.

32.2.6 Statistical Analysis

The data were divided into three groups according to the sex of patients, the history of erysipelas, and different stages of lesions. Volume of aspirated fat, liposuction rate, the volume of blood loss, and percent volume difference were compared.

Data were presented as mean ± standard deviation (Mean ± SD). Kolmogorov-Smirnov test was performed to verify that the parameters conformed to normal distribution. The means of the two samples were compared by applying *t-test* of independent samples. A corrected *t-test* was employed when there was a lack of variance. Fisher's exact probability method was utilized to test the rate. $P < 0.05$ was considered statistically significant. The data were analyzed using SPSS version 20.0 (IBM, Armonk, New York, USA).

32.3 Results

In this study, 30 cases were operated successfully without skin necrosis, subcutaneous effusion, infection, or other complications. The operation time was (159 ± 41.2) min (range 90–300). The volume of aspirated fat was (1920 ± 830) ml (range 900–3900). The estimated blood loss (EBL) was (730 ± 264) ml (range 160–1100).Intraoperative autotransfusion was performed in 6 patients. The liposuction rate was 12.1 ± 5.3 ml/mim (range 5.5–26.0). The appearance of the lymphedematous extremity significantly improved at 3 months follow-up. Preoperative BMI was 23.7 ± 4.0, and 3 months follow-up BMI was 23.3 ± 3.9. This difference was not statistically significant ($t = 0.390$, $P = 0.698$).

Percent volume differences at preoperation, postoperation, and 3 months follow-up were (31.4 ± 16.4)%, (6.6 ± 10.0)%, and (12.2 ± 10.7)%, respectively. Percent volume difference at postoperation and at 3 months follow-up

Table 32.1 Comparison of surgical results between male and female patients with primary lymphedema of lower extremities (Mean ± SD)

	Male	Female	*t*	*P* value
N	13	17	–	–
Volume of blood loss(ml)	855 ± 241	641 ± 246	2.377	0.025
Volume of aspirated fat (ml)	1576 ± 523	2182 ± 934	−2.029	0.046
Liposuction rate (ml/mim)	9.7 ± 2.3	13.8 ± 6.2	−2.448	0.023
Percent volume difference				
Preoperation (%)	38.8 ± 19.3	25.7 ± 11.4	−2.325	0.028
Postoperation (%)	15.1 ± 7.7	0.1 ± 5.8	6.073	0.000
3 month follow-up (%)	21.7 ± 8.9	4.9 ± 4.1	6.337	0.000

Table 32.2 Comparison of surgical results between erysipelas and non-erysipelas group with primary lymphedema of lower extremities (Mean ± SD)

	Erysipelas	Non-erysipelas	*t*	*P* value
N	9	21	–	–
Volume of blood loss(ml)	901 ± 106	662 ± 278	−3.398	0.002
Volume of aspirated fat (ml)	1422 ± 571	2133 ± 841	2.305	0.029
Liposuction rate (ml/mim)	8.8 ± 2.7	13.4 ± 5.6	2.311	0.028
Percent volume difference				
Preoperation (%)	26.4 ± 13.5	33.5 ± 17.3	1.083	0.288
Postoperation (%)	6.8 ± 7.3	6.5 ± 11.2	−0.088	0.930
3 month follow-up (%)	11.2 ± 9.6	12.6 ± 11.3	0.330	0.744

significantly decreased compared with that at preoperation ($P < 0.05$), but it increased at 3 months follow-up compared with that at postoperation.

The lipid volume and liposuction rate were higher in females than those in males; whereas the EBL, percent volume difference at preoperation, postoperation, and 3 months follow-up was higher in male than those in female (Table 32.1). The EBL was higher in the erysipelas group than in non-erysipelas group, whereas the volume of aspirated fat and liposuction rate was lower in the former group (Table 32.2). The volume of aspirated fat and liposuction rate were higher in Stage II than in Stage III group. In contrast, the EBL, percent volume difference at preoperation, postoperation and 3 months follow-up were lower in Stage II group (Table 32.3).

The feeling of heaviness and fatigue of the operative limb alleviated at 3 months follow-up compared with that at preoperation, whereas the feeling of tenderness and tightness worsened. There were no significant differences in stiffness, pain, numbness, and weakness between preoperation and 3 months follow-up (Table 32.4).

Table 32.3 Comparison of surgical results between stage II and stage III group with primary lymphedema of lower extremities (Mean ± SD)

	Stage II	Stage III	*t*	*P* value
N	14	16	–	–
Volume of blood loss (ml)	594 ± 235	856 ± 226	−3.097	0.004
Volume of aspirated fat (ml)	2292 ± 974	1593 ± 514	2.407	0.026
Liposuction rate (ml/min)	14.8 ± 6.4	9.6 ± 2.4	2.826	0.012
Percent volume difference				
Preoperation (%)	24.2 ± 11.8	37.7 ± 17.6	−2.433	0.022
Postoperation (%)	−1.6 ± 4.9	13.8 ± 7.4	−6.584	0.000
3 month follow-up (%)	3.6 ± 3.3	19.7 ± 9.1	−6.510	0.000

Table 32.4 Comparison of subjective sensation between preoperation and 3 months follow-up in 30 patients with primary lymphedema of the lower extremity [case (%)]

	Preoperation	3 month follow-up	χ^2	*P* value
Stiffness	10(33.3)	17(56.7)	3.300	0.069
Tightness	8(26.7)	16(53.3)	4.444	0.035
Heaviness	24(80.0)	16(53.3)	4.800	0.028
Tenderness	3(10)	11(36.7)	5.963	0.030
Pain	3(10)	10(33.3)	4.536	0.057
Numbness	11(36.7)	16(53.3)	1.684	0.194
Fatigue	21(70)	11(36.7)	6.696	0.010
Weakness	3(10)	5(16.7)	0.577	0.706

32.4 Discussion

Since 2009, the Department of Lymphatic Surgery at Beijing Shijitan Hospital Affiliated with Capital Medical University has adopted liposuction to treat lymphedema and has completed more than 2600 cases so far.

Thirty patients with primary unilateral lower extremity lymphedema were studied. Changes in limb volume and subjective feelings were assessed, as well as the intraoperative parameters and variables that may affect surgical outcome.

The percent volume difference was significantly lower at postoperation and 3 months follow-up than that at preoperation. The mean estimated blood loss (EBL) was 730 ml (range 160–1100 ml), which was much higher than the EBL of 292 ml when liposuction was done in obese patients [10]. The reason may be that there is abnormal hyperplasia of subcutaneous adipose tissue in lymphedematous limbs and that the proliferating adipose layer contains multiple fiber septators, which causes more difficulty in liposuction of lymphedematous limbs, aggravated peripheral vascular injury, and increased bleeding than conventional liposuction. Therefore, patients with anemia should be actively corrected before liposuction. Some patients may need to have packed red blood cells (pRBC) prepared before surgery. In this study, six patients were given autotransfusion.

Male had a significantly higher percent volume difference and EBL than female at preoperation, postoperation, and 3 months follow-up, but significantly lower volume of aspirated fat. This suggests that there may be differences between male and female in the occurrence and development of primary lower extremity lymphedema. Perhaps the abnormality of the lymphedematous lower extremity in male is more profound than that in female. In addition, subcutaneous tissue hyperplasia and fibrosis may aggravate as the disease progresses. We also found that the liposuction rate in male was significantly lower than that in female during the operation. That is, it was more difficult to extract fat in male. Moreover, the effect of different hormone levels between male and female on the composition of subcutaneous tissue [11, 12] as well as poor compliance of male may also account for the aforementioned differences, which still need to be further investigated.

Lymphedema is one of the risk factors for the occurrence of erysipelas [13]. Recurrent erysipelas can lead to subcutaneous tissue fibrosis, which in turn can aggravate lymphedema. In the study of Kosenkov [14], a correlation was found between occurrence of erysipelas and the degree of lymphedema, and they aggravated each other. In our study, the erysipelas group was noted to have higher EBL, less volume of aspirated fat, and lower liposuction rate than the non-erysipelas group. This suggests that patients with recurrent erysipelas may have more fibrosis in the subcutaneous tissue, which could increase the difficulty and risk of the surgery.

The percent volume difference of Stage III group was significantly higher than that of Stage II group at preoperation, postoperation, and 3 months follow-up, whereas the volume of aspirated fat and liposuction rate of Stage III group was significantly lower than those of Stage II group. In addition, EBL of Stage III group is greater than that of Stage II group. These results suggest that the longer the disease period, the more difficult the liposuction may become, and the more blood loss may ensue. It can be deduced that the surgical outcome may also be worse. The reason may be that the degree of fibrosis of subcutaneous tissue gradually elevates along the course of the disease. Sun et al.[15] also believe that skin hardness is positively correlated with the stage of lymphedema. Consequently, the outcome of liposuction and volume reduction in advanced limb lymphedema may not be as good as those in early lymphedema.

Regarding subjective feelings of the patients, the feeling of heaviness and fatigue of the affected limbs significantly reduced at 3 months follow-up compared with that at preoperation, but the feeling of tenderness and tension of the lymphedematous limb was more severe than that at preoperation. This may be related to the injury of subcutaneous nerves and inflammatory reactions after liposuction. It is worth noting that 56.7% of patients still felt stiff, and 53.3% felt tight and heavy 3 months after liposuction. The reason may be that the compression stocking fails to effectively improve lymphatic circulation despite significantly reduced volume of the lymphedematous limb after liposuction. The data also show that the percent volume difference increases significantly at 3 months follow-up after liposuction, which is consistent with the subjective sensory changes of the patients.

Qi et al. [16] compared the outcome of liposuction in 17 patients—7 upper limb lymphedema and 10 lower limb lymphedema. Substantial limb volume reduction was noted in all cases immediately after operation. This state of volume reduction remained 3–12 months with a mean of 6.01 months by applying low-stretch bandages or compression stockings. Subsequently, it returned to the preoperative volume level. This implies that liposuction combined with more effective postoperative measures to ameliorate lymphatic circulation could contribute to a better surgical outcome of extremity lymphedema.

In our study, all cases were treated with a second-stage surgery within 3 to 6 months after liposuction to improve lymphatic circulation. All cases are still being followed up.

In conclusion, liposuction demonstrates a certain positive effect on the treatment of lymphedema. Nevertheless, compared with traditional liposuction in plastic surgery, it is more risky and difficult and should be combined with more effective methods to improve lymphatic circulation in the early postoperative period. Moreover, gender differences, history of erysipelas, and stage of the disease should be taken into account during the treatment process, especially during the perioperative period.

Although liposuction is effective in the treatment of lymphedema, there are some complications of which we should take precautions. The common complications, prevention, and management are summarized as follows.

Hematoma, Seroma, and Lymph Cyst (Lymphocele): These are relatively common postoperative complications, mainly due to inappropriately loose compression bandages or poor drainage of the drains after surgery. They can also be caused by damage of relatively large blood vessels and lymph vessels during the operation. In order to prevent the occurrence of hematoma, seroma, and lymph cyst, it is crucial to know the course of the main blood vessels in the operative field. Pay close attention to the direction of movement of the cannula during liposuction to avoid damaging large blood vessels. Apply proper pressure when wrapping the operative limb with a compression bandage. For patients with a significant amount of subcutaneous drainage, JP drains can be left in place longer. If there is minimal amount of drainage after drain removal, squeeze out the drainage as much as possible by wrapping both hands around the limb at the drainage site and applying pressure. If there is moderate amount of drainage after drain removal, the fluid collection can be aspirated, and compression bandage is applied again. For subcutaneous drainage that repeatedly occurs for a long period of time, a pseudocyst usually has formed. At this time, cyst inactivation or cystectomy can be performed to promote better healing of the skin and subcutaneous tissue.

Skin Necrosis: The incidence of skin necrosis after liposuction of lymphedematous limbs is about 2–3%. The main reason for this complication is that the plain of suction is too shallow during the operation, which damages the subdermal vascular network, leading to impaired skin blood flow. Therefore, it is imperative NOT to let the side slits of the tip of the cannula face the skin surface and to repeat suction this way intraoperatively. Small area of skin necrosis usually heals by themselves after local dressing change. Alternatively, the skin edges can be pulled directly and sutured. For large areas of skin necrosis, skin grafting is required.

Uneven Skin Surface: The main reasons for this complication are that the liposuction cannula used is too thick, that the plane of liposuction is too close to the skin, that the fan-shaped suction technique is not utilized, and that careful inspection is not performed at the end of the operation. In order to prevent unevenness of the skin surface, choose an appropriate liposuction cannula when different body parts are operated and pay attention to the depth and direction of movement of the cannula during liposuction. Carefully examine the skin surface at the end of the operation. If any irregularities are found, further action should be taken until uniform and smooth skin surface is achieved.

Pigmentation: This is mainly due to excessive aspiration of the adipose tissue, leading to damage of the subdermal vascular network, which in turn causes skin ischemia. This can usually subside on its own.

Asymmetry of the Extremities: The direct cause of asymmetry after liposuction is that there is a discrepancy in the amount of fat aspirated from both limbs. Therefore, the circumference of both limbs should be accurately measured before and after surgery to ensure that the circumferences of both limbs match each other.

Decreased Skin Sensation: This is mainly due to damage to the sensory nerve endings of the skin during liposuction, which generally does not require intervention and can recover on its own.

Body Fluid Imbalance: It is a common complication of liposuction primarily because of injection of a large amount of tumescent solution and significant interstitial fluid loss during the operation. Blood electrolytes should be routinely checked after surgery so that any imbalance can be corrected in time once it is identified.

Others: The incidence of deep vein thrombosis, fat embolism, lidocaine intoxication, etc. is minimal. They can be managed with symptomatic treatment when they do occur.

References

1. Illouz YG. Une nouvelle technique pour les lipodystrophies localises. Rev Chir Esthet. 1980;4(1):19.
2. Brorson H. From lymph to fat: liposuction as a treatment for complete reduction of lymphedema. Int J Low Extrem Wounds. 2012;11(1):10–9. https://doi.org/10.1177/1534734612438550.
3. Boyages J, Kastanias K, Koelmeyer LA, et al. Liposuction for advanced lymphedema: a multidisciplinary approach for complete reduction of arm and leg swelling. Ann Surg Oncol. 2015;22(Suppl 3):S1263–70. https://doi.org/10.1245/s10434-015-4700-3.
4. Chang K, Xia S, Sun YG, et al. Liposuction combined with lymphaticovenous anastomosis for treatment of secondary lymphedema of the lower limbs: a report of 49 cases. [J]. Zhonghua Wai Ke Za Zhi. 2017;55(4):274–8. https://doi.org/10.3760/cma.j.issn.0529-5815.2017.04.008.
5. Xin JF, Sun YG, Xia S, et al. Application of liposuction in treating the primary end-stage lymphedema of lower extremities. Chin J Plast Surg. 2019;35(2):142–7. https://doi.org/10.3760/cma.j.issn.1009-4598.2019.00.000.
6. International Society of Lymphology. The diagnosis and treatment of peripheral lymphedema: 2013 Consensus Document of the International Society of Lymphology. Lymphology. 2013;46(1):1–11.
7. Brorson H, Hoijer P. Standardised measurements used to order compression garments can be used to calculate arm volumes to evaluate lymphoedema treatment. J Plast Surg Hand Surg. 2012;46(6):410–5. https://doi.org/10.3109/2000656X.2012.714785.
8. Nadler SB, Hidalgo JH, Bloch T. Prediction of blood volume in normal human adults. Surgery. 1962;51(2):224–32.
9. Budny PG, Regan PJ, Roberts AH. The estimation of blood loss during burns surgery. Burns. 1993;19(2):134–7. https://doi.org/10.1016/0305-4179(93)90036-8.
10. Swanson E. Does laser assistance reduce blood loss after liposuction? Aesthet Surg J. 2015;35(2):38–9. https://doi.org/10.1093/asj/sjv010.
11. de la Casa AM, Suarez SC, Rebollo RJ, et al. Cellulite's aetiology: a review. J Eur Acad Dermatol Venereol. 2013;27(3):273–8. https://doi.org/10.1111/j.1468-3083.2012.04622.x.
12. Xiao Z, Guo B, Gong J, et al. Sex-and age-specific percentiles of body composition indices for Chinese adults using dual-energy X-ray absorptiometry. Eur J Nutr. 2017;56(7):2393–406. https://doi.org/10.1007/s00394-016-1279-9.
13. Inghammar M, Rasmussen M, Linder A. Recurrent erysipelas – risk factors and clinical presentation. BMC Infect Dis. 2014;14:270. https://doi.org/10.1186/1471-2334-14-270.
14. Kosenkov AN, Narenkov VM, Abramov I. Erysipelas as the cause of lymphedema. Khirurgiia (Mosk). 2005;11:51–3.
15. Sun D, Yu Z, Chen J, et al. The value of using a Skin FibroMeter for diagnosis and assessment of secondary lymphedema and associated fibrosis of lower limb skin. Lymphat Res Biol. 2017;15(1):70–6. https://doi.org/10.1089/lrb.2016.0029.
16. Qi FZ, Yang YW, Gu JY, et al. The long term efficacy of the pure liposuction treatment for patiens with limb lymphoedema. Clin Med J China. 2008;15(1):89–91. https://doi.org/10.3969/j.issn.1008-6358.2008.01.028.

Part VIII

Curative Effect Assessment

Circumference Measurement

33

Zhengyun Liang, Elan Yang, and Xiao Long

Abstract

This chapter lists out a few curative assessments that are both economically efficient and induce minimal discomfort for patients diagnosed with lymphedema. Tape measurement is a common method to measure the limb circumferential girth with a simple tool that is easily accessible, and anyone can maneuver. Water plethysmography, using water displacement as a way to carry out the limb volume, is still considered to be the gold standard in limb volumetry. Three-dimensional photography is a relatively new imaging system that processes the limb volume information with computer software automation. Other measuring tools such as perometry, are also frequently used measurements of limb volume in the clinical setting due to their ease of use and consistency.

Keywords

Lymphedema assessments · Lymphedema tape measurement · Water plethysmography · Three-dimensional photography · Perometry

Circumference measurement or tape measurement or girth assessment is the most commonly used and fundamental method in the evaluation of lymphedema. All the tools needed to perform standard circumferential girth assessment is a flexible, non-stretch tape, which in some cases is modified with a spring load for tension accuracy [1]. Devoogdt et al. applied a stainless steel bar with tapeline fixed at every four centimeters as a new circumferential measurement device [2]. For upper extremity lymphedema assessment, the patient's arm is positioned straight and abducted 90 degree on a table, while measurements are taken with the patient's hip flexed at 90 degree and knee and foot extended in 0 position in lower limb evaluation [1, 3]. Measurement intervals differ from 3 cm to 12 cm, with 4 cm being considered more convenient for arms and 8 cm for lower limbs [4–6]. Multiple points are traditionally measured to fully assess limb edema following different protocols.

As absolute values are less valid and depend on body composition, they are conventionally converted into volumes and other indices [7]. Volume calculation visualized the edematous limb (s) as a series of truncated cones, cylinders, disks, rectangular, and trapezoidal solids with respective mathematical formulae [4]. Limb segment bearing more resemblance to truncated cone than cylinder shape, frustum formula, if possible, is highly recommended for volume monitoring [5]:

$$V = \frac{1}{3}\pi h\left(r_1^2 + r_2^2 + r_1 r_2\right)$$

(Where V is the segment volume; r_1 or r_2 respectively represents the radius of measure point 1 or point 2; h is the height of the segment or measurement interval)

Summing all the individual volume segments calculated by formulae such as above gives us approximate information of total limb volume. For unilateral lymphedema, indices such as absolute excess volume (affected limb−unaffected limb), excess volume in percent ((affected limb−unaffected limb)/unaffected limb×100), and relative value in percent (affected limb/unaffected limb×100) pre and posttherapy are widely adopted in evaluating excess fluid reduction [7, 8]. Another indispensable index is percentage reduction:

$$\%\text{reduction} = \frac{\Delta_{before\ therapy} - \Delta_{after\ therapy}}{\Delta_{before\ therapy}} \times 100$$

(Δ Represents volume difference between affected limb and unaffected limb.)

In bilateral lymphedema, change in volume in percent ((1 − volume after therapy/volume before therapy) × 100))

Z. Liang · E. Yang · X. Long (✉)
Department of Plastic and Reconstructive Surgery, Peking Union Medical College Hospital, Beijing, People's Republic of China

N. Liu (ed.), *Peripheral Lymphedema*, https://doi.org/10.1007/978-981-16-3484-0_33

should be calculated for each limb. Yamamoto et al. suggested the Lower Extremity Lymphedema (LEL) index and LV/BMI (affected leg volume divided by BMI) may be efficient in evaluating bilateral lower extremity lymphedema therapeutic effect [9, 10].

Among a wide range of instruments, clinicians favor tape measurement the most for its feasible and economical characteristics. Favorable as it is, girth assessment is not without limitations: (1) Volume change of hand and foot cannot be calculated due to rather irregular shape, and midline volume measurement is difficult to perform. (2) Comparison between individuals or groups is difficult because of variability. (3) There is a substantial risk for inter- and intra-observer variability and a poor reproducibility for it's poorly standardized.

33.1 Other Measurement Tools

33.1.1 Water Plethysmography

Strictly following Archimedes' principle, water plethysmography, also known as inverse volumetry, is widely recognized as the criterion standard for limb volume estimation [1, 3, 6, 11, 12]. With the limb of clinical interest immersed in a water tank, the amount of water displaced equals the limb volume. A specially designed volume meter with an overflow spout and a separate water container are the classic components of water volumetric device [12–15]. The overflow will be measured by a weighing scale or a cylindrical measure [4]. The weight (g) will then be converted into ml using the standard conversion of 1 kg of water being equal to 1000 ml. For arm plethysmography, the arm is brought down to the water-filled container slowly with the palm closely leaned against the wall and the tip of the middle finger lightly touching the bottom or individualized gradation line [8, 16]. Akin to arm plethysmography, the lower limb should be placed into the tank closely by the wall, and different spacers could be applied to the volume meter to compensate for different leg lengths. It is highly critical the extremity should be immersed at the same depth each time.

Water displacement with a high logical validity is a sensitive, inexpensive, and painless method for therapeutic assessment and follow-up. Compared to girth measurement, it takes into account the hand and foot volume. However, it is deemed impractical in daily clinical setting. The reasons are (1) The set-up is cumbersome and rather complicated dealing with water and tanks [6, 11]. (2) It is patient-unfriendly, for it requires the patient to hold completely still until the end of the measurement [12]. (3) It could be time-consuming and difficult to perform by one observer alone. (4) It may be contraindicated in the case of post-operative status, open wounds, ulcers, or other severe skin disorders [1, 12, 15]. (5) It's deemed unfit for midline (head and neck, breast, trunk, or genitalia) lymphedema volume measurement. Damstra et al. introduced a more user-friendly new apparatus for arm water volumetric with most of the disadvantages mentioned above absent, further studies on its practicality and reliability are in need, though [11].

33.1.2 Three-Dimensional Photography

Three-dimensional photography is a relatively new tool in limb volume estimation, which deploys a variety of 3D imaging systems to capture/scan the limb of interest and processes volume information with computer software automation. The Handyscan 3D REVscan system (Creaform, Levis, Quebec, Canada) [17], the 3D stereophotogrammetry system (3dMD Cranial, Atlanta, USA) [18] and the VECTRA XT surface photo imaging system (Canfield Imaging Systems, Fairfield, NJ) [19–23] are conventional standardized 3D systems currently used in volume evaluation, with VECTRA being the major focus of studies. VECTRA encompasses digital reflex cameras (three or six depending on a different version of VECTRA) divided into three stations in a triangulated configuration and speckle-pattern flash projectors, positioned stereoscopically within a unit, both of which fire simultaneously to obtain points in three dimensions when image capture commences [19, 21, 23] (Fig. 33.1). The cameras are only able to capture 3D images in 180°due to angles, thus anterior and posterior side images are traditionally taken. Images will be transmitted into VECTRA software, which automatically merges data to construct a 360°digital model and stipples the boundary of the selected area to calculate enclosed surface volume. Difference between pre- and post-treatment volumes can be displayed in absolute values or image color change by photographs contrast (an increase in quantity as light and a decrease as dark) [19]. In upper-extremity assessment, subjects are instructed to abduct the arm up to 90° and extend it horizontally into the defined measuring space with the palm facing down [21, 23]. Hands are conventionally excluded due to larger inaccuracy [23], while Landau et al. demonstrated that VECTRA volume determination of the hand (up to the ulnar styloid) taken with the fist closed correlated well with water volume measurements [22]. Prior to photo capturing, 30% and 80% of the arm length are drawn as cutoff lines, and reference points are set along the midline of the arm. Studies about VECTRA's application in lower limb lymphedema are scarce, resulting in a less standardized protocol. Tokumoto et al. proved that VECTRA would be useful in therapy follow-ups for the thigh region [19]. They also suggested three or more individualized, not movable marks such as a nevus or a scar should be predefined before evaluation.

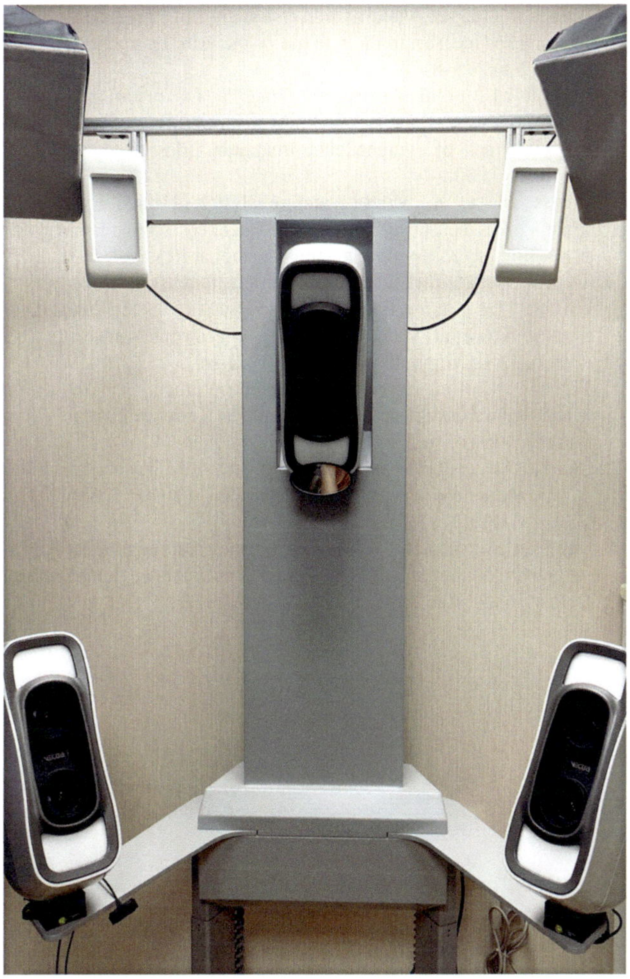

Fig. 33.1 VECTRA[xt] (https://www.canfieldsci.com/imaging-systems/vectra-xt-3d-imaging-system/)

Undoubtedly, three-dimensional photography, especially VECTRA, has many distinct advantages: 1. It has been applied in evaluating lymphedema of facial, pubic, and hypogastric sites [19] and deemed possibly applicable in the whole body region. 2. It is patient-friendly and time-efficient, the measurement for each point taking only milliseconds to conduct. 3. It provides precise and reliable information and high-spatial-resolution images with computer software doing all the processing and calculating. 4. The VECTRA assessment can be used on open wounds, cellulitis, or other skin lesions due to its non-contact nature. Sophisticated as this technology is, its flaws should not be neglected: 1. Special trainings on how to perform VECTRA are in need and lack of experience might give rise to poor selection of 3D photographs and lengthy procedures. 2. Reference points or cutoff lines marked by different examiners under different skin conditions might introduce large errors. 3. Relatively affordable as it is, VECTRA can still be costly and not accessible in every clinic.

33.1.3 Perometry

Perometry is considered to be an accurate, fast, and objective way to assess limb volume. It consists of a square frame with multiple infrared emitting diodes and infrared light detecters. As the frame is moved along the long axis of the limb, the limb and the dimensions interrupt light beams. Information of the interruption is converted into coordinates continuously, which will be used to reconstruct a 3D model and calculate limb volume by Perometer software [24, 25]. Over the years, diverse perometer systems are developed, applying different calculation formulae and measuring intervals. It has been used to measure arm and leg volume, foot and hand excluded, though, for its efficient, precise, and automatic properties [26–28]. Distinct as its merit is, perometer system has one fatal flaw: the equipment is costly and deemed unobtainable in daily practice.

References

1. Sander AP, et al. Upper-extremity volume measurements in women with lymphedema: a comparison of measurements obtained via water displacement with geometrically determined volume. Phys Ther. 2002;82(12):1201–12.
2. Devoogdt N, et al. A new device to measure upper limb circumferences: validity and reliability. Int Angiol. 2010;29(5):401–7.
3. Sawan S, et al. Lower-limb lymphedema and vulval cancer: feasibility of prophylactic compression garments and validation of leg volume measurement. Int J Gynecol Cancer. 2009;19(9):1649–54.
4. Hidding JT, et al. Measurement properties of instruments for measuring of lymphedema: systematic review. Phys Ther. 2016;96(12):1965–81.
5. Sitzia J. Volume measurement in lymphoedema treatment: examination of formulae. Eur J Cancer Care (Engl). 1995;4(1):11–6.
6. Brorson H, Hoijer P. Standardised measurements used to order compression garments can be used to calculate arm volumes to evaluate lymphoedema treatment. J Plast Surg Hand Surg. 2012;46(6):410–5.
7. Hidding JT, et al. Accuracy of a single measurement site for self-monitoring of patients with breast cancer at risk for lymphedema. Physiother Theory Pract. 2018:1–6.
8. Arin KG, Sumner AS, Håkan B. Lymphedema: presentation, diagnosis and treatment. Springer; 2015.
9. Yamamoto T, et al. Lower extremity lymphedema index: a simple method for severity evaluation of lower extremity lymphedema. Ann Plast Surg. 2011;67(6):637–40.
10. Yamamoto T, et al. Practicality of the lower extremity lymphedema index: lymphedema index versus volumetry-based evaluations for body-type-corrected lower extremity volume evaluation. Ann Plast Surg. 2016;77(1):115–8.
11. Damstra RJ, Glazenburg EJ, Hop WC. Validation of the inverse water volumetry method: A new gold standard for arm volume measurements. Breast Cancer Res Treat. 2006;99(3):267–73.
12. Gjorup C, Zerahn B, Hendel HW. Assessment of volume measurement of breast cancer-related lymphedema by three methods: circumference measurement, water displacement, and dual energy X-ray absorptiometry. Lymphat Res Biol. 2010;8(2):111–9.
13. Chen YW, et al. Reliability study of measurements for lymphedema in breast cancer patients. Am J Phys Med Rehabil. 2008;87(1):33–8.

14. Ergin G, et al. Effects of aqua-lymphatic therapy on lower extremity lymphedema: a randomized controlled study. Lymphat Res Biol. 2017;15(3):284–91.
15. Perrin M, Guex JJ. Edema and leg volume: methods of assessment. Angiology. 2000;51(1):9–12.
16. Edgar DW, Briffa NK, Wood FM. Whole arm water displacement volumetry is a reliable and sensitive measure: a pilot to assess acute postburn volume change. J Burn Care Res. 2016;37(6):e508–14.
17. Mestre S, et al. Validation of lower limb segmental volumetry with hand-held, self-positioning three-dimensional laser scanner against water displacement. J Vasc Surg Venous Lymphat Disord. 2014;2(1):39–45.
18. Hameeteman M, et al. 3D stereophotogrammetry in upper-extremity lymphedema: an accurate diagnostic method. J Plast Reconstr Aesthet Surg. 2016;69(2):241–7.
19. Tokumoto H, et al. Utilization of three-dimensional photography (VECTRA) for the evaluation of lower limb lymphedema in patients following lymphovenous anastomosis. Lymphat Res Biol. 2018.
20. Ardehali B, et al. Objective assessment of keloid scars with three-dimensional imaging: quantifying response to intralesional steroid therapy. Plast Reconstr Surg. 2007;119(2):556–61.
21. Erends M, et al. Validity and reliability of three-dimensional imaging for measuring the volume of the arm. Lymphat Res Biol. 2014;12(4):275–81.
22. Landau MJ, et al. Vectra 3D imaging for quantitative volumetric analysis of the upper limb: a feasibility study for tracking outcomes of lymphedema treatment. Plast Reconstr Surg. 2018;141(1):80e–4e.
23. Preuss, M., et al., Validity and reliability of three-dimensional imaging for measuring breast cancer-related lymphedema in the upper limb: a cross-sectional study. Lymphat Res Biol. 2018.
24. Tierney S, et al. Infrared optoelectronic volumetry, the ideal way to measure limb volume. Eur J Vasc Endovasc Surg. 1996;12(4):412–7.
25. Stanton AW, et al. Validation of an optoelectronic limb volumeter (Perometer). Lymphology. 1997;30(2):77–97.
26. Batista BN, et al. Agreement between perometry and sequential arm circumference measurements in objective determination of arm volume. J Reconstr Microsurg. 2018;34(1):29–34.
27. Sharkey AR, et al. Measuring limb volume: accuracy and reliability of tape measurement versus perometer measurement. Lymphat Res Biol. 2018;16(2):182–6.
28. Sun F, et al. Perometry versus simulated circumferential tape measurement for the detection of breast cancer-related lymphedema. Breast Cancer Res Treat. 2018;172(1):83–91.

Bioelectrical Impedance Analysis

34

Yunzhu Li, Elan Yang, and Xiao Long

Abstract

Measurement procedures for the determination of limb volumes objectify the success of treatments. There are currently many noninvasive measuring methods for assessing the results of treatments for lymphedema. Bioelectrical impedance analysis permits the assessment of lymphedema by directly measuring lymph fluid changes through the rate at which an electrical current travel through the body, which can serve as an objective, reliable comparison between the changes in lymph volume before and after treatment.

Keywords

Lymphedema assessments · Bioelectrical impedance analysis

34.1 Bioelectrical Impedance Analysis

The Bioelectrical impedance analysis (BIA) is a noninvasive measurement method of body water volume (Fig. 34.1). Originally applied to body composition assessment in the field of nutrition, BIA has been gradually utilized for lymphedema since the first attempt by Watanabe et al. [1].

34.1.1 How BIA Works

Its principle lies in the nature of bioelectrical impedance (Z), the vector sum of resistance (R), and reactance (X_c), both of which are frequency-dependent. R reflects the flow of current that passes through the body and is inversely correlated with the amount of water. X_c is caused by the delay in conduction when current passes through the cell membrane. The low frequency cannot penetrate the cell membranes. Hence, the measured value R_0 at zero frequency (or very low frequency) refers to the extracellular water (ECW). The high frequency is a perfect (or near-perfect) capacitor, thus, the measured value R_∞ at infinite (or very high frequency) is the total body water (TBW), a combination of ECW and intracellular water (ICW). However, practical limitations hold it back from clinical application. A possible solution is to set fix frequencies close to zero and infinite, such as 5 KHz and 500 KHz. There are several methods of BIA, including single-frequency BIA (SF-BIA), multi-frequency BIA (MF-BIA), and bioelectrical impedance spectroscopy (BIS). Nowadays, BIS is the most common approach in the clinical setting, measuring impedances at spectra of frequencies ranging from 5 to 1000 KHz and plotting them graphically. The generating relationships between R and body fluid will allow the values of R_0 and R_∞ (Both of which are unable to be measured directly) to be determined.

The human body resembles a set of cylinders (e.g., the trunk, the arms, and the legs), with the fixed length that can be measured and the diameter assumed to be relatively constant. In a cylindrical conductor the impedance (Z) is a function of the resistivity (ρ), the length (L), and the cross-sectional area of the conductor (A).

$$R = \rho \times (L/A)$$

The equation can be rearranged if the volume (V) is included.

$$V = \rho \times (L2/Z)$$

As demonstrated in the equation, L is squared, which means a minor alternation in the measured length will have a great impact on the estimated volume. To obtain a reliable value, it is vital to apply a reproducible method of locating the sites of the measurement electrodes. Bioimpedance

Y. Li · E. Yang · X. Long (✉)
Department of Plastic and Reconstructive Surgery, Peking Union Medical College Hospital, Beijing, People's Republic of China

N. Liu (ed.), *Peripheral Lymphedema*, https://doi.org/10.1007/978-981-16-3484-0_34

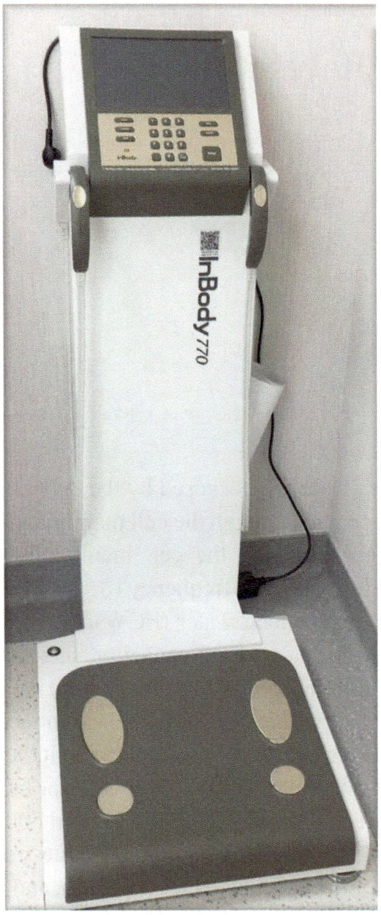

Fig. 34.1 The Inbody body composition analyzer is a noninvasive body composition analysis that provides a detailed breakdown of your weight in terms of muscle, fat, and water. (https://inbodyusa.com/)

Table 34.1 Recommended positions of electrodes

Electrode	Upper limbs	Lower limbs
Drive	The dorsal surface of the third metacarpal of the hand	The dorsal surface of the third metacarpal of the hand
Measurement	The dorsum of the wrist midway between the styloid processes	The dorsum of the ankles midway between the malleoli
Measurement	The dorsum of the wrist midway between the styloid processes	The dorsum of the ankles midway between the malleoli
Drive	The dorsal surface of the third metatarsal of the foot	The dorsal surface of the third metatarsal of the foot

measurements are usually taken following a standard tetrapolar arrangement, with the patient in the supine or standing position on a non-conducting surface. Four electrodes are applied, with two measurement electrodes positioned each at the end of the segment to be measured and two drive electrodes each positioned distal to the measurement electrodes.

The recommended positions of electrodes are listed here (Table 34.1).

Of note, the jewelry should be removed, and the skin at the electrode sites should be cleaned with an alcohol wipe prior to the test.

34.1.2 BIA and Lymphedema Diagnosis

Lymphedema is the accumulation of excessive lymph fluid in the extracellular space caused by abnormal lymphatic function, leading to chronic inflammation and fibrosis [2]. As a result, by measuring ECW, BIA measures the obstructive lymph theoretically. Early in 1992, Ward et al. found that BIA could produce a quantitative agreement with a clinical diagnosis of lymphedema and with the limb size calculated from circumferences [3]. BIA permits the assessment of lymphedema by directly measuring lymph fluid changes. The superiority of BIA in application especially lies in its early diagnosis of lymphedema, demonstrating better sensitivity than circumferential limb measurements. Several studies have proposed a cutoff of inter-limb impedance ratio to detect early lymphedema. Derived from the impedance values of the lymphedematous limb and the contralateral unaffected limb, the inter-limb impedance ratio is compared to normative values. Though not exactly the same, most proposed cut-offs fall in the range of the mean + 2SD to the mean + 3SD [4–6]. Set to the mean + 3SD, Cornish et al. observed a sensitivity of 100% and a specificity of 98% in their study of breast-cancer-related lymphedema (BCRL) [7]. More importantly, diagnosis of sub-clinical lymphedema using BIA means early intervention, reducing the subsequent development of lymphedema. A prospective trial including 186 patients who underwent axillary lymph node dissection (ALND) observed that 33% of patients were diagnosed with sub-clinical lymphedema and received early treatment [8]. During the 20-month follow-up, the incidence of clinically apparent BCRL reduced to 4.4% compared with the 36.4% in the control group. However, contrary results were also seen. Barrio et al. questioned its ability to quantify the change in volume differences between limbs [9]. They compared BIA against the "gold standard" volume displacement (VD) in a prospective cohort in patients following breast cancer surgery and found considerable discordance between BIA and VD measurements. Abnormalities in BIA are not well correlated with subsequent lymphedema development. Therefore, BIA does play a role in lymphedema diagnosis but should be used in an integrated diagnostic setting.

References

1. Watanabe R, et al. Evaluation of leg edema using a multifrequency impedance meter in patients with lymphatic obstruction. Lymphology. 1989;22(2):85–92.
2. Ryan TJ. Lymphatics and adipose tissue. Clin Dermatol. 1995;13(5):493–8.
3. Ward LC, et al. Multi-frequency bioelectrical impedance augments the diagnosis and management of lymphoedema in post-mastectomy patients. Eur J Clin Investig. 1992;22(11):751–4.
4. York SL, et al. Single frequency versus bioimpedance spectroscopy for the assessment of lymphedema. Breast Cancer Res Treat. 2009;117(1):177–82.
5. Ridner SH, et al. Bioelectrical impedance for detecting upper limb lymphedema in nonlaboratory settings. Lymphat Res Biol. 2009;7(1):11–5.
6. Hayes S, et al. Lymphedema secondary to breast cancer: how choice of measure influences diagnosis, prevalence, and identifiable risk factors. Lymphology. 2008;41(1):18–28.
7. Cornish BH, et al. Early diagnosis of lymphedema using multiple frequency bioimpedance. Lymphology. 2001;34(1):2–11.
8. Soran A, et al. The importance of detection of subclinical lymphedema for the prevention of breast cancer-related clinical lymphedema after axillary lymph node dissection; a prospective observational study. Lymphat Res Biol. 2014;12(4):289–94.
9. Barrio AV, Eaton A, Frazier TG. A prospective validation study of bioimpedance with volume displacement in early-stage breast cancer patients at risk for lymphedema. Ann Surg Oncol. 2015;22(Suppl 3):S370–5.

Skin Fibrometer and Lymph Scanner

35

Ziyou Yu

Abstract

Skin and subcutis have undergone a series of pathological changes due to sustained lymph stagnation in lymphedema. Current knowledge of the skin alterations in lymphedema based mainly on biopsies and histological evaluations of the lymphedematous tissues and detailed functions and texture changes of the affected skin has been overlooked in clinical examination of lymphedema. In this chapter, we introduced two recently developed instruments SkinFibroMeter and LymphScanner, for the noninvasive and quantitative assessment of skin properties in lymphedema. Quantification of skin properties changes could be a valuable supplement to the diagnosis and evaluation of chronic lymphedema.

Keywords

Lymphedema · Skin · Fibrosis · Stiffness · Percentage water content

35.1 Skin Fibrometer

Skin fibrosis is one of the characteristic features of lymphedema. The skin and subcutis usually becoming thickened or hardened with disease progress. Diagnosis and measurement of skin fibrosis play an important role for the pathophysiological evaluation of lymphedema. SkinFibroMeter (Delfin, Kuopio, Finland) is a device recently developed for assessing skin stiffness (SF). This device is portable and sensitive, consists of a 1 mm length indenter. The instrument is briefly pressed on the skin, and the indenter imposes a constant deformation when the reference plate of the probe is fully in contact with the skin. The skin resists deformation to the external force, and the SF value (Newton, N) is thus measured. SF value is an indicator of mechanical properties of the skin and can be used to reflect the presence and severity of skin fibrosis.

Recently, SkinFibroMeter has been used to evaluate the degree of fibrosis in secondary lymphedema [1, 2]. In our study, SF value was measured in the affected and contralateral control limb on five sites (Fig. 35.1). The average value in each limb was considered to indicate the overall SF value for the limb. We found the SF value was significantly higher in lymphedematous than control limbs (Fig. 35.2a). Given that baseline SF value may vary among patients, we used the contralateral control limb as a reference to calculate the "excess ratio" of the affected limb. The excess SF ratio was defined as (mean induration value of lymphedematous limb—mean induration value of the control limb)/mean induration value of the control limb*100%. Significant differences between different stages of lymphedema and strong correlations between the excess SF ratio and lymphedema stage were found (Fig. 35.2b, c), indicating decreased tissue compliance and increased skin fibrosis and hardening with disease progression. The results also reflect that tissue fibrosis progresses throughout the development of lymphedema and therefore plays a critical role in the pathophysiology of the disease.

Measurement of SF value provides diagnostic valuable information of the skin fibrosis in lymphedema. The evaluation of skin fibrosis may help in monitoring the progression of the disease. Assessing SF before and after therapeutic interventions could be helpful in selecting the optimal treatment regimen.

35.2 LymphScanner

Currently, Bioimpedance (BI) analysis is the widely used approach for measuring extracellular fluid (ECF) in lymphedema. However, this approach could only reflect the fluid

Z. Yu (✉)
Department of Plastic and Reconstructive Surgery, Shanghai Ninth People's Hospital, Shanghai Jiao Tong University School of Medicine, Shanghai, China

N. Liu (ed.), *Peripheral Lymphedema*, https://doi.org/10.1007/978-981-16-3484-0_35

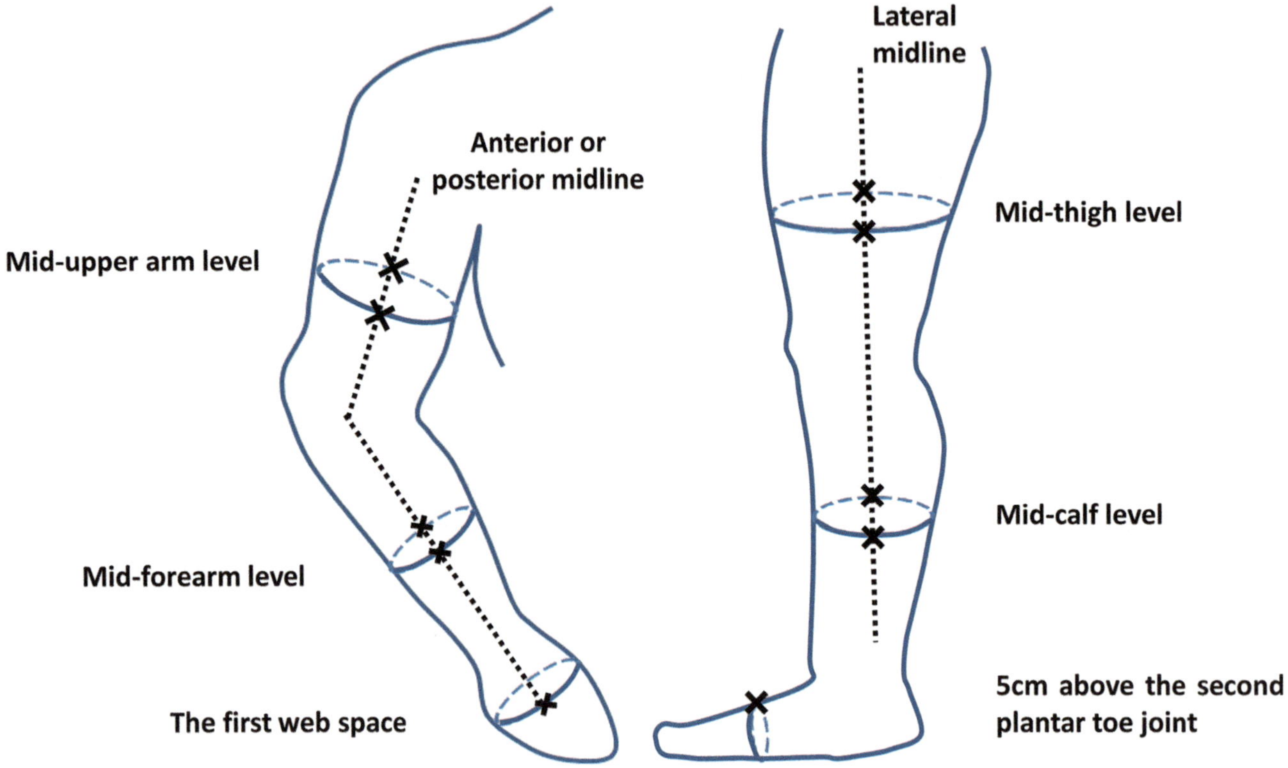

Fig. 35.1 Measured sites of the extremities. This figure is reproduced with permission from Yu Z, Liu N, Wang L, Chen J, Han L, Sun D. Assessment of Skin Properties in Chronic Lymphedema: Measurement of Skin Stiffness, Percentage Water Content, and Transepidermal Water Loss. Lymphatic research and biology. 2019

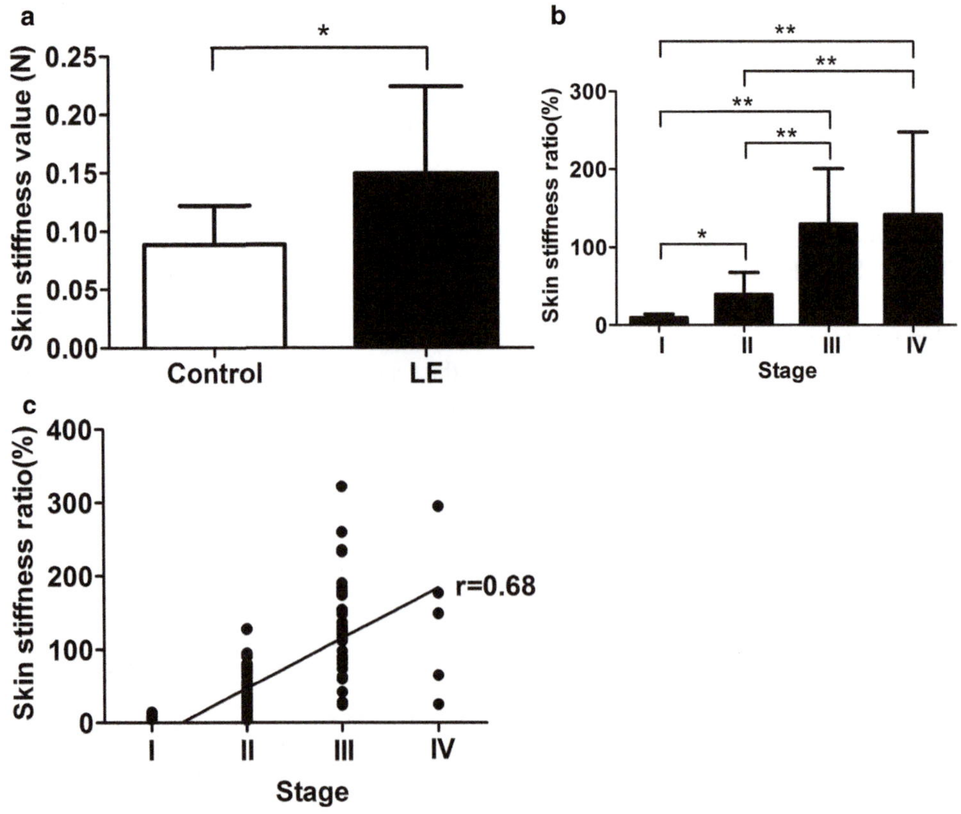

Fig. 35.2 SkinFibroMeter Measurement in secondary lymphedematous skin. SF value was significantly higher in lymphedematous than control limbs (**a**). Significant differences between different stages of lymphedema (**b**) and strong correlations between the excess SF ratio and lymphedema stage was found (**c**). $*p < 0.05$, $**p < 0.01$. This figure is reproduced with permission from Yu Z, Liu N, Wang L, Chen J, Han L, Sun D. Assessment of Skin Properties in Chronic Lymphedema: Measurement of Skin Stiffness, Percentage Water Content, and Transepidermal Water Loss. Lymphatic research and biology. 2019

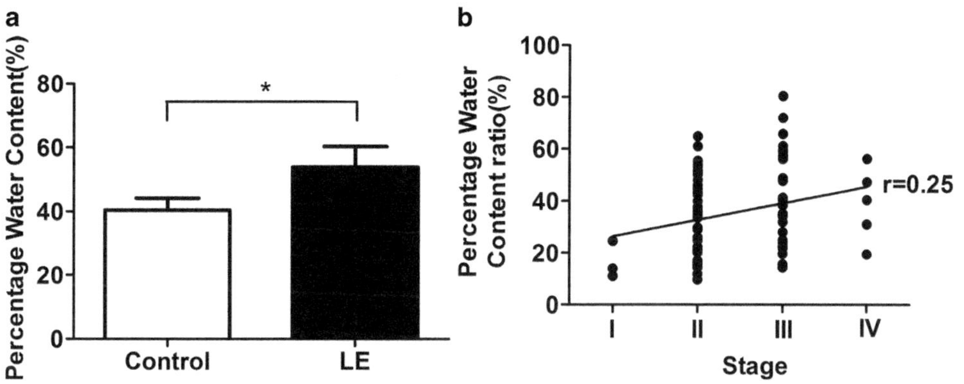

Fig. 35.3 LymphScanner Measurement in secondary lymphedematous skin. PWC value was significantly higher in lymphedematous than control limbs (**a**). Correlation analysis performed with PWC showed weak correlations with lymphedema stage (**b**). $^{*}p < 0.05$, $^{**}p < 0.01$. This figure is reproduced with permission from Yu Z, Liu N, Wang L, Chen J, Han L, Sun D. Assessment of Skin Properties in Chronic Lymphedema: Measurement of Skin Stiffness, Percentage Water Content, and Transepidermal Water Loss. Lymphatic research and biology. 2019

volume of the whole limb, localized changes may not be detected by BI measurement, thus causing false-negative results and insufficient sensitivity for detecting lymphedema [3]. Tissue dielectric constant (TDC) of human skin measured at a frequency of 300 MHz is directly proportional to skin water content, local tissue water is quantifiable using the TDC measurements and can be defined as percentage water content (PWC). Therefore, the PWC value reflects the amount of fluid accumulation in the measurement site. The previous study has shown that measurements of TDC are useful for documenting localized lymphedema and the early detection of incipient lymphedema [4, 5].

LymphScanner (Delfin, Kuopio, Finland) is a recently developed instrument used for evaluating local and regional edema by the TDC measurement. LymphScanner has a sensitive probe of a measurement depth up to 2.5 mm. Measurement is initiated by touching the probe to the skin, and the reading is reported as PWC on the screen. We have previously used LymphScanner for the evaluation of PWC in lymphedematous skin and proved this device is sensitive and convenient for detecting lymphedema [2]. Five sites of each limb were measured as described above. The mean PWC value of these five sites was calculated for each limb. We found PWC value was significantly higher in lymphedematous than control limbs (Fig. 35.3a). Although the value is significantly increased even in stage I lymphedema, the correlation analysis performed with PWC showed weak correlations with the lymphedema stage (Fig. 35.3b). This may due to the progressive accumulation of the fluid and increased thickness of the skin and subcutis with increased severity of LE, while LymphScanner with a measurement depth of 2.5 mm can only detect a certain layer of tissue. Once fluid accumulation beyond the maximum depth of measurement, LymphScanner may not be able to detect accurately.

As a noninvasive and quantitative measurement modality, LymphScanner shows high sensitivity for detection of early-stage lymphedema and measurement of the water content of superficial lymphedema. In addition, by rapid skin scanning, localized swelling or the extent of lymphedema can be easily assessed. In contrast, BI analysis measures the water volume change in the whole limb, thus could be more suitable in reflecting the severity and progression of the disease. These approaches may be combined for more comprehensive evaluation of tissue water change in lymphedema.

References

1. Sun D, Yu Z, Chen J, Wang L, Han L, Liu N. The value of using a SkinFibroMeter for diagnosis and assessment of secondary lymphedema and associated fibrosis of lower limb skin. Lymphat Res Biol. 2017;15(1):70–6.
2. Yu Z, Liu N, Wang L, Chen J, Han L, Sun D. Assessment of skin properties in chronic lymphedema: measurement of skin stiffness, percentage water content, and transepidermal water loss. Lymphat Res Biol 2019.
3. Qin ES, Bowen MJ, Chen WF. Diagnostic accuracy of bioimpedance spectroscopy in patients with lymphedema: A retrospective cohort analysis. J Plast Reconstr Aesthet Surg. 2018;71(7):1041–50.
4. Mayrovitz HN, Singh A, Akolkar S. Age-related differences in tissue dielectric constant values of female forearm skin measured noninvasively at 300 MHz. Skin Res Technol. 2016;22(2):189–95.
5. Mayrovitz HN, Davey S, Shapiro E. Suitability of single tissue dielectric constant measurements to assess local tissue water in normal and lymphedematous skin. Clin Physiol Funct Imaging. 2009;29(2):123–7.

Part IX

Lymphedema in Children

Lymphedema in Childhood

36

Cristóbal M. Papendieck

Abstract

The clinical and surgical analysis of lymphedema in pediatrics allows to appreciate (or identify) some very important aspects of this disorder. Eighty percent of lymphedemas in children are primary, and 80% of them are grade 0-I. 20% are secondary, all of them operable to some extent. The lifetime (+ 80 years) cost of treatment is huge and requires much consideration in terms of the decisions that may or must be taken (or not), particularly in a primary lymphedema that needs habilitation—as no rehabilitation is possible when something has never functioned, There is no such thing as agenesis of the lymphatic system because the lymph is the result of life.

Keywords

Primary lymphedema · Secondary lymphedema in pediatrics · LAD I · LAD II · Phlebolymphedema · Inflammatory aspects in primary lymphedema · Podoconiosis · Filariasis

It is estimated that 30% of patients with lymphedema are patients of pediatric age. Eighty percent of them have primary lymphedemas. Eighty percent of them have no diagnosis, or their diagnosis is unknown [1]. This is why they are said to be *orphan carriers*. Where are they? Who are they diagnosed by? Who cares for them and where? Such is the purpose of this analysis.

The sign of lymphedema is the consequence of a malfunction of the lymphatic system. It is a soft, painless, non-specific, non-inflammatory edema with a positive Stemmer sign and a positive or negative pitting test in primary lymphedemas; and with attached signs of its etiopathogenesis in secondary lymphedemas. We define lymphedema as primary when its cause lies in the lymphatic system itself. It is secondary when the cause is external to the system. In general, lymphedemas are suspected only clinically and must be identified by means of specific functional tests.

The lymphatic system may be involved in one, some, or all of its parts, which are specifically three:

The initial interstitial lymphatic capillary endothelium (which lacks basement membrane). Its development depends on the VEGF and its receptors, and their malfunctioning is the most frequent cause of primary lymphedema.

Lymphatic vessels of any diameter, in general, due to a malformation (lymphangiodysplasia, LAD I) [2], congenital hypoplasia, or hyperplasia in primary lymphedemas; and due to severing, trauma or compression acquired hypoplasia or hyperplasia in secondary lymphedemas.

Lymph nodes in all anatomical locations. Malformation (LAD II), hypoplasia or hyperplasia in primary lymphedemas, and severing or injury, hypoplasia or hyperplasia in secondary lymphedemas.

All primary causes are congenital, identified, identifiable or unknown at the time of the pediatric perinatal control.

The following are LAD I: lymphangioleiomyomatosis (LAM), lymphangiomatosis, lymphangioma, avalvulation, dysvalvulation, lymphangioneurosis, narrowing, ectasia (Fig. 36.1).

The following are LAD II: fibrosis (either capsular, subcapsular, or central), intranodal angiomatoid malformation.

In addition, hyperplasia or hypoplasia should be included. The lymphatic system expresses life; it is indispensable in vertebrates; it is indispensable in all tissues. Agenesia is not possible.

There are hyperplastic lymphatic systems in primary lymphedemas.

Lymphedema is interstitial, with or without lymphatic hypertension at the vascular level. It is defined by the initial

C. M. Papendieck (✉)
Angiopediatrics Foundation. Frontiers of Lymphology Group, Buenos Aires, Argentina

N. Liu (ed.), *Peripheral Lymphedema*, https://doi.org/10.1007/978-981-16-3484-0_36

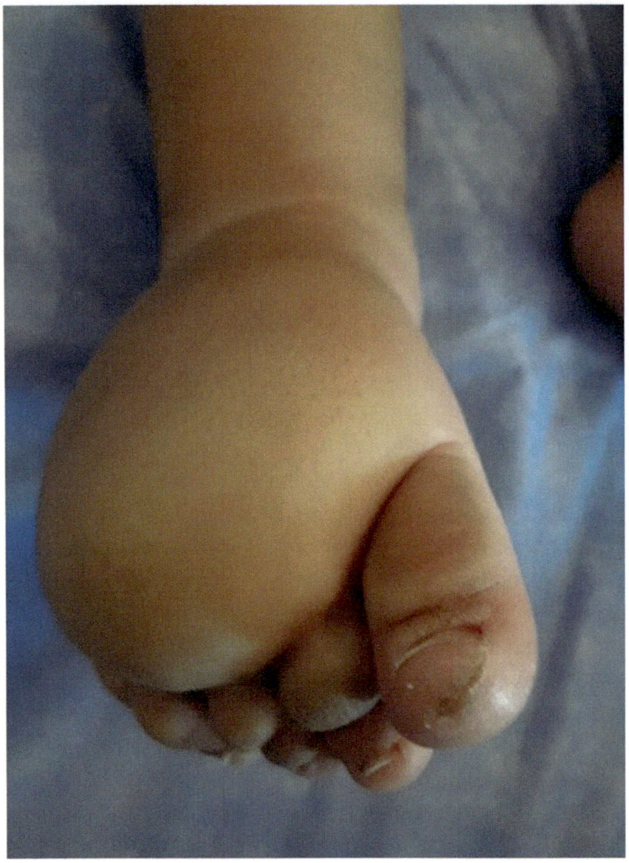

Fig. 36.1 Foot of an infant with primary lymphedema grade I–II

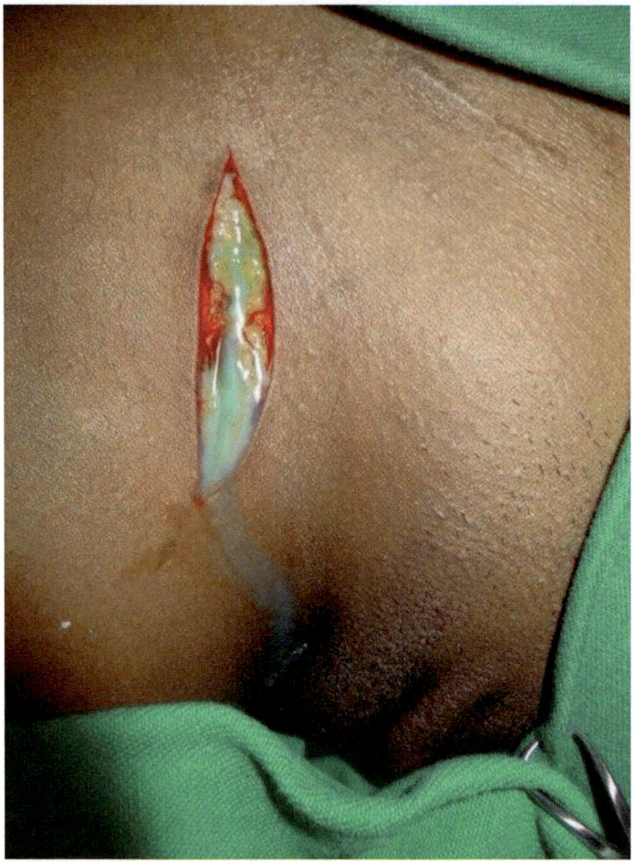

Fig. 36.2 Lymphatic transvascular and interstitial reflux in a girl

interstitial capillary endothelium, or the anatomical or functional nodal obstruction, or reflux of the interstitial systemic lymph, or reflux of jejuno ileal lymph, lymph-chyle (Fig. 36.2), to the insufficient lymphatic system or through aberrant paths (diverted flow).

Eighty percent of primary lymphedemas has no diagnosis in pediatrics for their expression as grade 0 or eventually 1. Another 10% expresses as great combined vascular syndromes or overgrowth syndromes, or important systemic conditions, or generalized lymphatic disorders or malformations (LAD I + II) (grade III) [3]. Lastly, the remaining 10%, grade I and II lymphedemas, express exclusively as conditions of the lymphatic system in 140 diseases or syndromes in pediatrics.

Primary lymphedemas, if the context allows, express as such continuously in the adult patient, at which time they account for 20% of lymphedemas.

It is complicated to forecast survival in children with lymphedema as a single condition or in the context of multisystem disorders. The complications of these syndromes and lymphedema itself, such as infections (*Erysipelas*) and oncological aspects due to chronic interstitial hypertension, have an influence there.

Not all malformations of the lymphatic system express as primary lymphedema. Some, never…

Molecular biology has identified numerous mutations specifically involving the lymphatic system. For example, Milroy's disease, the lymphedema-distichiasis syndrome, and the hypotrichosis-lymphedema-telangiectasia syndrome. In addition, more than 20 syndromes [4] have been identified with which primary lymphedema coexists [5]. For example, some leukemias, Turner's and Noonan's syndromes, among others, are frequent in pediatrics and/or are associated with other vascular malformations, in combination or not. Other examples are CLOVES, Klippel and Trenaunay, and other syndromes [6]. And also, syndromes with a generalized lymphatic malformation and others such as the Gorham (Stout) and/or Haferkamp syndromes.

Primary lymphedema is chronic and progressive. It may entail a progressive increase in adipogenesis. Adipose overgrowth…) This condition may be congenital and require neonatal observation. It is difficult to establish whether this is a syndromic lipomatous overgrowth or a consequence of interstitial hypertension. If this were the case, the primary lymphedema would need at least 8 months to trigger the phe-

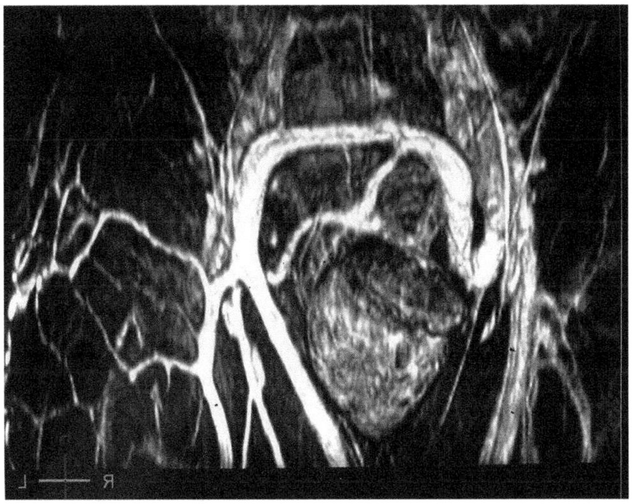

Fig. 36.3 Image of the A–V time in an AMRI (angio MRI) where the occlusion of the left iliac vein and a spontaneous congenital Palm bypass can be observed. The vascular system has been balanced, but a contralateral Palma procedure remains to be performed with a lymphovenous or nodal anastomosis, due to a secondary, and eventually primary, lymphedema

nomenon. This may explain the absence of a pitting test in some primary or secondary lymphedemas.

Anatomical pathology studies of lymph node micro biopsies in primary lymphedemas have revealed that the inflammatory phenomenon is practically a constant. This is an important finding with no rational explanation to date. Biopsies have all been performed as an initial step of a lymphovenous anastomosis in pediatrics. An important fact.

Generally, primary lymphedema in the limbs is asymmetric. It does not involve bone growth. Therefore, digital X-ray measurements are a relevant differential diagnostic element in, for example, asymmetric growth syndromes such as Wiedemann Beckwith's.

Secondary lymphedema in pediatrics is identified by its etiology or etiopathogenesis in addition to the sign of lymphedema, to which inflammatory phenomena, in some cases, acute or chronic phenomena in other, should be added depending on the etiology.

Possibly, the most frequent cause of secondary lymphedema is truncal venous hypertension (Fig. 36.3), segmental or regional to congenital or acquired lymphedema. Phlebolymphedema? This context is often observed in overgrowth syndromes as, for example, secondary and primary lymphedema, or as iatropathology, mainly vascular access procedures for different causes occurring in neonatology and complex cardiovascular surgery in particular.

Other causes of secondary lymphedema may be amniotic bands, filariasis, podoconiosis, radiation therapy, radical surgery, drug addiction (puffy hand syndrome), hair tourniquet, and other syndromes, chronic infections, vaccines, and pharmacological causes (chronic and specific medications), among other.

36.1 Diagnosis

All diagnostic methods or techniques are possible in pediatrics. Many need general anesthesia, and some are complex because of the time required to conduct them. It is important to have information on the time of lymphatic circulation, level of obstruction, valve disorders, and lymph node and vascular hypoplasia and hyperplasia. Magnetic resonance imaging is very useful to identify grade 0–I lymphedemas and more specifically to identify lymph node accessibility for anastomosis and/or diagnostic purposes.

The genetic assessment should be a constant, but it is not always possible. The anatomical pathology evaluation of lymph nodes (minimally invasive biopsies at the time of a lymphovenous anastomosis) is a routine procedure that provides basic information and lymph node information of vascular malformations or anomalies and/or associated conditions.

36.2 Treatment

The treatment can and must observe all national and international consensus protocols [7, 8] (ISL, ESL, LF, LA, and other). The physician's ability and experience in managing the chronic progressive condition in a child is also important. Still today, patients wonder if lymphedema is contagious, if they can fly wearing bandages, if they can exercise, if they have a genetic disease, and so on. Where can they be treated? There are no specific pediatric centers for vascular rehabilitation. However, if a child needs hospitalization, it should be in a pediatric facility—although these centers do not expect to receive patients with elephantiasis, lymphangiomatosis of the tongue, or chylous reflux of genitalia, to name a few.

Primary lymphedemas must undergo habilitation. What has never existed cannot be rehabilitated. Technically, the purpose is the same, but the outcome is not. The sooner, the better. Not all surgical techniques require postoperative vascular rehabilitation. Other procedures require inelastic compression for life, which is not compatible with a child's psychophysical care and integration.

With regard to the surgical techniques to use, it all depends on experience and a right diagnosis. Anything done in pediatrics is for the rest of the life. The fundamental issue is not the anastomosis itself but healing and functional recovery. Not all supermicro anastomoses that work are enough. Lymphovenous anastomoses are all valid, the same as lymph node transfer, especially in secondary lymphedema. Regarding local or regional venous hypertension, this aspect should be solved or reduced before conducted a lymphovenous anastomosis. If this is not possible, the option may be a cross lymphatic "rescue" using a Palma bypass on a lymph node with the usual technique (Fig. 36.4) [9].

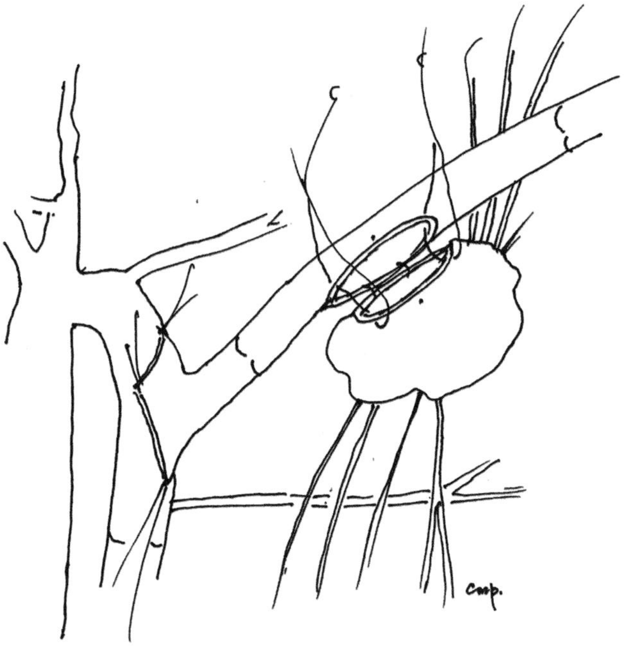

Fig. 36.4 Diagram of a crossed inguinal lymphovenous anastomosis. Crossed lymphatic rescue

36.3 Conclusion

Pediatric lymphedema is a great clinical-surgical chapter in medicine. But it is an orphan condition. It requires clinical practice, particularly in terms of syndrome and disorder diagnosis, as well as experience to decide what the priorities and technical choices are. Pediatric patients always require the participation of at least one parent during all the stages of the treatment, which is chronic. It demands time, transportation, support, and technology. This is not possible in all regions or cities, and the climate deserves special considerations. It is complicated to organize hospital care in general because it is an orphan condition in many senses.

References

1. Papendieck CM. Linfedema en pediatria. Clasificacion y etiopatogenia. Rev Hosp Niños B Aires. 2003;46(201):14–2.
2. Papendieckc M. Lymphatic dysplasias in pediatrics. Int Angiol. 1999;18:6–9.
3. ISSVA. Vascular anomalies classification. Amsterdam; 2018.
4. Barbosa ML, Papendieck CM. Linfangioadenodisplasias en pediatria. Patologia Vascular. 2000;6(4):323–7.
5. Hennekam RC. Syndromic lymphatic maldevelopment. 4° International Conference NLN, Orlando; 2000.
6. Papendieck CM. El pie de la sombra. Dialogo entre Historia, Arte y Enfermedad. Rev Hosp Niños (B. Aires). 2014; 56(255):221–236.
7. International Society of Lymphkigy (ISL) The diagnosis and treatment of peripheral lymphedema. Consensus document. Lymphology. 2013;46:1–11.
8. Ciiucci JL. 5° Consenso Larinoamericano para el tratamiento del Linfedema. San Nicolas 2014. Ed. Nayarith. Buenos Aires. Argentina.
9. Papendieck CM, Barbosa ML, Amore M, Ruy MA, et al. A new combined operative technique using crossed inguinal lymphatic rescue for pediatric patients with mixed lymphatic and venous malformation. Lymphology. 2017;50(3):141–7.

Part X

Prevention of Tumor Treatment Related Lymphedema

37 Prevention of Lymphedema After Breast Cancer Surgery

Dehong Zou

Abstract

The pathogenesis of upper limb lymphedema on the affected side of breast cancer after surgery is unknown. The most effective preventive measure at present is sentinel lymph node biopsy instead of axillary lymph node dissection, especially for early breast cancer. Secondly, to avoid upper limb injury on the affected side, especially various forms of the excessive load; seeking out high-risk factors for lymphedema, detection of early lymphedema, and early CDT-based intervention should be paid attention to; Application of microsurgical techniques to reconstruct lymphatic drainage pathways while axillary lymph node dissection has attractive prospects. The basic research on the pathogenesis of lymphedema and its transformation into prevention and treatment measures are worth looking forward to.

Keywords

Lymphedema · Prevention · Breast neoplasm · Sentinel lymph node biopsy · Axillary lymph node dissection

37.1 Introduction

The pathogenesis of lymphedema in the upper limbs of the affected side of breast cancer after surgery is unknown, with a high incidence and difficult treatment. It severely troubles the affected limb's sensation, movement, shape and psychology, living, work, and social aspects. Lymphedema is prone to recurrent skin and soft tissue infections and repeated infections of skin and soft tissues of affected limbs, edema and infection are causal, and a vicious circle eventually develops into elephantiasis. A few may have malignant skin changes, which significantly affect the quality of life of patients and therefore constitute a social issue that cannot be ignored, such as breast cancer. It is also a medical problem urgently to be overcome worldwide [1, 2].

Lymphedema has obvious symptoms and signs after breast cancer surgery, and the diagnosis is relatively easy. The most common causes are axillary lymph node dissection (ALND) and postoperative limb injury. A preliminary clinical diagnosis can be obtained with a history of breast cancer surgery and swelling of the upper limbs (Fig. 37.1a, b, c). The problem is that treatment is difficult, there is no hope for cure, and the course is long, so prevention is especially important.

Breast cancer surgery includes procedures like classic radical mastectomy, modified radical mastectomy, breast-conserving radical surgery, especially sentinel lymph node biopsy (SLNB) instead of ALND. Classic radical mastectomy designed for locally advanced breast cancer emphasizes massive resection, including all of the breast and a certain range of chest wall skin and subcutaneous tissue of the chest wall, pectoralis major, pectoralis minor, all lymph nodes, and the surrounding fat tissues in the axilla (Fig. 37.2a). The incidence of lymphedema after breast cancer surgery has been reported as high as 60%. Modified radical mastectomy preserves the pectoralis major and/or pectoralis minor, which is based on traditional radical mastectomy (Fig. 37.2b). Breast-conserving mastectomy is a clean removal of breast tumors while retaining the breast (combined with postoperative radiotherapy) (Figs. 37.2c, d, 37.3a, c, d). Sentinel lymph node biopsy (SLNB) is a procedure in which the axillary sentinel lymph node (SLNs) are removed and pathologically examined during the operation. If tumor cells are identified in the SLN, ALND is performed. If no, then no lymph node dissection is required (Fig. 37.3a, b, d). SLNB has been used in early breast cancer operations to replace ALND, and the incidence of postoperative lymphedema is below 7% [3].

Until now, the most effective treatment for lymphedema after breast cancer surgery with clinical evidence support is

D. Zou (✉)
Department of Breast Surgery, Cancer Hospital of University of Chinese Academy of Sciences (Zhejiang Cancer Hospital), Hangzhou, China

N. Liu (ed.), *Peripheral Lymphedema*, https://doi.org/10.1007/978-981-16-3484-0_37

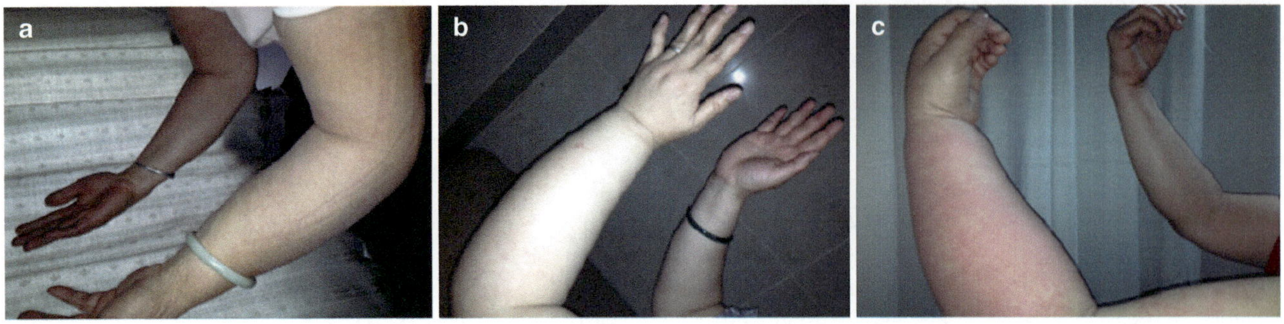

Fig. 37.1 (**a**) Lymphedema of the left upper limb, 4 months after left breast cancer. (**b**) Lymphedema of the left upper limb, 3 years after left breast cancer surgery. (**c**) Left upper limb lymphedema with acute lymphangitis, 7 years after left breast cancer surgery

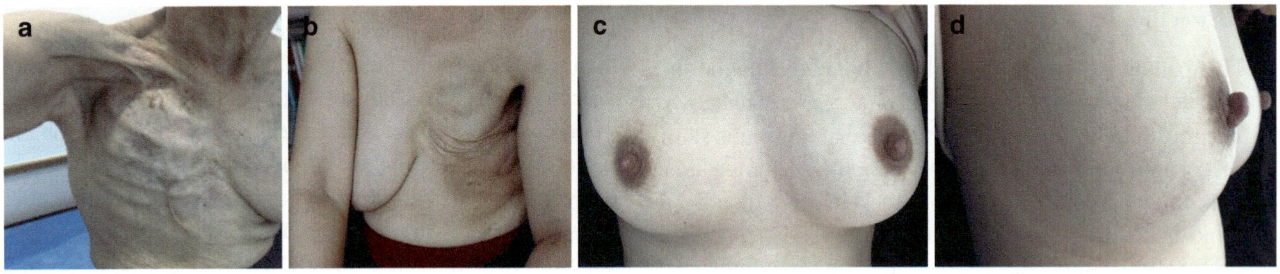

Fig. 37.2 (**a**) After traditional radical mastectomy of right breast cancer, axillary lymph node dissection, pectoralis major and pectoralis minor resection. (**b**) After a modified radical mastectomy of left breast cancer, axillary lymph node dissection, and pectoralis major and pectoralis minor muscle retention. (**c**) Front view of right breast cancer after breast-conserving and sentinel lymph node biopsy. (d) Lateral view of right breast cancer after breast-conserving and sentinel lymph node biopsy

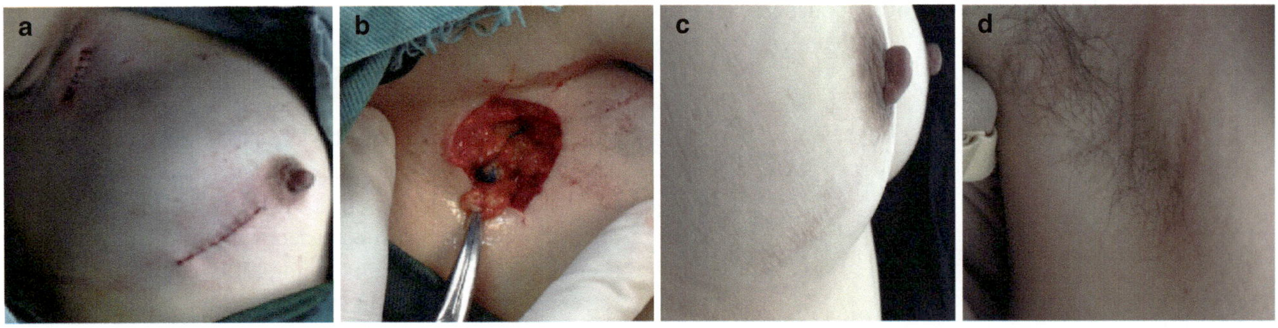

Fig. 37.3 (**a**) After breast-conserving and sentinel lymph node biopsy for right breast cancer, (**b**) Breast-conserving sentinel lymph node biopsy for right breast cancer with a small range of axillary injuries. (**c**) Right Breast incision scar, 1 year after breast-conserving surgery for breast cancer. (**d**) Right Axillary incision scar, 1 year after breast-conserving surgery and sentinel lymph node biopsy for breast cancer

complete decongestive therapy (CDT). Various forms of surgical treatment, especially microsurgery techniques, seem to have application prospects, but requirements for surgical equipment and technique are high, and the long-term effect is still uncertain. And CDT is still necessary before and after surgery. The CDT implementation process is time-consuming and labor-intensive, especially the use of bandages needs to be maintained for life. Developing countries might have poor accessibility due to the high cost of bandage materials. Prevention is important considering the dilemma of treatment and efficacy. However, the actual mechanism of lymphedema is not fully understood, and there are large differences in individual factors. For the prevention of etiology (primary prevention), Means are limited. What we urgently need and can do at present include: detecting early breast cancer, SLNB as a replacement of ALND in early breast cancer surgery, avoiding upper limb injury after breast cancer surgery. Preventive surgery and conservative intervention measures such as CDT worth further exploration. Personalized prevention based on hypertension and diabetes management, Body Mass Index control, deserves high attention.

37.1.1 Detection of Early Breast Cancer

About the prevention of lymphedema after breast cancer surgery, the first common problem is obviously the prevention of breast cancer. In the breast cancer prevention strategy, primary prevention is mainly to prevent the occurrence of tumors based on the cause of the disease. At present, it is almost impossible to implement because of the unknown cause of the disease. However, pay attention to the high-risk factors for breast cancer, especially good individual behavior factors. Adequate physical exercise, a reasonable diet to avoid obesity, marriage, and childbirth of the right age and breastfeeding are worth promoting [4]. Secondary prevention is mainly to take preventive measures for early detection, early diagnosis, and early treatment of breast cancer, early breast cancer detection is the basis or prerequisite for the effective prevention of lymphedema after breast cancer surgery. Tertiary prevention is a palliative treatment for patients with advanced clinical and recurrence and metastasis to reduce pain and prolong life, including palliative treatment of upper limb cancerous lymphedema caused by breast cancer recurrence and metastasis.

Early breast cancer surgery requires only sentinel lymph node biopsy and comprehensive breast-preserving treatment, which preserves the integrity of the breast and axillary to the greatest extent, thereby reducing damage to the axillary lymph network structure and upper limb lymphatic drainage function, the incidence of postoperative lymphedema is effectively reduced to less than 7%, while patients with locally advanced breast cancer inevitably need to undergo axillary lymph node dissection, the incidence of postoperative lymphedema is 15%–45% or even higher.

Early breast cancer is relative to locally advanced breast cancer (mammary invasive carcinoma with the largest diameter greater than 5 cm or axillary lymph node metastasis) or distant metastases. The definition and judgment criteria are still controversial. From the perspective of lymphedema prevention, breast cancer without Ipsilateral axillary lymph node metastasis can be considered as early breast cancer. Due to economic and cultural reasons, medical insurance, hierarchical medical treatment systems, and comprehensive management models are not complete in developing countries. More than half of the breast cancer patients treated clinically are beyond the early stage. It is not uncommon that patients only went to the doctor when they accidentally found a large breast lump or felt swollen axillary lymph nodes. Therefore, preventive education such as early diagnosis and early treatment of tumors is continuously carried out in the whole society, and regular self-examination methods of breasts are recommended in healthy people of appropriate age, which can detect 2–3 cm breast mass, while the probability of lymph node metastasis at this stage is relatively low. Regular breast check-ups, breast cancer screenings from any public welfare programs would be very beneficial to patients. If nipple eczema-like erosion, nipple retraction, nipple discharge, or any other abnormalities is found, it is strongly recommended to seek early diagnosis. If necessary, going to a specialized cancer hospital or a general one with a specialized breast disease health department may found an early breast cancer without lumps by a ultrasound, mammography, and magnetic resonance examination, and may avoid missed diagnosis, misdiagnosis, or non-standardized treatment of early breast cancer, which is important for lymphedema prevention.

37.1.2 SLNB as a Replacement of ALND

Sentinel lymph node refers to the first stop of lymph nodes that tumor lymphatics pass through. It can be located by dye or isotope to mark and take biopsy. Sentinel lymph node metastasis status can effectively indicate the metastasis status of draining lymph nodes. Sentinel lymph node biopsy is negative, and the drainage area can be stopped Lymph node dissection.

The direct factors for the occurrence of upper limb lymphedema on the ipsilateral side after breast cancer surgery are axillary lymph node dissection, and total axillary lymph node dissection causes extensive destruction of the axillary lymph network, severe impairment of lymphatic drainage of the upper limbs, and occurrence of lymphedema after decompensation. SLNB can replace ALND in breast cancer surgery, which preserves the anatomical integrity of the axillary lymph network to the greatest extent and reduces the incidence of lymphedema most effectively. The incidence of lymphedema in the upper limbs of the affected side of breast cancer patients has been reduced from about 45% (ALND) to less than 7% (SLNB) [3, 4]; The greatest significance of SLNB is to protect more than 70% early breast cancer patients without lymph node metastasis from ALND, thereby minimizing the occurrence of postoperative lymphedema [5, 6] (Figs. 37.3a, b, c, d, 37.4a, b, c, d).

Breast cancer axillary lymph node biopsy technology is mature and easy to operate. Sentinel lymph node biopsy can be successfully performed regardless of the use of dyes or isotopes or a combination of the two methods. The success rate of skilled operators can reach more than 95%, and the false-negative rate is less than 5%. The incidence of lymphedema after sentinel lymph node biopsy is reported in the literature of about 1–7%, most of which are related to the irregularity of sentinel lymph node biopsy such as the excessive removal of lymph nodes for biopsy, the scope of the operation too large, and the number of biopsy lymph nodes too large. Due to lack of understanding of the significance of SLNB, lack of confidence in the SLNB method, unnecessary fear of false negatives and false positives, Some surgeons

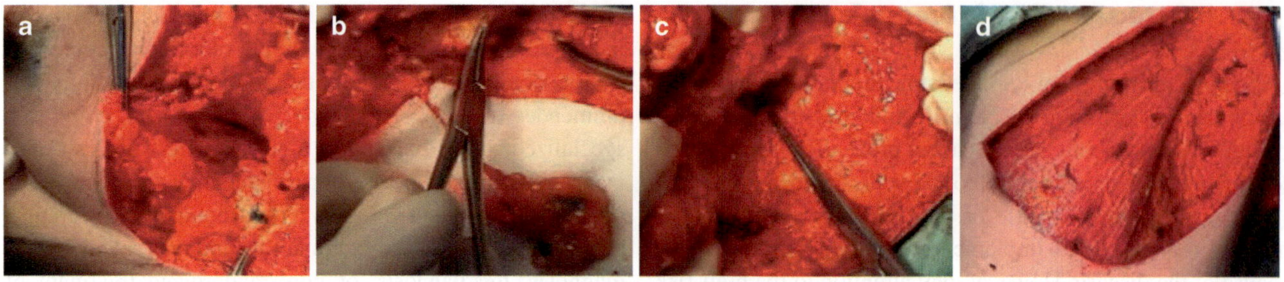

Fig. 37.4 (**a**) A blue-stained sentinel lymph nodes during surgery. (**b**) Sentinel lymph node dissection along blue-stained lymphatic vessels. (**c**) Local defect after a sentinel lymph node resection. (**d**) Chest wall fascia integrity is impaired after a mastectomy, and axillary fascia integrity damage is relatively minor

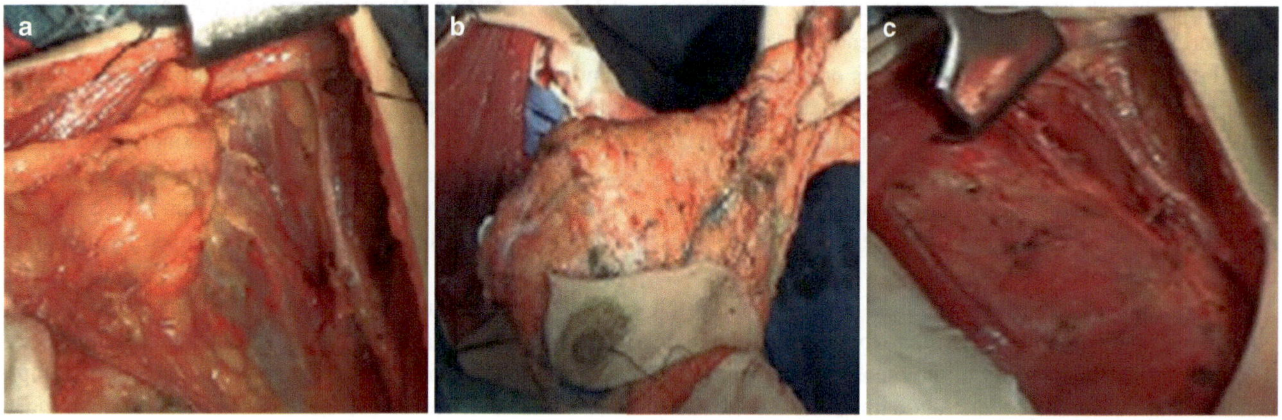

Fig. 37.5 (**a**) Dissection of axillary lymph nodes, lymph nodes below the axillary vein, and peripheral fat removal. (**b**) Breast and axillary lymph node dissection specimen. (**c**) Axillary injury range after mastectomy and axillary lymph node dissection

excessively remove non-sentinel lymph nodes around sentinel lymph nodes that have been successfully identified, the number is even as many as 7–10, which has destroyed a large area Anatomy of the axillary lymphatic network. It is generally believed that the number of axillary sentinel lymph node biopsies is 1–3. It needs to be combined with specific circumstances. If the sentinel lymph node tracking fails, the axillary lymph node closest to the breast may be taken as the target lymph node for biopsy, the markedly enlarged lymph node found near the successfully labeled SLN should be cut off for inspection. So far, there are still some surgeons who will perform ALND instead of SLNB in early-stage breast cancer operation, especially in economically underdeveloped areas, which needs to be highly concerned.

37.1.3 Considerations for ALND

Although axillary lymph node dissection can directly lead to postoperative lymphedema, patients with non-early stage breast cancer or early-stage SLNB positive or axillary lymph node recurrence after treatment still need to undergo axillary lymph node dissection. The extent of axillary clearance, the number of lymph nodes removed, and the incidence of lymphedema are directly proportional. For patients who need axillary lymph node dissection, there is no exact way to prevent the occurrence of postoperative lymphedema. Studies on the dynamics of upper limb lymphatic reflux and axillary vein function in patients with lymphedema suggest that postoperative axillary stenosis and restricted vasomotor activity may be related to the occurrence of upper limb lymphedema [7, 8]. It should usually be noted that: the scope of axillary lymph node dissection, especially the upper and lateral boundaries, should not exceed the lateral border of the latissimus dorsi muscle and the axillary vein junction, to avoid an excessive anatomical range, the removal of the subcutaneous fat tissue from the root of the affected side and the drainage of the lymphatic network of the upper limb; the range of ALND, especially the upper and lateral edges, should not exceed the lateral border of the latissimus dorsi and axillary vein, to avoid excessive anatomical range, without affecting the axillary lymph node dissection. At the same time, we must pay attention to the protection of the integrity of the axillary veins and the outer fascia close to the axillary veins to avoid the so-called skeletonization of the axillary veins previously required for axillary surgery, so as to avoid excessive adhesion of the axillary veins and surrounding tissues. Assuring the patency and diastolic function (Fig. 37.5a, b, c).

As for the advantages and disadvantages of preserving the intercostobrachial nerve in ALND and whether it can reduce the incidence of lymphedema, there is no credible evidence yet. It is speculated that Although a certain segment or level of lymphatic pathway exists if the lymphatic vessels at the level lose their diastolic rhythm due to loss of innervation, the lymphatic vessels continue to expand or contract, it will also cause lymphatic reflux disorder in the corresponding drainage area and cause edema. Axillary vein injury and axillary vein lumen stenosis caused by axillary surgery, postoperative hemorrhage, axillary infection, etc. cause fibrosis of the affected area, which may affect the regeneration of the lymphatic network and collateral circulation in the surgical area, Can ultimately affect the lymphatic reflux of the upper limbs, which should be avoided. At the same time, care must be taken to avoid incomplete axillary clearance, residual metastatic lymph node, lymphedema caused by axillary recurrence early after surgery, or edema caused by reoperation.

37.1.4 Avoidance of Postoperative Injuries in Ipsilateral Upper Limb

There are many injury factors for patients who received ALND, and the most common clinically is the excessive load on the affected upper limb, especially sudden excessive force such as lifting, pulling, and pushing during labor or exercise. Frequent or repeated exertion can result in cumulative strain, for example, a shoemaker who used a not-very-heavy hammer repeatedly, edema occurred six months after that. Lymphedema is prone to occur after Skin injuries and secondary infections, such as bruises, stabs, cuts, scratches induced Dermal lymphangitis or cellulitis of the affected upper limbs. Others, such as edema that occurs after receiving an infusion or blood transfusion on the affected limb, should be avoided. However, SLNB and breast-conserving surgery at the same time for patients with early breast cancer rarely affects the load-bearing capacity of the affected upper limb; In patients receiving SLNB and mastectomy, the affected upper limb can receive blood transfusion, infusion, and blood pressure measurement.

Breast cancer patients may not develop edema immediately after ALND. Most lymphedema occurs within 1 to 2 years after axillary dissection, some 7 years or long. In fact, more than half of the patients did not develop lymphedema of the ipsilateral upper limb after radical mastectomy or have late-onset many years afterward, while edema developed soon after excessive weight strain. Mastectomy disrupts the fascia continuity or integrity of the chest wall, upper limbs, and armpits, which inevitably affects the load-bearing capacity of the upper limb. But a small number of patients have performed farm work or daily chores without any protective measures on the affected upper limb, e.g., carrying a load of more than 20 kg in mountain climbing, with no signs of edema.

It is speculated that the lymphatic network, extensively damaged after axillary lymph node dissection of breast cancer, will be Repaired through body compensation mechanism to varying degrees, and most patients will not immediately have edema; when the affected upper limb is injured, such as a strain, it will be destroyed again after Surgical trauma. The compensatory repair of the lymphatic network will eventually fail to repair, and decompensated edema appears. Due to differences in individual factors, such as the fragile lymphatic drainage network structure, Less compensable lymphatic drainage pathways, or the high load of lymphatic drainage before surgery, surgical trauma and postoperative injury may be more likely to induce lymphedema [7–10]. Animal experimental research found that after regional lymph node resection, lymphatic regeneration was seen subcutaneously in the surgical area, additional collateral circulation was established, and the interrupted lymphatic drainage pathway was reopened [11, 12]. Clinical imaging studies have also shown compensatory hyperplasia of lymphatic collecting ducts in the limbs of the diseased side [13]. In addition, more than one patient reported that swimming exercise can significantly reduce the edema and swelling discomfort and that the edema and swelling discomfort during swimming interruption is obvious and worth noting.

37.1.5 Preventive Surgery—LYMPHA

The most promising preventive surgery is LYMPHA (the lymphatic microsurgical preventive healing approach). In 2009, Boccardo, Campisi reported that in breast cancer ALND, microvascular anastomosis can be performed. It is a microsurgical technique to create a shunt between the upper arm lymphatic channel and the branch of the axillary vein to reconstruct the upper arm lymphatic return pathway. This approach of the lymphatico-venous bypass has a high success rate and can effectively prevent the occurrence of lymphedema.

However, the reported results show that the incidence rate of edema is still 12.5% among patients with significant risk factors for lymphedema (BMI index greater than 30%). Some other reports suggest that the application of the current technology is a safe, effective, and feasible method that is worth looking forward to. However, the application of this technology still needs more case accumulation and longer follow-up evidence to support.

In addition to the high restrictions on equipment and technical requirements, attention should also be paid to the selection of indications, such as whether the preventive surgery is more suitable for patients with high-risk factors for lymphedema [14–17].

37.1.6 About ARM

Axillary reverse mapping (ARM) is a technique using lymph tracing technology to identify lymph nodes that belong to the upper limb lymphatic system in the axilla. When axillary lymph nodes are dissected, we hope to retain the lymph nodes by ARM to reduce damage to the upper limb lymphatic drainage pathway, thus the purpose of preventing lymphedema of the upper limbs is obtained. It is easy to perform in the modified radical mastectomy of breast cancer, and it is not easy to find the target lymph nodes in breast-conserving and sentinel lymph node biopsy. The axillary lymph vessels and lymph nodes are distributed in a network pattern, and they have assumed the functions of breast lymphatic drainage and upper limb lymphatic drainage at the same time, so upper limb lymphedema occurs after axillary lymph node dissection during radical mastectomy. When performing ALND, even if the lymph node by ARM is found Non-metastatic through a Fine needle aspiration cytology and is retained, the retention of the lymph node does not guarantee that the subsequent lymph drainage path will not be damaged, not to mention lymph nodes are not sure if there is metastasis and Metastatic lymph nodes or suspicious Metastatic ones must be removed, so only the implementation of ARM without lymphatic anastomosis and recanalization may not achieve the goal of preventing lymphedema [18–20].

37.1.7 Lymph Node Compound Flap Transplant

There are procedures to restore the impaired lymphatic transport function through transplantation. That is, to remove subcutaneous soft tissue with vascular pedicles and lymph nodes, of different masses, from the inguinal region or the adjacent chest wall and axillary region of the unaffected side; then transplant to the affected axilla or arm. It intends to regenerate the lymph system to serve as a "pump." This type of procedure has been used to treat upper extremity lymphedema after breast cancer surgery or to try to prevent lymphedema from occurring during autologous tissue flap transplantation for breast reconstruction such as transverse rectus abdominis myocutaneous flap (TRAM). However, due to insufficient reported cases, ineffective evaluation criteria, and inadequate follow-up time, it is not certain whether repairing the local lymphatic pathway would induce a higher risk of lymphedema in distant limb sites. Whether it can be used in the clinic as a preventive surgery in the future still needs to be studied [21, 22].

It is believed that surgical preventive surgery for limb lymphedema will increase gradually, but what is currently lacking is a dynamic comparison of the imaging changes of lymphatic drainage pathways before and after surgery in patients undergoing preventive surgery and images of lymphatic drainage pathways between patients with different risks of edema. The selection of surgical indications needs to be cautious, because any surgical measures inevitably damage the normal tissue structure and function of the body, including minimally invasive surgery.

37.1.8 Non-Surgical Preventive Interventions

Some studies have conducted an evaluation scheme to identify patients who are more likely to lymphedema. For patients at high risk, early conservative intervention, including a combination of traditional Chinese and Western medicine, can prevent the occurrence or slow down the development of edema. For example, Bioelectrical Impedance Analysis can be used for the Measurement of Local Tissue Water between the patient's two upper limbs or the same upper limb before and after surgery. If the difference reaches 3%, then preventive measures should be taken, like CDT, wearing a compression sleeve or apply intermittent pneumatic compression, etc. Theoretically speaking, methods for lymphedema treatment can be used for prevention as well. But the existing prevention and prediction models lack effectiveness and practicability and need further research and improvement [23, 24].

Basic education on the prevention and treatment of lymphedema can reduce the chance of unnecessary upper limb injury and thus effectively reduce the incidence of lymphedema, which cannot be ignored. But you should also pay attention, not to over-protection, such as no strict restrictions on flying, hot spring bath, sauna, etc.

The occurrence of lymphedema after breast cancer surgery may be the result of a combination of multiple factors, and any one treatment or prevention method cannot solve all problems. Prevention should be based on different factors at the preoperative, intraoperative, and postoperative stages, and individualized preventive measures should be taken according to local conditions, and multiple methods are required [25]. Basic clinical research has found that the pathophysiology of primary or secondary lymphedema involves changes in genes, inflammatory cells, and cytokines [26–28]. As basic research continues, the pathogenesis of lymphedema after breast cancer surgery will be further elucidated. In the future, it may be possible to find clinically significant abnormalities at the gene and molecular levels and obtain therapeutic targets. Biological drugs, including targeted drugs and gene therapy technology, are expected to be applied for the prevention and treatment of lymphedema to benefit the majority of patients.

References

1. Shaitelman MF, Cromwell KD, Rasmussen JC, Stout NL, Armer JM, Lasinski BB, et al. Recent progress in the treatment and prevention of cancer-related lymphedema. CA Cancer J Clin. 2015;65:55–81.
2. Cal A, Bahar Z. Women's Barriers to prevention of lymphedema after breast surgery and home care needs: a qualitative study. Cancer Nurs. 2016;39(6):E17–25.
3. Sayegh HE, Asdourian MS, Swaroop MN, Brunelle CL, Skolny MN, Salama L, et al. Diagnostic methods, risk factors, prevention, and management of breast cancer-related lymphedema: past, present, and future directions. Current Breast Cancer Reports. 2017;9(2):111–21.
4. Ridner SH, Dietrich MS, Stewart BR, Armer JM. Body mass index and breast cancer treatment-related lymphedema. Support Care Cancer. 2011;19:853–7.
5. He Xiang-Ming I, Li-Yuz C, Bo C, Yan-hong L, Xing-feil Y, Jianfen N, et al. Methylene blue combined with sonography for SLNB replacing ALND in the operation for early-stage breast cancer. Bullet Chin Cancer. 2015;24(7):603–6.
6. Zhang X, He X, Tang B, Yang H, Ding X, Yu Y, et al. Risk factors of lymphedema on affected side of upper limb after breast cancer surgery—report from a single center of China. Int J Clin Exp Med. 2017;10(1):1592–601.
7. Pain SJ, Vowler S, Purushotham AD. Axillary vein abnormalities contribute to development of lymphoedema after surgery for breast cancer. Br J Surg. 2005;92:311–5.
8. Cintolesi V, Stanton AWB, Bains SK, Emma C, Michael Peters A, Purushotham AD, et al. Constitutively enhanced lymphatic pumping in the upper limbs of women who later develop breast cancer-related lymphedema. Lymphat Res Biol. 2016;14(2):51–61.
9. Liu NF, Lu Q, Jiang ZH, Wang CG, Zhou JG. Anatomic and functional evaluation of the lymphatics and lymph nodes in diagnosis of lymphatic circulation disorders with contrast magnetic resonance lymphangiography. J Vasc Surg. 2009;49(4):980–7.
10. Unno N, Nishiyama M, Suzuki M, Tanaka H, Yamamoto N, et al. A novel method of measuring human lymphatic pumping using indocyanine green lfluorescence lymphography. J Vasc Surg. 2010;52(4):946–52.
11. Suami H, Scaglioni MF. Lymphatic territories (lymphosomes) in the rat: an anatomical study for future lymphatic research. Plast Reconstr Surg. 2017;140(5):945–51.
12. Ito R, Suami H. Lymphatic territories (lymphosomes) in swine: an animal model for future lymphatic research. Plast Reconstr Surg. 2015;136(2):297–304.
13. Liu NF, Yan ZX, Wu XF, Luo Y. Magnetic resonance lymphography demonstrates spontaneous lymphatic disruption and regeneration in obstructive lymphedema. Lymphology. 2013;46(2):56–63.
14. Hahamoff M, Gupta N, Munoz D, Lee BT, Clevenger P, Shaw C, et al. A lymphedema surveillance program for breast cancer patients reveals the promise of surgical prevention. J Surg Res. 2019;244:604–11.
15. Agrawal J, Mehta S, Goel A, Pande PK, Kumar K. Lymphatic Microsurgical Preventing Healing Approach (LYMPHA) for prevention of breast cancer-related lymphedema – a preliminary report. Indian J Surg Oncol. 2018;9(3):369–73.
16. Feldman S, Bansil H, Ascherman J, Grant R, Borden B, Henderson P, et al. Single institution experience with Lymphatic Microsurgical Preventive Healing Approach (LYMPHA) for the primary prevention of lymphedema. Ann Surg Oncol. 2015;22(10):3296–301.
17. Boccardo F, Casabona F, DeCian F, DeCian F, Friedman D, Murelli F, et al. Lymphatic Microsurgical Preventing Healing Approach (LYMPHA) for primary surgical prevention of breast cancer-related lymphedema: over 4 years follow-up. Microsurgery. 2014;34(6):421–4.
18. Tummel E, Ochoa D, Korourian S, Betzold R, Adkins L, McCarthy M, et al. Does axillary reverse mapping prevent lymphedema after lymphadenectomy? Ann Surg. 2017;265(5):987–92.
19. Beek MA, Gobardhan PD, Klompenhouwer EG, Rutten HJ, Voogd AC, Luiten EJ. Axillary reverse mapping (ARM) in clinically node positive breast cancer patients. Eur J Surg Oncol. 2015;41(1):59–63.
20. Tausch C, Baege A, Dietrich D, Vergin I, Heuer H, Heusler RH, et al. Can axillary reverse mapping avoid lymphedema in node positive breast cancer patients? Eur J Surg Oncol. 2013;39(8):880–6.
21. Lan M, Peng Z, Zang H, Yang K, Liu Y, Li G, et al. Operating microscope with near infrared imaging function for indocyanine green lymphography in prevention of lymphedema with lymphaticovenous anastomosis immediately after mastectomy and axillary dissection. Microsurgery. 2017;37(4):354–5.
22. Nicoli F, Orfaniotis G, Lazzeri D, Lim SY, Kiranantawat K, Chen P-Y, et al. The latissimus dorsi-groin-lymph node compound flap: a comprehensive technique with three features including skin coverage, restoration of motor function, and prevention of upper limb lymphedema. Microsurgery. 2016;36(8):689–94.
23. Mazor M, Smoot BJ, Mastick J, Mausisa G, Paul SM, Kober KM, et al. Assessment of local tissue water in the arms and trunk of breast cancer survivors with and without upper extremity lymphoedema. Clin Physiol Funct Imaging. 2019 Jan;39(1):57–64.
24. Bakar Y, Tuğral A, Üyetürk Ü. Measurement of local tissue water in patients with breast cancer-related lymphedema. Lymphat Res Biol. 2018;16(2):160–4.
25. Devoogdt N, Van Kampen M, Geraerts I, Coremans T, Christiaens MR. Different physical treatment modalities for lymphoedema developing after axillary lymph node dissection for breast cancer: a review. Eur J Obstet Gynecol Reprod Biol. 2010;149(1):3–9.
26. Liu NF, Yu ZY, Sun D, Lou Y. Rare variants in LAMA5 gene associated with FLT4 and FOXC2 mutations in primary lymphedema may contribute to severity. Lymphology. 2016;49(4):192–204.
27. Yu ZY, Sun D, Luo Y, Liu NF. Abnormal mural cell recruitment in lymphatic capillaries: a common pathological feature in chronic lymphedematous skin? Microcirculation. 2016;23(7):495–502.
28. Liu NF, Yu ZY, Lou Y, Sun D. A Milroy case with FLT4/VEGFR3 mutation and an unusual skin biopsy. Br J Dermatol. 2019;180(1):223–4.

Prevention of Pelvic Malignancies and Related Lymphedema

38

Hanmei Lou, Xiaoxian Xu, and Yuxin Zhang

Abstract

Pelvic malignancies are a group of tumors with common characteristics. Secondary lower limb lymphedema (LLL) is a common complication that cannot be completely avoided after treatment of pelvic malignancies. Factors related to the onset of LLL are as follows: patient-related factors, treatment-related factors, and tumor-related risk factors, etc. LLL will affect the quality of life of survivors. Prevention of LLL can be started from the following points: the improved treatment method, such as reduction the scope of lymph node resection, early diagnosis, and increased awareness of patients and medical staff.

Keywords

Pelvic malignancies · Secondary lower limb lymphedema · High risk factor · Prevention · Quality of life

38.1 General Situation of Pelvic Malignancies Related Lymphedema

38.1.1 Incidence of Pelvic Malignancies

Pelvic malignancies are tumors that occur in organs within the pelvic cavity, mainly including genitourinary malignancies (prostate and bladder cancer), intestinal malignancies (colon and rectal cancer), and gynecological malignancies (cervical cancer, endometrial cancer, ovarian cancer, vulvar cancer, vaginal cancer), based on the GLOBOCAN 2018 estimates of cancer incidence and mortality produced by the International Agency for Research on Cancer (IARC). The incidence of colon and rectal cancer, prostate cancer, and cervical cancer ranks third, fourth, and eight, respectively. Among female malignant tumors, colon and rectal cancer, cervical cancer, uterine cancer, and ovarian cancer ranks second, fourth, sixth, and eighth [1]; the complication and quality of life between urinary, intestinal, and gynecological malignancies after treatment have commonness, which eventually deserves further attention.

38.1.2 Lymphatic Drainage and Treatment Characteristics of Pelvic Malignancies

The main ways of female pelvic lymphatic drainage are: tumors of the vulva and lower third of the vagina mainly spread by the superficial inguinal pathway to the inguinofemoral nodes. Carcinomas of the cervix, endometrium, ovary, and upper two-thirds of the vagina often spread by the lateral pelvic pathway, which drains lymph from the pelvic organs to the medial chain of the external iliac lymph node group. Lymphatic fluids are drained by the hypogastric pathway from most of the pelvic organs along the visceral branches of the hypogastric vessels to the junctional lymph nodes. The presacral pathway is a channel where tumors of the lower pelvic tumors spread posteriorly via the perirectal lymphatic vessels, along the uterosacral ligament, to the presacral space. Another pathway is from the uterine corpus and the ovaries along the ovarian vessels to the paraaortic and paracaval basins between the renal vessels and the inferior mesenteric artery [2].

The treatment for pelvic malignant tumors is a comprehensive model mostly based on surgery, combined with radiotherapy and chemotherapy. Lymphatic metastasis is the main way of colorectal cancer, cervical cancer, endometrial cancer, vulvar cancer, and vaginal cancer. According to the

H. Lou (✉) · X. Xu
The Cancer Hospital of the University of Chinese Academy of Sciences (Zhejiang Cancer Hospital), Institute of Basic Medicine and Cancer (IBMC), Chinese Academy of Sciences, Hangzhou, Zhejiang, China
e-mail: louhm@zjcc.org.cn

Y. Zhang
The Second Clinical Medical College, Zhejiang Chinese Medical University, Hangzhou, Zhejiang, China

N. Liu (ed.), *Peripheral Lymphedema*, https://doi.org/10.1007/978-981-16-3484-0_38

pattern of lymphatic metastasis with tumors at different sites, performed pelvic lymphadenectomy or biopsy, paraaortic lymph node resection or biopsy, superficial inguinal lymphadenectomy. And most patients need adjuvant radiotherapy after surgery, the lymph node drainage area was considered as the tumor target received radiation at the prescribed dose (45–50GY).

Surgery or radiotherapy will directly damage the regional lymphatic drainage system, resulting in an imbalance between production and transport of lower limb lymph fluid to the systemic circulation, so cause accumulation of protein-rich fluid in the tissue interstitium, and the fluid pass through capillary circulation into space by ultrafiltration and enter the lymphatic system, finally get into the systemic circulation. Lower limb lymphedema (LLL) emerges when the filtration rate exceeds the ability of the lymphatic system fluid balance, and then the interstitium changes and gradually develops into swelling of the limbs, enlargement of fat cells, and irreversible fibrosis, causing a vicious cycle. Based on the above diseases and treatment characteristics, LLL is a common complication after treatment of pelvic malignant tumors such as urinary, intestinal, and gynecological malignant tumors. The most closely related, the most common, and the most studied is gynecological cancer.

38.1.3 Incidence of Pelvic Malignancies-Associated LLL

The research on LLL secondary to pelvic malignancies is generally retrospective. The standard for LLL detection has not been well established. Perimeter and volume measurement are common diagnostic methods but time-consuming. Lack of uniform assessment and diagnosis has led to difficulty in identifying the true rates of LLL. At present, the true incidence of LLL and its impact are not clear, big data statistics are lacking, and reports are inconsistent. LLL ranges between 2.4% and 41% after pelvic lymph node dissection in patients with gynecologic malignancies [3]. In a retrospective cohort of 264 patients who underwent pelvic lymphadenectomy with or without paraaortic lymphadenectomy for gynecologic cancer, the rate of LLL was 23.1% at one year after surgery [4]. In a cohort of 591 patients who underwent total hysterectomy and pelvic lymphadenectomy for endometrial cancer, the overall prevalence of lower limb lymphedema of 47% at 6.2 years of follow-up [5]. Patient-reported LLL was 35% in patients undergoing endometrial cancer, but only 22% of patients were diagnosed with LLL (6); there is indeed a missed diagnosis of LLL in the clinic. A multicenter study from France included two prospective trials of sentinel lymph node biopsy for cervical cancer (SENTICOL I and II), with 248 patients who underwent total hysterectomy between 2005 and 2012, prospectively recorded postoperative complications, the main complications were urinary infection and LLL, the incidence of LLL was 14.5%, lower than other reports [6].

The American Gynecologic Oncology Group (GOG) conducted a clinical study of LLL related to patients with gynecological malignancies (GOG244), 1054 women were enrolled, including endometrial cancer, cervical cancer, and vulvar cancer. In a 2-year study, 14% reported an LLL diagnosis, while lime volume change (LVC) ≥10% accounted for 34%, LLL differed depending on the site of the disease: 22% in the endometrial cancer group, 32% in the cervical cancer group, and 49% in the vulvar cancer group, consistent with literature report. The incidence of lymphedema of the lower extremity (LLE) was highest in the vulvar group. The LLE rate in the cervical cancer group is higher than in the endometrial cancer group [7].

Other pelvic malignancies related to lymphedema for which data were available in a systematic review [8], which performed meta-analysis of the literature to derive estimates of lymphedema incidence among various pelvic malignancies. Among the 1060 combined patients with genitourinary cancers, those with penile cancer (n = 244), prostate cancer (n = 549), and bladder cancer (n = 267), the incidence of lymphedema was 21%, 4%, and 16%, respectively. 11% were identified for whole genitourinary cancers, less than the incidence of lymphedema observed for gynecological malignancies (20%), which is interpreted as the influence from that approximately 70% of the patients in these studies reported to have undergone pelvic lymph node dissections and/or radiation therapy, which is a lower percentage of genitourinary cancer patients undergoing adjunctive radiation therapy (27%).

Onset time of LLL secondary to pelvic malignant tumors is diversity. 75% occur within the first year after treatment, 19% occur within 1–2 years, and 6% occur within 2–5 years [9]. 40% is temporary, 60% is continuous, and some patients will run a chronic course for 20–30 years [10]. The clinical manifestations of LLL are swelling, pain, feel heavy of unilateral or bilateral lower limbs, or even repeated infection, dysfunction, impact on quality of life [11]. Patients will feel frustrated and angry. They often complain about very serious psychosocial health problems, such as sexual decline and isolated by society. It is urgent need to obtain the true incidence of LLL, develop effective educational materials and programs to improve the management of lymphedema.

To date, most studies on secondary lymphedema have focused on upper extremity lymphedema secondary to breast cancer treatment. In recent years, more and more attention has been paid to complications related to pelvic malignancies. It is also very important to control, evaluate and prevent the risk factors of LLL associated with pelvic malignancies, which can provide accurate knowledge points in the prevention and treatment of LLL.

38.2 Factors Related to the Onset of LLL

38.2.1 Patient-Related Factors

Body mass index (BMI) is generally considered to be significant predictive factors for LLL. There was a positive correlation between LLL and overweight in endometrial cancer and ovarian cancer, but it is not obvious in cervical cancer [4, 5, 9, 12], It is possible that the treatment of cervical cancer occupies a large proportion of undermining the lymphatic system, which conceals the effect of BMI. Studies show that the incidence of LLL in patients with cervical cancer ≥60 years and < 60 years is 17.1% and 12.4%, respectively. Generally, the physical activity ability of the elderly is low and more likely result in postoperative complications [13]. Race and smoking have no obvious correlation with LLL [4]. There are also a few studies report that the correlation between LLL and BMI, age is not obvious [14].

38.2.2 Treatment-Related Factors

38.2.2.1 Lymph Node Resection

It is generally believed that the extent and number of lymphadenectomy are related to LLL. The incidence of LLL in patients with pelvic lymph node dissection is 27.9%, and those without lymph node dissection is 5.8% [10, 15–17]. Studies show that cut-off point >10 [18], >21 [19], >25 [20] and >31 [21] lymph nodes resection is significant risk factor for LLL. Obviously, as the number of lymph nodes removed increases, the incidence of LLL increases, but the most significant boundary value is not clear. The circumflex iliac lymph nodes (CILNs) are located at the farthest end of the extra iliac lymph node between the deep circumflex vein and the femoral canal. CILNs resection is a high-risk factor for LLL in gynecological malignant tumor [11, 22–24] A retrospective study reported 140 patients who preservation of CILNs compared with 189 patients who had CILNs removed, the incidence of LLL was 6.4% and 37%, respectively ($P < 0.0001$), in the preserved group, lymphoscintigraphy showed that lymph fluid flowed into CILNs from the deep inguinal nodes, in the nonpreserved group, the accumulation of radiotracer in the lower leg increased and the inguinal nodes could not be imaged [23].

Does minimally invasive surgery help reduce the incidence of LLL? There is no evidence suggest that the incidence of LLL will be higher by laparotomy than minimally invasive surgery [25].

38.2.2.2 Tumor Location

The incidence of LLL postoperative is different for different malignant tumor of the pelvis, vulvar cancer 30–70% [26], cervical cancer 0–55.9% [27, 28], endometrial cancer 1.2–47.0% [5, 18], ovarian cancer 4.7–40.8% [9, 26]. Scope and location of lymphadenectomy of tumors are different. Ovarian cancer and endometrial cancer are treated by staging surgery, which is not a complete lymph node dissection for every patient. Sometimes only part of the lymph nodes are removed. Usually, cervical cancer will receive pelvic lymphadenectomy. Superficial inguinal lymph node dissection is performed for vulvar cancer and vaginal cancer that involve the one-third of the lower vagina. Superficial inguinal lymph node dissection and pelvic lymphadenectomy are more likely to cause LLL, all of this may lead to significantly different rates of LLL.

38.2.2.3 Radiotherapy

There is a close relationship between pelvic radiotherapy postoperative and LLL [21, 29]. Radiotherapy interferes with the healing of injured lymphatic vessels, resulting in fibrosis of lymphatic vessels at all levels, which will further promote the development of LLL. Surgery combined with radiotherapy is a common gynecological malignant tumor treatment model, which has a significantly increased incidence of LLL, when compared with surgery alone (44.4%vs.15.8%) [30] or compared with radiotherapy alone (15% vs. 6%) [31]. Another report shows the incidence of LLL was not high in patients receiving radical radiotherapy alone (4.96%) [32]. In general, the higher the dose of radiation, the more serious and frequent side effects, but the specific relationship between LLL and pelvic radiotherapy is not clear.

38.2.2.4 Other Factors

LLL can cause recurrent cellulitis or lymphangitis in the lower limbs, and the infection can aggravate LLL. Studies have shown that cellulitis is a risk factor for LLL. If LLL patients have a secondary infection, that will bring further damage to the lymphatic system and aggravate edema [11, 23]. If infection cannot be effectively controlled, it will be a vicious circle. Lymphocytic cysts have the same etiological basis as LLL, excessive lymphocysts, or secondary infections will aggravate lower extremity edema. It will be necessary for patients with compression symptoms and secondary infections treated with cyst drainage and anti-infection timely.

38.2.3 Tumor-Related Risk Factors

In patients with advanced cancer and multiple lymph node metastasis, the damage to the lymphatic vessels due to cancer and treatment will be more extensive, and LLL is more likely to occur.

38.2.4 Genetic Factors

Researches show that some primary lymphedema has a genetic etiology. Lymphangiogenesis is regulated by many cytokines. Researchers at the University of Pittsburgh have been searching for possible genetic components of secondary lymphedema, more mutations in the gene connexin-47 were found in patients with secondary lymphedema among 188 cases of breast cancer between 2000 and 2010. Connexin-47 is considered to be an important cause of valve development in normal lymphatic vessels, whose absence may cause dysfunction of lymphatic system. This study challenges the traditional view that secondary lymphedema in cancer patients is due to lymphatic transport dysfunction caused by cancer treatment. More precisely, susceptible genetic factors may also play an important role [33].

Vascular endothelial growth factor (VEGF) is considered as another genetic factor. Reviews show that VEGF plays a central role in the mitogenic substance that initiates and regulates the growth of vascular structure. VEGF-C and VEGF-D combined with VEGF receptor-3 (VEGFR-3) dominate the growth and development of the lymphatic system. VEGFR-3 is only expressed in the endothelial tissues of the lymphatic vessels [34]. The gene defect of VEGF-C is the root cause of some forms of primary lymphedema. Exogenous VEGF-C can up-regulate the receptor VEGFR-3 and promote lymphangiogenesis and has the ability of the growth factor to ameliorate tissue edema. A test of postsurgical lymphedema in the mouse tail model showed that the therapeutic impact of added VEGF-C is markedly attenuated in the presence of the monoclonal anti-VEGFR-3 neutralizing antibody. The central role of the VEGFR-3 receptor and its ligands in the development and therapeutic resolution of lymphedema is needed more research [35].

38.3 Prevention of LLL

In summary, patients with risk factors like pelvic lymphadenectomy, more pelvic lymph nodes being resected, adjuvant pelvic radiotherapy, paraaortic lymph node dissection [36], high BMI, and old age need more attention for LLL. A variety of early interventions including preventive surgery can be used in patients who are most likely to develop LLL.

38.3.1 Improved the Treatment Method

38.3.1.1 Reduction the Scope of Lymph Node Resection

In the early stage of cervical cancer, endometrial cancer, and vulvar cancer, sentinel lymph node biopsy (SLN) is expected as effective and less invasive surgical technique to replace pelvic lymph node or superficial inguinal lymph node dissection. SLN biopsy greatly reduced the scope of lymphadenectomy, preserved the lymph nodes without metastasis, and maintained the integrity of the local lymph system. Now the level of evidence for SLN biopsy is increasing in the national comprehensive cancer network guidelines. In clinical practice, patients can be carefully selected for SLN biopsy instead of lymph node dissection to reduce unnecessary damage to the lymphatic system, thus effectively reducing the incidence of postoperative LLL. SLN mapping alone has been shown to decrease the risk of lymphedema in breast cancer [8]. Patients undergoing SLN biopsy have a lower incidence of LEL than patients undergoing total lymphadenectomy (1.3% vs 18.1%, $P = 0.0003$) in researches, including endometrial cancer and very limited data on other pelvic cancers, in which SLN mapping was considered as a standard treatment for staging early endometrial cancer [37].

The study to assess patient-reported LLL after SLN mapping for endometrial cancer concluded that SLN mapping was independently associated with a significantly lower prevalence of patient-reported LLL, while high BMI and adjuvant EBRT were associated with results on the contrary [38]. Many literatures indicated that circumflex lymph nodes resection was considered a major risk of LLL, so the resection should be cautious due to its low rate of metastasis [11, 22–24].

38.3.1.2 Appropriate Range of Radiation Field

The extent of radiation has also been shown to be related to the risk of LLL. A study compared the conventional standard with the reduced field radiotherapy for cervical cancer patients with intermediate-risk pathological factors, the curative effects were the same, but the reduced field radiotherapy significantly decreased the incidence of vaginal stenosis and LLL. Therefore, shrinking the radiotherapy field for patients with a low expected rate of recurrence in the lymph node area in order to reduce the irradiation to the lymphatic drainage region may be considered to reduce the incidence of LLL [39].

38.3.1.3 Early Diagnosis for LLL

The most effective strategy for preventing LLL is early diagnosis of stage 0 and 1 lymphedema, it is easy to control and reverse the edema in that stages. There are many reasons for the missed diagnosis of LLL, including factors from medical care and patient. Beesley et al. reported that of the 802 patients with gynecological tumors without a diagnosis of LLL, 15% had some symptoms that deserved further evaluation [9]. In GOG 244 study, GCLQ evaluated 20 types of LLL-related symptoms through effective patient-reported outcomes (PROs) in 914 patients, discerned the presence or absence of patient-reported diagnosis of LLL, and revealed the predictive value of the Questionnaire Score. Results show that the GCLQ symptom set questionnaire score is closely related to limb volume change (LVC) ≥10% and LLE from the PROs

($P < 0.001$), but the LVC changes may not necessarily infer LLL. The GCLQ is simple and easy to implement, screening patients before and after treatment using GCLQ combined with LVC can help predict and diagnose early LLL for early intervention, which can positively impact the quality of these women's lives. In this study, at least eight lymph nodes resected, GCLQ total score change ≥4, patient-reported diagnosis of LLE and LVC ≥ 10% were the significant risk factors of LLL [7].

38.3.1.4 Surgical Intervention for LLL

Generally speaking, patients initially diagnosed with LLL should be treated with conservative treatments first, and if these approaches fail, more invasive approaches such as surgery should be considered. However, some believe that a "therapy time window" may be missed if surgery is considered as "the last defense" in the treatment of lymphedema, this is especially true when successful surgery has to rely on the residual function of the lymphatic system. In patients with advanced lymphedema, ICG lymphangiography often shows that there are no superficial lymphatic vessels available for bypass transplantation. The remaining lymphatic vessels may be damaged by being flooded by excessive accumulation of lymph, which leads to local fibrosis, so they may no longer be suitable for bypass surgery [40]. Therefore, most surgeons recommend surgical treatment for patients with stage II or early-stage III lymphedema. The future direction of lymph surgery will allow the design of personalized surgical management strategies to meet the needs of individual cancer patients better. Jøgensen et al. reported that prophylactic lymphovenous anastomosis and shunts were effective and may be suitable for properly selected patients undergoing lymphadenectomy, although its wider applicability is not yet known [41].

38.3.1.5 Etiology Treatment (Potential Treatment)

As previously described, exogenous VEGF-C has the ability of the growth factor to ameliorate tissue edema. And upregulate the receptor VEGFR-3 and promote lymphangiogenesis [35]. Adipose-derived stem cells (ADSCs) were transplanted into a mouse rat tail lymphedema model. LYVE-1 immunohistochemically number of lymphatic vessels and cells expressing VEGF-C- or VEGFR3- significantly increased in the transplanted groups ($p < 0.05$) [42]. A research group was able to show better lymphatic regeneration when used in combination with autologous lymph node transplantation in animal models [43]. It was proved at laboratory and animal level that the close relationship between the development and therapeutic resolution of lymphedema and VEGF-C and its receptor. With further clinical transformation research, VEGF-C may be a potential gene therapy target for LLL.

38.3.2 Increased Awareness of Patients and Medical Staff

38.3.2.1 Health Education

Survey showed that the average time from the onset of lymphedema to treatment was 3.6 years [33], and 75% of patients developed LLL within the first year after cancer treatment. Due to the patients' lack of knowledge about LLL and the lack of attention paid to LLL, the diagnosis and treatment were delayed. In one study of endometrial cancer, only 8% of the patients received preoperative education about the risk of LLL [14]. Most of the patients had not received any oral or text information about LLL before discharge, even if the patients who had received relevant information were not satisfied with and understood the information provided. Health education and guidance for patients should include the symptoms, risk factors, and preventive measures of LLL. Educating patients about the symptoms may facilitate early diagnosis. Patients should be told to form good behavior habits or purposeful behaviors to prevent postoperative LLL, such as keeping weight in the normal range and proper exercise. In addition, medical staffs should pay sufficient attention to LLL, as awareness of the curative efficacy of malignant tumors has risen to the point that quality of life and survival are equally important.

38.3.2.2 Early Intervention

Unfortunately, the data that allowed us to identify truly effective, preventative postoperative measures is very limited. A randomized trial showed that prophylactic physiotherapy significantly reduced the risk of chronic lymphedema in breast cancer patients undergoing surgery, from 25% to 7% ($P = 0.010$) [44].

A pilot cohort of 56 patients was treated with customized compression garments vs. conventional care in a small randomized study, results showed that the prophylactic use of these garments reduced the incidence of clinically and objectively measured lower extremity lymphedema (13.3% vs 7.7%) ($P = 0.496$), although the data did not reach statistical difference, but when the patients wearing custom low compression clothing for 6 weeks while having risk reduction education, may help reduce the risk of developing LLL [45].

Complete decongestive therapy (CDT) is most widely used in the treatment of lymphedema, which mainly includes:1. Daily care including raising the injured limb and functional exercise of the affected limb; 2.Compression therapy: Using elastic bandages, elastic socks, gradient pressure stockings to give compression to the affected limb and control the circumference depending on the massage effect produced by the elastic socks during the movement to produce the therapeutic effect to the affected limb. 3. Manual lymphatic drainage: apply a certain pressure with bare hands according to the path of lymphatic return to perform centripetal or centrifugal lymphatic tube massage on the affected limb, which will stimulate normal lymph ducts and promote limb edema recedes. It should be performed by a specialist nurse or professional massage therapist as the standardized CDT to have a long-term effect on reducing edema volume in LLL after gynecological malignancies treatment [46].

38.4 Conclusion

LLL is one of the common complications after treatment of gynecological cancer, which will reduce the quality of life of the survivors. Such measures as effective prevention, LLL control, and encouraging patients and medical staff to participate in the management process of LLL should be taken into consideration and paid more attention to. Standardized methods for identifying high-risk patients and improved education are extremely required for patients, and medical staff early diagnosis and timely interventions are the key strategies for LLL. Study showed that PROs can improve early diagnosis and monitor treatment response. We could use it as an easy measurement. With cultivating risk awareness of patients, early diagnosis of LLL, and appropriate comprehensive treatment, we can reduce the incidence of LLL, perform effective treatment of lymphedema and then, improve the quality of life of patients who suffered from LLL secondary to the treatment of pelvic malignancies.

References

1. Bray F, Ferlay J, Soerjomataram I, Siegel RL, Torre LA, Jemal A. Global cancer statistics 2018: GLOBOCAN estimates of incidence and mortality worldwide for 36 cancers in 185 countries. CA Cancer J Clin. 2018;68(6):394–424.
2. Pano B, Sebastia C, Ripoll E, Paredes P, Salvador R, Bunesch L, et al. Pathways of lymphatic spread in gynecologic malignancies. Radiographics. 2015;35(3):916–45.
3. Bakar Y, Tuğral A. Lower extremity lymphedema management after gynecologic cancer surgery: a review of current management strategies. Ann Vasc Surg. 2017;44:442–50.
4. Kuroda K, Yamamoto Y, Yanagisawa M, Kawata A, Akiba N, Suzuki K, et al. Risk factors and a prediction model for lower limb lymphedema following lymphadenectomy in gynecologic cancer: a hospital-based retrospective cohort study. BMC Women's Health. 2017;17(1).
5. Yost KJ, Cheville AL, Al-Hilli MM, Mariani A, Barrette BA, McGree ME, et al. Lymphedema after surgery for endometrial cancer. Obstet Gynecol. 2014;124(2, PART 1):307–15.
6. Balaya V, Mathevet P, Magaud L, Delomenie M, Bonsang-Kitzis H, Ngo C, et al. Predictive factors of severe perioperative morbidity of radical hysterectomy with lymphadenectomy in early-stage cervical cancer: a French prospective multicentric cohort of 248 patients. Eur J Surg Oncol. 2019;45(4):650–8.
7. Carter J, Huang HQ, Armer J, Carlson JW, Lockwood S, Nolte S, et al. GOG 244 – The LymphEdema and Gynecologic cancer (LEG) study: The association between the gynecologic cancer lymphedema questionnaire (GCLQ) and lymphedema of the lower extremity (LLE). Gynecol Oncol. 2019;155(3):452–60.
8. Cormier JN, Askew RL, Mungovan KS, Xing Y, Ross MI, Armer JM. Lymphedema beyond breast cancer. Cancer. 2010;116(22):5138–49.
9. Beesley V, Janda M, Eakin E, Obermair A, Battistutta D. Lymphedema after gynecological cancer treatment. Cancer. 2007;109(12):2607–14.
10. Achouri A, Huchon C, Bats AS, Bensaid C, Nos C, Lécuru F. Complications of lymphadenectomy for gynecologic cancer. Eur J Surg Oncol (EJSO). 2013;39(1):81–6.
11. Hareyama H, Hada K, Goto K, Watanabe S, Hakoyama M, Oku K, et al. Prevalence, classification, and risk factors for postoperative lower extremity lymphedema in women with gynecologic malignancies: a retrospective study. Int J Gynecol Cancer. 2015;25(4):751–7.
12. Münstedt K, Wagner M, Kullmer U, Hackethal A, Franke FE. Influence of body mass index on prognosis in gynecological malignancies. Cancer Causes Control. 2008;19(9):909–16.
13. Kashima K, Yahata T, Fujita K, Tánaka K. Analysis of the complications after radical hysterectomy for stage IB, IIA and IIB uterine cervical cancer patients. J Obstet Gynaecol Res. 2010;36(3):555–9.
14. Salani R, Preston MM, Hade EM, Johns J, Fowler JM, Paskett EP, et al. Swelling among women who need education about leg lymphedema: a descriptive study of lymphedema in women undergoing surgery for endometrial cancer. Int J Gynecol Cancer. 2014;24(8):1507–12.
15. Sekse RJ, Gjengedal E, Raheim M. Living in a changed female body after gynecological cancer. Health Care Women Int. 2013;34(1):14–33.
16. Mehra G, Weekes A, Vantrappen P, Visvanathan D, Jeyarajah A. Laparoscopic assisted radical vaginal hysterectomy for cervical carcinoma: morbidity and long-term follow-up. Eur J Surg Oncol. 2010;36(3):304–8.
17. Paskett ED, Dean JA, Oliveri JM, Harrop JP. Cancer-related lymphedema risk factors, diagnosis, treatment, and impact: a review. J Clin Oncol. 2012;30(30):3726–33.
18. Abu-Rustum NR, Alektiar K, Iasonos A, Lev G, Sonoda Y, Aghajanian C, et al. The incidence of symptomatic lower-extremity lymphedema following treatment of uterine corpus malignancies: a 12-year experience at Memorial Sloan-Kettering Cancer Center. Gynecol Oncol. 2006;103(2):714–8.
19. Bae HS, Lim MC, Lee JS, Lee Y, Nam BH, Seo SS, et al. Postoperative lower extremity edema in patients with primary endometrial cancer. Ann Surg Oncol. 2016;23(1):186–95.
20. Fuller J, Guderian D, Kohler C, Schneider A, Wendt TG. Lymph edema of the lower extremities after lymphadenectomy and radiotherapy for cervical cancer. Strahlenther Onkol. 2008;184(4):206–11.
21. Todo Y, Yamamoto R, Minobe S, Suzuki Y, Takeshi U, Nakatani M, et al. Risk factors for postoperative lower-extremity lymphedema in endometrial cancer survivors who had treatment including lymphadenectomy. Gynecol Oncol. 2010;119(1):60–4.
22. Beesley VL, Rowlands IJ, Hayes SC, Janda M, O'Rourke P, Marquart L, et al. Incidence, risk factors and estimates of a woman's risk of developing secondary lower limb lymphedema and lymphedema-specific supportive care needs in women treated for endometrial cancer. Gynecol Oncol. 2015;136(1):87–93.
23. Hareyama H, Ito K, Hada K, Uchida A, Hayakashi Y, Hirayama E, et al. Reduction/prevention of lower extremity lymphedema after pelvic and para-aortic lymphadenectomy for patients with gynecologic malignancies. Ann Surg Oncol. 2012;19(1):268–73.
24. Abu-Rustum NR, Barakat RR. Observations on the role of circumflex iliac node resection and the etiology of lower extremity lymphedema following pelvic lymphadenectomy for gynecologic malignancy. Gynecol Oncol. 2007;106(1):4–5.

25. Salehi S, Avall-Lundqvist E, Brandberg Y, Johansson H, Suzuki C, Falconer H. Lymphedema, serious adverse events, and imaging 1 year after comprehensive staging for endometrial cancer: results from the RASHEC trial. Int J Gynecol Cancer. 2019;29(1):86–93.
26. Lim MC, Lee JS, Nam BH, Seo SS, Kang S, Park SY. Lower extremity edema in patients with early ovarian cancer. J Ovarian Res. 2014;7:28.
27. Abu-Rustum NR, Gemignani ML, Moore K, Sonoda Y, Venkatraman E, Brown C, et al. Total laparoscopic radical hysterectomy with pelvic lymphadenectomy using the argon-beam coagulator: pilot data and comparison to laparotomy. Gynecol Oncol. 2003;91(2):402–9.
28. Biglia N, Librino A, Ottino MC, Panuccio E, Daniele A, Chahin A. Lower limb lymphedema and neurological complications after lymphadenectomy for gynecological cancer. Int J Gynecol Cancer. 2015;25(3):521–5.
29. Kim JH, Choi JH, Ki EY, Lee SJ, Yoon JH, Lee KH, et al. Incidence and risk factors of lower-extremity lymphedema after radical surgery with or without adjuvant radiotherapy in patients with FIGO stage I to stage IIA cervical cancer. Int J Gynecol Cancer. 2012;22(4):686–91.
30. Tanaka T, Ohki N, Kojima A, Maeno Y, Miyahara Y, Sudo T, et al. Radiotherapy negates the effect of retroperitoneal nonclosure for prevention of lymphedema of the legs following pelvic lymphadenectomy for gynecological malignancies: an analysis from a questionnaire survey. Int J Gynecol Cancer. 2007;17(2):460–4.
31. Matsuura Y, Kawagoe T, Toki N, Tanaka M, Kashimura M. Long-standing complications after treatment for cancer of the uterine cervix–clinical significance of medical examination at 5 years after treatment. Int J Gynecol Cancer. 2006;16(1):294–7.
32. Wang N, Li-Chun W, Jian-Ping L, Wei-Wei L, Juan-Yue L, Ying Z, et al. Comparison of concurrent chemoradiotherapy followed by radical surgery and high-dose-rate intracavitary brachytherapy: a retrospective study of 240 patients with FIGO stage IIB cervical carcinoma. Onco Targets Ther. 2014;
33. Finegold DN, Baty CJ, Knickelbein KZ, Perschke S, Noon SE, Campbell D, et al. Connexin 47 mutations increase risk for secondary lymphedema following breast cancer treatment. Clin Cancer Res. 2012;18(8):2382–90.
34. Saito Y, Nakagami H, Kaneda Y, Morishita R. Lymphedema and therapeutic lymphangiogenesis. Biomed Res Int. 2013;2013:1 6.
35. Jin DP, An A, Liu J, Nakamura K, Rockson SG. Therapeutic responses to exogenous VEGF-C administration in experimental lymphedema: immunohistochemical and molecular characterization. Lymphat Res Biol. 2009;7(1):47–57.
36. Chang WI, Kang HC, Wu HG, Kim HJ, Jeon SH, Lee M, et al. Lower extremity lymphedema in gynecologic cancer patients: propensity score matching analysis of external beam radiation versus brachytherapy. Cancers. 2019;11(10).
37. Geppert B, Lonnerfors C, Bollino M, Persson J. Sentinel lymph node biopsy in endometrial cancer-Feasibility, safety and lymphatic complications. Gynecol Oncol. 2018;148(3):491–8.
38. Leitao MM, Zhou QC, Gomez-Hidalgo NR, Iasonos A, Baser R, Mezzancello M, et al. Patient-reported outcomes after surgery for endometrial carcinoma: Prevalence of lower-extremity lymphedema after sentinel lymph node mapping versus lymphadenectomy. Gynecol Oncol. 2020;156(1):147–53.
39. Yeo RMC, Chia YN, Namuduri RPD, Yap SP, Soong YL, Yam PKL, et al. Tailoring adjuvant radiotherapy for stage IB–IIA node negative cervical carcinoma after radical hysterectomy and pelvic lymph node dissection using the GOG score. Gynecol Oncol. 2011;123(2):225–9.
40. Suami H, Chang DW. Overview of surgical treatments for breast cancer-related lymphedema. Plast Reconstr Surg. 2010;126(6):1853–63.
41. Jørgensen MG, Toyserkani NM, Sørensen JA. The effect of prophylactic lymphovenous anastomosis and shunts for preventing cancer-related lymphedema: a systematic review and meta-analysis. Microsurgery. 2018;38(5):576–85.
42. Yoshida S, Hamuy R, Hamada Y, Yoshimoto H, Hirano A, Akita S. Adipose-derived stem cell transplantation for therapeutic lymphangiogenesis in a mouse secondary lymphedema model. Regen Med. 2015;10(5):549–62.
43. Schindewolffs L, Breves G, Buettner M, Hadamitzky C, Pabst R. VEGF-C improves regeneration and lymphatic reconnection of transplanted autologous lymph node fragments: an animal model for secondary lymphedema treatment. Immun Inflamm Dis. 2014;2(3):152–61.
44. Torres Lacomba M, Yuste Sanchez MJ, Zapico Goni A, Prieto Merino D, Mayoral del Moral O, Cerezo Tellez E, et al. Effectiveness of early physiotherapy to prevent lymphoedema after surgery for breast cancer: randomised, single blinded, clinical trial. BMJ (Clinical research ed). 2010;340:b5396.
45. Hnin YK, Ong LX, Tsai CC, Ong SS, Yee SG, Choo BA, et al. Does initial routine use of a compression garment reduce the risk of lower limb lymphedema after gynecological cancer treatment? A randomized pilot study in an Asian institution and review of the literature. Lymphology. 2018;51(4):174–83.
46. Kim YB, Hwang JH, Kim TW, Chang HJ, Lee SG. Would complex decongestive therapy reveal long term effect and lymphoscintigraphy predict the outcome of lower-limb lymphedema related to gynecologic cancer treatment? Gynecol Oncol. 2012;127(3): 638–42.

GPSR Compliance

The European Union's (EU) General Product Safety Regulation (GPSR) is a set of rules that requires consumer products to be safe and our obligations to ensure this.

If you have any concerns about our products, you can contact us on ProductSafety@springernature.com

In case Publisher is established outside the EU, the EU authorized representative is:

Springer Nature Customer Service Center GmbH
Europaplatz 3
69115 Heidelberg, Germany

Batch number: 10731524

Printed by Printforce, the Netherlands